Physical Therapy *of the*
Shoulder

CLINICS IN PHYSICAL THERAPY

ALREADY PUBLISHED

HAND REHABILITATION • Christine A. Moran, M.S. R.P.T., guest editor

SPORTS PHYSICAL THERAPY • Donna Bernhardt, M.S. R.P.T., A.T.C., guest editor

THERAPEUTIC CONSIDERATIONS FOR THE ELDERLY • Osa Littrup Jackson, Ph.D., guest editor

PHYSICAL THERAPY MANAGEMENT OF ARTHRITIS • Barbara Banwell, M.A., P.T., and Victoria Gall, M.Ed., P.T., guest editors

PHYSICAL THERAPY OF THE GERIATRIC PATIENT, 2ND ED. • Osa L. Jackson, Ph.D., R.P.T., guest editor

PHYSICAL THERAPY FOR THE CANCER PATIENT • Charles L. McGarvey III, M.S., P.T., guest editor

GAIT IN REHABILITATION • Gary L. Smidt, Ph.D., guest editor

PHYSICAL THERAPY OF THE HIP • John L. Echternach, Ed.D., guest editor

PEDIATRIC NEUROLOGIC PHYSICAL THERAPY, 2ND ED. • Suzann K. Campbell, Ph.D., P.T., F.A.P.T.A., guest editor

PHYSICAL THERAPY MANAGEMENT OF PARKINSON'S DISEASE • George I. Turnbull, M.A., P.T., guest editor

PULMONARY MANAGEMENT IN PHYSICAL THERAPY • Cynthia Coffin Zadai, M.S., P.T., guest editor

PHYSICAL THERAPY ASSESSMENT IN EARLY INFANCY • Irma J. Wilhelm, M.S., P.T., guest editor

PHYSICAL THERAPY OF THE LOW BACK, 2ND ED. • Lance T. Twomey, Ph.D., and James R. Taylor, M.D., Ph. D., guest editor

TEMPOROMANDIBULAR DISORDERS, 2ND ED. • Steven L. Kraus, P.T., guest editor

PHYSICAL THERAPY OF THE CERVICAL AND THORACIC SPINE • Ruth Grant, B.P.T., M.App.Sc., Grad. Dip. Adv. Man. Ther.

PHYSICAL THERAPY FOR TRAUMATIC BRAIN INJURY • Jacqueline Montgomery, P.T., guest editor

PHYSICAL THERAPY OF THE FOOT AND ANKLE, 2ND ED. • Gary C. Hunt, M.A., P.T., O.C.S., and Thomas G. McPoil, Ph.D., P.T., A.T.C.

PHYSICAL THERAPY OF THE KNEE • Robert E. Mangine, M.Ed., P.T., A.T.C.

FORTHCOMING VOLUME IN THE SERIES

CLINICAL DECISION MAKING IN PEDIATRIC NEUROLOGIC PHYSICAL THERAPY, 3RD ED. • Suzann K. Campbell, Ph.D., P.T., F.A.P.T.A.

Physical Therapy *of the*
Shoulder

THIRD EDITION

Edited by
Robert A. Donatelli, Ph.D., P.T., O.C.S.

Instructor
Division of Physical Therapy
Department of Rehabilitation Medicine
Emory University School of Medicine
Atlanta, Georgia
National Director of Sports Rehabilitation
Physiotherapy Associates
Memphis, Tennesse

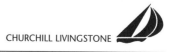

CHURCHILL LIVINGSTONE

A *Harcourt Health Sciences Company*
New York, Edinburgh, London, Philadelphia

CHURCHILL LIVINGSTONE
A *Harcourt Health Sciences Company*

The Curtis Center
Independence Square West
Philadelphia, Pennsylvania 19106

Library of Congress Cataloging-in-Publication Data

Physical therapy of the shoulder / edited by Robert A. Donatelli.—
3rd ed.
    p. cm.—(Clinics in physical therapy)
  Includes bibliographical references and index.
  ISBN 0-443-07591-3 (alk. paper)
  1. Shoulder—Wounds and injuries. 2. Shoulder—Wounds and
injuries—Treatment. 3. Shoulder—Wounds and injuries—Physical
therapy. I. Donatelli, Robert. II. Series.
  [DNLM: 1. Shoulder—injuries. 2. Shoulder Joint—injuries.
3. Physical Therapy—methods. WE 810 P578 1997]
RD557.5.P48 1997
617.5'72062—dc20
DNLM/DLC   96–29475

© **Churchill Livingstone Inc. 1997, 1991, 1987**

Distributed in the United Kingdom by Churchill Livingstone, Robert Stevenson House, 1–3 Baxter's Place, Leith Walk, Edinburgh EH1 3AF, and by associated companies, branches, and representatives throughout the world.

Medical knowledge is constantly changing. As new information becomes available, changes in treatment, procedures, equipment and the use of drugs become necessary. The editors/authors/contributors and the publishers have, as far as it is possible, taken care to ensure that the information given in this text is accurate and up to date. However, readers are strongly advised to confirm that the information, especially with regard to drug usage, complies with the latest legislation and standards of practice.

The Publishers have made every effort to trace the copyright holders for borrowed material. If they have inadvertently overlooked any, they will be pleased to make the necessary arrangements at the first opportunity.

Printed in the United States of America

Last digit is the print number: 7 6 5

I would like to dedicate this book to my late father, Revy Donatelli, and to my mother, Rose Donatelli. They provided the guidance, motivation, and love to help me through my college years, enabling me to pursue a career in physical therapy. I would also like to dedicate the book to my sister, Linda Schultheiss, and to my brother, Jerry Donatelli, for their friendship, love, and support.

Contributors

Mark S. Albert, M.Ed., P.T., A.T.C, S.C.S.
Part–time Instructor, Department of Physical Therapy, College of Health Sciences, Georgia State University; Clinical Specialist, Physiotherapy Associates, Atlanta, Georgia

Robert Cantu, M.M.Sc., P.T., M.S.C.
Assistant Professor, Institute of Physical Therapy, St. Augustine, Florida; Clinical Director, Physiotherapy Associates, Atlanta, Georgia

Deborah Seidel Cobb, M.S. P.T.
Physical Therapist, Physiotherapy Associates, Atlanta, Georgia

David J. Conaway, D.O.
Associate Clinical Professor, Department of Orthopaedics, West Virginia College of Osteopathic Medicine, Lewisburg, West Virginia; Honorary Clinical Instructor, Graduate Program in Physical Therapy, Division of Allied Heath Professions, Department of Rehabilitation Medicine, Emory University School of Medicine; Past Chairman, Department of Surgery, Northlake Regional Medical Center; Staff Orthopaedic Surgeon, Dekalb Medical Center, Northlake Regional Medical Center, Eastside Medical Center, Atlanta, Georgia; Orthopaedic Surgeon, Killian Hill Orthopaedic and Sports Medicine Clinic, Lilburn, Georgia

Jeff Cooper, M.S., A.T.C.
Athletic Trainer, The Phillies, Philadelphia, Pennsylvania; Consultant, Physiotherapy Associates, Atlanta, Georgia

Karen E. Davis, M.P.T., A.T.C.
Physical Therapist, Physiotherapy Associates, Jonesboro, Georgia

Robert A. Donatelli, Ph.D., P.T., O.C.S.
Instructor, Division of Physical Therapy, Department of Rehabilitation Medicine, Emory University School of Medicine, Atlanta, Georgia; National Director of Sports Rehabilitation, Physiotherapy Associates, Memphis, Tennessee

Peter I. Edgelow, M.A., P.T.
Senior Staff Therapist, Physiotherapy Associates; Graduate Residency in Orthopaedic Physical Therapy, Kaiser Permanente, Hayward, California

Todd S. Ellenbecker, M.S., P.T., S.C.S., C.S.C.S.
Clinic Director, Physiotherapy Associates-Scottsdale Sports Clinic, Scottsdale, Arizona

Robert L. Elvey, P.T.
Senior Lecturer, School of Physiotherapy, Curtin University of Technology, Perth, Western Australia, Australia

Blanca Zita Gonzalez-King, P.T., C.H.T.
Clinic Director, Physiotherapy Associates, Jonesboro, Georgia

John C. Gray, P.T.
Assistant Instructor, Ola Grimsby Institute; Clinical Specialist, Department of Physical Therapy, Sharp Rees–Stealy, San Diego, California; Fellow, American Academy of Orthopaedic Manual Physical Therapists

Bruce H. Greenfield, M.M.Sc., P.T., O.C.S.
Instructor, Division of Physical Therapy, Department of Rehabilitation Medicine, Emory University School of Medicine, Atlanta, Georgia

Ola Grimsby, P.T.
Chairman of the Board, Ola Grimsby Institute, San Diego, California

Toby Hall, P.T.
Clinical Consultant, School of Physiotherapy, Curtin University of Technology, Perth, Western Australia, Australia

Marie A. Johanson, M.S., P.T., O.C.S.
Clinic Director, Physiotherapy Associates, Peachtree City, Georgia

Kathryn Levit, M.Ed., O.T.R.
Partner, Making Progress, Alexandria, Virginia; Adjunct Clinical Faculty, Massachusetts General Hospital Institute of Health Professions, Boston, Massachusetts; Coordinator/Instructor, Neurodevelopmental Treatment Association, Inc., Chicago, Illinois

Angelo J. Mattalino, M.D.
Medical Director, Southwest Sports Medicine and Orthopaedic Surgery Clinic, Ltd., Scottsdale, Arizona; Medical Director, Baseball Research and Rehabilitation Center/Physiotherapy, Tempe, Arizona

George M. McCluskey III, M.D.
Staff Orthopaedic Surgeon, The Hughston Clinic; Staff Orthopaedic Surgeon, Hughston Sports Medicine Hospital, Columbus, Georgia

Timothy J. McMahon, P.T.
Clinical Instructor, Division of Physical Therapy, Department of Medicine, Emory University School of Medicine, Atlanta, Georgia; Assistant Director, Physiotherapy Associates, Lilburn, Georgia

Helen Owens, M.S., P.T.
Owner, Orthopedics Physical Therapy Services, Lockport, Illinois

Susan Ryerson, P.T.
Partner, Making Progress, Alexandria, Virginia; Adjunct Clinical Faculty, Massachusetts General Hospital Institute of Health Professions, Boston, Massachusetts, Coordinator/Instructor, Neurodevelopmental Treatment Association, Inc., Chicago, Illinois

Dorie B. Syen, M.S., O.T.R., C.H.T.
Rehabilitation Projects Coordinator, Georgia Baptist Medical Center, Atlanta, Georgia

Lori A. Thein, M.S., P.T., S.C.S., A.T.C.
Associate Lecturer, Department of Kinesiology, University of Wisconsin School of Education; Senior Clinical Therapist, Sports Medicine Center, University of Wisconsin Clinics Research Park, Madison, Wisconsin

Timothy Uhl, M.S., P.T., A.T.C.
Director of Physical Therapy, Human Performance and Rehabilitation Center, Columbus, Georgia

Joseph S. Wilkes, M.D.
Associate Clinical Professor, Department of Orthopaedics, Emory University School of Medicine; Orthopedist, The Hughston Clinic; Medical Director, Piedmont Hospital Sports Medicine Institute, Atlanta, Georgia; Orthopedic Consultant, United States Luge Association, Lake Placid, New York

Michael J. Wooden, M.S., P.T., O.C.S.
Instructor, Division of Physical Therapy, Department of Rehabilitation Medicine, Emory University School of Medicine; National Director, Clinical Research, Physiotherapy Associates, Memphis, Tennessee

Preface

Normal function of the shoulder is critical for recreational activities, occupational performance, and activities of daily living. Given the importance of normal shoulder biomechanics, it is not surprising that changes in shoulder mechanics, altered kinematics, and anatomic deficits contribute to shoulder pathomechanics. Our role as physical therapists is to assess the intricate shoulder mechanics to determine abnormal movement patterns before we begin our treatment program.

Many rehabilitation students and clinicians are uncertain in assessing shoulder pathomechanics and in establishing treatment protocols for different shoulder pathologies. This shortcoming is due to the variety of treatment approaches to the shoulder and the complexity of the shoulder and upper quarter interrelationships.

In keeping up to date with new and innovative treatment techniques, surgical procedures, and evaluation methods for the shoulder, this third edition of *Physical Therapy of the Shoulder* has become a totally new book. We have expanded the third edition to 20 chapters from 16. There are 18 new authors and 10 new chapters.

The third edition has been divided into five sections; Mechanics of Movement and Evaluation, Neurologic Considerations, Special Considerations, Treatment Approaches, and Surgical Considerations. Case studies are presented throughout the text.

Chapter 1 emphasizes the clinical mechanics of shoulder movement. The mechanical components of shoulder elevation are described and divided into phases. Jeff Cooper, a new author for this edition who is the athletic trainer for the Philadelphia Phillies, does an excellent job in describing the mechanics of pitching and injuries related to the sport. Chapter 3 reviews the traditional approach of Cyriax's differential soft tissue evaluation of the shoulder and all the special tests.

I am honored to include Ola Grimsby, John Gray, Robert Elvey, Toby Hall, and Peter Edgelow as chapter authors in the third edition. Their contributions to the Neurologic Considerations section are excellent. The chapters on Interrelationship of the Spine and Shoulder Girdle, Neural Tissue Evaluation and Treatment, and Neurovascular Consequenses of Cumulative Trauma Disorders Affecting the Thoracic Outlet demonstrate the importance of understanding the interrelationship between the musculoskeletal and neurologic systems. Chapter 7 was completely rewritten with a more clinical approach to brachial plexus lesions.

The Special Considerations section reviews the most common pathologies and dysfunctions of the shoulder. In Chapter 12 John Gray demonstrates the importance of understanding how other systems in the body can refer pain to the shoulder. Mobilization, strengthening exercises (including isokinetics), and myofascial techniques are discussed in the Treatment Approaches section. All four chapters in this section include figures accurately demonstrating treatment techniques. The Surgical Considerations section features new information on the most common surgical procedures for shoulder instabilities, rotator cuff repairs, and total joint replacements.

Any rehabilitation professional entrusted with the care and treatment of mechanical and pathologic shoulder dysfunction will benefit from this book. We trust that the third edition of *Physical Therapy of the Shoulder* will meet the reader's expectation of comprehensive, clinically relevant presentations that are well documented, contemporary, and personally challenging to the student and clinician alike.

Robert A. Donatelli, Ph.D., P.T., O.C.S.

Contents

1

Functional Anatomy and Mechanics

ROBERT A. DONATELLI

One of the most common peripheral joints to be treated in the physical therapy clinic is the shoulder joint. The physical therapist must understand the anatomy and mechanics of this joint to most effectively evaluate and design a treatment program for the patient with shoulder dysfunction. This chapter will describe the pertinent functional anatomy of the shoulder complex and relate this anatomy to the functional movements, stability, and muscle activity.

The shoulder joint is better termed the shoulder *complex*, because a series of articulations are necessary to position the humerus in space (Fig. 1.1). Most authors, when describing the shoulder joint, discuss the acromioclavicular joint, sternoclavicular joint, scapulothoracic articulation, and glenohumeral joint.[1-4] Dempster relates all of these areas by using a concept of links. The integrated and harmonious roles of all of the links are necessary for full normal mobility.[5]

The glenohumeral joint sacrifices stability for mobility. The shoulder is capable of moving in over 16,000 positions, which can be differentiated by 1° in the normal person.[6] The mobility of the shoulder is dependent upon proximal stability of the humerus and scapula. The position of the humerus and scapula must change throughout each movement in order to maintain stability.[6]

Osteokinematic and Arthrokinematic Movement

Analysis of shoulder movement emphasizes the synchronized movement of four joints: the glenohumeral, scapulothoracic, sternoclavicular, and acromioclavicular joints.[2,4,7,8] As the humerus moves into elevation, movement must occur at all four joints. Elevation of the arm can be observed in three planes: the frontal plane (abduction), sagittal plane (flexion), and plane of the scapula (scaption).[8,9] Movement of the long bones of the arm into elevation is referred to as osteokinematics. Arthrokinematics describes the intricate movement of joint surfaces: rolling, spinning, and sliding.[10]

OSTEOKINEMATIC MOVEMENT

Scaption-Abduction

Abduction of the shoulder in the frontal or coronal plane has been extensively researched.[4,8,11-17] Poppen and Walker[15] and Johnston,[8] suggest that the true plane of movement in the shoulder joint occurs in the plane of the scapula. The scapula plane (scaption) is defined as elevation of the shoulder in a range

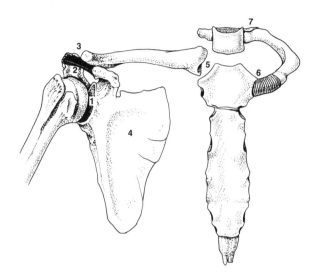

FIGURE 1.1 *The components of the shoulder joint complex.* (1) *Glenohumeral joint.* (2) *Subdeltoid joint.* (3) *Acromioclavicular joint.* (4) *Scapulothoracic joint.* (5) *Sternoclavicular joint.* (6) *First costosternal joint.* (7) *First costovertebral joint.*

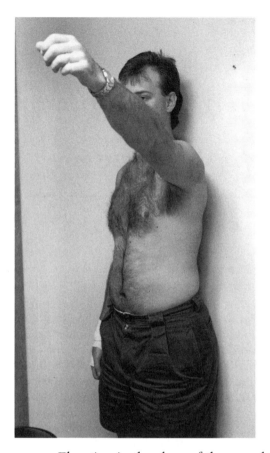

FIGURE 1.2 *Elevation in the plane of the scapula.*

between 30° and 45° anterior to the frontal plane (Figs.1.2 and 1.3).[15]

Kondo et al.[18] devised a new method for taking radiographs to define scaption during elevation. The medial tilting angle was used to describe scaption. Medial tilting angle refers to the tilting of the scapula toward the sagittal plane. As the medial tilting angle increases, there is a movement of the scapula around the thoracic cage. Kondo et al.[18] demonstrated that the medial tilting angle was constant at 40° anterior to the frontal plane throughout the range of 150° of elevation.

Several authors believe that the plane of the scapula is clinically significant because the length-tension relationship of the shoulder abductors and rotators are optimum in this plane of elevation.[8,15] Research has demonstrated that the length of the muscle determines the amount of stretch applied to the individual sarcomeres, enabling them to exert maximum tension.[19] The length–tension curves obtained from normal muscles show that maximum tension is developed when the muscle length is approximately 90% of its maximum length.[19] Conversely, when the muscle is fully shortened, the tension developed is minimal.[20,21] Therefore, the optimal lengthened position of the muscle tendon will facilitate optimal muscle contraction.[22]

Several studies have compared the torque production of different shoulder muscle groups when tested in scaption versus other body planes.[23–27] Soderberg and Blaschak[23] and Hellwig and Perrin[24] demonstrated no significant differences in the peak torque of the glenohumeral rotators between scaption and other body planes. These studies used 45° and 40° anterior to the frontal plane, respectively, for the scaption test position. Greenfield et al.[25] reported greater torque production of the external rotators when tested in scaption versus the coronal plane. Fur-

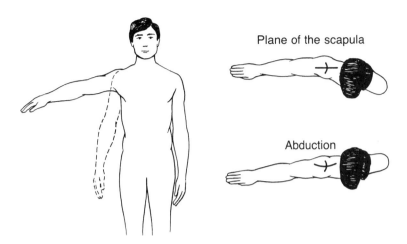

Plane of the scapula

Abduction

FIGURE 1.3 *Abduction in the plane of the scapula.*

thermore, Tata et al.[26] reported higher ratios of abduction to adduction and external to internal torque when tested in the scapular plane at 30° and 35° anterior to the frontal plane, respectively. Whitcomb et al.[27] found no significant difference between torque produced by the shoulder abductors in the coronal and scapular planes, using a scaption position 35° anterior to the frontal plane.

The studies cited indicate that the external rotators are the only muscle group that demonstrated a significant increase in torque production in the scaption plane 30° anterior to the frontal plane. The pectoralis major and the latissimus muscles groups are not attached to the scapula. Therefore, it would seen reasonable that when comparing the torque output of the internal rotators, the change in position of the scapula should not effect the optimal length-tension relationship. Thus, the internal rotators exhibit no change in the torque output when testing in different planes of movement.

In addition to optimal muscle length-tension relationship in the plane of the scapula, the capsular fibers of the glenohumeral joint are relaxed.[8] Poppen and Walker[14] demonstrated that in scaption there is an increase in joint congruity, allowing for greater joint stability. Therefore, for reasons of glenohumeral stability, avoidance of impingement, and balance of muscle action, scaption may be the plane in which shoulder

trauma is minimal, and the most advantageous plane for strength training programs.

Flexion

The movement of flexion has been less thoroughly investigated. Flexion is movement in the sagittal plane. Full flexion from 162° to 180° is possible only with synchronous motion in the glenohumeral, acromioclavicular, sternoclavicular, and scapulothoracic joints.[14] The movement is similar to that of abduction.

ARTHROKINEMATIC MOVEMENT

The motion occurring at joint surfaces is arthrokinematic motion, of which there are three types: rolling, gliding, and rotation (Fig. 1.4) Rolling occurs when various points on a moving surface contact various points on a stationary surface. Gliding occurs when one point on a moving surface contacts multiple points on a stationary surface. When rolling or gliding occur, there is a significant change in the contact area between the two joint surfaces. The third type of arthrokinematic movement, rotation, occurs when one or more points on a moving surface contact one point on a stationary surface. There is little displacement between the two joint surfaces in rotation.

All three arthrokinematic movements can

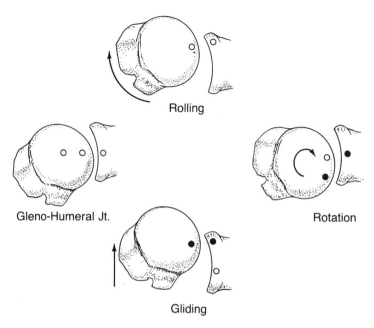

FIGURE 1.4 *Arthrokinematic motion occurring at the glenohumeral joint: rolling, rotation, and gliding.*

occur at the glenohumeral joint, but they do not occur in equal proportions. These motions are necessary for the large humeral head to take advantage of the small glenoid articulating surface.[16] Saha investigated the contact area between the head of the humerus and the glenoid with abduction in the plane of the scapula[14] and found that the contact area on the head of the humerus shifted up and forward while the contact area on the glenoid remained relatively constant, indicating a rotation movement. Poppen and Walker measured the instant centers of rotation for the same movement.[15] They found that in the first 30°, and often between 30° and 60°, the head of the humerus moved superiorly in the glenoid by 3 mm, indicating rolling or gliding. At more than 60°, there was minimal movement of the humerus, indicating almost pure rotation.[15]

Normal arthrokinematic movements occur only in the presence of normal periarticular connective tissue, extensibility, and integrity and muscle function. A stiff shoulder has limited capsular flexibility and altered muscle function. In order to reestablish harmonious movement within the shoulder complex the therapist must rehabilitate the connective tissue by restoring its extensibility, and restore the normal balance of muscles.

Rotations of the Humerus

Concomitant external rotation of the humerus is necessary for abduction in the coronal plane.[4,8,10,14,17] Some investigators have postulated that this motion is necessary for the greater tuberosity to clear the acromion and the coracoacromial ligament.[1,2,17] Saha reports that there is sufficient room between the greater tuberosity and the acromion to prevent bone impingement. External rotation also remains necessary for full coronal abduction even after the acromion and the coracoacromial ligament are surgically removed. Saha has reasoned that external rotation is necessary to prevent the humeral head from impinging on the glenoid rim.[16]

Rajendran,[28] using cadaveric glenohumeral joints, demonstrated automatic external rotation of the humerus is an essential component of active as well as passive elevation of the arm through abduction. Even in the absence of extra-articular influences such as the coracoacromial arch and glenohumeral muscles, external rotation of the humerus was spontaneous. An Kn et al.[29] used a magnetic tracking system to monitor the three-dimensional orientation of the humerus with respect to the scapula. Appropriate coordinate transformations were then performed for the calculation of glenohumeral joint rotation. Maximum elevation in all planes anterior to the scapular plane required external axial rotation of the humerus.

Furthermore, Otis et al.[30] demonstrated that external rotation of the humerus allows the insertion of the subscapularis tendon to move laterally, resulting in an increase in the distance from the axis of elevation in the scapula plane. An increase in the moment arm enhances the ability of the superior fibers of the subscapularis to participate in scaption. Conversely, internal rotation of the humerus increases the moment arm of the superior fibers of the infraspinatus, enhancing the ability of the muscle to participate in scaption. Flatow et al.[31] reported that acromial undersurface and rotator cuff tendons are in closest proximity between 60° and 120° of elevation. Conditions limiting external rotation or elevation may increase rotator cuff compression. Rajendran and Kwek[32] described how the course of the long head of the biceps will influence external rotation of the humerus, which in turn prevents tendon impingement between the greater tuberosity and the glenoid labrum, and allows glenohumeral elevation to move to completion. Brems[33] reports that external rotation is possibly the most important functional motion that the shoulder complex allows. Loss of external rotation could result in significant functional disability.

Static Stabilizers of the Glenohumeral Joint

The stability of the glenohumeral joint is dependent on the integrity of soft tissue and bony structures such as the labrum, glenohumeral ligaments, capsular ligaments, and the bony glenoid.[34] The glenohumeral joint contributes the greatest amount of motion to the shoulder because of its ball and socket configuration. Saha[35] confirmed the ball and socket joint of the glenohumeral articulation in 70 percent of his specimens. In the remaining 30 percent, the radius of curvature of the humeral head was greater than the radius of curvature of the glenoid. Thus, the joint was not a true enarthrosis.[16] Saha[16] further described the joint surfaces, especially on the head of the humerus, to be very irregular and to demonstrate a great amount of individual variation.

The head of the humerus is a hemispherical convex articular surface that faces superior, medial, and posterior. This articular surface is inclined 130° to 150° to the shaft of the humerus and is retroverted 20° to 30°[3] The retroversion, and the posterior tilt of the head of the humerus and the glenoid, cultivate joint stability (Fig. 1.5). This retroversion of the head of the humerus corresponds to the forward inclination of the scapula, so that free pendulum movements of the arm do not occur in a straight sagittal plane but at an angle of 30° across the body.[36] This corresponds to the natural arm swing evident in ambulation.

The head of the humerus is large in relation to the glenoid fossa; therefore only one-third of the humeral head can contact the glenoid fossa at a given time.[1,36] The glenoid fossa is a shallow structure deepened by the glenoid labrum. The labrum is wedgeshaped when the glenohumeral joint is in a resting position, and changes shape with various movements.[37] The glenoid and the labrum combine to form a socket with a depth up to 9 mm in the superior–inferior direction and 5 mm in the anteroposterior direction.[38] The functional significance of the labrum is questionable. Most authors agree that the labrum is a weak supporting structure.[37,39] The function of the labrum has also been described as a "chock block" preventing humeral head translation.[38] Moseley and Overgaard[37] considered the labrum a redundant fold of the capsule composed of dense fibrous connective tissue but generally de-

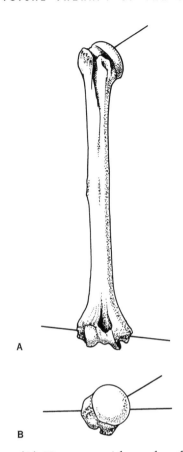

A

B

FIGURE 1.5 (A) *Humerus with marker through the head-neck and a second marker through the epicondyles.* **(B)** *Retroversion of the humerus as seen from above.*

void of cartilage except in a small zone near its osseous attachment.

The glenohumeral joint has been described by Matsen et al.[40] as a "suction cup" because of the seal of the labrum and glenoid to the humeral head. This phenomenon is caused by the graduated flexibility of the glenoid surface, which permits the glenoid to conform and seal to the humeral head. Compression of the head into the socket expels the synovial fluid to create a suction that resists distraction. A negative intra-articular joint pressure is produced by the limited joint volume.[41] Matson et al.[40] illustrated the importance of an intact glenoid labrum in establishing a concavity compression stabilization.

The compressive load is provided by dynamic muscle contraction.

The glenoid fossa faces laterally. Freedmand and Munro[42] found that the glenoid faced downward in 80.8 percent of the shoulders that they studied with radiographs. Saha[35] found a 7.4° retrotilt of the glenoid in 73.5 percent of normal subjects. The retrotilt is a stabilizing factor to the glenohumeral joint. Both the humeral and glenoid articular surfaces are lined with articular cartilage. The cartilage is the thickest at the periphery on the glenoid fossa and at the center of the humeral head.[16]

The capsule and ligaments reinforce the glenohumeral joint. The capsule attaches around the glenoid rim and forms a sleeve around the head of the humerus, attaching on the anatomical neck. The capsule is a lax structure; the head of the humerus can be distracted one-half inch when the shoulder is in a relaxed position.[43] The capsule is reinforced anteriorly and posteriorly by ligaments and muscles. There is no additional support inferiorly, causing weakness of this portion of the capsule. This inferior portion of the capsule lies in folds when the arm is adducted. The redundant portion of the capsule adheres to itself and limits motion in adhesive capsulitis.[36]

The anterior capsule is reinforced by the glenohumeral ligaments. The support that these ligaments lend to the capsule is insignificant.[44] Also, these ligaments are not consistently present in each individual.

Turkel et al.[45] described the inferior glenohumeral ligament as the thickest and most consistent structure. The inferior glenohumeral ligament attaches to the glenoid labrum. Turkel et al.[45] determined the relative contribution to anterior stability by testing external rotation in different positions. The subscapularis resisted passive external rotation in the adducted position more than any other anterior structure (Fig. 1.6) In patients with internal rotation contracture and pain after anterior repair for recurrent dislocation of the shoulder, surgical release of the subscapularis increased the external rotation range of motion an average of 27°[46] Turkel et al.[45] demonstrated at 45° abduction that external rotation was resisted by the subscapularis, mid-

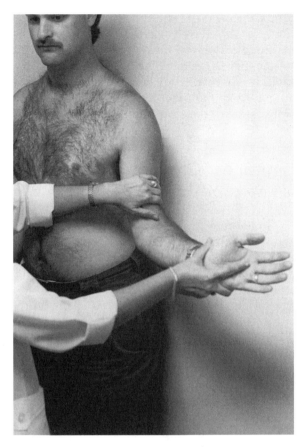

FIGURE 1.6 *External rotation of the humerus in the adducted position. The most stabilizing structure to this movement is the subscapularis muscle.*

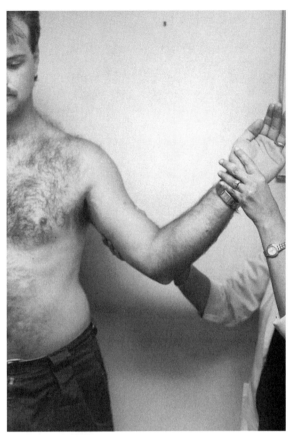

FIGURE 1.7 *External rotation of the humerus at 45° abduction. The most stabilizing structures for this movement are the middle and inferior ligaments and subscapularis muscle.*

dle glenohumeral ligament, and superior fibers of the inferior ligament (Fig. 1.7). At 90° of abduction, external rotation was restricted by the inferior glenohumeral ligament (Fig. 1.8).

Itoi et al.[47] concluded that the long head of the biceps (LHB) and short head of the biceps (SHB) have similar functions as anterior stabilizers of the glenohumeral joint with the arm in abduction and external rotation. Furthermore, the role of the LHB and SHB increased with shoulder instability. Warner et al.[48] studied the capsuloligamentous restraints to superior and inferior translation of the glenohumeral joint. The primary restraint to inferior translation of the adducted shoulder was the superior glenohu-

meral ligament. The coracohumeral ligament appeared to have no significant suspensory role. Abduction to 45° and 90° demonstrated the anterior and posterior portions, respectively, of the glenohumeral ligament to be the main static stabilizers resisting inferior translation.

Guanche et al.[49] studied the synergistic action of the capsule and the shoulder muscles. A reflex arch from mechanoreceptors within the glenohumeral capsule to muscles crossing the joint was identified. Stimulation of the anterior and the inferior axillary articular nerves elicited electromyographic (EMG) activity in the biceps, subscapularis, supraspinatus, and infraspinatus muscles. Stimulation of the posterior axillary ar-

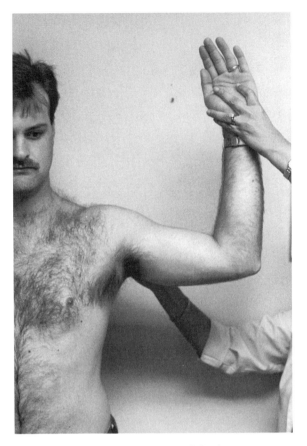

FIGURE 1.8 *External rotation of the humerus at 90° abduction. The most stabilizing structure for this movement is the inferior ligament.*

ticular nerve elicited EMG activity in the acromiodeltoid muscle.

The coracohumeral ligament is the strongest supporting ligament of the glenohumeral joint. Fibers of the capsule and coracohumeral ligament blend together and insert into the borders of the supraspinatus and subscapularis.[50] The coracohumeral ligament limits external rotation and elevation of the humerus.[50] Release of the coracohumeral ligament increased external rotation both with the arm held in adduction and at 90° of abduction.[50]

Between the supporting ligaments and muscles lie synovial bursa or recesses. Anteriorly there are three distinct recesses.[51] The superior recess is the subscapular bursa, which normally communicates with the shoulder joint. The inferior recess is referred to as the axillary pouch, and the middle synovial recess lies posterior to the subscapularis tendon. Arthrograms of frozen shoulders in relatively early stages, before glenohumeral abduction is completely restricted, show obliteration of the anterior glenoidal bursa.[51]

Dynamic Stabilizers of the Glenohumeral Joint

The major muscles that act on the glenohumeral and scapulothoracic joints may be grouped into the scapulohumeral, axiohumeral, and axioscapular muscles. The muscles of the scapulohumeral group, which include the rotator cuff muscles, originate on the scapula and insert on the humerus. The rotator cuff muscles insert on the tuberosities and along the upper two-thirds of the humeral anatomic neck.[10] The subscapularis muscle is often overlooked in shoulder dysfunction. It has the largest amount of muscle mass of the four rotator cuff muscles.[4] As previously noted, passive external rotation range of motion with the arm neutral (adducted) is resisted by the subscapularis muscle. Many times trigger points develop within the subscapularis muscle secondary to trauma or microtrauma, resulting in restrictions in external rotation in neutral and limited glenohumeral elevation. Travell and Simons[52] believe that a trigger point within the subscapularis may sensitize the other shoulder girdle musculature into developing secondary and satellite trigger points, leading to major restrictions in glenohumeral jointmotion.

The rotator cuff muscles have been described as steerers of the head of the humerus on the glenoid.[16] The subscapularis, latissimus dorsi, teres major, and teres minor act as humeral depressors.[16,53] The arthrokinematics (rolling, spinning, and sliding) of the glenohumeral joint result from the action of the steerers and the depressors of the humeral head. Translation of the humeral head is of clinical interest in most shoulder disorders. At the glenohumeral joint, the amount and direction of translation define the type of instability. Wuelker et al.[54] demonstrated that translation of the humeral head during elevation of the glenohumeral joint between 20° and 90° averaged 9 mm superiorly and 4.4 mm anteriorly. Translation of the humeral head during active elevation may be diminished by the coordinated activity of the rotator cuff muscles. This active control of the translation forces provides dynamic stability to the glenohumeral joint. Perry[55] describe 17 muscle groups providing a dynamic interactive stabilization of the composite movement of the thoraco–scapular–humeral articulation.

Abnormal glenohumeral translation is observed most often in overhead throwing athletes. Loss of coordinated balance between accelerating, decelerating, and stabilizing muscle function may produce microtraumatic injuries and possibly instability of the glenohumeral joint. Further examination of the dynamic stabilizers in the throwing athlete will be discussed in Chapter 2.

The deltoid muscle makes up 41% of the scapulohumeral muscle mass.[4] This muscle, in addition to its proximal attachment on the acromion process and the spine of the scapula, also arises from the clavicle. The distal insertion is on the shaft of the humerus at the deltoid tubercle. The mechanical advantage of the deltoid is enhanced by the distal insertion and the evolution of a larger acromion process.[4] The deltoid is a multipennate and fatigue-resistant muscle. This may explain its rare involvement in shoulder pathology.[56] The deltoid and the clavicular head of the pectoralis major muscles have been described as prime movers of the glenohumeral joint because of their large mechanical advantage.[4] Michiels and Bodem[57] demonstrated that deltoid muscle action is not restricted to the generation of an abducting moment in the shoulder joint. The clavicular and scapular regions of the deltoid muscle group afford stability to the glenohumeral joint.

Itoi et al.[47] reported that the biceps muscle group becomes more important than the rotator cuff muscles as stability from the capsuloligamentous structure decreases. The anterior displacement of the humeral head under 1.5 kg force was significantly decreased by both the long and short head of the biceps loading in all capsular conditions when the arm was in 60° or 90° of external rotation and abduction.

Sternoclavicular Joint

The sternoclavicular (SC) joint is the only articulation that binds the shoulder girdle to the axial skeleton (Fig. 1.9). This is a sellar joint, with the sternal articulating surface greater than the clavicular surface, providing stability to the joint.[10] The joint is also stabilized by its articular disc, joint capsule, ligaments, and reinforcing muscles.[5,58] The disc binds the joint together and divides the joint into two cavities. The capsule surrounds the joint and is thickest on the anterior and posterior aspects. The section of the capsule from the disc to the clavicle is more lax, therefore allowing more mobility here than between the disc, sternum, and first rib.[10] The interclavicular ligament reinforces the capsule anteriorly and inferiorly. The costoclavicular ligament connects the clavicle to the first rib.[10] The SC joint gains increased stability from muscles, especially the sternoclydomastoid, sternohyoid, and sternothyroid.[58]

Acromioclavicular Joint

At the other end of the clavicle is the acromioclavicular (AC) joint. This articulation is characterized by variability in size and shape of the clavicu-

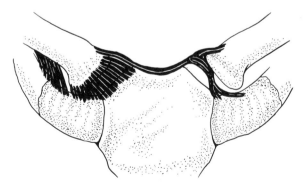

FIGURE 1.9 *The upper and lower attachments of the meniscus and upper and lower ligaments of the sternoclavicular joint.*

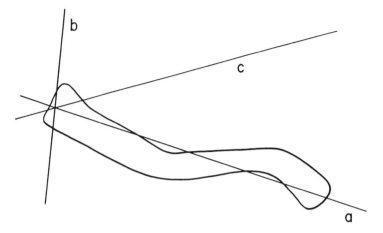

FIGURE 1.10 *Axes of motion of the clavicle. (a) Longitudinal axis of rotation. (b) Vertical axis for protraction and retraction. (c) Horizontal axis for elevation and depression. The sternal end of the scapula is on the left. (From Schenkman and Rugo de Cartaya,[65] with permission.)*

lar facets and the presence of an intra-articular meniscus.[58] The AC joint capsule is more lax than the sternoclavicular joint; thus a greater degree of movement occurs at the AC joint, contributing to the increased incidence of dislocations.[58] There are three major supporting ligaments to the AC joint. The conoid and trapezoid ligaments are collectively called the coracoclavicular ligament and the acromioclavicular ligament. It is through the conoid and trapezoid ligaments that scapula motion is translated to the clavicle.[5]

Rotation of the clavicle is the major movement at the AC joint. Steindler[59] describes AC joint rotation occurring around three axes. Longitudinal axial rotation, vertical axis for protraction and retraction, and horizontal axis for elevation and depression (Fig. 1.10) are all controlled and facilitated by the conoid, trapezoid, and acromioclavicular ligaments.

Scapulothoracic Joint

The scapulothoracic joint is not an anatomic joint, but it is an important physiologic joint that adds considerably to motion of the shoulder girdle. The scapula is concave, articulating with a convex girdle.[1,55] The scapula is without bony or ligamentous connections to the thorax, except for its attachments at the acromioclavicular joint and coracoacromial ligament. The scapula is primarily stabilized by muscles. The importance of the scapula rotators has been established as an essential ingredient to glenohumeral mobility and stability (Fig. 1.11). The stable base, and therefore the mobility of the glenohumeral joint, is largely dependent on the relationship of the scapula and the humerus. The scapula and humerus must accommodate the ever-changing positions during shoulder movement in order to maintain stability.[6]

Functional Biomechanics

As previously noted, shoulder elevation is defined as the movement of the humerus away from the side, and it can occur in an infinite number of body planes.[41]

Shoulder elevation can be divided into three phases. The initial phase of elevation is 0° to 60° degrees. The middle or "critical phase" is 60° to 140°. The final phase of elevation is 140° to 180°. Specific to each phase of movement, precise muscle function and joint kinematics allow normal pain-free motion. Analysis of the precise

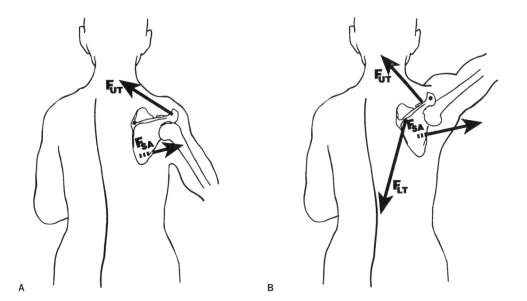

FIGURE 1.11 *Force couple of muscles acting at scapula* **(A)** *Axis of scapular rotation from 0° to 30°.* **(B)** *Axis of scapular rotation from 30° to 60° (F_{UT}, force of upper trapezius; F_{LT}, force of lower trapezius; F_{SA} force of serratus anterior.) (Modified from Schenkman and Rugo de Cartaya,[65] with permission.)*

components critical for each phase of shoulder elevation will determine the success of clinical management of shoulder dysfunction.

INITIAL PHASE OF ELEVATION: 0° TO 60°

All three arthrokinematic movements occur at the glenohumeral joint, but they do not occur in equal proportions. These movements—roll, spin, and glide—are necessary for the large humeral head to take advantage of the small glenoid articulating surface.[16] Saha[60] and Sharkey and Marder[61] investigated the contact area between the head of the humerus and the glenoid with elevation in abduction and in scaption. The studies found that the contact area on the head of the humerus was centered at 30° and shifted superiorly 1.5 mm by 120°. Poppen and Walker[14] also studied the instant centers of rotation for abduction. They reported that in the first 30° and often between 30° 60° of abduction, the head of the humerus moved superiorly in the glenoid by 3 mm, indicating that rolling or gliding of the head had occurred. The EMG activity of the su-

praspinatus muscle indicates an early rise in tension, producing a compressive force to the glenohumeral joint surface.

The deltoid muscle also demonstrates EMG activity in the initial phase of elevation. The subscapularis, infraspinatus, and teres minor muscles are important stabilizers of the humerus in the initial phase of elevation.[3] Kadaba et al.[53] report EMG activity of the upper and lower portions of the subscapularis muscle recorded by intramuscular wire electrodes. During the initial phase of elevation, EMG activity of the upper subscapularis was greater at the beginning of the range, while that in the lower subscapularis increased as the elevation reached 90°.[53] A significant amount of force is generated at the glenohumeral joint during abduction.[4,15] In the early stages of abduction, the loading vector is beyond the upper edge of the glenoid.[62]

During the initial stage of elevation, the pull of the deltoid muscle produces an upward shear of the humeral head.[3] This shearing force peaks at 60° of abduction and is counteracted by the transverse compressive forces of the rotator cuff muscles.[3,15] The primary function of the subscapularis muscle is to depress the humeral head, counteracting the superior migrating force of the deltoid.[53] At 60° (abduction), the downward (short rotator) force was maximal at 9.6 times the limb weight or 0.42 times the body weight.[2,15] The subscapularis, infraspinatus, and latissimus dorsi muscle have small lever arms that form 90° angles to the glenoid face, producing compressive forces to the joint.

Movement of the scapula is permitted by movement in the AC and SC joints. Shoulder abduction is accompanied by clavicular elevation. Sternoclavicular elevation is most evident during the initial phase of arm elevation. There are 4° SC movement for each 10° of shoulder abduction.[4] The acromioclavicular joint moves primarily before 30° and after 135°.[4]

The instantaneous center of rotation (ICR) of the scapula during the initial phase of elevation is located at or near the root of the scapula spine in line with the SC joint.[63] The initial phase of arm elevation is referred to by Poppen and Walker[15] as the setting phase; scapula rotation occurs about the lower midportion. The relative contribution from scapular rotation during the initial phase of elevation is considerably less than from glenohumeral motion. Bagg and Forest[63] estimated a 3.29 to 1 ratio of glenohumeral to scapulothoracic mobility during the initial phase of elevation. The upper trapezius and lower serratus anterior muscles provide the necessary rotatory force couple to produce upward scapular rotation during the early phase of arm abduction.[63]

MIDDLE OR CRITICAL PHASE OF ELEVATION: 60° TO 100°

The middle or critical phase of elevation is initiated by excessive force at the glenohumeral joint. As previously noted, the shearing force of the deltoid muscle is maximum at 60° elevation (Fig. 1.12). Wuelker et al.[54] simulated muscle forces under the coracoacromial vault. The forces at the glenohumeral joint were recorded and applied to the shoulder muscles at a constant ratio approximating physiologic conditions of shoulder

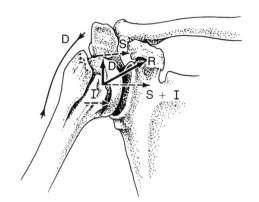

FIGURE 1.12 *In the early stages of glenohumeral abduction, the deltoid reactive force (D) is located outside the glenoid fossa. This force is counteracted by the transverse compressive forces of the supraspinatus (S) and infraspinatus (I) muscles. The resultant reactive force (R) is therefore more favorably placed within the glenoid fossa for joint stability.*

elevation: deltoid, 43 percent supraspinatus, 9 percent; subscapularis, 26 percent; and infraspinatus/teres minor, 22 percent (Fig. 1.13). Peak forces under the coracoacromial vault occurred between 51° and 82° of glenohumeral joint elevation. These force values may represent the pathomechanics of shoulder impingement.

The resultant acting forces, which are stabilizing to the joint, are maximum at 90° of elevation,[3] with shear and compressive forces equal.[64] As the arm reaches the end of the critical phase, the resultant force and the shearing forces of the deltoid are almost zero.[3,15]

Dynamic stability of the glenohumeral joint is established by the balance of shearing and compressive forces. In the early part of the critical phase, dynamic stability must be initiated before further progression of pain-free movement can occur. As previously noted, the lower fibers of the subscapularis muscle showed more activity at 90° of abduction.[53] The deltoid muscle reaches maximum EMG activity at about 110° of abduction and maintains a plateau level of activity.[3] Supraspinatus EMG activity peaks at 100° of elevation and rapidly diminishes thereafter.[3] The subscapularis activity decreases substan-

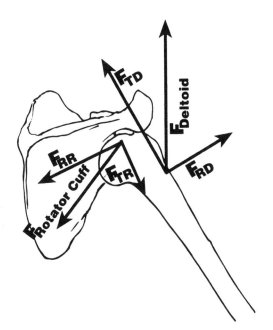

FIGURE 1.13 *Force couple of deltoid and rotator cuff muscles. Rotatory forces, acting on opposite sides of axis of motion, combine to produce upward rotation. Translatory forces cancel each other out. (F_{RR} rotatory force of rotator cuff; F_{TR}, translatory force of rotator cuff; F_{RD}, rotatory force of deltoid; F_{TD}, translatory force of deltoid.) (Modified from Schenkman and de Cartaya,[65] with permission.)*

humeral motion to every degree of scapular motion from 20.8° to 81.8° scaption. The humeral component decreased to 0.71° for scaption between 81.8° and 139.1°. Therefore, the greatest relative amount of scapular rotation occurs between 80° and 140° of arm abduction.[63] The ratio of glenohumeral to scapulothoracic motion has been calculated to be 0.71 to 1 during the middle phase of elevation.[64] Doody et al.,[12] along with Freedman and Munro,[42] proposed that the significant role of the scapular rotators during the critical phase of elevation is secondary to the relatively long moment arms of the upper trapezius, lower trapezius, and lower serratus anterior muscles. Therefore, during the middle phase of elevation, the scapula rotators provide an important contribution to elevation of the humerus in the plane of the scapula.

Movement of the scapula is permitted by movement of the acromioclavicular and sternoclavicular joints. The relative contribution of these two joints changes throughout the range of motion depending on where the instant center of rotation (ICR) lies.[63] During the middle phase of abduction, the ICR of the scapula begins to migrate towards the AC joint. Clavicular elevation about the SC joint, coupled with scapular rotation about the AC joint, facilitates normal scapular mobility. Motion can occur at the AC joint with less movement occurring at the SC joint, because of the clavicular rotation around its long axis.[4] The double-curved clavicle acts like a crankshaft permitting elevation and rotation at the AC end. The rotation of the scapula about the AC joint is initiated between 60° and 90° of elevation.[63] Clavicular elevation is completed between 120° and 150° of humeral abduction.[63] Clavicular elevation at the AC joint permits maximum scapular rotation. At approximately 150° of elevation the ICR of the scapula is in line with the AC joint.[63]

tially after 130° of elevation, supporting the concept that anterior ligament stability is critical beyond 130° of elevation.[3]

The head of the humerus demonstrates an excursion of 1 to 2 mm of a superior and inferior glide on the glenoid surface.[14] The movement of the humeral head in a superior and inferior direction after 60° of elevation indicates that a roll and glide is occurring in opposite directions, resulting in a spin of the bone. As previously noted, external rotation of the humerus is critical for elevation (abduction) of the arm.

Bagg and Forrest[63] evaluated 20 subjects and found three distinctive patterns of scapulohumeral movement. Each pattern had three phases with varying ratios of humeral to scapular movement. The most common pattern had 3.29° of

FINAL PHASE OF ELEVATION: 140° TO 180°

During the final phase of elevation, the ratio of glenohumeral to scapulothoracic motion is 3.49 to 1, indicating relatively more glenohumeral motion.[63] The ICR of the scapula has relocated upward and laterally. The rotatory force arm of the upper trapezius muscle has reduced in length, and the role of this muscle is now supportive to the scapula.[64] The new location of the ICR of the scapula allows the middle trapezius to become a prime mover for downward scapular rotation.[64] The lower trapezius and the serratus anterior muscles continue to increase in activity during the final phase of elevation, acting as an upward rotator and opposing the forces of the upper and middle trapezius.[63]

As the humerus elevates towards the end of the elevation range of motion, it must disengage itself from the scapula. As previously noted, the ratio of glenohumeral to scapulothoracic motion is 3.49 to 1. Good extensibility of the latissimus, pectoralis major, teres major, teres minor, infraspinatus, and subscapularis muscles is important in order to allow the humerus to dissociate itself from the scapula. Often with passive humeral elevation, a bulge of the scapula is noted laterally. The bulge is usually the inferior angle, secondary to increased protraction of the scapula. Lack of elongation of these muscles prevents the normally dominant movement of the humerus at the end of the elevation range. I often observe tightness of the subscapularis muscle, teres major muscle, or both.

Furthermore, observation of limited passive humeral elevation may exhibit elevation of the chest cavity. If muscles connecting the humerus and rib cage are not flexible enough, movement will occur at both ends. The latissimus and pectoralis major muscles connect the humerus to the rib cage. Lack of dissociation of the rib cage from the humerus will result in excessive rib cage mobility in passive terminal elevation.

Summary of Shoulder Phases of Movement

The initial phase of elevation occurs predominantly at the glenohumeral joint. A 3-mm superior glide of the humeral head has been observed in the initial phase of elevation. The activity of the deltoid muscle produces this superior shearing force at the glenohumeral joint. The activity of the supraspinatus, infraspinatus, teres minor, and subscapularis muscles counteract the forces of the deltoid muscle, creating a resultant force that is stabilizing to the joint and necessary for full pain-free movement to continue. The resultant force in the normal glenohumeral joint is maximum at 90° of elevation. The early phase of scapula movement is described as the setting phase, with the majority of movement occurring at the glenohumeral joint.

The middle phase of elevation is referred to as the critical phase. At the beginning of the critical phase, maximum shearing forces of the deltoid muscle occur. The ratio of glenohumeral to scapulothoracic movement shifts, emphasizing the latter. The increased scapula movement is established by the activity of the upper and lower trapezius and lower anterior serratus muscles. The arthrokinematic movement of the head of the humerus on the glenoid has been observed as an inferior and superior glide of 1.5 mm.

During the final phase of elevation, the movement is once again dominated by the glenohumeral joint. Good extensibility of the latissimus, pectoralis major, teres major, teres minor, and subscapularis muscles is necessary to allow the increased and unconstrained movement of the humerus away from the scapula.

Summary

Patients with shoulder dysfunction are routinely treated in the physical therapy clinic. An understanding of the anatomy and biomechanics of this joint can help provide the physical therapist with a rationale for evaluation and treatment. Most studies involving shoulder anatomy and biomechanics reveal a common pattern along with a wide variation among subjects. The physical therapist should keep this variation in mind when treating an individual patient.

Treatment may be directed toward restoring mobility, providing stability, or a combination of the two. The shoulder is an inherently mobile complex, with various joint surfaces adding to the freedom of movement. The shallow glenoid with its flexible labrum and large humeral head provides mobility. At times, this vast mobility occurs at the expense of stability. The shoulder relies on various stabilizing mechanisms, including shapes of joint surfaces, ligaments, and muscles to prevent excessive motion. Nearly 20 muscles act on this joint complex in some manner, and at various times can be both prime movers and stabilizers. Harmonious actions of these muscles are necessary for the full function of this joint.

Acknowledgments

We give special thanks to Martha Kaput Frame for her contributions to this chapter.

References

1. Kent BE: Functional anatomy of the shoulder complex. A review. Phys Ther 51:867, 1971
2. Lucas D: Biomechanics of the shoulder joint. Arch Surg 107:425, 1973
3. Sarrafian SK: Gross and functional anatomy of the shoulder. Clin Orthop Rel Res 173:11, 1983
4. Inman VT, Saunders M, Abbott LC: Observations on the function of the shoulder joint. J Bone Joint Surg 26A:1, 1944
5. Dempster WT: Mechanism of shoulder movement. Arch Phys Med Rehabil 46A:49, 1965
6. Moseley JB et al: EMG analysis of the scapular muscles during a shoulder rehabilitation program. Am J Sports Med 20:128, 1992
7. Bechtol C: Biomechanics of the shoulder. Clin Orthop 146:37, 1980
8. Johnston TB: Movements of the shoulder joint: plea for use of "plane of the scapula" as plane of reference for movements occurring at humeroscapula joint. Br J Surg 25:252, 1937
9. Townsend H, Jobe F, Pink M, Perry J: Electromyographic analysis of the glenohumeral muscles during a baseball rehabilitation program. Am J Sports Med 19:264, 1991
10. Warwick R, Williams P (eds): Gray's Anatomy. 35th British Ed. WB Saunders, Philadelphia, 1973
11. Calliet R: Shoulder Pain. FA Davis, Philadelphia, 1966
12. Doody SG, Freedman L, Waterland JC: Shoulder movements during abduction in the scapular plane. Arch Phys Med Rehabil 51d: 595, 1970
13. Saha AK: Mechanics of elevation of glenohumeral joint. Acta Orthop Scand 44: 6688, 1973
14. Poppen NK, Walker PS: Forces at the glenohumeral joint in abduction. Clin Orthop 135:165, 1978
15. Poppen NK, Walker PS: Normal and abnormal motion of the shoulder. J Bone Joint Surg 58A: 195, 1976
16. Saha AK: Theory of Shoulder Mechanism: Descriptive and Applied. Charles C Thomas, Springfield, IL, 1961
17. Codman EA: The Shoulder. Thomas Dodd, Boston, 1934
18. Kondo M, Tazoe S, Yamada M: Changes of the tilting angle of the scapula following elevation of the arm. In Gateman JE, Welsh RP (eds): Surgery of the Shoulder. Philadelphia, CV Mosby, 1984
19. Williams PE, Goldspink G: Changes in sarcomere length and physiological properties in immobilized muscle. J Anat 127: 459, 1978
20. Tabury JC, Tabary C, Tardieu C et al: Physiological and structural changes in the cat's soleus muscle due to immobilization at different lengths by plaster casts. J Physiol 224:231, 1972
21. Tardieu C, Huet E, Bret MD et al: Muscle hypoextensibility in children with cerebral palsy, 1. Clinical and experimental observations. Arch Phys Med Rehabil 63:97, 1982
22. Lucas D: Biomechanics of the shoulder joint. Arch Surg 107:425, 1973
23. Soderberg GJ, Blaschak MJ: Shoulder internal and external rotation peak torque production through a velocity spectrum in differing positions. J Orthop Sports Phys Ther 8:518, 1987
24. Hellwig EV, Perrin DH: A comparison of two positions for assessing shoulder rotator peak torque: the traditional frontal plane versus the plane of the scapula. Isokin Exerc Sci 1:202, 1991
25. Greenfield BH, Donatelli R, Wooden MJ, Wilkes J: Isokinetic evaluation of shoulder rotational strength between the plane of the scapula and the frontal plane. Am J Sports Med 18:124, 1990
26. Tata EG, Ng L, Kramer JF: Shoulder antagonistic strength ratios during concentric and eccentric muscle actions in the scapular plane. J Orthop Sports Phys Ther 18:654, 1993
27. Whitcomb LJ, Kelley MJ, Leiper CI: A comparison

of torque production during dynamic strength testing of shoulder abduction in the coronal plane and the plane of the scapula. J Orthop Sports Phys Ther 21:227, 1995

28. Rajendran K: The rotary influence of articular contours during passive glenohumeral abduction. Singapore Med J 33:493, 1992

29. An KN, Browne AO, Korinek S et al: Three-dimensional kinematics of glenohumeral elevation. J Orthop Res 9:143, 1991

30. Otis JC, Jiang CC, Wickiewicz TL et al: Changes in the moment arms of the rotator cuff and deltoid muscles with abduction and rotation. J Bone Joint Surg 76-A:667, 1994

31. Flatow EL, Soslowsky LJ, Ticker JB: Excursion of the rotator cuff under the acromion: patterns of subacromial contact. Am J Sports Med 22:779, 1994

32. Rajendran K, Kwek BH: glenohumeral abduction and the long head of the biceps. Singapore Med J 32:242, 1991

33. Brems JJ: Rehabilitation following total shoulder arthroplasty. Clin Orthop 307:70, 1994

34. Terry GC, Hammon D, France P et al. The stabilizing function of passive shoulder restraints. Am J Sports Med 1991;19:26–34

35. Saha AK: Dynamic stability of the glenohumeral joint. Acta Orthop Scand 42:491, 1971

36. Kessell L: Clinical Disorders of the Shoulder. 2nd Ed. Churchill Livingstone, Edinburgh, 1986

37. Moseley HP, Overgaard B: The anterior capsular mechanism in recurrent anterior dislocations of the shoulder: morphological and clinical studies with special reference to the glenoid labrum and glenohumeral ligaments. J Bone Joint Surg 44B:913, 1962

38. Bowen MK, Russell FW: Ligamentous control of shoulder stability based on selective cutting and static translation experiments. Clin Sports Med 10:757, 1991

39. Reeves B: Experiments in the tensile strength of the anterior capsular structures of the shoulder in man. J Bone Joint Surg 50B:858, 1968

40. Matsen FA, Lippitt SB, Slidles JA et al: Stability. In Matson FA, Lippitt SB, Slides JA et al. (eds): Practical Evaluation and Management of the Shoulder. WB Saunders, Philadelphia, 1993

41. Pagnani MJ, Galinat BJ, Warren RF. Glenohumeral instability. In DeLee JC, Drez D, (eds): Orthopaedic Sports Medicine: Principles and Practice. WB Saunders, Philadelphia, 1993

42. Freedman L, Munro RH: Abduction of the arm in the scapular plane: scapular and glenohumeral movements. A roentgenographic study. J Bone Joint Surg 48A:1503, 1966

43. Kapanji IA: The Physiology of the Joints—Upper Limb, Vol 1. Churchill Livingstone, New York, 1970

44. Basmajian J: The surgical anatomy and function of the arm-trunk mechanism. Surg Clin North Am 43:1475, 1963

45. Turkel SJ, Panio MW, Marshall JL, Girgis FG: Stabilizing mechanisms preventing anterior dislocation of the glenohumeral joint. J Bone Joint Surg 63A:1208, 1981

46. MacDonald PB, Hawkins RJ, Fowler PJ, Miniaci A: Release of the subscapularis for internal rotation contracture and pain after anterior repair for recurrent anterior dislocation of the shoulder. J Bone Joint Surg 74A:734, 1992

47. Itoi E, Kuechle DK, Newman SR, Murrey BF, Am Koy et al: Stabilizing function of the biceps in stable and unstable shoulders. J Bone Joint Surg Br 75:546, 1993

48. Warner JJ, Deng XH, Warren RF, Torzilli PA: Static capsuloligamentous restraints to superior–inferior translation of the glenohumeral joint. Am J Sports Med 20:675, 1992

49. Guanche C, Knatt T, Solomonow M et al: The synergistic action of the capsule and the shoulder muscles. Am J Sports Med 23:1995

50. Harryman DT, Sidles JA, Harris SL, Matsen FA: The role of rotator interval capsule in passive motion and stability of the shoulder. J Bone Joint Surg 74A:53, 1992

51. Kummell BM: Spectrum of lesions of the anterior capsular mechanism of the shoulder. Am J Sports Med 7:111, 1979

52. Travell J, Simons D: Myofascial Pain and Dysfunction. The Trigger Point Manual. Williams & Wilkins, Baltimore, 1993

53. Kadaba MP, Cole MF, Wooten P et al: Intramuscular wire electromyography of the subscapularis. J Orthop Res 10:394, 1992

54. Wuelker N, Schmotzer H, Thren K, Korell M et al: Translation of the glenohumeral joint with simulated active elevation. Clin Orthop 309:193, 1994

55. Perry J: Muscle control of the shoulder. p. 17. In Rowe CR (ed): The Shoulder. Churchill Livingstone, New York, 1988

56. Hagberg M: Electromyographic signs of shoulder muscular fatigue in two elevated arm positions. Am J Phys Med 60:111, 1981

57. Michiels I, Bodem F: The deltoid muscle: an electromyographical analysis of its activity in arm abduction in various body postures. Int Orthop 16: 268, 1992

58. Moseley HF: The clavicle: its anatomy and function. Clin Orthop Res 58:17, 1968

59. Steindler A: Kinesiology of the Human Body Under Normal and Pathological Conditions. Charles C Thomas, Springfield, IL, 1955

60. Saha AK: Mechanism of shoulder movements and a plea for the recognition of "zero position" of glenohumeral joint. Clin Orthop 173:3, 1983

61. Sharkey NA, Marder RA: The rotator cuff opposes superior translation of the humeral head. Am J Sports Med 23:270, 1995

62. Himeno S, Tsumura H: The role of the rotator cuff as a stabilizing mechanism of the shoulder. In Bateman S, Welch P (eds): Surgery of the Shoulder. CV Mosby, St. Louis, 1984

63. Bagg DS, Forrest WJ: A biomechanical analysis of scapular rotation during arm abduction in the scapular plane. Am J Phys Med Rehabil 67:238, 1988

64. Bagg DS, Forrest WJ: Electromyographic study of the scapular rotators during arm abduction in the scapular plane. Am J Phys Med 65:111, 1986

65. Schenkman M, Rugo de Cartaya V: Kinesiology of the shoulder complex. J Orthop Sports Phys Ther 8:438, 1987

2

Throwing Injuries

J E F F   C O O P E R

To throw a baseball with high velocity and with great accuracy is a skill that escapes the majority of the population. Those who have accomplished this skill often demonstrate a heightened neuromuscular system and have invested many hours of sport-specific training. This unique athletic act has produced a wide array of disabilities that have been reported in the literature. These disabilities include neurologic entrapments and compression syndromes, acromioclavicular joint degeneration, primary impingement, secondary impingement due to instabilities, instabilities due to derangement of the glenoid, SLAP (superior labrum anterior to posterior) lesions, subdeltoid bursitis, biceps tendinitis, subluxing bicipital tendon, undersurface tears of the rotator cuff, full-thickness tears of the rotator cuff, lesions of the humeral head, fracture of the humerus, fracture of the coricoid, posterior capsular syndrome, and muscle imbalances.[1–10]

Injury to the glenohumeral complex as a result of the overhand throw is most often the result of repetitive microtrauma. Chronic overuse causes the healing process to fall behind that of the rate of stress. Macrotrauma injuries such as fractures of the humerus have been reported; however, they represent a very small percentage of the disabilities associated with the overhand throw.

Overhand Throwing

The biomechanical and electromyographic activity of the overhand throw has been investigated[11–17] to give us a relative model of function in a controlled environment. It is assumed that the forces recorded during these data collections are less than those produced in a competitive arena. Electromyographic sequence activity appears fairly consistent regardless of generated velocities. The overhand throw as it relates to pitching has been divided into the following phases: (1) windup, (2) early cocking, (3) late cocking, (4) acceleration, and (5) follow-through.

WINDUP

The windup is an activity that is highly individualized. Its purpose is to organize the body beneath the arm to form a stable platform. As with all overarm activities, it is vital that the body perform in sequential links to enable the hand to be in the correct position in space to complete the assigned task. The hand can be placed in an infinite number of localities, and it is essential that the scapulahumeral rhythm places it in an optimum setting for the task of propulsion. The drawing of the humerus into the moment center of the glenoid fossa is accomplished during the first 30° of elevation as the arm is brought upward by the deltoid and supraspinatus. Throughout the windup phase there is no consistent pattern of muscle activity due to these many individual styles.

EARLY COCKING

Early cocking is the period of time when the dominant hand is separated from the gloved hand, and ends when the forward foot makes

19

contact with the mound. The scapula is retracted and maintained against the chest wall by the serratus anterior. The humerus is brought into position of 90° of abduction and horizontal extension, with a minimal external rotation of approximately 50°. This is accomplished with the activation of the anterior, middle, and posterior deltoid. The external rotators of the cuff are activated toward the end of early cocking, with the supraspinatus being more active than the infraspinatus and the teres minor as it steers the humeral head in the glenoid. The biceps brachii and brachialis act on the forearm to develop the necessary angle of the elbow.

As the body moves forward, the humerus is supported by the anterior and middle deltoid as the posterior deltoid pulls the arm into approximately 30° of horizontal extension. At this time the static stability of the humeral head becomes dependent upon the anterior margin of the glenoid, notably the inferior glenohumeral ligament and the inferior portion of the glenoid labrum.

LATE COCKING

Late cocking is the interval in the throwing motion when the foot makes contact with the mound, and ends when the humerus begins internal rotation. During this time the humerus is moved into a position more forward in relation to the trunk and begins to come into alignment with the upper body. The extreme of external rotation, an additional 125° is achieved to provide positioning for the power phase or acceleration.

Supraspinatus, infraspinatus, and teres minor are active in this phase but become quiet once external rotation is achieved. Deceleration of the externally rotating humerus is accomplished by the contraction of the subscapularis. It remains active until the completion of late cocking. The serratus anterior and the clavicular head of the pectoralis major have their greatest activity during deceleration. The biceps brachii aids in maintaining the humerus in the glenoid by producing compressive axial load. At the end of this phase the triceps begins activity providing compressive axial loading to replace the force of the biceps. The capsule becomes wound tight in preparation of acceleration.

ACCELERATION

Acceleration is a ballistic action lasting less than one-tenth of a second. The ball is accelerated from 4 miles per hour to a speed of 85 plus miles per hour.[11] This rapid acceleration produces angular velocities that have been reported as high as 9,198°/s.[16] The scapula is protracted and rotated downward and held to the chest wall by the serratus anterior. The arm continues into forward flexion and is marked by a maximum internal rotation of the humerus. The humerus travels forward in 100° of abduction but adducts about 5° just prior to release. The lattismus dorsi and pectoralis major develop the power to the forward-moving shoulder. The subscapularis activity is at maximum levels as the humerus travels into medial rotation. The triceps develops strong action in accelerating the extension of the elbow.

The forces developed in this instant reflect the body's amazing ability to develop power and encase itself in a protective mechanism. Pappas et al.[16] reported peak accelerations approaching 600,000°/s. Gainor et al.[5] reported 14,000 inch pounds of rotatory torque produced at the shoulder. This torque develops 27,000 inch pounds of kinetic energy in the humerus.

Control of the ball is lost approximately midway through the acceleration phase, when the humerus is positioned slightly behind the forward-flexing trunk and at a angle of about 110° of external rotation. The hand follows the ball after release and is unable to apply further force.

FOLLOW-THROUGH

Follow-through is the time beginning with the release of the ball. Within the first tenth of a second the humerus travels across the midline of the body and develops a slight external rotation before finishing in internal rotation. This is a very active phase for all glenohumeral muscles as the arm is decelerated. The deltoid and upper trapezius have strong activity as does the lattisimus dorsi. The infraspinatus, teres minor, supraspinatus, and subscapularis are all active as eccentric loads are produced. The biceps develops peak activity in decelerating the forearm and imposes a traction force within the glenohumeral joint.

The task of documenting the sequence of muscle activity during the act of pitching has allowed the musculature acting upon the glenohumeral joint during this act to be divided into two groups.[12] The first group of muscles are those that are most active during the second and third phases of throwing, early and late cocking. They are least active during the acceleration phase. The deltoid, trapezius, external rotators, supraspinatus, infraspinatus, teres minor, and biceps brachii comprise this first group.

The second group of muscles are those used primarily for the fourth phase of throwing, acceleration. These muscles are necessary to protract the scapula, horizontal forward flex and internally rotate the humerus, and extend the elbow. This group consists of the subscapularis, serratus anterior, pectoralis major, lattismus dorsi, and triceps brachii. The first phase of throwing is not included in either group due to its nonspecific generalized activity.

Professional Versus Amateur Pitchers

Gowan et al.[12] conducted a study to determine if the muscle-firing sequence of professional pitchers was significantly different from that of amateur pitchers. No significant differences were noted in the first three phase of the pitch, the windup, early and late cocking. There were no significant differences in the follow-through, where muscle activity was described as general.

During the acceleration phase, professional pitchers recorded increased activity of the pectoralis major and lattisimus dorsi. There was also increased activity in the serratus anterior muscle. The professional pitchers had decreased activity in the supraspinatus, infraspinatus, and teres minor during the acceleration. Professional pitchers used the subscapularis predominately

during acceleration and internal rotation. Activity in the biceps brachii was also lower in the professionals that in the amateurs.

Electromyographic Activity in the Injured Thrower

Those athletes who were diagnosed as subacromial impingers demonstrated differences in their electromyographic studies compared with uninjured throwers.[18] During the second phase of throwing, early cocking, the injured athletes continued deltoid activity while the healthy athletes had deceased deltoid activity. A lower level of supraspinatus activity was also noted during this time period. During early cocking and late cocking, the internal rotators, subscapularis, petoralis major, and latissimus dorsi had decreased activity. The serratus anterior followed this pattern and was less effective. It was theorized that the combination of these differences may lead to increased external rotation, superior humeral migration, and impaired scapular rotation. All or some of these factors may be an underlying cause for the initial problem or a factor in the continuum of the syndrome.

Throwing athletes who have been hampered by glenohumeral instabilities were compared to normal athletes in a similar fashion. This series[19] tested the activity of the biceps, middle deltoid, supraspinatus, infraspinatus, pectoralis major, subscapularis, latissimus dorsi, and serratus anterior. Noted were differences in every muscle except the middle deltoid. The authors suggest that the mildly increased activity of the biceps and supraspinatus may be compensatory for the laxity present in the anterior capsule. The infraspinatus developed a pattern of activity during early cocking, reduced activity during late cocking, and again increasing in the follow-through. As noted with the impingement group, the internal rotators, consisting of the subscapularis, pectoralis major, and lattisimus dorsi, had decreased activity, which was marked in the early cocking phase. The serratus anterior showed decreased activity as well.

The authors concluded that these changes in muscle activity allowed decreased internal rotation force needed in both late cocking and acceleration. Reduced activity demonstrated in controlling the scapula by the serratus anterior allowed the glenoid to be placed in a compromising position during late cocking, increasing the stress upon the labrum and capsule.

Microtraumas can be associated with deficiencies in a muscle or muscle group failing to aid in the stabilizing of the glenohumeral joint or failing to become active in the proper sequence during the distinct phases of throwing. Lack of flexibility can be a factor leading to disability, particularly in the deceleration phase, when tremendous eccentric forces are developed.

The Instability Continuum

Repetitive stretching of the anterior static stabilizers may be the most damaging pathology to the throwing athlete. The development of small occult anterior translations of the humerus upon the glenoid during late cocking and early acceleration has a cumulative effect most often manifested as anterior shoulder pain. As the anterior stabilizers of the glenohumeral joint are progressively overwhelmed, the rotator cuff attempts to compensate for the loss of stability. They are eventually overcome. The scapular rotators react to provide a stable base for the glenohumeral joint, become innervated out of sequence, and begin to fail.[20] This pattern of disability is described by Jobe and Pink as one of instability permitting subluxation, and subluxation permitting impingement of the rotator cuff against the acromion and coracromial ligament and the eventual disruption of the muscle. This sequence of events has been termed the instability continuum.[21]

Athletes with anterior shoulder pain are classified into four groups. Group 1 presents pure impingement without a detectable instability. They will test positive for a Neer or Hawkins sign, or for both. They prove negative to an apprehension test for instability. Group 2 includes those athletes who demonstrate instability due to chronic labral microtrauma with secondary impingement. This group presents signs of posterior labrum defects with anterior capsule and ligamentous involvement. There may be tears in the undersurface of the supraspinatus and/or infraspinatus muscles. These athletes will present a positive impingement sign and have pain but not apprehension when subjected to the apprehension test. Their pain will be relieved with the relocation test.

Group 3 athletes present instability due to hyperelasticity with impingement. Hyperelasticity is defined as the ability to passively touch the thumb to the forearm and/or the ability to hyperextend the elbow more than 10°. The metacaropophalangeal joint can hyperextend more than 90° and the interphalangeal joint can hyperextended in excess of 60°.[22,23] A positive impingement sign will be presented but the athletes will not be apprehensive when tested. Their pain is relieved with the relocation test.

Group 4 present instability without impingement. They have acquired their instability from a traumatic event—a dislocation. These athletes have a negative impingement test, positive apprehension test, and pain relief with relocation.

Groups 2 and 3 comprise the majority of throwing athletes with anterior shoulder pain. These athletes are often unaware of the subtle anterior translations occuring within their glenohumeral joint. Their complaint is usually that of pain upon the transition from late cocking to acceleration or a loss of velocity with a feeling of general shoulder weakness.

The Biceps Labral Complex

The role of the long head of the biceps tendon has long been the stepchild of glenohumeral mechanism. Often dismissed as only a minor player at the shoulder as a humeral head depressor, it was recognized for its role as an elbow stabilizer and decelerator. In the last decade, since the shoulder has been thoroughly investigated via the athroscope, we have gained a new appreciation for this structure.

Andrews et al.[2] examined a population of 73 throwing athletes and observed that 60 percent of this group had tears in the anterosuperior labrum and another 23 percent had tears in both the anterosuperior and posterosuperior portion. In a subgroup of baseball pitchers, this lesion was associated with a partial tear of the supraspinatus in 73 percent of the athletes. A smaller group of 7 percent demonstrated a partial tear of the long head of the biceps. Andrews et al. hypothesized that the incident of injury to this region of the glenoid labrum was due to the tremendous eccentric stresses placed on the biceps in an attempt to decelerate the arm during the follow-through phase of the overhand throw.

A correlation of patient history revealed 95 percent of the patients reported pain during the overhand throw and 45 percent of the population reported a popping or catching sensation. On physical exam, the popping was evident in the position of full abduction and full flexion as the upper arm was aligned with the ear in 79 percent of the athletes. None of the population demonstrated a significant weakness of either the rotator cuff or biceps tendon. This lesion gives the athlete a sensation of instability; however, this instability does not exist anatomically.

In a retrospective totaling 2,375 arthoscopic evaluated shoulders, Snyder et al.[24] reported 140 cases with superior glenoid labrum injuries. These represented only 6 percent of the sample population. Ninety-one percent of this group was male. The involvement of the dominant shoulder versus the nondominant shoulder was greater than two to one.

No radiographic findings could be correlated to the pathology. No clinical exam was considered to be specific for the superior labrum. About half of the patients described a painful catching or popping, which was consistent with Andrews et al. Only about one-third demonstrated a positive biceps tension test.

Fifty-five percent of these shoulders were categorized as having a type II SLAP lesion consisting of detachment of the superior labrum and biceps tendon from the glenoid rim. Of these shoulders, only 28 percent were isolated from a rotator cuff injury or other labral problems.

Rodosky et al.[22] investigated the role of the long head of the biceps and its attachment to the superior labrum in a laboratory model of the glenohumeral joint positioned in abduction and external rotation as experienced by the overhand thrower. They hypothesized that the presence of the long head of the biceps acted to help limit the external rotating shoulder. The biceps compressed the humeral head against the glenoid resisting the rotation. The long head of the biceps withstood higher external rotational forces without the inferior glenohumeral ligament experiencing a greater strain. This suggested that the biceps has a role in the provision of anterior stability. The glenohumeral joint demonstrated a heightened torsional stiffness as force was increased through the long head.

When a surgical SLAP lesion was created, the strain produced upon the inferior glenohumeral ligament was significantly increased. This model suggests that the shoulder is thus dependent upon the long head of the biceps to provide dynamic stability to the glenohumeral joint in the cocking, acceleration, and follow-through phases. This dynamic stability ensures a consistent stress upon the inferior glenohumeral ligament. The long head acts as a continuum provider of axial tension as a protective mechanism for the humerus and the inferior glenohumeral ligament. Once the integrity of the glenohumeral joint is reduced due to occulant subluxations, the long head of the biceps becomes a larger player in the attempt to achieve stabilization to the glenohumeral joint.

The data of Snyder et al.[24] suggest that the SLAP lesion occurs in a very limited number of cases among the general population. However, this trauma must be among the suspected diagnoses of the overhand throwing athlete with shoulder problems due to the theoretical injury mechanism. Because there is no clear imaging or clinical test for this lesion, it is presently diagnosed via the arthoscope. Pathology of the biceps labral complex should be considered in throwing athletes who report popping or clicking of the glenohumeral joint and can reproduce these symptoms in the forward-flexed and extreme abduction position.

Anterior Capsular Labrum Reconstruction

The relocation test places stress in a direction posterior to the humeral head when the glenohumeral joint is place in the apprehension position of 90° of abduction, horizontal extension, and external rotation. This maneuver relieves the stress on the anterior structures and is considered positive when the athlete's pain is relieved. A distinct factor on examination is that those who continue to have pain when subjected to the relocation test suffer from impingement. Athletes with instability will tolerate maximum external rotation without discomfort during this maneuver.

Rubenstein et al.[23] reported the results of an anterior capsular labrum reconstruction procedure. Of his population of 36 baseball players, 20 were pitchers. Of this group, 15 were determined to have excellent results (measured by the modified Rowe test score that included return to previous level of play as a criterion). A subgroup of 13 professional pitchers yielded 6 who had excellent results.

An important rehabilitation issue related in this study was the time between surgery and the return to throwing. Those players who began their throwing program at 5 months postsurgery had a better outcome than those who began at 7 months.

Montgomery and Jobe[25] reported the results of an advanced surgical procedure comprised of a horizontal capsulotomy and suture anchors. Thirty-two subjects were included in this study with a subgroup of 13 pitchers. Clinical examination revealed 44 percent of the athletes had a positive Neer sign, 48 percent had a positive Hawkins sign, and 100 percent demonstrated a positive relocation test. Of the 13 pitchers, 9 returned to their previous level of play. Included in the group of pitchers were 7 of professional ranks. Of this group, 6 (86 percent) returned to their previous level of professional baseball. Sixteen percent[26] of the entire study group reported posterior postoperative shoulder pain. Three of these athletes returned for an arthroscopic labrum debridement.

Rehabilitation

The knowledge gained over the past decade in the rehabilitation of the overhand throwing athlete has allowed the athletic trainer/therapist to design improved preventative protocols. These protocols have made not only a significant impact in the prevention of disabilities but have played an important role in the reduction of severity and time loss by the athlete. As the surgeon's knowledge expands and it is supported with the technical tools necessary to repair previously undiagnosed lesions, a whole generation of athletes have been given a second opportunity. Overhand-throwing athletes who were previously cast aside due to interarticular structural damage can now entertain surgical options once a period of conservative care has proven fruitless. Athletes must understand that return to play demands that the rehabilitation will be a continuing process, and at no point should they think they have obtained a cure. If athletes anticipate a cure, they will revert to the previous stress cycle, predisposing themselves to injury.

The goals of the rehabilitation process should include (1) the reduction of inflammation and pain, (2) the return of normal shoulder motion, (3) an increase in strength and endurance, (4) a reestablished synchrony of motion, (5) cardiovascular conditioning, and (6) a progressive return to throwing.

Clinically the control of inflammation and pain is often aided by the combined use of subthreshold electrical muscle stimulation and ice. The surface electrodes should be large and should be placed in a fashion to course both the anterior and posterior joint line to develop the desired effect within the glenohumeral joint. The shoulder is placed in the loose packed position and encased in ice for a period of 20 minutes. This protocol is often repeated four to six times a day.

Normal shoulder motion is established by the use of passive proprioceptive neuromuscular facilitation patterns. This provides the additional benefit of educating the athlete on the expected angles and rotations necessary for the active phase. Particular attention is paid to stretching the posterior capsule to regain the adaptive shortening associated with the overhand thrower.[27] A home range-of-motion (ROM) program is instituted via an over-the-door pulley system, and the athlete is encouraged to use this and a posterior capsule stretch six periods during the day.

Jobe and Pink[21] have suggested that the sequence of muscle strengthening begin with the scapular pivoters and glenohumeral protectors. Once a solid foundation has been established in these areas, the strengthening should progress to the humeral positioners, and then to the propeller muscles or accelerators. The scapular glides[28] taught passively in the ROM phase now become active. As noted in the EMG data, the serratus anterior is active throughout most of the overhand throw, and therefore it is important to include this component of the rehabilitation process at the beginning of each treatment. The serratus is not often trained in an endurance mode, but this should be a priority in establishing desired scapular control. The glenohumeral protectors or the muscles of the rotator cuff are strengthened in association with the scapular pivoters. The sequence of muscle strengthening and endurance usually progresses through PNF, isotonics, concentric/eccentric resistive cords, concentric isokinetics, and eccentric isokinetics, to stretch-shortening exercises. Often an attempt to apply the accelerated lessons learned from the lower kinetic chain to that of the upper extremity cheat a solid, methodical isotonic strength base.

The isotonic program in Appendix 2.1 is included for a reference. Townsend,[17] Moseley,[29] and their associates explored the commonly used exercises used by many throwing athletes and attempted to establish specific muscle function and the peak activity arc for each. Because the experimental model used light weights at low intensity and low speed, the full benefit of this element of the rehabilitation program may not be apparent.

First, these exercises are not performed into the arc of greatest benefit if one limits the exercise to what is commonly referred to as below the plane. The majority of the exercises qualify at the extremes of the available range of motion. Second, a less than adequate resistance is employed to elicit the desired muscular response. Third, the use of a high repetition program has not been explored using these exercises. Fourth, the exercises lend themselves easily to an eccentric, or deceleration program. When the athletic trainer/therapist provides the concentric component of the exercise, the resistance of the eccentric component can be significantly increased. It is paramount that this negative base be established prior to the introduction of stretch-shortening exercises. Fifth, a goal of any rehabilitation program is to make the patient or athlete independent. Isotonic dumbbell exercises, resistive cords, and to some extent stretch-shortening exercises can be placed in an independent arena. Isotonic exercises are easily monitored and lend themselves to be measured outside of the clinic.

As shoulder rehabilitation builds upon PNF, isotonic dumbbells, and resistive cords into eccentric loading, it is important to gain knowledge of eccentric exercises as a means of muscle training (Appendix 2.2). Progression into the stretch-shortening exercises is preceded by PNF, isotonics, and eccentric exercises. The use of the Body Blade (Hymanson, Playa Del Rey, CA) in conditioning the upper extremity is an excellent tool to aid in the transition to the more dynamic exercises. Stretch-shortening exercises are usually instituted in the same general time frame as an early throwing program. The progression of these exercises always begins with bilateral routines before attempting single-extremity exercises. Extreme care must be take to protect the stability of the glenohumeral with adequate muscle strength before stretch-shortening exercises are performed in the vulnerable abducted, horizontally extended, and externally rotated position.

The reestablishment of synchrony of motion is developed through a throwing program that emphases long throwing (Appendix 2.3). The act of long throwing builds arm strength by overloading the specific demands necessary for a pitcher who is required to compete at a range of 60 feet and 6 inches. Long throwing provides an element of deceleration in a slightly longer form (time), which is necessary to develop the required eccentrics applied upon the glenohumeral joint. By progressively increasing the distances of throwing, the additional stress is applied at a consistent rate.

Cardiovascular conditioning should be an aspect of the rehabilitation process continued and built upon from the preinjury protocol. Because 46.7 percent of the velocity developed by the throwing arm is developed by the lower body and trunk,[30] it is important to focus upon the conditioning of these segments as part of the entire rehabilitation process. The lower extremities are the larger consumers of oxygen within the muscloskeletal system. If the lower extremities fail in their conversion of oxygen, the entire system becomes less efficient. This failure to perform compounds the stresses in the recovery cycle.

Two programs are provided (Appendices 2.4 and 2.5 D and E) for the progression of the overhand-throwing athlete to a level of competition. Appendix 2.5 represents a more aggressive protocol and can be used in rehabilitations that have a shorter focus in relation to return to play. Appendix 2.4 is suitable for the extended rehabilitation periods and often used for a preseason conditioning program.

CASE STUDY 1

After an uneventful 5-week spring training conditioning period, the pitcher removed himself from his first game after five completed innings. He complained of nonspecific anterior shoulder pain. Upon examination, his range of motion was within normal limits, with the exception of reduced internal rotation that was accompanied with pain. He presented a positive Hawkins sign.

MRI was performed, and abnormalities of the inferior aspect of the anterior glenoid were noted; however, this was consistent with an MRI of 13 months earlier. There were also small degenerative cysts present in the humeral head, and there was evidence of posterior capsular laxity. The player's inflammation was controlled with nonsteroidal anti-inflammatory medica-

tion, EMS, and ice. His prophylatic conditioning program was adjusted to below-plane exercises and supplemented with a PNF series with particular attention paid to the scapular glides and diagonal patterns with a shortened lever. His posterior capsule stretching was accelerated.

Five days postinjury the pitcher attempted to throw on the side to determine his roster status. After completing 42 throws with discomfort, it was necessary to place him on a disabled list, which removed him from the active roster. Eleven days postinjury the player again attempted to throw from the mound and was successful in completing 72 pitches without discomfort. Fourteen days postinjury the player pitched five innings totaling 55 pitches in a minor league game without difficulty and reported no difficulties the following day.

Nineteen days from the original complaint, the player started a major league game, completed five innings, and continued in the five-man rotation until again complaining of similar anterior shoulder pain after six starting assignments. At this time his forward flexion was reduced by 10° in his dominant arm. His external rotation was reduced by 15° and his internal rotation showed a marked reduction, presenting only a L2 dominant compared to T4 nondominant. His posterior capsule remained restricted in spite of the active stretching. There was no joint laxity, a negative apprehension sign, and a negative relocation sign.

The pitcher made one more start, in which he pitched into the sixth inning, but he left the game due to a lack of velocity. Two days later he was unable to throw. Upon examination he demonstrated a subtle anterior subluxation for the first time. There was a popping sensation with pain when he was abducted with external rotation and forced into extension. A radiograph and bone scan were conducted and they were interpreted as normal. An arthroscopic examination was performed, and the following were noted. An undersurface cuff tear was seen in the supraspinatus, which was small, linear, and debrided. The anterior labrum was frayed and also debrided. The posterior labrum was frayed and also debrided. There was a trough defect on the posterior humeral head, indicating anterior subluxation. There was inflammation about the biceps tendon but no evidence of a SLAP lesion. There was an absence of a middle glenohumeral ligament. The subacromial space was normal.

Ten days post injury his range of motion was within normal limits and his internal range of motion had increased by four vertebrae. At one month postinjury the player began a two days on, one day off throwing program in an attempt to return to the mound. Ten days later he threw 40 pitches from the mound. His throwing activities increased, which included throwing batting practice at 7 weeks and pitching in a minor league contest in the ninth week. He continued to pitch in the minor leagues on a 5-day rotation, building arm strength and velocity. At 12 weeks he was ready to return to the major league roster.

The following season the athlete repeated the cycle of early season difficulties and lack of velocity associated with an anteriorly unstable shoulder. After another extended period of rehabilitation, he was again able to return to a major league mound, but was unable to develop the necessary velocity to be competitive. He had progressed into the instability continuum and will be forced to decide if he will undergo an anterior capsular labrum reconstruction or retire.

CASE STUDY 2

During the fourth month of the championship season a starting pitcher complained of discomfort in his throwing shoulder medial to the joint line. He was examined by the attending orthopedist, which yielded no concise diagnosis, but was prescribed a course of general therapy. Due to scheduling, the pitcher did not have to compete for a period of 11 days. On his next start he was able to perform without reservation and pitched well into the game. In his next start 6 days latter, he threw a pitch in the fourth inning that resulted in tremendous pain. The athlete was immediately unable to actively forward flex or abduct his arm. He was examined the following day by the attending orthopedist and a bone scan was ordered. This test resulted in the discovery of an avulsion fracture of the coracoid process.

After a 6-week period of relative inactivity the athlete began a rehabilitation process of active range of motion, scapular glides, and isotonic exercises. Bone scans were repeated at 2, 5, and 7 months. The following season the athlete participated in every scheduled start, compiling a total of 230 innings.

Acknowledgments

I would like to thank Jim Richards, PhD, and Dan Elkins, ATC, for their assistance with the photography.

References

1. Altchek DW, Warren RF, Wickiewicz TL et al: Arhroscopic labral debridement: a three-year follow-up study. Am J Sports Med 20:702, 1992
2. Andrews JR, Carson WG et al: Glenoid labrum tears related to the long head of the biceps. Am J Sports Med 13:337, 1985
3. Black KP, Lombardo JA: Suprascapular nerve injuries with isolated paralysis of the infraspinatus. Am J Sports Med 18:225, 1990
4. Branch T, Partin C et al: Spontaneous fractures of the humerus during pitching: a series of 12 cases. Am J Sports Med 20:468, 1992
5. Gainor BJ, Piotrowski G et al: The throw: biomechanics and acute injury. AJSM 8:114, 1980
6. Garth WP, Allman FL, Armstrong WS: Occult anterior subluxations of the shoulder in noncontact sports. Am J Sports Med 15:579, 1987
7. Jobe FW, Kvitne RS: Shoulder pain in the overhand or throwing athlete. Othopaed Rev 18:963, 1989
8. Ringel SP, Treihaft M et al: Suprascapular neuropathy in pitchers. Am J Sports Med 18:80, 1990
9. Schachter CL, Canham PB, Mottola MF: Biomechanical factors affecting Dave Dravecky's return to cometitive pitching: a case study. J Orthop Sports Phys Ther 16:2, 1992
10. Simon ER, Hill JA: Rotator cuff injuries: an update. J Orthop Sports Phys Ther 10:394, 1989
11. Dillman CJ, Fleisig GS, Andrews JR: Biomecha-

nics of pitching with emphasis upon shoulder kinematics. JOBST 18:402, 1993

12. Gowan ID, Jobe FW, Tibone JE et al: A comparative electromyographic analysis of the shoulder during pitching. Am J Sports Med 15:586, 1987

13. Jobe FW, Tibone JE, Perry J, Moynes D: An EMG analysis of the shoulder in throwing and pitching: a preliminary report. Am J Sports Med 11:3, 1983

14. Jobe FW, Moynes DR, Tibone JE, Perry J: An EMG analysis of the shoulder in pitching: a second report. Am J Sports Med 12:218, 1984

15. Moynes DR, Perry J, Antonelli DJ, Jobe FW: Electromyographic and motion of the upper extremity in sports. Phys Ther 66:1905, 1986

16. Pappas AM, Zawacki RM, Sullivan, TJ: Biomechanics of baseball pitching: a preliminary report. Am J Sports Med 14:216, 1985

17. Townsend H, Jobe F, Pink M et al: Electromyographic analysis of the glenohumeral muscles during a baseball rehabilitation program. Am J Sports Med 19:264, 1991

18. Miller L et al: p. 741. In Nicholas J, Hershman E (eds): The Upper Extremity in Sports Medicine. Mosby, St. Louis, 1990

19. Glousman R, Jobe F, Tibone J et al: Dynamic Electromyographic analysis of the throwing shoulder with glenohumeral instability. J Bone Joint Surg 70A:220, 1988

20. Jobe FW, Giangarra CE, Kvitne RS et al: Anterior capsulolabral reconstruction of the shoulder in athletes in overhand sports. Am J Sports Med 19:428, 1991

21. Jobe FW, Pink M: Classification and treatment of shoulder dysfunction in the overhead athlete. J Orthop Sports Phys Ther 18:427, 1993

22. Rodosky MW, Harner CD, Fu FH: The role of the long head of the biceps muscle and superior glenoid labrum in anterior stability of the shoulder. Am J Sports Med 22:121, 1994

23. Rubenstein DL, Jobe FW, Glousman RE et al: Anterior capsulolabral reconstruction of the shoulder in athletes. JSES 1:229, 1992

24. Snyder SJ, Banas MP, Karzel RP: An analysis of 140 injuries to the superior labrum. JSES 4:243, 1995

25. Montgomery WM, Jobe FW: Functional outcomes in athletes after modified anterior capsulolabral reconstruction. Am J Sports Med 22:352, 1994

26. Blackburn TA, McLeod WD, White B et al: EMG analysis of posterior rotator cuff exercises. Athl Training 25:40, 1990

27. Pappas AM, Zawacki RM, McMarthy CF: Rehabilitation of the pitching shoulder. Am J Sports Med 14:223, 1985

28. Engle RP, Canner GC: Posterior shoulder instability: Approach to rehabilitation. J Orthop Sports Phys Ther June 1989:488

29. Moseley J, Jobe F, Pink M et al: EMG analysis of the scapular muscles during a shoulder rehabilitation program. Am J Sports Med 20:128, 1992

30. Toyoshima S, Hoshikawa T, Miyashita M et al: Contribution of the body parts to throwing performance, p. 169. In Nelson RC, Morehouse CA (eds): Biomechanics. Vol. 4. Balitimore, University Park Press, 1974

31. Cain PR, Mutschler TA et al: Anterior stability of the glenohumeral joint: a dynamic model. Am J Sports Med 15:144, 1987

APPENDIX 2.1

Muscle Activity Elicited by Common Shoulder Conditioning Exercises

The anterior stability of the glenohumeral joint is enhanced by the dynamics of the rotator cuff.[31] Blackburn et al.[26] examined the supraspinatus, infraspinatus, and teres minor via electromyographic analyses to determine which of 23 shoulder exercises elicited the greatest muscle activity. They demonstrated that externally rotating the humerus during prone exercise increased EMG activity to the highest levels. Specific to the teres minor, arm extension with external rotation produced the best isolation.

Prone Horizontal Abduction at 100° with External Rotation (Fig. 2.1)

Prone Horizontal Abduction at 90° with External Rotation (Fig. 2.2)

Prone Extension with External Rotation (Fig. 2.3)

Prone Horizontal Abduction at 90° and 90° of Elbow Flexion with External Rotation (Fig. 2.4)

Independently, Townsend,[17] Moseley,[29] and their associates examined the dynamic exercise routines most commonly instituted for conditioning of the shoulder in the throwing athlete. By coupling electromyography and cinematography they developed a baseline for individual muscle activity in relation to specific patterned movements. They compared the active signal to that of a manual muscle test. Each movement

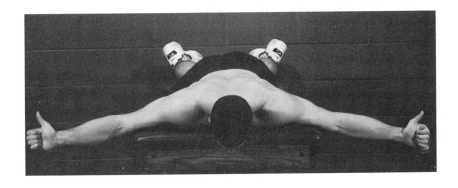

FIGURE 2.1

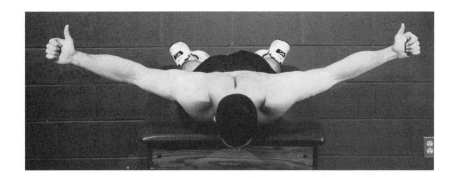

FIGURE 2.2

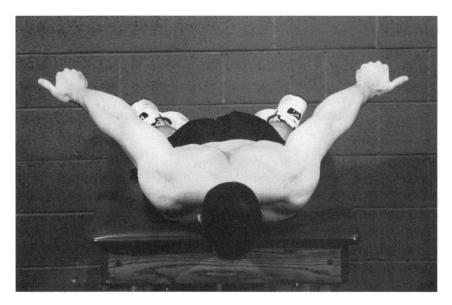

FIGURE 2.3

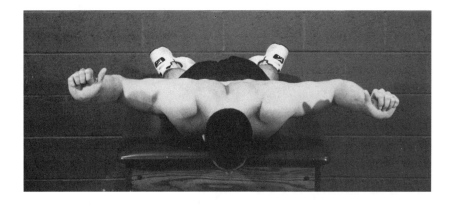

FIGURE 2.4

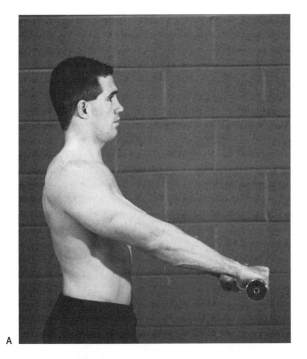

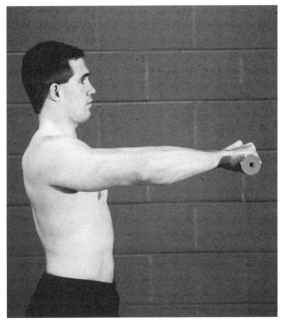

FIGURE 2.5 **(A–C)**

was divided into 30° arcs of motion. For a muscle to qualify for a movement, it had to develop EMG activity greater than 50 percent of the manual muscle test, and this activity would have to occur over three consecutive arcs of motion. Each peak activity arc (PAA) was also noted. This criterion held true for all tested motions except the press-up, shrug, and push-up. The press-up and shrug motion was divided into two halves of upward motion, three seconds of a end range hold, and two halves of the downward motion. The push-up range was based on the amount of elbow flexion beginning with full extension to 30° of flexion and descending in 30° arcs. The results of these studies are incorporated in the descriptions of the movements that follow.

Forward Flexion (Fig. 2.5)

Starting position: A standing posture with the weights in hands with palms to the sides. *Movement*: With elbows straight, lift the weights forward until they are above shoulder height. *Qualified muscles*: Middle serratus anterior 1 (PAA 120°–150°), lower serratus anterior 3 (120°–150°), anterior deltoid 3 (PAA 120–150°), supraspinatus 3 (PAA 90°–120°), subscapularis 3 (PAA 120°–150°), middle deltoid 4 (PAA 90°–120°), lower trapezius 4 (PAA 120–150°), infraspinatus 5 (PAA 90°–120°).

Abduction (Fig. 2.6)

Starting position: A standing posture with the weights in the hands with palms to the sides. *Movement*: With elbows straight, lift the weights away from the sides to a height above the shoulder. *Qualified muscles*: Lower trapezius 1 (PAA 90°–150°), middle serratus anterior 1 (PAA 120°–150°), lower serratus anterior 2 (PAA 120°–150°), rhomboids 3 (PAA 90°–150°), infraspinatus 4 (PAA 90°–120°), subscapularis 4 (PAA 120°–150°), anterior deltoid 5 (PAA 90°–120°), upper trapezius 6 (PAA 90°–120°), middle deltoid 8.

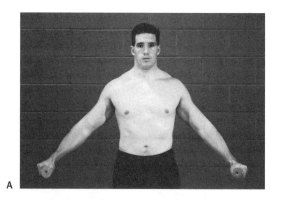

A

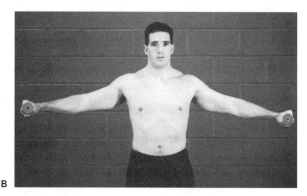

B

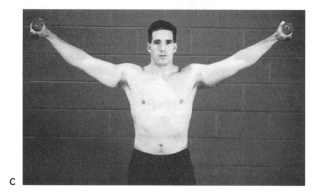

C

FIGURE 2.6 (A–C)

Shrug (Fig. 2.7)

Starting position: A standing posture with the weights in the hands with palms to the sides. *Movement*: The shoulders are elevated. *Qualified muscles*: Levator scapulae 3 (PAA at extreme range). *Note*: Avoid for the multidirectional instability patient. Apply traction for the primary impinger.

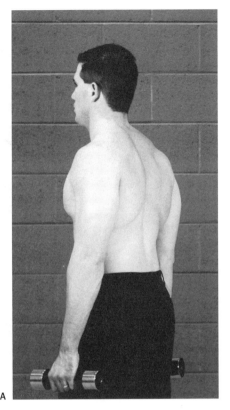 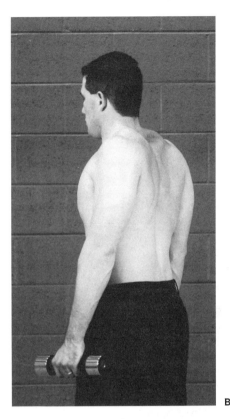

FIGURE 2.7 **(A & B)**

Scaption: Internal Rotation (Fig. 2.8)

Starting position: A standing posture with weights in hand with the thumbs turned in toward thighs. *Movement*: With elbows straight, lift the weights in a manner to maintain a plane of 30° forward of vertical. Lift to the height above the shoulders. *Qualified muscles*: Anterior deltoid 1 (PAA 90°–150°), middle deltoid 1 (PAA 90°–120°), subscapularis 1 (PAA 120°–150°), supraspinatus 2 (PAA 90°–120°).

Scaption: External Rotation (Fig. 2.9)

Starting position: A standing posture with weights in hand with thumbs turned away from the thighs. *Movement*: With the elbows straight, lift the weights in a manner to maintain a plane of 30° forward of vertical. Lift to the completion of the range of motion. *Qualified muscles*: Lower

serratus anterior 1 (PAA 120°–150°), rhomboids 2 (PAA 120°–150°), anterior deltoid 2 (PAA 90°–120°), middle serratus anterior 3 (PAA 120°–150°), supraspinatus 4 (PAA 90°–120°), middle deltoid 5 (PAA 90°–120°), upper trapezius 5 (PAA 120°–150°), infraspinatus 6 (PAA 90°–120°), lower trapezius 6 (PAA 120°–150 deg.), levator scapulae 6 (PAA 120°–150°).

Military Press (Fig. 2.10)

Starting position: A standing posture with weights in hand positioned at the height of the shoulders. *Movement*: Press weights upward to the completion of the range of motion. *Qualified muscles*: Supraspinatus 1 (PAA 0°–90°), subscapularis 2 (PAA 60°–90°), upper trapezius 2 (PAA 150°–peak), anterior deltoid 4 (PAA 60°–90°), middle serratus anterior 4 (PAA 150°–peak),

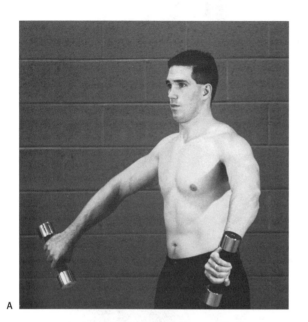

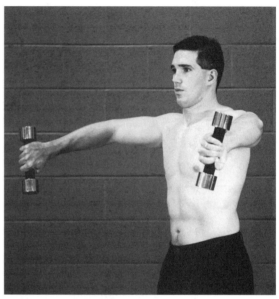

FIGURE 2.8 (A–C)

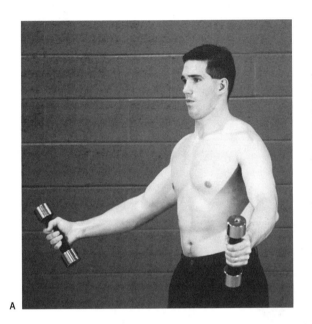

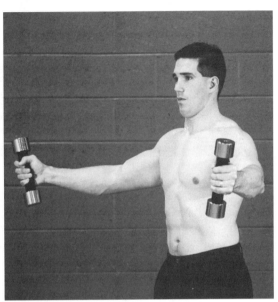

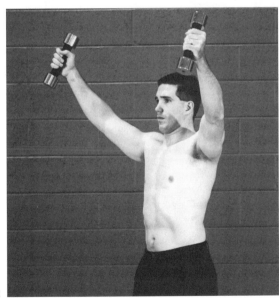

A

B

C

FIGURE 2.9 **(A–C)**

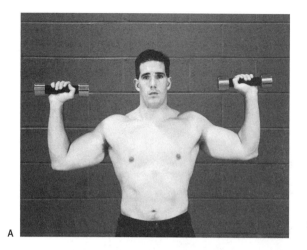 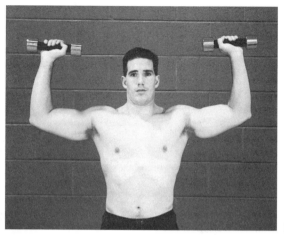

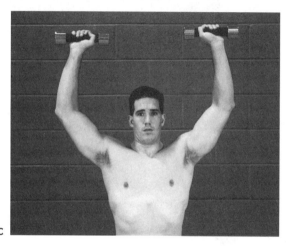

FIGURE 2.10 (A–C)

lower serratus anterior 6 (PAA 120°–150°), middle deltoid 7 (PAA 90°–120°).

Horizontal abduction: Internal Rotation (Fig. 2.11)

Starting position: From a standing position, bend forward at the waist until the upper body approaches parallel to the floor. The weights are held in an extended elbow position and internally rotated. *Movement*: The weights are lifted to just above the shoulder. *Qualified muscles*: Posterior deltoid 1 (PAA 90°–120°), middle trapezius 1 (PAA 90°–peak), rhomboids 1 (PAA 90°–peak), middle deltoid 2 (PAA 90°–120°), levator scapulae 2 (PAA at extreme range), infraspi-

natus 3 (PAA 90°–120°), teres minor 3 (PAA 90°–120°), upper trapezius 4 (PAA 90°–peak), lower trapezius 5 (PAA 90°–peak).

Horizontal abduction: External Rotation (Fig. 2.12)

Starting position: From a standing position, bend forward at the waist until the upper body approaches parallel to the floor. The weights are held in an extended elbow position and externally rotated. *Movement*: The weights are lifted to just above the shoulder. *Qualified muscles*: Infraspinatus 1 (PAA 90°–120°), posterior deltoid 2 (PAA 90°–120°), teres minor 2 (PAA 60°–90°), middle trapezius 2 (PAA 90°–peak), upper trape-

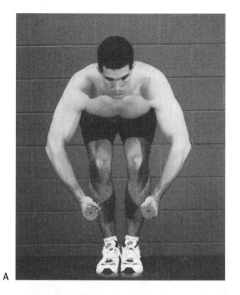
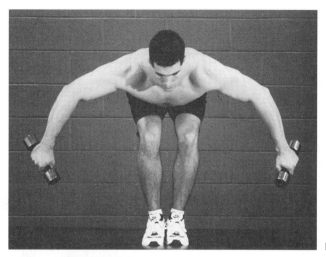
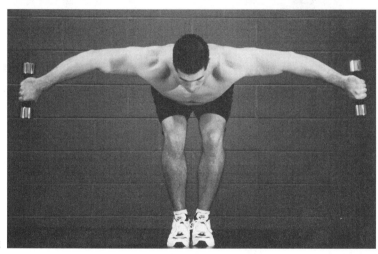

A

B

C

FIGURE 2.11 (A–C)

zius 3 (PAA at extreme range), lower trapezius 3 (PAA 90°–peak), middle deltoid 3 (PAA 90°–120°), levator scapulae 4 (PAA at extreme range).

The weights are lifted back past the hips. *Qualified muscle*: Middle trapezius 3 (PAA neutral–30°), posterior deltoid 4 (PAA 90°–120°), levator scapulae 5 (PAA at extreme range).

Extension (Fig. 2.13)

Starting position: From a standing position, bend forward at the waist until the upper body is close to parallel to the floor. The weights are held in an extended elbow position. *Movement*:

Rowing (Fig. 2.14)

Starting position: From a standing position, bend forward at the waist until the upper body is close to parallel to the floor. The weights are held in an extended elbow position. *Movement*:

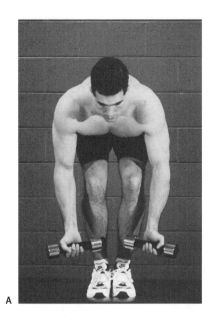

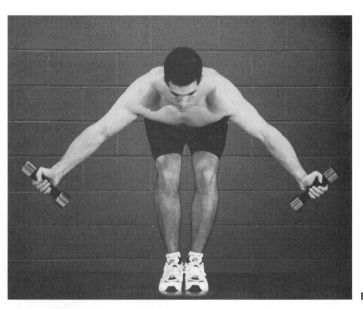

A

B

C

FIGURE 2.12 **(A–C)**

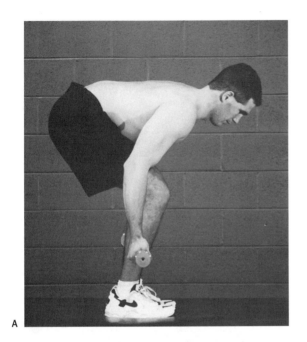

A

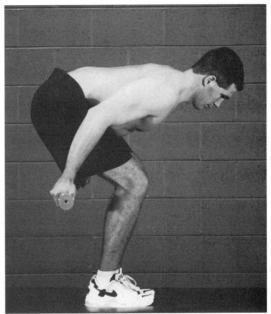

B

C

FIGURE 2.13 **(A–C)**

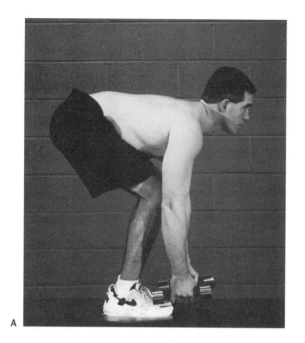

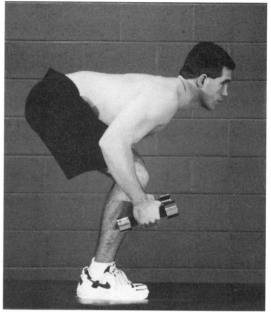

C

FIGURE 2.14 **(A–C)**

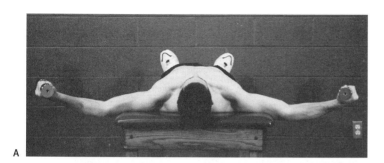

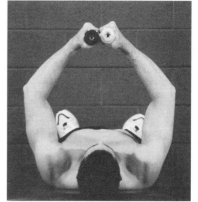

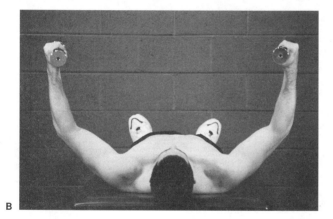

FIGURE 2.15 (A–C)

Leading with the elbows, the weights are lifted to the chest. *Qualified muscles*: Upper trapezius 1 (PAA 90°–120°), levator scapulae 1 (PAA at extreme range), lower trapezius 2 (PAA 120°–150°), posterior deltoid 3 (PAA 90°–120°), middle trapezius 4 (PAA 90°–120°), rhomboids 4 (PAA at extreme), middle deltoid 6 (PAA 90°–120°).

Horizontal adduction (Fig. 2.15)

Starting position: From a back-lying position, the arms are extended out to the sides to the height of the shoulders. *Movement*: The weights are lifted with a slight flexed elbow position to the midline. *Qualified muscle*: None. It is suggested that the resistance used in the experimental model may not have been of sufficient weight to elicit the necessary response to determine qualified muscle.

Bench press (Fig. 2.16)

Starting position: From a back-lying position, the elbows are at the side and flexed so the weights are next to the shoulders. *Movement*: The weights are pressed into an extended vertical arm position. *Qualified muscle*: None. It is suggested that the resistance used in the experimental model may not have been of sufficient weight to elicit the necessary response to determine qualified muscle.

Straight arm press (Fig. 2.17)

Starting position: From a back-lying position, the arms are extended in a vertical position. *Movement*: The weights are pressed into an elevated position with the motion occuring at the shoulder. *Qualified muscles*: Not rated.

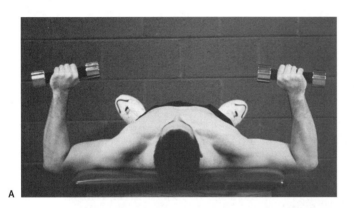

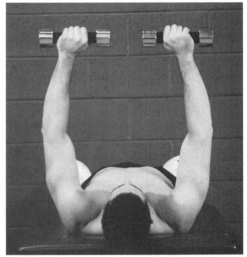

FIGURE 2.16 (A–C)

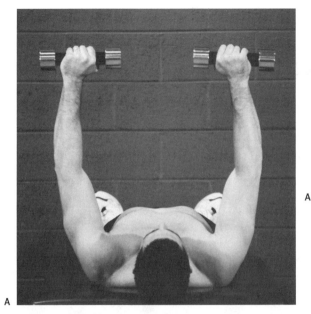

A

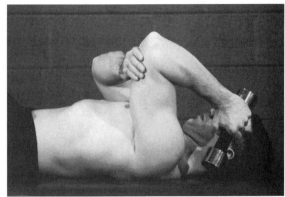

A

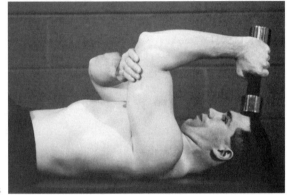

B

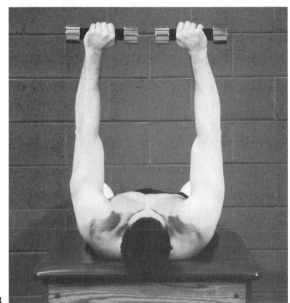

B

FIGURE 2.17 (A & B)

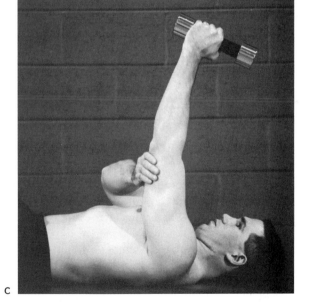

C

FIGURE 2.18 (A–C)

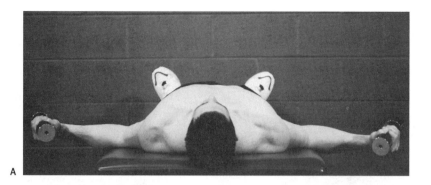

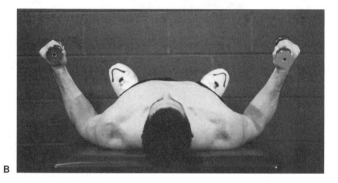
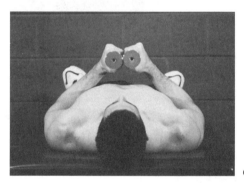

FIGURE 2.19 (A–C)

Triceps (Fig. 2.18)

Starting position: From a back-lying position, the arms are extended to the vertical, elbows flexed. *Movement*: The weights are lifted to an extended vertical arm positions. *Qualified muscles*: Not rated.

Internal rotation (Fig. 2.19)

Starting position: From a back-lying position, the arms are held at the side the elbows are flexed and externally rotated. *Movement*: The weights are lifted to the midline maintaining a flexed elbow. *Qualified muscles*: None. It is suggested that the resistance used in the experimental model may not have been of sufficient weight to elicit the necessary response to determine qualified muscle. *Note*: To limit external rotation and humeral head translation, this exercise may be performed in a sidelying position.

External rotation (Fig. 2.20)

Starting position: From a sidelying position, the elbow is flexed to 90° and the forearm is externally rotated. *Movement*: The weight is lifted from the midline to a vertical position. *Qualified muscles*: Teres minor 1 (PAA 60°–90°), infraspinatus 2 (PAA 60°–90°), posterior deltoid 5 (PAA 60°–90°). *Note*: The extreme range of external rotation should be limited to avoid anterior translation of the humeral head.

Press-up (Fig. 2.21)

Starting position: From a sitting position, the hands are placed next to the hips. *Movement*: By extending the elbows, the hips are lifted from the sitting position. *Qualifying muscles*: Pectoralis major 1 (PAA upper half of range), pectoralis minor 1 (PAA at extreme range), latissimus dorsi 1 (PAA at extreme for hold).

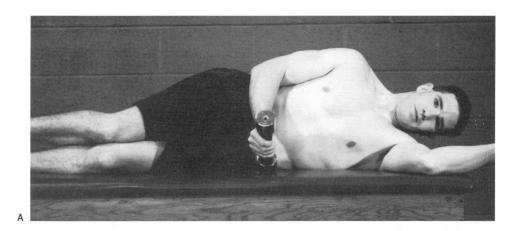

A

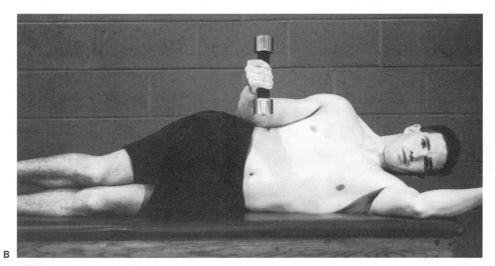

B

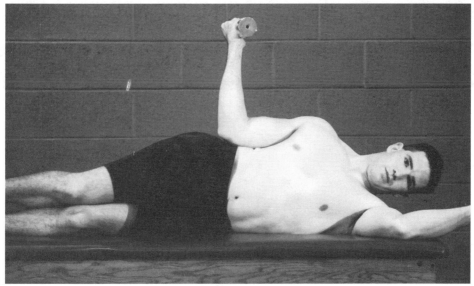

C

FIGURE 2.20 (A–C)

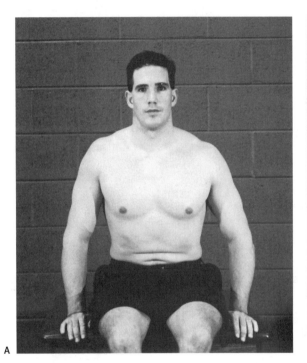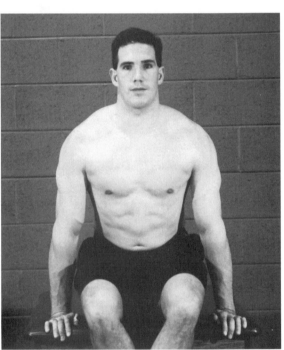

FIGURE 2.21 **(A & B)**

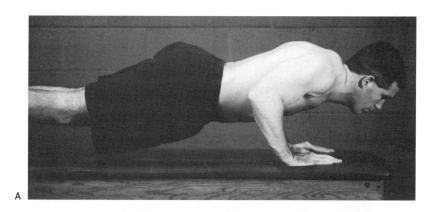

A

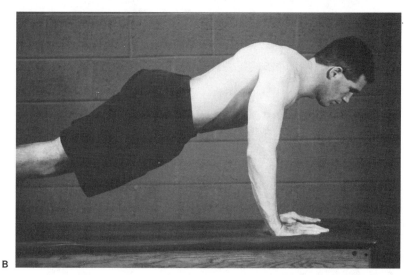

B

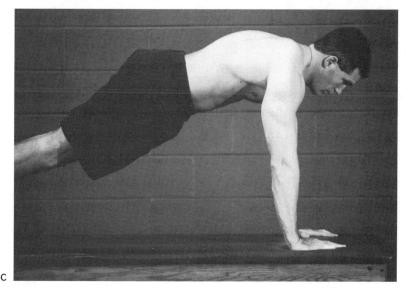

C

FIGURE 2.22 (A–C)

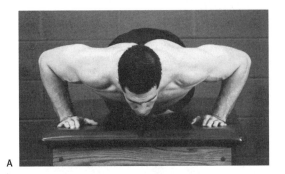

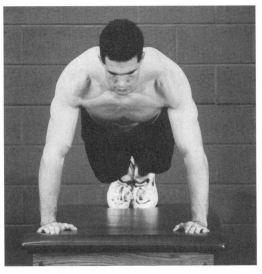

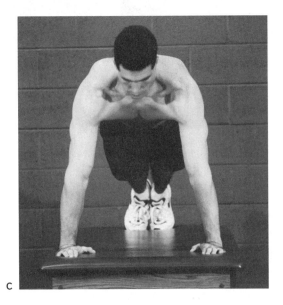

FIGURE 2.23 (A–C)

Push-up (Fig. 2.22)

Starting position: In a prone position, the hands are placed at the width of the shoulders, elbows flexed. *Movement*: By extending the elbows, the body is elevated from the surface. *Qualified muscles* (hands together): Infraspinatus 8 (PAA 90°–60°); (hands apart): Pectoralis major 2 (PAA 60°–30°), pectoralis minor 3 (PAA second to last arc), lower serratus anterior 5 (PAA isometric to chest near floor), middle serratus anterior 6 (PAA last arc).

Push-up plus (Fig. 2.23)

Starting position: In a prone position, the hands are placed at the width of the shoulders, elbows flexed. *Movement*: By extending the elbows, the body is elevated from the surface. Upon completion of elbow extension, the body is furthered elevated at the shoulder. *Qualified muscles*: Pectoralis minor 2 (PAA plus movement), lower serratus anterior 3 (PAA beginning movement), middle serratus anterior 5 (PAA plus movement).

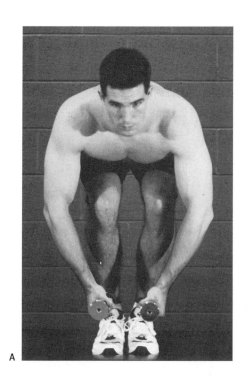

A

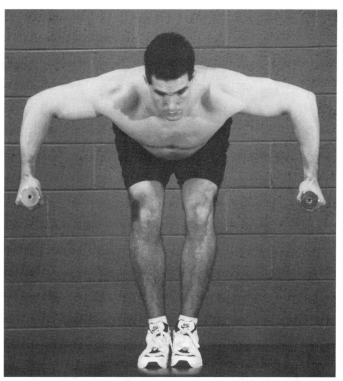

B

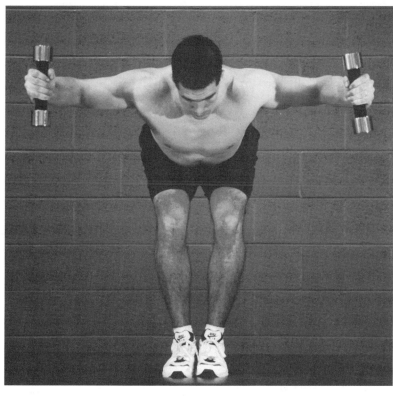

C

FIGURE 2.24 **(A–C)**

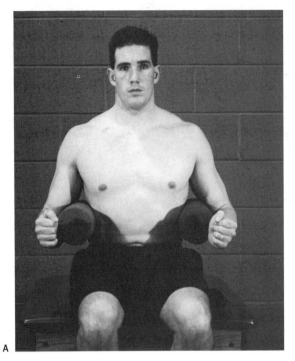
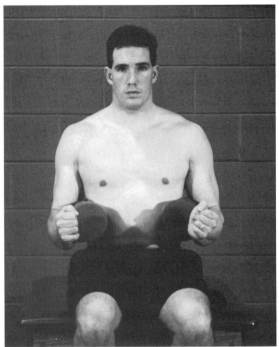

A

B

FIGURE 2.25 **(A & B)**

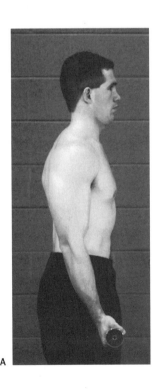
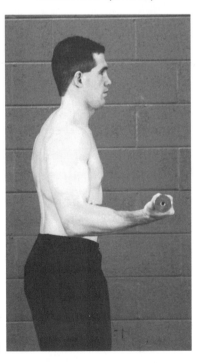
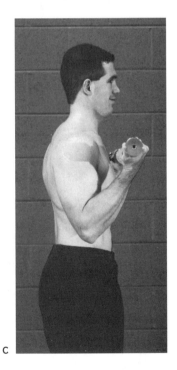

A

B

C

FIGURE 2.26 **(A–C)**

ADDITIONAL EXERCISES

Horizontal abduction: External rotation:Isolated: (Fig. 2.24)

Starting position: From a standing position, bend forward at the waist until the upper body approaches parallel to the floor. The weights are held in an extended elbow position in a neutral position. *Movement*: Leading with the elbows, the upper arms are brought into the horizontal abducted position, and then the weights are brought into the externally rotated position.

Pillow squeeze (Fig. 2.25)

Starting position: Place a rigid pillow between the upper arm and the chest wall. *Movement*: Squeeze the pillows with the upper arm against chest wall.

Biceps curl (Fig. 2.26)

Starting position: From a standing position, with the weights in hand with palms to the sides. *Movement*: The elbows are flexed, bringing the weights toward the shoulders.

APPENDIX 2.2

Upper Extremity Conditioning Program

Date:	WEIGHT AND REPETITIONS						
Forward Flexion							
Abduction							
Shrug							
Scaption @ IR							
Scaption @ ER							
Military Press							
Hor. Abd. @ IR							
Hor. Abd. @ ER							
Extension							
Rowing							
Hor. Adduction							
Bench Press							
Straight Arm Press							
Triceps							
Internal Rotation							
External Rotation							
Hor. Abd. XR–Iso.							
Press-up							
Push-up							
Push-up Plus							
Pillow Squeeze							
Biceps Curls							
Wrist Flexion							
Wrist Extension							
Pro/Supination							
Ulnar Deviation							
Radial Deviation							
Throwing Level							

APPENDIX 2.3

Nine-Level Rehabilitation Throwing Program

This program is designed for athletes to work at their own pace to develop the necessary arm strength to begin throwing from a mound. The athlete is to throw two days in a row and then rest for one day. It is not important to progress to the next throwing level with each outing. It is preferred that a number of outings at the same level be completed before progressing. It is important to throw with comfort, which may necessitate moving back a level on occasion.

LEVEL	THROWS/FEET				THROWS/FEET		THROWS/FEET	
One	25	25	25	60				
Two	25	25	50	60				
Three	25	25	75	60				
Four	25	25	50	60	25			90
Five	25	25	50	60	25			120
Six	25	25	50	60	25			150
Seven	25	25	50	60	25			180
Eight	25	25	50	60	25			210
Nine	25	25	50	60	25			240

APPENDIX 2.4

Rehabilitation Pitching Program

LEVELS	THROWS/FEET		THROWS/MOUND/FLAT	THROWS/FEET	
1	25	25	50 Mound	25	90
2	25	25	60 Flat	25	120
3	25	25	50 Mound	25	150
4	25	25	60 Mound	25	120
5	25	25	70 Flat	25	150
6	25	25	60 Mound	25	180
7	25	25	70 Mound	25	150
8	25	25	60 Flat	25	180
9	25	25	80 Mound	25	210
10	25	50	70 Mound	25	240
11	25	50	80 Mound	25	180
12	25	50	90 Mound	25	210
13	25	50	90 Mound	25	240
14	25	50	80 Mound	25	180
15	25	50	100 Mound	25	210
16	25	50	100 Mound	25	240
17	25	50	<60 Mound		
18	25	50	100 Mound	25	240
19	25	50	<60 Mound	25	240
20	Batting practice		10 Minutes		
21	25	50	<60 Mound	25	240
22	Batting practice		15 Minutes		
23	25	50	<60 Mound	25	240
24	Game:		<60 Mound	45 Pitches	
	25	50	Warm up		

APPENDIX 2.5

Short-Focus Throwing Rehabilitation Programs

1. 25 at 60 ft, 25 at 90 ft, 15 at 60 ft.
2. 25 at 90 ft, 25 at 120 ft, 15 at 90 ft.
3. 3 min. at 90 ft, 3 min. at 120 ft, 3 min. at 150 ft, 3 min. at 90 ft.
4. 2 min. at 90 ft, 2 min. at 120 ft, 3 min. at 150 ft, 2 min. at 120 ft, 2 min. at 90 ft.
5. 2 min. at 90 ft, 2 min. at 120 ft, 1 min. at 150 ft, 2 min. at 120 ft, 2 min. at 90 ft.
6. 2 min. at 90 ft, 2 min. at 120 ft, 2 min. at 150 ft, 1 min. at 180 ft, 2 min. at 150 ft, 2 min. at 120 ft, 2 min. at 90 ft.

THROWING MOUND PROGRAM

1. 5 min. long toss, 5 min. mound, aerobic—bike.
2. Aerobic work—10 min. bike, 10 sprints, 10 min. bike.
3. 5 min. long toss, 7 min. mound, aerobic—bike.
4. Aerobic work—10 min. bike, 10 sprints, 12 min. bike.
5. 5 min. long toss, 10 min. mound, aerobic—bike.
6. Aerobic work—10 min. bike, 10 sprints, 15 min. bike.
7. 5 min. long toss, 12 min. mound, aerobic—bike.
8. Day off.
9. Batting practice—2 innings (30 pitches).
10. Aerobic work—10 sprints, 20 min. bike.
11. Normal day.

3

Differential Soft Tissue Diagnosis

MARIE A. JOHANSON

BLANCA ZITA GONZALEZ-KING

Efficient and effective patient care is always dependent on the clinician's ability to perform a systematic evaluation. The evaluation serves to identify all tissues involved in dysfunction, the current stage and progression of the dysfunction, and the baseline parameters on which to judge treatment efficacy. Soft tissue diagnosis of the shoulder joint includes evaluation of the glenohumeral, stemoclavicular, acromiclavicular, and scapulothoracic articulations, as well as the cervical spine and related upper quarter structures.

We will discuss each component of the shoulder evaluation including the patient interview, cervical screening, observation, mobility, musculotendinous strength, palpation, and special tests. The soft tissue diagnosis is derived from assessment of information obtained from each component of the evaluation. The chapter concludes with a case study that illustrates the ongoing assessment process that accompanies each component of the evaluation.

Patient Interview

The purposes of the patient interview are to identify the patient's symptoms, determine the history of the patient's current problem, identify co-existing medical factors that may affect either the current problem or its treatment, and estab-

lish the probable irritability level of the problem. The irritability level is a measure of how easily symptoms may be provoked and relieved.[1] The two major components of the patient interview are (1) the history of the patient's problem(s), and (2) the location, nature, and behavior of symptoms.

HISTORY

Initially, the clinician must establish the onset and progression of the patient's problem by asking *when* the problem started and *how* it began. The problem will likely fall into one of two major categories: macrotrauma or microtrauma. A macrotrauma is an injury resulting from a specific trauma. A microtrauma is an injury resulting from repetitive stress to tissues, and is characterized by an insidious onset of symptoms. The categorization of macrotraumas and microtraumas serves to guide the clinician most efficiently through the remainder of the history and the physical exam.

Whenever a macrotrauma is suspected, the clinician must determine the mechanism of injury to aid in the identification of the injured structure(s). Awareness of possible gross disruption of tissue (such as fractures and dislocations) may alert the examiner to exert caution during passive range of motion and special tests,

TABLE 3.1. *Medical conditions that may refer pain to the shoulder complex*

BODY SYSTEM	RIGHT SHOULDER	LEFT SHOULDER	RIGHT OR LEFT SHOULDER
Cardiovascular		Typical angina pectoralis	Atypical angina pectoralis
		Myocardial infarction (rarely may refer to right shoulder)	Pericarditis
Pulmonary			Pleurisy
Gastrointestinal	Gallstones	Pancreatitis	Pulmonary neoplasm
	Acute or chronic cholecystitis	Pancreatic carcinoma	
	Hepatitis	Hiatal hernia	

thereby preventing further trauma to injured tissues. Many postoperative patients may be grouped with macrotrauma injuries.

When a microtrauma is suspected, the clinician must identify the patient's daily activities and postures to determine both intrinsic and extrinsic factors that may contribute to the problem. Intrinsic factors are physical characteristics that predispose an individual to microtrauma injuries, such as a hooked (or type III) acromion process[2] or strength deficits of the rotator cuff muscles.[3,4] Extrinsic factors are external conditions under which an activity is performed that predispose an individual to microtrauma injuries, such as training errors.

The patient interview should also identify demographic information that may aid in the soft tissue diagnosis, as well as past and present medical conditions that may affect the current problem or its treatment. Additionally, any current medications that may mask pain or otherwise affect the patient's current problem should be ascertained. Because many disease processes may result in referral of pain to the shoulder region (most notably, diseases of the cardiovascular, pulmonary, and gastrointestinal systems),[5–7] the clinician can ill afford exclusion of medical conditions that may explain shoulder pain (Table 3.1). Finally, the clinician should establish any previous treatment received by the patient and its result on the frequency and intensity of symptoms as well as functional abilities.

LOCATION, NATURE, AND BEHAVIOR OF PAIN

Definition of the boundaries of the patient's pain and other symptoms will establish the extent of the examination. All injured structures that potentially produce pain within the boundaries of the patient's pain, whether it be local pain or referred pain, will need to be considered.

The nature of the pain may assist in identifying the structures at fault, and this can be determined by asking the patient to describe the pain or symptoms. Deep, dull, and poorly localized pain has been attributed to visceral structures as well as deep ligamentous, deep muscular, and bony structures.[5] A superficial pain described as sharp or burning in quality has been attributed to skin, tendon, or bursal tissue.[8] A patient may report "throbbing" or "pulsing" pain when suffering from a vascular injury. Reports of such symptoms as paresthesias or numbness may indicate irritation or injury of a nerve.

Though subjective reports of the nature of pain are not usually reliable enough to be considered, when combined with the location of pain, some patterns may assist in the differentiation of local and referred pain. Referred pain is suspected when the patient reports a deep burning or deep aching pain with indefinite boundaries, while local pain is suspected when the pain is superficial with clear boundaries.[8]

The behavior of pain may assist in identifying injured structures, and it also can predict the irritability level of the problem. The following questions are routine in exploring the behavior of pain:

1. Is the pain constant?
2. What activities or positions provoke or increase the pain?
3. What activities and positions relieve or decrease the pain?

4. Does the pain level vary with the time of day or night?

Cyriax[8] recommends three questions regarding the location and behavior of pain in order to establish the irritability level of a shoulder dysfunction:

1. Does it hurt to lie on the affected side at night?
2. Does the pain extend below the elbow?
3. Is there pain at rest?

According to Cyriax,[8] affirmative answers to all three questions indicates a high irritability level. Affirmative answers to one or two of the questions indicates a moderate irritability level, while negative answers to all three questions indicates a low irritability level. The irritability level may be used to predict the tolerance of the patient to subsequent evaluation and treatment procedures.

Maitland[1] recommends a specific set of questions regarding the behavior of pain to establish the irritability level of the problem. Once an activity or position that provokes symptoms has been identified, subsequent queries address that specific activity or position:

1. How long can the activity or position be maintained before the pain begins or increases (time 1 or T1)?
2. How long can the activity or position be continued before the pain level becomes unbearable and the activity or position must cease (T2)?
3. How long does it take for the pain to return to its baseline level after cessation of the activity or position (T3)?

Relatively short periods for T1 and T2, coupled with a relatively long period for T3, indicate a high irritability level. Conversely, relatively long periods for T1 and T2, coupled with a relatively short period for T3, indicate a low irritability level.

Generally, mechanical musculoskeletal pain varies throughout the day and is related to activities or positions. Therefore, constant pain not so related may alert the clinician to pain associated with medical disease processes.

Cervical Screening

The prevalence of cervical spine problems and the pain referral patterns of the cervical spine combine to necessitate the inclusion of routine screening for cervical pathology during examination of any shoulder patient. Cervical radiculopathy due to irritation or compression of the C5 spinal nerve root often results in referred pain over the lateral aspect of the proximal arm. Because most glenohumeral joint structures are innervated by the C5 and C6 spinal nerves, the lateral proximal aspect of the arm is also a very common pain location for the patient with a shoulder dysfunction. (A notable exception is the acromioclavicular joint, which is innervated by the C4 spinal nerve. An injury to this joint usually results in pain specifically over the AC joint.) Therefore, it is imperative to examine every patient for both shoulder and cervical dysfunction.

A cervical spine screening begins with active cervical movements. If active movements are normal, passive pressures at the ends of active movement are performed. The clinician determines if pain is produced during these tests, and if so, locates the pain produced. To confirm suspicion of changeable shoulder pain potentially referred from the cervical spine, compression and distraction tests of the cervical spine can be done. Neurologic screening may further inform the examiner of the integrity of the cervical spinal nerves[9–11] (Table 3.2) and spinal cord. Additionally, palpation of structures within the anterior and posterior triangles of the cervical spine may provide information on referral of pain from muscular structures common to the cervical spine and shoulder complex, or from cervical articular structures (palpation will be discussed later in the chapter). See Chapter 4 for further discussion of the inter-relationship of the cervical spine and the shoulder.

TABLE 3.2. *Neurologic screening of cervical spinal nerves*

SEGMENT	MOTOR	SENSORY	REFLEX
C1–2	Neck flexion	Skull	None
C3	Neck side bending	Lateral neck and jaw	None
C4	Scapular elevation	Top of shoulder	None
C5	Shoulder abduction, elbow flexion	Proximal lateral arm	Biceps
C6	Elbow flexion, wrist extension	Thumb and index finger	Brachioradialis
C7	Finger extension, elbow extension	Middle finger	Triceps
C8	Finger flexion	Ulnar aspect of forearm and hand	None
T1	Finger abduction	Medial arm	None

Observation

Observation of the patient in both static and dynamic situations can reveal information about the patient's condition. The three basic components of examination by observation are assessment of (1) symmetry, (2) posture, and (3) dynamic activities of daily living (ADL), sports, and work activities.

SYMMETRY

An assessment of symmetry can give clues to areas of dysfunction, although the clinician must be aware that some degree of asymmetry is normal. In fact, significant degrees of asymmetry can be perfectly normal for some individuals, such as athletes in one-handed sports.[11] Generally, an assessment of symmetry includes both soft tissue and bony contours.

Anteriorly, the clinician can observe changes in the thoracic inlet area (such as bony abnormalities of the clavicle, acromioclavicular or sternoclavicular joint, or areas of ecchymosis or edema in the supraclavicular fossa), and in the muscle contours of the deltoid and pectoral muscle groups. Posteriorly, muscle atrophy of the supraspinatus, infraspinatus, and teres minor may be seen, and gross differences in the position of the scapula may be noted. Due to specific sports activities, some individuals may have hypertrophied muscles on their dominant side, resulting in the appearance of muscle atrophy on the nondominant side.

POSTURE

An assessment of posture includes scrutiny of the anterior, posterior, and lateral views in the standing position, as well as identification of the patient's sitting and sleeping postures.

Anterior View

From an anterior view, the clinician can assess the position of the head on the neck in the frontal and transverse planes (cervical side bending or rotation) and the superior-inferior position of the glenohumeral joint. A relative inferior position of the humeral head on one side may be seen from this view, although atrophy of the deltoid can give a false impression of inferior subluxation.

Lateral View

From the lateral side, the positions of the head on the cervical spine and of the cervical spine relative to the torso may be seen, the degree of thoracic spine kyphosis assessed, and sagittal plane position of the glenohumeral joint observed (anteroposterior position of the humeral head). Two common problems most easily seen from this view are an anteriorly displaced position of the humeral head and forward head posture. Forward head posture is characterized by excessively protracted and laterally rotated scapulae, internal rotation of the glenohumeral joint, increased kyphosis of the upper thoracic spine, decreased lordosis of the midcervical spine, and increased backward bending of the upper cervical spine.[12] Forward head posture is more prevalent in patients with microtrauma shoulder injuries than in the uninjured population.[13] The increase in scapular protraction that occurs with forward head posture decreases the subacromial space,[14] and may predispose an individual to some shoulder dysfunctions such as impingement syndrome.

Posterior View

From the posterior view, the clinician can again ascertain the position of the head on the cervical spine and the cervical spine relative to the torso in the frontal and transverse planes. The positions of the scapulae may be compared as to superior-inferior and medial-lateral placement, as well as in degree of "winging." Scapular "winging" is defined as the movement of the medial border of the scapula away from the chest wall.[11] Some depression of the shoulder gridle on the dominant side is normal, presumably due to greater activity of the dominant side resulting in greater extensibility of the joint capsules and ligaments.[11] The position of the scapula can be further assessed by palpation of the bony landmarks (see the palpation section later in the chapter).

Objective Clinical Measures of Scapular Position

Diveta et al.[15] evaluate protraction of the scapulae by taking two linear measurements with a string (Fig. 3.1). The distance in centimeters from the root of the scapular spine to the inferior angle of the acromion (scapular width) is divided into the distance from the third thoracic segment to the inferior angle of the acromion (scapular protraction). The resulting ratio provides a measurement of scapular protraction corrected for scapular size (normalized scapular protraction). A larger ratio indicates a greater degree of scapular protraction.

Diveta et al.[15] report good to excellent intrarater reliability of the scapula width and scapula protraction measurements (ICCs of 0.94 and 0.85, respectively), and fair intrarater reliability of the normalized scapula protraction measurement (ICC of 0.78). However, some controversy in the literature regarding the reliability of the normalized scapula protraction measurement has subsequently emerged. Neiers and Worrell[16] report good to excellent intrarater reliability of the scapula width and scapula protraction measurements, but poor intrarater reliability of the normalized scapula protraction measurement (ICC of 0.34). Gibson et al.[17] report excellent intrarater and interrater reliability of the scapula protraction measurement (ICCs of 0.91 to 0.95), but did not study the normalized scapula protraction measurement. Greenfield et al.[13] compared the clinical method of measuring normalized scapula protraction described by Diveta et al.[15] to identical measurements taken from radiographs. No statistically significant differences in values obtained between the two methods were reported, lending credence to Diveta's clinical measurement of normalized scapular protraction. Greenfield et al.[13] also reported excellent intrarater and interrater reliability of the normalized scapular protraction measurement (ICCs of 0.97 and 0.96, respectively).

The position of the scapula in the frontal plane (relative degree of scapular abduction or lateral rotation) can be obtained using the first of three test positions that comprise the lateral slide test described by Kibler[18] (see the section on musculotendinous strength later in the chapter).

Mobility

Examination of mobility of the shoulder complex generally begins with a scrutiny of active range of motion (AROM) in the cardinal planes, the plane of the scapula, and during functional movements, followed by passive range of motion (PROM), and accessory motion. Information derived from mobility testing includes extensibility of contractile and noncontractile tissues, functional capabilities, irritability level, and differentiation of muscle weakness and/or pain from joint or muscle restrictions.

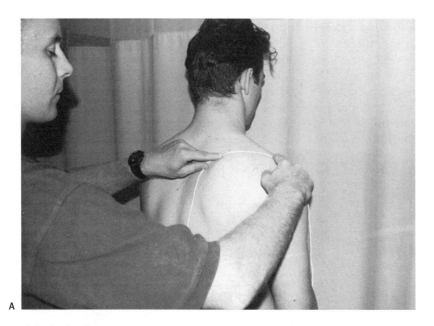

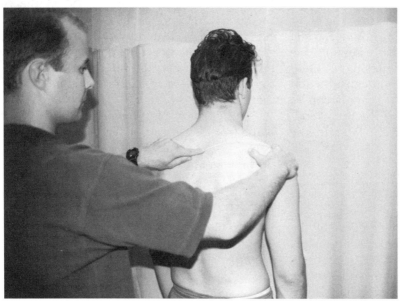

FIGURE 3.1 **(A)** *Measurement of scapular width. (***B***) Measurement of scapular protraction.*

ACTIVE RANGE OF MOTION

The evaluation of active range of motion encompasses multiple components of function. When AROM is limited, one or more of the following is possible: limited joint mobility, muscle weakness, or unwillingness of the patient to complete the motion due to pain, apprehension, or other reasons. Therefore, diagnosis of soft tissue dysfunction at the shoulder from active movements alone is difficult, as the examiner is unable to isolate the contribution of specific muscle groups and joints of the shoulder complex to the limitation in movement.

Active range of motion can reveal abnormal movement patterns, and can predict for the examiner what functional abilities and disabilities the patient is likely to exhibit.

Generally, AROM of the involved side is compared to the uninvolved side, although some degree of asymmetry may be normal. Often, the dominant side will exhibit less AROM than the nondominant side.[11] Conversely, apparent symmetry in AROM may be achieved by excessive movements in adjacent joints to compensate for the restriction of a given joint (see the following sections on cardinal planes and plane of the scapula).

Cardinal Planes

Generally, cardinal plane active movements of the shoulder complex grant less information regarding specific patterns of joint restrictions than do cardinal plane passive movements. However, significant decreases in AROM compared to PROM in the cardinal planes can distinguish weakness or pain as a primary functional limitation from true joint restriction. Normal ROM in the cardinal planes is 160° to 180° of flexion, 45° to 60° of extension, 170° to 180° of abduction, 70° to 80° of internal rotation, 80° to 90° of external rotation, 30° to 45° of horizontal abduction, and 135° to 140° of horizontal adduction.[19]

Cyriax[8] advocated active abduction testing to discern the presence of a "painful arc." Cyriax[8] defines a painful arc as "pain encountered midrange that disappears before the end of range" and indicates compression of subacromial structures. Painful arcs are often used clinically to assist in the diagnosis of impingement syndromes.[20,21]

When observing AROM, the examiner must be careful to identify abnormal patterns of movement even when the gross quantity of movement is normal. For example, a patient may substitute excessive scapular adduction for active glenohumeral external rotation in 0° of abduction (Fig. 3.2), or substitute excessive scapular elevation and external rotation for glenohumeral elevation during active elevation (Fig. 3.3).

Plane of the Scapula

Active elevation in the plane of the scapula offers an excellent assessment of scapulohumeral rhythm and scapular stability. The movement can be grossly observed through the three phases of elevation (see Ch. 1) for symmetry and the expected biomechanical events.

INITIAL PHASE OF ELEVATION (0° TO 60°).
Some oscillation of the scapula is normally observed through the first 30° to 60° of motion. After 30° to 60°, the scapula should stabilize against the thoracic wall and begin to laterally rotate. Movement of the glenohumeral joint should exceed movement of the scapulothoracic joint through the initial phase of elevation.[4,22] An inability to complete the initial phase of elevation most often indicates severe restrictions of the glenohumeral joint, severe pain and/or apprehension reported by the patient, and in rare cases may also indicate severe restriction of the sternoclavicular joint.

MIDDLE PHASE OF ELEVATION (60° TO 140°).
The middle phase of elevation is clinically the most common phase of dysfunction. During this phase, the amount of scapular rotation exceeds the amount of glenohumeral motion.[22] Due to deltoid muscle activity, upward shear force at the glenohumeral joint peaks, and is counteracted by activity of the rotator cuff musculature.[23,24] If scapular rotation is decreased on the patient's involved side, it may be due to limitation at the acromioclavicular and/or sternoclavicular joints, which restrict clavicular elevation and rotation. A limitation of scapulothoracic rotation may also be due to tightness of the levator scapula muscle, weakness of the serratus anterior and upper and lower trapezius muscles, or both. Weakness of the scapular muscles, or "scapular instability," is most often apparent during the eccentric phase of elevation, and may be observed as winging of the scapula or excessive oscillations of the scapula. This may become more accentuated after multiple repetitions of elevation.

Excessive scapular rotation on the involved

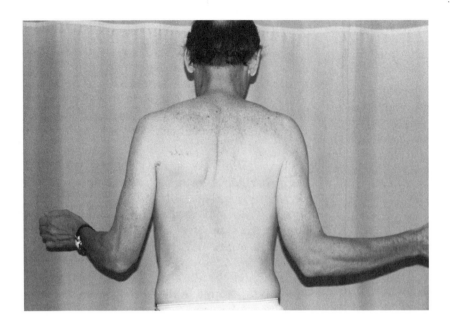

FIGURE 3.2 *Excessive left scapular adduction exhibited by a patient with limited left glenohumeral external rotation at 0° of abduction during active range of motion testing.*

side may indicate weakness of the rotator cuff muscles (inability to counteract the upward shear force of the deltoid), or restrictions of the anterior and inferior glenohumeral capsule. During the middle phase of elevation, the presence of a painful arc may indicate impingement of subacromial structures.

FINAL PHASE OF ELEVATION (140° TO 180°). During the final phase of elevation, movement of the glenohumeral joint significantly exceeds that of the scapulothoracic joint.[22] Therefore, the examiner can observe a "disassociation" of the humerus from the scapula that requires good extensibility of the teres major, subscapularis, pec-

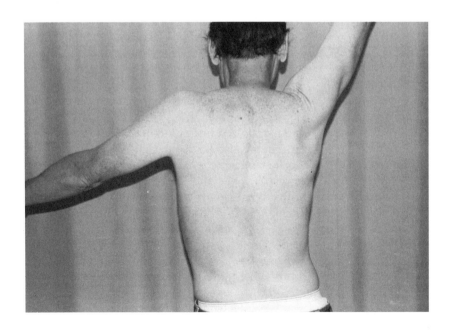

FIGURE 3.3 *Excessive left scapular elevation and external rotation exhibited by a patient with limited glenohumeral elevation during active range of motion testing.*

toralis major, latissimus dorsi, teres minor, and infraspinatus muscles.

Functional Movements

Three functional movements can predict the patient's ability to perform the activities of daily living. As with AROM, active functional movements concurrently test joint mobility, muscle strength, and willingness of the patient to complete the motion.

HANDS BEHIND NECK. Combined glenohumeral elevation and external rotation, and scapular rotation into the middle phase of elevation are required to complete this movement. Inability to perform this movement indicates inability to groom, inability to shave the axilla, inability to manipulate objects overhead, and inability to throw.

HANDS BEHIND BACK. Combined glenohumeral extension, adduction and internal rotation, and scapular distraction are required to complete this movement. Limitation indicates inability to fasten a brassiere, zipper clothes, or tuck in shirts or blouses posteriorly, and reach back pockets.

HAND TO OPPOSITE SHOULDER. Combined glenohumeral flexion and horizontal adduction are required to complete this movement. Limitation indicates an inability to manipulate objects across the body or provide adequate follow-through with many sports maneuvers such as a golf swing, tennis forehand, or baseball pitch.

PASSIVE RANGE OF MOTION

Passive range of motion allows the examiner to identify specific restrictions at each joint, to distinguish muscle restriction from restriction of noncontractile tissue, to evaluate the quality of resistance at the end of the range of motion (endfeel), and to discern patterns of restrictions that may indicate specific soft tissue problems. Additionally, the probable irritability level of the patient can be established and serve as one guide

in the selection of initial stretching or strengthening techniques.

Although differences in PROM between the involved and uninvolved sides are generally good indications of abnormal mobility, the clinician needs to be aware that some asymmetries may be normal. For example, high-level baseball pitchers are expected to exhibit greater external rotation PROM and lesser internal rotation PROM of their dominant shoulder.[25]

As with AROM, the examiner must be alert for motions of the involved side that only appear to have full mobility because of excessive motion at adjacent joints. For example, when the subscapularis, pectoralis major, and latissimus dorsi muscles lack flexibility or when the inferior glenohumeral capsule is restricted, the patient may substitute excessive lateral rotation of the scapula (Fig. 3.4) or excessive extension of the trunk (Fig. 3.5) to achieve full shoulder elevation. Passive glenohumeral extension may also obscure a limitation in passive glenohumeral internal rotation at 90° of abduction (Fig. 3.6).

Irritability Level

Cyriax[8] advocates use of the sequence of pain and resistance during passive movement testing to establish indications and contraindications for stretching of a joint. If pain is encountered in the range of motion prior to resistance, a high level of irritability is likely, and stretching is contraindicated. If pain and resistance are encountered at the same time, a moderate irritability level is likely, and any stretching should be performed gently and with caution. If resistance occurs during passive movement before pain, or if no pain is encountered, then a low irritability level is likely and the patient is expected to tolerate stretching well. The clinical use of Cyriax's sequence of pain and resistance has not been well studied. One recent study of the use of the sequence in patients diagnosed with osteoarthritis of the knee showed poor reliability. The authors attributed this to very short intervals between onset of pain and resistance, which precluded clinical measurement through manual palpation.[26] Reliability of the pain and resis-

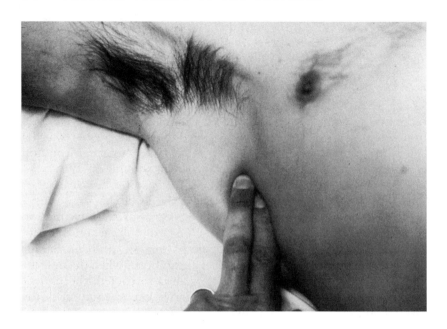

FIGURE 3.4 *Excessive lateral rotation (lateral "bulge") of the right scapula during passive range of motion testing in abduction exhibited by a patient with glenohumeral capsular restriction.*

tance sequence in other patient populations is unknown.

Maitland[1] also advocates a method to establish irritability level during passive range of motion testing. The method is somewhat more complex and requires the examiner to graph the following four occurrences during PROM testing:

1. The point in the range of motion where resistance is first detected (resistance 1 or R1)
2. The point in the range of motion where no further movement can be achieved due to passive resistance (R2)
3. The point in range of motion where pain is first reported by the patient (pain 1 or P1)
4. The point in range of motion where no further movement can be achieved due to pain (P2)

Maitland[1] asserts that when pain is the patient's primary problem, P1 will precede R1, and pain rather than resistance will usually limit the motion. When pain is the patient's primary problem, mobilization techniques to increase joint mobility are contraindicated. Conversely, when stiffness is the patient's primary problem, pain may or may not be encountered before resistance, but resistance rather than pain will limit the motion. When stiffness is the patient's primary problem, mobilization and stretching techniques to increase mobility are indicated.

End-feel

The use and interpretation of endfeel is controversial due to individual variation and questionable reliability.[26] Cyriax[8] describes 6 end-feels (3 normal and 3 abnormal) and Paris and Loubert[27] describe 15 end-feels (5 normal and 10 abnormal). However, clinicians may more simply define a normal end-feel as an expected resistance of muscle or periarticular tissue at the end of full PROM, and define abnormal end-feel as an unexpected passive resistance of intra-articular or extra-articular structure(s), or pain that limits PROM prior to expected end range.

Specific Patterns of Restrictions

Several specific patterns of passive restrictions may assist in the soft tissue diagnosis of shoulder problems. Arguably the most often

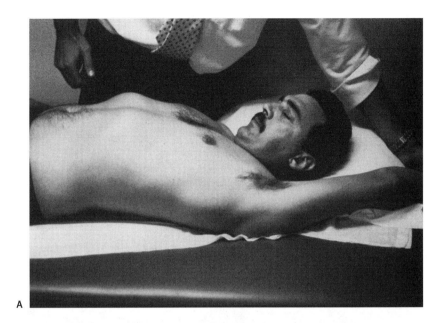

A

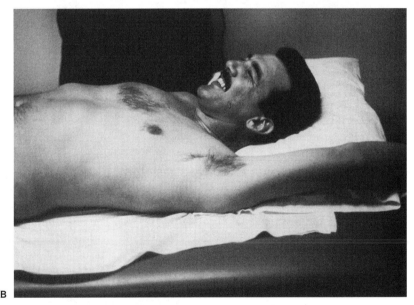

B

FIGURE 3.5 (A) *Excessive extension of the trunk during passive elevation testing in a patient with subscapularis muscle tightness.* **(B)** *Same patient after extensibility of the subscapularis is restored.*

cited is Cyriax's capsular pattern of restriction that aids in the diagnosis of frozen shoulder (see Ch. 10).[8]

FROZEN SHOULDER OR ADHESIVE CAPSULITIS. As described by Cyriax,[8] the capsular pattern of restriction is characterized by a restriction of the glenohumeral joint that is greatest in external rotation, lesser in abduction, and least in internal rotation. The authors have observed a modification of Cyriax's capsular pattern. The greatest restriction at the glenohumeral joint is external rotation in 0° of abduction. Abduction to 90° combined with external rotation is the next most restricted range, and internal rotation at 90° of abduction the least restricted range of mo-

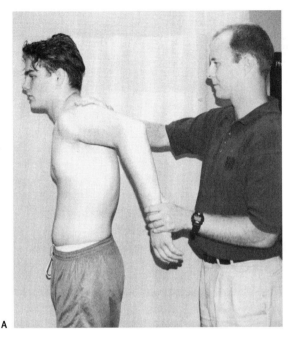
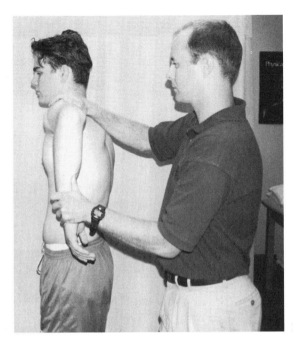

FIGURE 3.6 **(A)** *Substitution of glenohumeral extension for glenohumeral internal rotation in a patient with restriction of the posterior capsule.* **(B)** *Same patient after extensibility of the posterior capsule is restored.*

tion. See Chapter 1 for further discussion of anatomic restrictions at the glenohumeral joint.

TIGHT POSTERIOR CAPSULE. Limited glenohumeral internal rotation and horizontal adduction indicate a restriction of the posterior capsule. Posterior capsule tightness is often found in patients with anterior glenohumeral instability with secondary impingement.[28]

SUBSCAPULARIS MUSCLE TIGHTNESS. Subscapularis tightness will result in a greater limitation of glenohumeral external rotation in 0° of abduction than in 45° to 90° of abduction.[29]

MIDDLE AND INFERIOR GLENOHUMERAL LIGAMENT TIGHTNESS. Restriction of the middle and inferior glenohumeral ligaments and capsule will result in greater limitation of glenohumeral external rotation in 45° to 90° of abduction than in 0° of abduction.[29]

ACCESSORY MOTION

An assessment of accessory motion at the sternoclavicular, acromioclavicular, scapulothoracic, and glenohumeral joints identifies the presence and direction of hypomobilities and hypermobilities of the noncontractile structures (primarily the capsule and ligaments) of a joint. When hypomobilities are identified, mobilization techniques to restore the mobility may be employed (see Ch. 15); for hypermobilities, strengthening exercises to improve joint stability may be employed (see Ch. 14).

Musculotendinous Strength

A careful assessment of the musculotendinous structures is of vital importance for soft tissue diagnosis. This is particularly true of the glenohumeral and scapulothoracic joints, because they function with little stability provided by

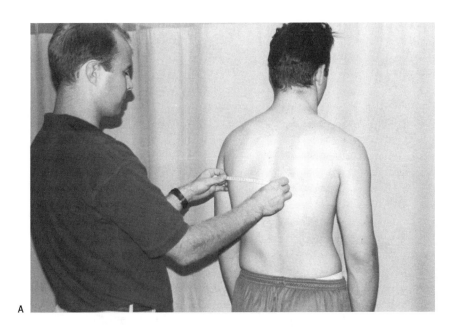

A

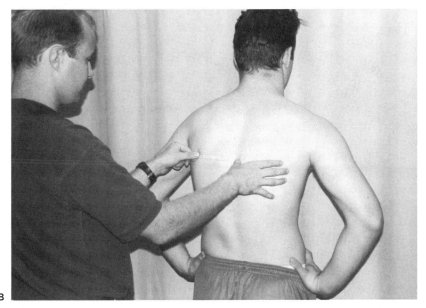

B

FIGURE 3.7 *Lateral slide test. Measurement of distance from inferior angle of scapula to the nearest thoracic segment.* **(A)** *Patient's arms resting at sides.* **(B)** *Patient's hands on hips (thumbs pointing posteriorly). (Figure continues.)*

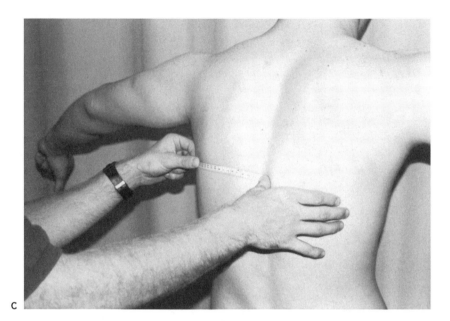

FIGURE 3.7 *(continued)* **(C)** *Glenohumeral joints 90° abducted and internally rotated.*

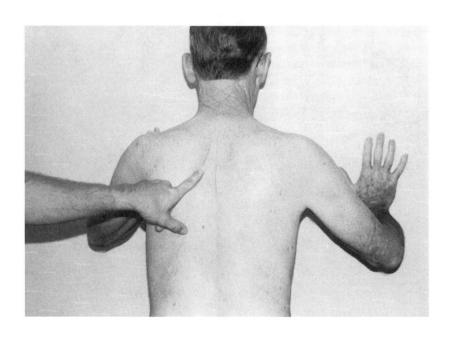

FIGURE 3.8 *Wall push-up. Patient with mild left serratus anterior muscle weakness exhibits mild "winging" of left scapula.*

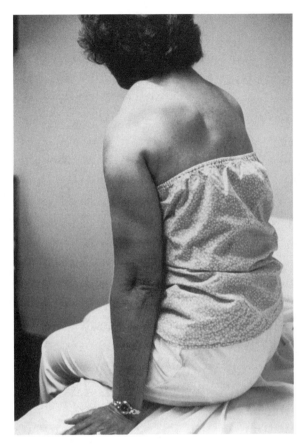

FIGURE 3.9 *Sitting press-up. Patient with long thoracic nerve palsy exhibits severe winging of the left scapula.*

TABLE 3.3. *Diagnosis based on resistive tests*

FINDING OF RESISTIVE TEST	LESION
Strong and painless	Normal
Strong and painful	Minor muscle lesion
	Minor tendon lesion
Weak and painful	Gross macrotraumatic lesion such as fracture
	Partial rupture of muscle or tendon
Weak and painless	Muscle or tendon rupture
	Neurologic dysfunction

(Adapted from Cyriax,[8] with permission.)

shoulder dysfunction, all performed with the glenohumeral joint in a neutral position: shoulder adduction, abduction, external rotation, internal rotation, and elbow flexion and extension. Many clinicians include shoulder flexion and extension as well. According to Cyriax,[8] pain that occurs during the muscle contraction is more likely to indicate a lesion within a muscle belly, while pain that occurs upon release of the contraction is more likely to indicate a lesion within a tendon. Additionally, each possible combination of pain and weakness can aid in soft tissue diagnosis (Table 3.3).

When one or more resistive tests are strong and painful, Cyriax[8] also advocates identifying the muscle or tendon at fault. This is done by confirming or excluding a given muscle/tendon with other resistive tests that also activate the same contractile unit (Table 3.4). According to Cyriax,[8] resistive tests of the primary function of a muscle are expected to produce the most pain.

MANUAL MUSCLE TESTING

Manual muscle testing provides information regarding the degree of resistance that a musculotendinous unit is able to generate. The reader is referred to texts on manual muscle testing for specific protocols.[30,31] Some of the classic manual muscle testing positions for the shoulder musculature have been modified in recent years, in response to EMG studies identifying positions that optimally recruit a given muscle. Test positions for the supraspinatus muscle are one exam-

inert structures relative to other joints. Unless contraindicated following known rupture or surgical disruption of tendon or muscle, an assessment of musculotendinous strength generally will include resistive tests, manual muscle testing, and often, scapular stability tests. Isokinetic strength testing may also be included if more specific information is desired regarding absolute strength values, comparison of involved to uninvolved strength values, and strength ratios of muscle groups (see Ch. 19).

RESISTIVE TESTS

Resistive tests may be defined as isometric muscle tests for strength and provocation of pain. Cyriax[8] advocates six resistive tests to assess

TABLE 3.4. *Identification of specific muscle/tendon lesion with resistive tests*

POSITIVE RESISTIVE TEST	MUSCLE/TENDON	FINDINGS OF ADDITIONAL RESISTIVE TESTS
Shoulder abduction	Deltoid	Positive flexion (anterior deltoid)
		Positive extension (posterior deltoid)
	Supraspinatus	Negative flexion
		Negative extension
Shoulder adduction	Pectoralis major	Positive flexion
		Positive horizontal adduction
	Teres minor	Positive external rotation
	Latissimus dorsi	Positive extension
		Positive internal rotation
	Teres major	Positive extension
		Positive internal rotation
Shoulder external rotation	Teres minor	Positive adduction
	Infraspinatus	Negative adduction
	Supraspinatus	Positive abduction
Shoulder internal rotation	Subscapularis	Negative adduction
	Pectoralis major	Positive adduction
		Positive horizontal adduction
	Latissimus dorsi	Positive adduction
		Positive extension
	Teres major	Positive adduction
		Positive extension

(Modified from Cyriax,[8] with permission.)

TABLE 3.5. *Response of specific upper quarter muscles to dysfunction*

MUSCLE GROUP	POSTURAL MUSCLES (TIGHTEN)	PHASIC MUSCLES (WEAKEN)
Axioscapular muscles	Upper trapezius	Rhomboid major and minor
	Levator scapulae	Middle trapezius
	Pectoralis minor	Lower trapezius
		Serratus anterior
Scapulohumeral muscles	Subscapularis	Deltoid
		Supraspinatus
		Infraspinatus
		Teres minor
Axiohumeral muscles	Pectoralis major (clavicular portion)	
Cervical and stomatognathic muscles	Sternocleidomastoid	Longus colli
	Suboccipitals	Longus capitus
	Scaleni	Infrahyoid
	Suprahyoid	

(Data from Janda and Schmid[32] and Jill and Janda.[33])

TABLE 3.6. *Palpation of upper quarter structures*

REGION	STRUCTURE	SOFT TISSUE INJURY OR POSTURAL FAULT	FINDING
Anterior cervical triangle	Suprahyoid muscles	FHP	Tight, TP's
	Infrahyoid muscles	FHP	TP's
	Anterior tubercles of transverse processes	FHP	Tender (insertion of anterior scalene)
	Longus colli	FHP	TP's
Posterior cervical triangle	Sternocleidomastoid muscle	FHP	Tight, TP's
	Anterior and middle scalene muscles	FHP	Tight, TP's
		TIS	Tight, tender, edema
	First rib	FHP	Elevated, tender
	Upper trapezius muscle	FHP	Tight, TP's
		Scapular instability	Tight, TP's
	Cervical facet joints	Facet strain	Tender, edema, thickened
	Posterior tubercles of transverse processes	FHP	Tender (attachment of levator scapulae muscles)
	Clavicle	Scapular protraction	Elevated

FHP, forward head posture; TIS, thoracic inlet syndrome; TP, trigger point.

ple (see the section on special tests later in the chapter).

Muscle imbalances are a common intrinsic factor in shoulder microtrauma injuries.[3,4] A muscle imbalance may be defined as a weak agonist, a tight agonist, or a combination of the two. Janda and Schmid[32] and Jull and Janda[33] believe that muscles respond in a predictable pattern to an altered state of mechanics in both microtrauma and macrotrauma. Jull and Janda[33] developed a classification system of skeletal muscle based on response to dysfunction. Muscles that shorten and tighten in dysfunction are classified as postural muscles, while those that lengthen and weaken in dysfunction are classified as phasic muscles. This classification system can expedite the evaluation of shoulder musculature by predicting which muscles to routinely manually muscle test and which to routinely evaluate for flexibility (Table 3.5).

A muscle imbalance of the rotator cuff generally involves tightness of the subscapularis and weakness of the infraspinatus, teres minor, and supraspinatus. This results in anterior instability of the glenohumeral joint when in a position of external rotation and abduction.[34] Muscle imbalance of the scapula often involves both tight-

ness of the levator scapulae and weakness of the serratus anterior and lower trapezius muscles; combined, these limit elevation of the acromion and potentially contribute to an impingement syndrome.

SCAPULAR STABILITY TESTS

Normal function of the shoulder complex demands adequate scapular stability. Thus, in addition to manual muscle testing, specific scapular stability tests may assist in soft tissue diagnosis.

Lateral Slide Test

Kibler[18] described the lateral slide test to evaluate the function of the muscles that stabilize and/or externally rotate the scapula (upper and lower trapezius, serratus anterior, and rhomboid major and minor). A measurement is taken from the inferior angle of the scapula to the nearest thoracic segment in three different glenohumeral joint positions (Fig. 3.7). Kibler[18] asserts that a difference of 1 cm or greater in the second and third positions is associated with microtrauma injuries of the shoulder. Gibson et

TABLE 3.7. *Palpation of structures of the shoulder complex*

REGION	STRUCTURE	SOFT TISSUE INJURY OR POSTURAL FAULT	FINDING
Scapular region	Acromion process	Impingement syndrome	Tender
		Scapular elevation or protraction	Elevated
	Inferior angle of scapula	Scapular abduction	Lateral
		Scapular protraction	Elevated
	Suprascapular notch	Suprascapular nerve entrapment	Tender
	Spine of scapula	Scapular protraction	Excessively angled in frontal plane
	Levator scapulae insertion on scapula	FHP	Tight, TP's
		Cervical strain	Tight, TP's
		Decreased scapular rotation	Tight
	Supraspinatus muscle	All rotator cuff pathologies	Atrophy
		Suprascapular nerve entrapment	Atrophy
		Anterior instability	Atrophy
	Infraspinatus and teres minor muscles	All rotator cuff pathologies	Atrophy
		Supraspinatus nerve entrapment	Atrophy (infraspinatus)
		Anterior instability	Atrophy
	Quadrangular space	Axillary nerve entrapment	Tender
	Rhomboid major/minor muscles	Scapular instability	Atrophy, TP's
	Lower trapezius muscle	Scapular instability	Atrophy
Axillary region	Pectoralis major muscle	Scapular protraction	Tight
		Frozen shoulder	Tight
	Pectoralis minor muscle	Scapular protraction	Tight, tender, TP's
	Corocoid proces	Scapular protraction	Tender (insertion of pectoralis minor)
		TIS	Tender
	Subscapularis muscle	Muscle imbalance rotator cuff	Tight, tender, TP's
Articular structures	Sternoclavicular joint	Dislocation	Malalignment
		Sprain	Tender
	Acromioclavicular (AC) joint	Dislocation	Malalignment
		Sprain	Tender
	Coracoacromial ligament	Impingement syndrome	Tender
		AC joint sprain	Tender
	Coracoclavicular ligaments	AC joint sprain	Tender
	Humeral head	Anterior subluxation	Positioned anteriorly
		Tight posterior capsule	Positioned anteriorly
	Lesser tubercle humerus	Tight subscapularis	Tender
		Subscapularis bursitis	Tender
	Greater tubercle humerus	Impingement syndrome	Tender, thickened
		Subacromial bursitis	Tender, edema, thickened
		Supraspinatus or infraspinatus tendonitis	Tender, thickened
	Long head biceps tendon	Bicipital tendonitis	Tender, edema, thickened

FHP, forward head posture; TIS, thoracic inlet syndrome; TP, trigger point.

al[17] studied the reliability of the lateral slide test measuring with a string from the T8 segment to the inferior angle of the scapula, and reported intrarater ICCs of 0.81 to 0.94 and interrater ICCs of 0.18 to 0.69. Therefore, although a useful measurement for each clinician, the lateral slide test may not be suitable for comparison between clinicians.

Functional Tests of Scapular "Winging"

Direct observation of scapular "winging" is not possible in the classic supine position for manual muscle testing of the serratus anterior muscle.[30,31] The examiner may observe scapular winging due to weakness of the serratus anterior muscle by observing active elevation (see the section on mobility later in the chapter), wall push-ups (Fig. 3.8), or sitting press-ups (Fig. 3.9).

ISOKINETIC TESTING

Many commercially available isokinetic testing devices are now manufactured and can be utilized to obtain more specific parameters of strength. The reader is referred to Chapter 16 for further information on isokinetic strength testing.

Proprioception and Kinesthesia

Until recently, proprioceptive and kinesthetic abilities received more attention in rehabilitation of lower extremity injuries than upper extremity injuries. Proprioception is defined as the ability to perceive position, weight, and resistance of objects in relation to the body. Kinesthesia is defined as the ability to sense the extent, direction, or weight of body movement. In addition to visual, vestibular, and cutaneous input, receptors in the joint capsule, ligaments, and labrum provide proprioceptive and kinesthetic information.

Published studies on shoulder proprioceptive and kinesthetic testing have used specialized testing apparatus.[35,36] Davies and Dickoff-Hoffman[37] advocate clinical angular joint replication testing with an electronic digital inclinometer. They report for normal males average mean differences of plus or minus 2.4° to 3.0° for seven shoulder joint positions between known angles and subject replication of known angles.

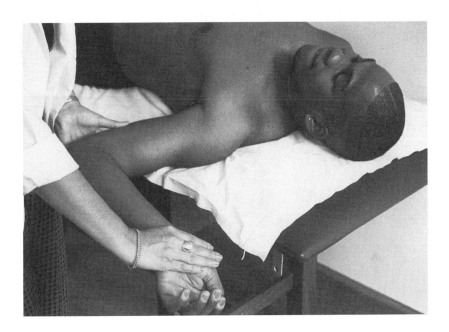

FIGURE 3.10 *Apprehension test.*

Because proprioception and kinesthesia are compromised following anterior shoulder dislocation,[35,38] exercises designed to improve proprioception and kinesthesia seem logical, at least in rehabilitation of macrotraumatic injuries that are likely to disrupt the capsular, ligamentous, or labral structures.

Palpation

Direct manual palpation of specific structures is performed to evaluate tissue tension, structure size, temperature, swelling, static position, crepitus, and provocation of pain. A systematic procedure for palpation of tissues is advised to facili-

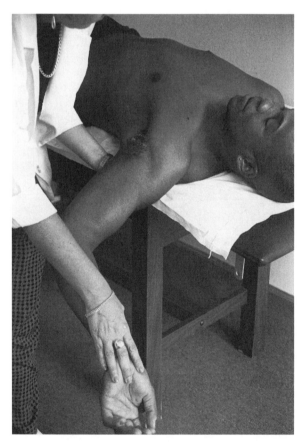

FIGURE 3.11 *Jobe subluxation test.*

tate an efficient yet comprehensive evaluation. In general, palpation of the anterior and posterior cervical triangles may be more important in patients with postural abnormalities, while palpation of glenohumeral articular structures may be more important when glenohumeral macrotrauma is suspected. Because many structures of the shoulder complex are normally tender to palpation, comparison of findings to the uninvolved side is crucial. Additionally, similar palpation findings are common to many shoulder dysfunctions, so palpation may be the least valuable component in diagnosis of soft tissue dysfunction. Structures commonly palpated by region are shown in Tables 3.6 and 3.7, along with the possible dysfunction(s) when palpation findings are positive.

Special Tests

Special tests may be included in evaluation of the shoulder complex to confirm or exclude the presence of specific shoulder soft tissue dysfunctions. In this section we will describe the more commonly performed special tests for glenohumeral instabilities, labral tears, impingement syndrome, musculotendinous dysfunctions, and rupture of the transverse humeral ligament.

GLENOHUMERAL STABILITY TESTS

Glenohumeral stability tests are performed to assess the integrity of the capsular and ligamentous structures. The tests may be used to confirm both unidirectional and multidirectional instabilities.

Apprehension Test

The patient is placed in a supine position. The shoulder is then positioned in 90° of abduction and full external rotation (Fig. 3.10). The examiner provides overpressure into external rotation. Provocation of pain and apprehension indicate anterior instability.[39,40] The apprehension test may also be performed with the patient in a sitting position.

Jobe Subluxation Test

The patient is placed in a supine position. The arm is then positioned off the edge of the examining table and the glenohumeral joint placed in 90° of abduction and 90° of external rotation (Fig. 3.11). The examiner grasps the patient's forearm with one hand to maintain the test position and the posterior humeral head with the other hand. The examiner then gently applies an anteriorly directed force to the posterior humeral head. Pain and apprehension indicate a positive test for anterior instability.[41] Provocation of pain without apprehension may denote either primary impingement or mild anterior instability with secondary impingement.[41]

Jobe Relocation Test

This test may aid in the differentiation of a primary impingement from a primary instability with a secondary impingement.[41] The shoulder is positioned in 90° of abduction and 90° of external rotation, identical to the apprehension test. If pain and apprehension are provoked, the examiner then applies a posteriorly directed force to the anterior aspect of the humeral head (Fig. 3.12). Reduction of pain and apprehension while "relocating" the humeral head posteriorly is considered a positive test, and indicates primary anterior instability rather than primary impingement.

Glenohumeral Load and Shift Test

The patient is seated and the examiner is positioned behind the patient on the ipsilateral side (Fig. 3.13). The examiner stabilizes the scapula with the proximal hand and grasps the humeral head with the distal hand. The humeral head is directed superiorly and medially to approximate the glenoid fossa ("loaded"). While maintaining the "loaded" position, both anterior and posterior stresses are applied and the amount of translation is noted.[42] Abnormal displacement of the humerus may be categorized as follows:

1. *5 to 10 mm of displacement*: the humeral head rides up the glenoid slope, but not over the rim.
2. *10 to 15 mm of displacement*: the humeral head rides up and over the glenoid rim, but

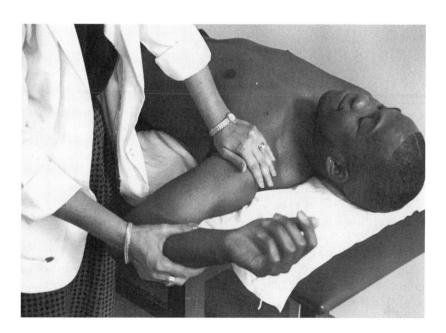

FIGURE 3.12 *Jobe relocation test.*

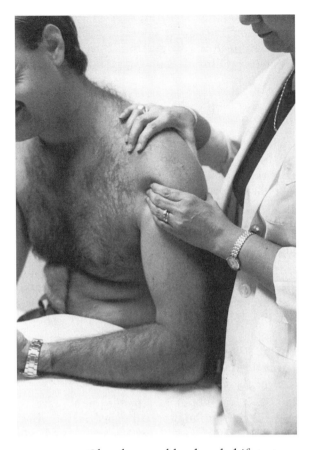

FIGURE 3.13 *Glenohumeral load and shift test.*

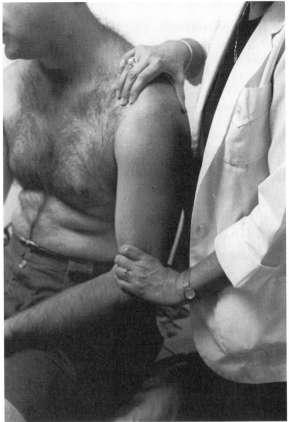

FIGURE 3.14 *Sulcus sign.*

spontaneously reduces when stress is removed.

3. *More than 15 mm of displacement*: the humeral head rides up and over the glenoid rim and remains dislocated when the stress is removed.

Sulcus Sign

The patient is seated with the arm at the side in a neutral position (Fig. 3.14). The examiner applies a distraction force to the humerus.[43] Excessive inferior translation with a sulcus defect between the acromion and humeral head indicates a positive test. The patient may report a subjective response of subluxation as well. The sulcus sign is indicative of multidirectional instability and is reported in centimeters of humeral head displacement from the inferior surface of the acromion.

Sulcus Sign at 90°

The patient is in a seated position, and the arm is abducted to 90° and placed on the examiner's shoulder (Fig. 3.15). The examiner applies a caudally directed force to the proximal humerus. Excessive inferior translation with the sulcus defect between the humeral head and acromion constitutes a positive test and indicates inferior glenohumeral instability.[44]

LABRAL INTEGRITY TESTS

Labral tests are performed to detect tears in the anterior or superior labrum. The common labral integrity tests are the clunk test and the **SLAP** (superior labrum anteroposterior) lesion test.

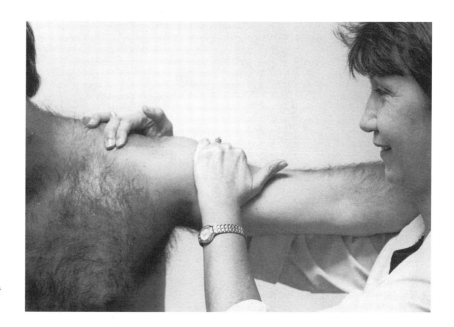

FIGURE 3.15 *Sulcus sign at 90°.*

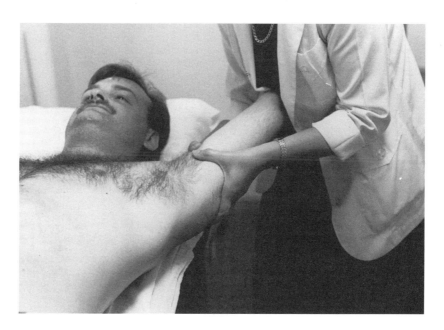

FIGURE 3.16 *Clunk test.*

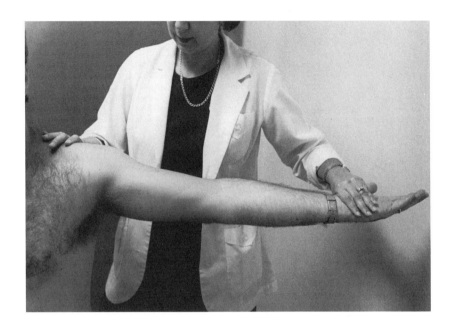

FIGURE 3.17 *Superior labrum anteroposterior (SLAP) lesion test.*

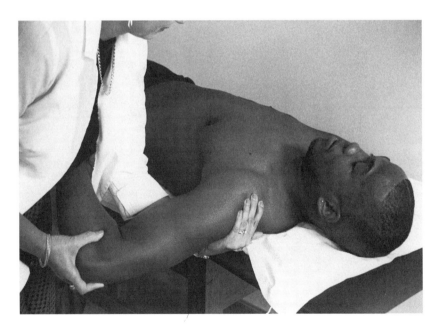

FIGURE 3.18 *Locking test.*

Clunk Test

The patient is supine and the humerus is shifted anteriorly and posteriorly while simultaneously circumducting the humerus and bringing the humerus into full abduction (Fig. 3.16). During these maneuvers, a "clunk" sound and pain, usually located between 90° of abduction and full abduction (anteroinferior aspect of glenohumeral joint), are positive clinical signs of a Bankart lesion.[45,46]

Superior Labrum Anteroposterior (SLAP) Lesion Test

The patient is sitting with the humerus in 90° of abduction, the elbow extended, and the forearm fully supinated. Resistance to abduction is applied (Fig. 3.17). Pain, a "clunk" sound, or

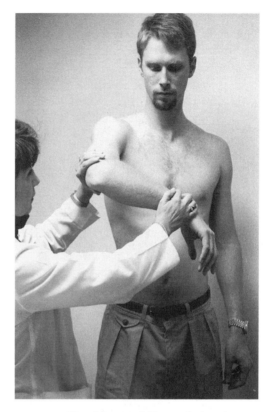

FIGURE 3.20 *Hawkins and Kennedy impingement test.*

pseudo-catching may implicate a SLAP lesion with a possible tear of the long head of the biceps tendon.[44,47]

IMPINGEMENT TESTS

Impingement tests are designed to approximate the greater tubercle of the humerus and the acromion, thereby compressing the subacromial structures. Common special tests that assist in the confirmation of a diagnosis of impingement syndrome include the locking test, the Neer and Welsh impingement test, and the Hawkins and Kennedy impingement test.

Locking Test

As described by Maitland,[48] the examiner stabilizes and depresses the scapula with the proximal hand while the distal hand internally rotates and slightly extends the humerus. The

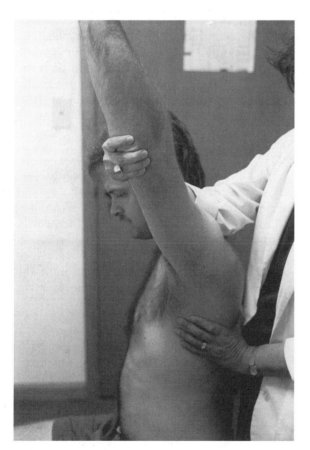

FIGURE 3.19 *Neer and Welsh impingement test.*

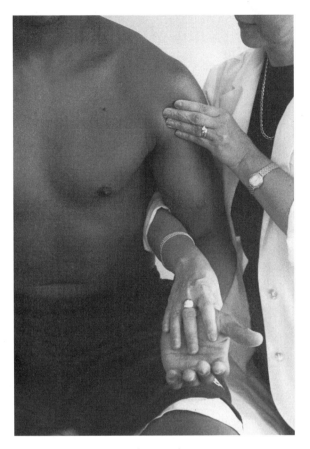

FIGURE 3.21 *Yergason's test.*

humerus is then abducted until firm joint resistance is detected (Fig. 3.18). Provocation of pain indicates a positive test for impingement of the supraspinatus tendon.[49]

Neer and Welsh Impingement Test

The patient is seated while the examiner stands. Scapular external rotation is blocked with one hand while the other hand raises the arm in forced flexion, causing approximation of the greater tuberosity and the acromion (Fig. 3.19).[50] Pain implicates impingement of the supraspinatus and long head of the biceps tendons.

Hawkins and Kennedy Impingement Test

The patient may either be sitting or standing. The humerus is placed in 90° of flexion and then internally rotated (Fig. 3.20).[47,51] The maneuver

is accomplished by exerting force through the forearm to bring the distal glenohumeral joint into internal rotation. Pain implicates supraspinatus tendon impingement.

MUSCULOTENDINOUS UNIT TESTS

Musculotendinous unit tests are designed to identify dysfunction of specific muscles and tendons. Tests specifically for bicipital tendinitis include Yergason's test and Ludington's test. The supraspinatus tests serve as resistive tests, thereby evaluating both musculotendinous strength and pain provocation. The Gilcrest sign and the Drop Arm test both assess the function of multiple muscles and tendons.

Yergason's Test

The patient is seated, the elbow is placed in 90° of flexion, and the forearm is pronated (Fig. 3.21). The examiner palpates the long head of the biceps tendon with the proximal hand while resisting supination and elbow flexion with the distal hand.[47,52] Provocation of pain over the anteromedial aspect of the shoulder is a positive sign of bicipital tendinitis.

Gilcrest Sign

The Gilcrest sign evaluates the eccentric activity of the biceps, supraspinatus, and deltoid muscles. The patient fully flexes the arm while holding 5 pounds, and then lowers the arm in the frontal plane in an externally rotated position (Fig. 3.22). Pain and inability to control the arm motion is a positive sign of dysfunction of the long head of the biceps, the supraspinatus, or the deltoid muscle.[47,53]

Ludington's Test

The patient's hand is placed on top of the head forcing the glenohumeral joint into abduction and external rotation (Fig. 3.23). The patient contracts the biceps muscle isometrically by pressing the hand against the head. Symptom reproduction in the bicipital groove is a positive sign for bicipital tendinitis.[47,54]

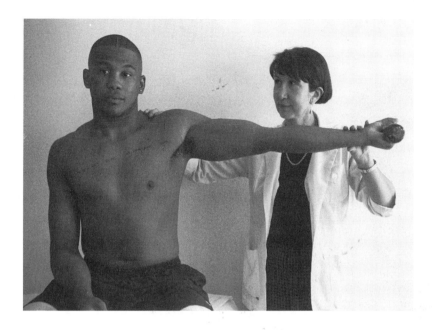

FIGURE 3.22 *Gilcrest sign.*

Drop Arm Test

The patient may either be seated or standing. The arm is passively raised above 90° of abduction. The patient then actively lowers the arm to 90° of abduction in internal rotation (Fig. 3.24).

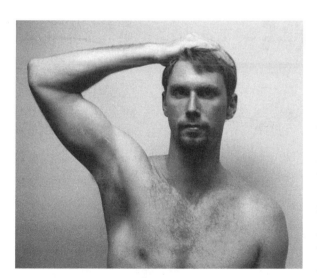

FIGURE 3.23 *Ludington's test.*

If the patient's arm approaches 90° and "drops," the test is positive for a full-thickness rotator cuff tear.[55,56]

Supraspinatus Test

The humerus is placed in 90° of elevation in the plane of the scapula and full internal rotation (Fig. 3.25). The examiner applies resistance to elevation while the patient attempts to maintain the position.[57,58] The examiner then grades the strength of the supraspinatus muscle and notes any pain provoked by the test.

Alternate Supraspinatus Test

The patient is prone with the arm to be tested resting off the side of the plinth. The patient horizontally abducts the arm at 100° of abduction in external rotation and the examiner applies resistance at the end of range (Fig 3.26).[59] The examiner then grades the strength of the supraspinatus muscle.

TRANSVERSE HUMERAL LIGAMENT TESTS

Special tests are also described to identify ruptures of the transverse humeral ligament. One common test is the Lippman test.

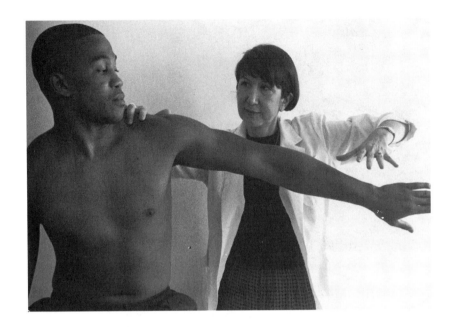

FIGURE 3.24 *Drop arm test.*

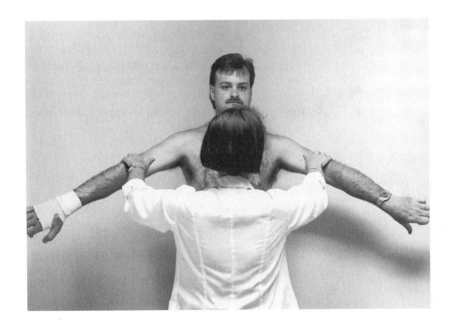

FIGURE 3.25 *Supraspinatus test.*

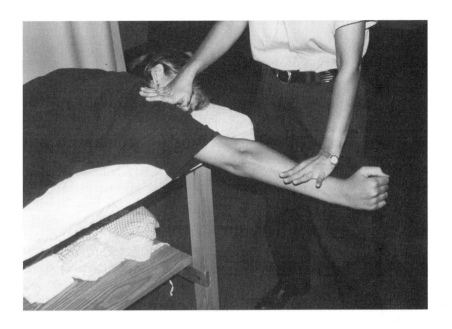

FIGURE 3.26 *Alternate supraspinatus test.*

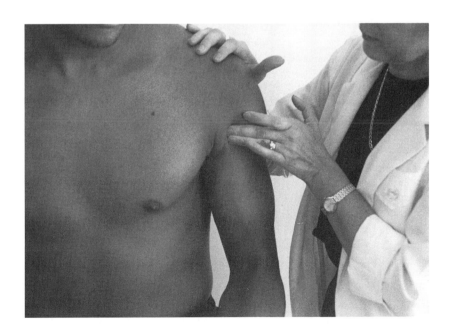

FIGURE 3.27 *Lippman test.*

Lippman Test

The patient's elbow is placed in flexion and the examiner palpates the long head of the biceps tendon within the bicipital groove (Fig. 3.27). The examiner then attempts to displace the long head of the biceps tendon by exerting lateral and medial manual forces to the tendon.[11] Ability to displace the tendon from the bicipital groove indicates a rupture of the transverse humeral ligament. A sharp pain without tendon displacement indicates bicipital tendinitis.

CASE STUDY

This case study demonstrates the use of each component of evaluation on a specific patient. A general plan of care concludes the case study; however, the reader is referred to subsequent chapters for more specific descriptions of treatment programs. Although specific diagnoses are withheld until the exam is complete, assessment is an ongoing process, and therefore a summary of ongoing assessments is included following each portion of the evaluation.

PATIENT INTERVIEW

HISTORY

The patient reports an onset of left shoulder pain beginning approximately 4 months ago. She is unable to identify a specific mechanism of injury. Her routine activities include carrying and storing luggage as a part of her occupation, and recreational tennis and swimming. The patient moved to a new home with a swimming pool 6 months ago and began swimming laps (freestyle) two or three times per week. She is currently taking a nonsteroidal antiinflammatory medication (Daypro) for her shoulder problem, and reports some improvement in her symptoms with this medication.

DEMOGRAPHIC INFORMATION

The patient is a 47-year-old flight attendant. She is married and has two teenaged children. She is left-hand dominant.

COEXISTING PROBLEMS

The patient has a 20-year history of irritable bowel syndrome for which she takes an antispasmodic medication (Bentyl). She also reports occasional bilateral neck pain and stiffness, for which she takes Advil. No other problems are reported.

LOCATION, NATURE, AND BEHAVIOR OF PAIN

The patient reports pain over the lateral aspect of the proximal half of the arm. The pain never extends below the elbow or above the subacromial area. Some discomfort in the medial left scapular area extends distally to the T4 level, proximally to the C5 level, does not cross midline, and extends laterally to the acromial area of the scapula.

The patient describes the arm pain as aching in nature and the scapular pain as tightness and soreness. The arm pain is intermittent. The pain is provoked by swimming, serving and backhand strokes in tennis, reaching behind her back, and lifting luggage overhead for storage while working. She reports waking with aching in the left arm after sleeping on the shoulder. During freestyle swimming, the pain begins towards the end of her 30 minute swim, but does not stop her from finishing. Resting the arm by the side eases the pain after about 10 minutes.

CONCLUSIONS BASED ON PATIENT INTERVIEW

1. The pain stems from microtrauma, based on the history of the problem's onset and the introduction of a new activity (swimming) 2 months prior to the onset of pain.

2. Irritability level is generally low because the patient meets only one of Cyriax's[8] three criteria for high irritability, and because she reports a relatively long T1, no T2, and relatively short T3, based on Maitland's[1] criteria.

3. The coexisting medical problem of irritable bowel syndrome is not known to refer pain to the shoulder and is unlikely to need further

consideration. Coexisting cervical symptoms will need special attention during the subsequent examination, due to common referral of pain to the shoulder region and common involvement in upper quarter dysfunctions.

4. Progressive degenerative joint dysfunctions are common in the patient's age group.

CERVICAL SCREENING

Compared to left rotation and left side bending, cervical right rotation and right side bending are slightly limited, with reports of stiffness at end range. Forward bending is full with stiffness at end range, and backward bending, left rotation, and left side bending are within normal limits (WNL). Passive overpressures into cervical right rotation and right side bending provoke mild discomfort in the left midcervical region, but no left arm or scapular pain. Cervical compression does not provoke pain.

CONCLUSIONS BASED ON CERVICAL SCREENING

1. Muscle tightness or cervical facet restriction is likely, limiting right cervical rotation and right side bending.

2. Cervical spine tests do not reproduce left arm or scapular symptoms.

3. Palpation of the anterior and posterior triangles of the cervical spine should be included in the palpation portion of the examination.

OBSERVATION OF SYMMETRY AND POSTURE

Anteriorly, a slight left head tilt and mild atrophy of the left deltoid can be observed. Laterally, moderate forward head posture, apparent excessive protraction of the left scapula, and a slight anterior position of the left humeral head are noted in comparison to the right side. Posteriorly, a slight left head tilt, a slight depression of the left scapula, and mild atrophy of the left infraspinatus and teres minor muscles are observed.

CLINICAL MEASURE OF SCAPULAR POSITION

A measurement of scapular protraction using the method described by Diveta et al[15] (see Fig. 3.1) demonstrates a 0.5-cm difference in scapular protraction, greater on the left side.

OTHER POSITIONS AND ACTIVITIES

The patient normally alternates between sleeping on the right and left sides with the arm in an adducted position. She now attempts to stay mostly on the right side because she wakes with discomfort when in left sidelying. Arm swing during ambulation is normal. The patient keeps the left shoulder near its neutral position when donning or doffing clothing to avoid a combination of abduction and external rotation. A videotape of her tennis lessons taken by her coach demonstrates lack of follow-through on her tennis forehand and poor positioning for her backhand.

CONCLUSIONS BASED ON OBSERVATION

1. Forward head posture supports the previous decision to include evaluation of the upper quarter in the ongoing assessment.

2. Left head tilt supports the previous assessment of possible left cervical facet or muscular tightness.

3. The 0.5-cm difference in scapular position is unlikely to be clinically significant.

4. Depression of left scapula is likely normal because this is the patient's dominant side.

5. Improper biomechanics of tennis strokes may be either an extrinsic factor in her dysfunction or a compensation for the dysfunction.

MOBILITY

ACTIVE RANGE OF MOTION

Cardinal plane movements exhibit limitation in internal rotation and horizontal adduction to 50° and 110°, respectively, with pain at end ranges over the lateral arm. A painful arc is present during active abduction. In the plane of the scapula, normal glenohumeral to scapulothoracic rhythm is observed during concentric activity through all three phases of elevation. After 7 to 8 repetitions, some mild "winging" of the left scapula and some oscillations of the left scapula are seen in the middle phase of elevation during eccentric activity.

Functional movement tests demonstrate the ability of the patient to put her left hand behind her neck, although there is mild arm discomfort during the maneuver. The patient is unable to put her hand behind her back (left thumb reaches the sacroiliac joint compared to the T7 segment on the right side), and is unable to put her left hand on the opposite shoulder. She reports left lateral arm pain during both maneuvers.

PASSIVE RANGE OF MOTION

Cardinal plane PROM of the left glenohumeral joint exhibits limitation of internal rotation to 60° and horizontal adduction to 115°. External rotation in 0° of abduction is slightly limited compared to the right side. Other motions are full, with mild left lateral arm pain at the end range of external rotation in 90° of abduction.

During passive internal rotation, resistance is encountered prior to pain, and resistance, not pain, prevents further movement. During passive horizontal adduction, pain and resistance are encountered concurrently at 110° and pain/muscle guarding (rather than joint resistance) are felt to further limit movement at 115°.

ACCESSORY MOBILITY

When compared to the right side, anteroposterior gliding of the left humerus is mildly restricted and posteroanterior gliding is slightly increased. During accessory mobility testing, caution is taken to begin the tests with the humeral head in a neutral position, because the patient's left humeral head is slightly anteriorly positioned when compared to the right side. If this caution is not taken, a false-positive restriction of the anterior capsule and a false-positive laxity of the posterior capsule may result. Passive scapular distraction is slightly limited on the left.

CONCLUSIONS BASED ON MOBILITY

1. Limited active and passive internal rotation and horizontal adduction of the glenohumeral joint indicate tightness of the posterior capsule.

2. With repeated movements, apparent scapular instability during the eccentric phase of elevation in the plane of the scapula may indicate weakness of the scapular rotators and/or stabilizers.

3. Limitations of functional movements indicate that the patient is unable to perform daily activities such as fastening a brassiere, tucking in blouses posteriorly, or performing tennis strokes with correct body mechanics. The functional movement limitations correlate to AROM findings of limited glenohumeral internal rotation and horizontal adduction.

4. PROM findings indicate that joint restriction, rather than muscle weakness or pain, primarily limits glenohumeral internal rotation and horizontal adduction. The PROM findings correlate to the functional movement limitations.

5. Irritability level is low (based on internal rotation PROM) and moderate (based on horizontal adduction PROM), using the method of assessing irritability from either Cyriax[8] or Maitland.[1]

6. Posterior capsule tightness and mild anterior capsule laxity may predispose the patient to an impingement syndrome.[28]

7. A muscle imbalance of the rotator cuff is likely, due to probable tightness of the subscapularis muscle (based on the PROM limitation of external rotation in 0° of abduction concurrent with full external rotation in 90° of abduction), as well as the slight restriction of passive scapular distraction.

MUSCULOTENDINOUS STRENGTH

RESISTIVE TESTS

Resisted shoulder external rotation and abduction are weak without pain.

MANUAL MUSCLE TESTING

Significant findings during manual muscle testing are as follows:

	Left	Right
GH external rotators	4−/5	4+/5
GH abductors	4−/5 (pain)	4/5
Supraspinatus	3+/5 (pain)	4/5
Serratus anterior	4−/5	5/5
Lower trapezius	4−/5 (pain)	5/5

SCAPULAR STABILITY TESTING

During the third component of the lateral slide test,[18] a 1.5-cm greater measurement is obtained on the left side (see Fig. 3.7). Mild left scapular "winging" is observed during wall push-ups (see Fig. 3.8).

ISOKINETIC TESTING

The shoulder external and internal rotators are tested in 30° of elevation in the plane of the scapula to avoid pain that may be encountered if tested in 90° of abduction. Test speeds of 60° and 180° per second are chosen. The peak torque ratio of the external rotators to internal rotators is 40% on the left and 60% on the right at 60° per second.

CONCLUSIONS BASED ON MUSCULOTENDINOUS STRENGTH TESTING

1. According to Cyriax,[8] weak and painless resistive tests indicate a muscle or tendon rupture or neurologic dysfunction (see Table 3.3). However, based on this patient's generally low irritability level and relatively high functional level, it is most likely that the neutral position for resistive testing does not provoke the patient's pain, and that muscle atrophy rather than gross macrotrauma explains the weakness.

2. There is a muscle imbalance of the rotator cuff based on the weakness of the external rotators and supraspinatus found with resistive tests, manual muscle testing, and isokinetic testing, combined with the previous finding of probable subscapularis muscle tightness.

3. The patient exhibits weakness and instability of the scapular muscles based on the lateral slide test, manual muscle testing, and previously observed oscillations of the scapula during the middle phase of elevation (with repeated testing of eccentric activity).

PALPATION

There are no significant findings to palpation of the structures within the anterior triangle of the cervical spine. Palpation of the posterior triangle of the cervical spine reveals tightness and tenderness of the left anterior and middle scalene muscles, tightness and trigger points of the left upper trapezius muscle, and tenderness of the left posterior tubercles of the transverse processes of C3 and C4.

During palpation of the scapular region, positive findings include a depressed left acromion and inferior angle of the scapula, tightness, tenderness, and trigger points at the insertion of the left levator scapulae muscle, and atrophy of the left supraspinatus, infraspinatus, and teres minor muscles. At the axillary region, mild tightness and trigger points are palpable over the left subscapularis muscle. Palpation of the articular structures shows tenderness over the anterior aspect of the left acromion, a slightly anteriorly positioned left humeral head, tenderness over the lesser and greater tubercles of the left humerus, and tenderness over the left long head of the biceps tendon.

CONCLUSIONS BASED ON PALPATION

1. The findings support previous conclusions of imbalance of the rotator cuff muscles and mild anterior subluxation of the left humeral head.

2. Tenderness over the greater and lesser humeral tubercles, anterior acromion, and long head of the biceps tendon are consistent with impingement syndrome.

3. Tightness and tenderness of the levator scapulae, anterior and middle scalene, and upper trapezius on the left are consistent with forward head posture, left head tilt, and limited left cervical rotation and side bending, and subjective tightness at the end range of cervical flexion.

SPECIAL TESTS

Stability test results are a positive left apprehension test, positive relocation test, and a mildly positive left anterior load-shift test. The Neer and Welsh[50] and Hawkins and Kennedy[51] impingement tests are positive. In this case, the locking test[48] is deferred due to painfully restricted glenohumeral internal rotation PROM. The supraspinatus test[57,58] is positive for pain and weakness. The Gilcrest sign[47,53] is also positive on the left.

CONCLUSIONS BASED ON SPECIAL TESTS

1. The previous assessment of slight laxity of the anterior glenohumeral joint capsule is further supported by the load-shift test.

2. Impingement tests are positive.

3. The apprehension and relocation tests suggest that the patient's impingement is secondary to a mild anterior glenohumeral subluxation.[39–41]

4. Pain and weakness of the supraspinatus support the findings of impingement and muscle imbalance of the rotator cuff.

5. Positive Gilcrest sign may suggest the involvement of both the long head of the biceps tendon and the supraspinatus tendon in the impingement syndrome.

ASSESSMENT

1. Microtrauma injury characterized by anterior subluxation of the glenohumeral joint with secondary impingement.[39–41]

2. Intrinsic factors in this patient's microtrauma injury include muscle imbalance of the rotator cuff (weakness of the posterior cuff muscles results in failure to counteract the upward shear forces of the deltoid muscle),[23,24] tightness of the posterior glenohumeral capsule and mild laxity of the anterior glenohumeral capsule (decreases the subacromial space),[28] and weakness of the scapular external rotators (weakness of the lower trapezius and serratus anterior muscles may alter the plane of the surface of the glenoid and change the length–tension relationship of the rotator cuff muscles).

3. Extrinsic factors in this patient's microtrauma injury include initiation of a free-style swimming program (repetitive elevation in internal rotation that may predispose to impingement), recreational tennis (tennis serves involve positioning of the shoulder in combined abduction and external rotation, and combined flexion and internal rotation), and an occupation that requires overhead lifting.

TREATMENT PLAN

Sequential treatment goals and a general treatment plan to accomplish the goals are shown in Table 3.8. The reader is referred to subsequent chapters for specific treatment programs.

Summary

As emerging trends in the health care delivery systems demand greater efficiency from health care providers, the need for a thorough evaluation is more vital than ever. A systematic evaluation is the most effective tool to establish soft tissue diagnoses and prioritization of the patient's problems, which can then direct the clinician to the most efficient treatment plan. The components of evaluation for the shoulder complex have each been discussed, and a case study has illustrated the process of assessment based on a specific patient's evaluation findings.

TABLE 3.8. *Sequential treatment goals and treatment plan*

TREATMENT GOAL	TREATMENT PLAN
Decrease activity-induced pain and inflammation	Ice following swimming nd therapeutic exercises
Correct scapular muscle imbalance	Stretching exercises for the levator scapulae muscle
	Strengthening exercises for the serratus anterior and lower trapezius muscles
Correct rotator cuff muscle imbalance	Stretching exercises for the subscapularis muscle
	Strengthening exercises for the supraspinatus, infraspinatus, and teres minor muscles
Increase strength of shoulder elevators	Strengthening exercises for the deltoid muscle
Return to pain-free occupational and recreational overhead activity	Proprioceptive/kinesthetic training
	Functional exercises
	Plyometric exercises
	Consult with tennis coach regarding biomechanics of tennis strokes

Acknowledgments

The authors wish to thank Marie-Josette Murray for her very valuable editorial assistance.

References

1. Maitland GD: Vertebral Manipulation. 5th Ed. Butterworths, London, 1986
2. Bigliani LU, Morrison DS, April EW: The morphology of the acromion and its relationship to rotator cuff tears. Orthop Trans 10:216, 1986
3. Fu FH, Hamer CD, Klein AH: Shoulder impingement syndrome: a critical review. Clin Orthop Rel Res 269:162, 1991
4. Kamkar A, Irrgang JJ, Whitney SL: Nonoperative management of secondary shoulder impingement syndrome. J Orthop Sports Phys Ther 17:212, 1993
5. Boissonnault WG: Examination in Physical Therapy Practice: Screening for Medical Disease. Churchill Livingstone, New York, 1991
6. Berkow R, Fletcher AJ: The Merck Manual of Diagnosis and Therapy. 15th Ed. Vol. 1. Merck Sharp and Dohme Research Laboratories, Rahway, NJ 1987
7. Berkow R, Fletcher AJ: The Merck Manual of Diagnosis and Therapy. 15th Ed. Vol 2. Merck Sharp and Dohme Research Laboratories, Rahway, NJ, 1987
8. Cyriax J: Textbook of Orthopaedic Medicine. 8th Ed. Vol 1. Bailliere Tindall, London, 1982
9. White AA, Panjabi MM: Clinical Biomechanics of the Spine. 2nd Ed. Lippincott-Raven Philadelphia, 1990
10. Hoppenfeld S: Physical Examination of the Spine and Extremities. Appleton-Century-Crofts, Norwalk, CT, 1976
11. Magee DJ: Orthopaedic Physical Assessment. 2nd Ed. WB Saunders, Philadelphia, 1992
12. Greenfield B: Upper quarter evaluation: structural relationships and interdependence. p. 43. In Donatelli R, Wooden MJ (eds): Orthopaedic Physical Therapy. 1st Ed. Churchill Livingstone, New York, 1989
13. Greenfield B, Catlin PA, Coats PW et al: Posture in patients with shoulder overuse injuries and healthy individuals. J Orthop Sports Phys Ther 21:287, 1995
14. Solem-Bertoft E, Thuomas KA, Westerberg CE: The influence of scapular retraction and protraction on the width of the subacromial space. Clin Orthop Rel Res 296:99, 1993
15. Diveta J, Walker ML, Skibinski B: Relationship between performance of selected scapular muscles and scapular abduction in standing subjects. Phys Ther 70:470, 1990
16. Neiers L, Worrell TW: Assessment of scapular position. J Sports Rehabil 2:20, 1993
17. Gibson MH, Goebel GV, Jordan TM et al: A reliability study of measurement techniques to determine static scapular position. J Orthop Sports Phys Ther 21:100, 1995
18. Kibler WB: Role of the scapula in the overhead throwing motion. Contemp Orthop 22:525, 1991
19. Rothstein JM, Roy SH, Wolf SL: The Rehabilita-

tion Specialist's Handbook. FA Davis, Philadelphia, 1991

20. Hawkins RJ, Abrams JS: Impingement syndrome in the absence of rotator cuff tear (stages 1 and 2). Orthop Clinics Nor Amer 18:373, 1987

21. Simon ER, Hill JA: Rotator cuff injuries: an update. J Orthop Sports Phys Ther 10:394, 1989

22. Bagg SD, Forrest WJ: A biomechanical analysis of scapular rotation during arm abduction in the scapular plane. Am J Phys Med Rehab 67:238, 1988

23. Poppen NK, Walker PS: Forces at the glenohumeral joint in abduction. Clin Orthop Rel Res 135: 165, 1978

24. Sharkey NA, Marder RA: The rotator cuff opposes superior translation of the humeral head. Am J Sports Med 23:270, 1995

25. Abrams JS: Special shoulder problems in the throwing athlete: pathology, diagnosis, and nonoperative management. Clin Sports Med 10:839, 1991

26. Hayes KW, Petersen C, Falconer J: An examination of Cyriax's passive motion tests with patients having osteoarthritis of the knee. Phys Ther 74: 697, 1994

27. Paris SV, Loubert PV: Foundations of Clinical Orthopaedics. Institute Press, St. Augustine, 1990

28. Harryman DT, Sidles JA, Clark JM et al: Translation of the humeral head on the glenoid with passive glenohumeral motion. J Bone Jt Surg 72A: 1332, 1990

29. Turkel SJ, Panio MW, Marshall JL et al: Stabilizing mechanisms preventing anterior dislocation of the glenohumeral joint. J Bone Jt Surg 63A: 1208, 1981

30. Daniels L, Worthingham C: Muscle Testing: Techniques of Manual Examination. 4th Ed. WB Saunders Company, Philadelphia, 1980

31. Kendall FP, McCreary EK, Provance PG: Muscles: Testing and Function. 4th Ed. Williams & Wilkins, Baltimore, 1993

32. Janda V, Schmid HJ: Muscles as a pathogenic factor in back pain. Paper presented at the 4th conference of the International Federation of Manipulative Therapy, Christchurch, New Zealand, 1988

33. Jull GA, Janda V: Muscles and motor control in low back pain: assessment and management. p. 253. In Grant R (ed): Physical Therapy of the Cervical and Thoracic Spine. Churchill Livingstone, New York, 1989

34. Cain PR, Mutschler TA, Fu FH et al: Anterior sta-

bility of the glenohumeral joint. Am J Sports Med 15:144, 1987

35. Smith RL, Brunolli J: Shoulder kinesthesia after anterior glenohumeral joint dislocation. Phys Ther 69:106, 1989

36. Allegrucci M, Whitney SL, Lephart SM et al: Shoulder Kinesthesia in Healthy Unilateral Athletes Participating in Upper Extremity Sports. J Orthop Sports Phys Ther 21:220, 1995

37. Davies GJ, Dickoff-Hoffman S: Neuromuscular testing and rehabilitation of the shoulder complex. J Orthop Sports Phys Ther 18:449, 1993

38. Lephart SM, Borsa PA, Warner JP et al: Proprioceptive sensation of the shoulder in healthy, unstable, surgically repaired shoulders. J Should Elbow Surg 3:371, 1994

39. Davis GJ, Gould JA, Larson RL: Functional examination of the shoulder girdle. Phys Sportsmed 6: 82, 1981

40. Yahara ML: Shoulder. p. 159. In Richardson JK, Igharsh ZA (eds): Clinical Orthopaedics Physical Therapy. WB Saunders, Philadelphia, 1994

41. Kvitne RS, Jobe FW: The diagnosis of anterior instability in the throwing athlete. Clin Ortho Rel Res 291:117, 1993

42. Silliman J, Hawkins RJ: Classification and physical diagnosis of instability of the shoulder. Clin Orthop Rel Res 291:7, 1993

43. Gerber C, Ganz R: Clinical assessment of instability of the shoulder. J Bone Jt Surg 66B:551, 1984

44. Caspari R, Gleisser WB: Arthroscopic manifestations of shoulder subluxation and dislocation. Clin Orthop Rel Res 291:54, 1993

45. Andrews JR, Gillogly S: Physical examination of the shoulder in throwing athletes. In Zarina B, Andrews JR, Carson WG (eds): Injuries to the Throwing Arm. WB Saunders, Philadelphia, 1985

46. Walsh DA: Shoulder evaluation of the throwing athlete. Sports Med Update 4:24, 1989

47. Davies GD, DeCarlo M: Examination of the shoulder complex. Sports Physical Therapy Session, Home Study Course, 1995

48. Maitland GD: Peripheral Manipulation. 2nd Ed. Butterworths, London, 1977

49. Boissomault WG, Janos S: Dysfunction, evaluation, and treatment of the shoulder. p. 169. In Donatelli R, Wooden MJ (eds): Orthopaedic Physical Therapy. 2nd Ed. Churchill Livingstone, New York, 1993

50. Neer CS III: Impingement lesions. Clin Orthop Rel Res 173:70, 1983

51. Hawkins RJ, Kennedy JC: Impingement syndrome in athletes. Am J Sports Med 8:151, 1980

52. Yergason RM: Supination sign. J Bone Jt Surg 13: 160, 1931

53. Davis GJ, Gould JA, Larson RL: Functional examination of the shoulder girdle. Phys Sportsmed 6: 82, 1981

54. Ludington NA: Rupture of the long head of the biceps flexor cubite muscle. Ann Surg 77:358, 1923

55. Mosely HF: Disorders of the shoulder. Clin Symposia 12:1, 1960

56. Hoppenfeld S: Physical Examination of the Spine and Extremities. Appleton-Century Crofts, Norwalk, CT 1976

57. Jobe FW, Tebone JE, Perry J, Maynes D: An EMG analysis of the shoulder in throwing and pitching. Am J Sports Med 11:3, 1983

58. Jobe FW, Jobe C: Painful athletic injuries of the shoulder. Clin Orthop Rel Res 173:117, 1983

59. Worrell TW, Corey BJ, York SL et al: An analysis of supraspinatus EMG activity and shoulder isometric force development: Med Sci Sports Exerc 24:744, 1992

4

Interrelationship of the Spine to the Shoulder Girdle

OLA   GRIMSBY

JOHN   C.   GRAY

One of the most difficult and challenging aspects of the orthopedic physical therapist's work is to determine the primary tissue in lesion. This is particularly true when evaluating the shoulder. Pain and/or dysfunction in the shoulder may arise from intrinsic or extrinsic pathology (spine and related structures, or viscera).[1-14] The therapist needs to recognize that pain in the shoulder may be referred from the cervical spine[2,4-14]; that shoulder dysfunction in the form of adhesive capsulitis, tendinitis, or bursitis may be initiated by the spine[10,11,14-17]; and that there may be simultaneous spine and shoulder pathology.[11,14] For these reasons it is important to understand the interrelationship between the spine and the shoulder girdle. This chapter will review the anatomic, neurologic, and biomechanic relationships between the spine and the shoulder. The chapter will close with a review of cervical pathologies causing shoulder pain, and a case study will be presented.

Musculoskeletal Relationship

One of the most direct relationships between the spine and the shoulder girdle is through muscle, tendon, and fascial attachments. In fact, seven muscles of the shoulder, the rotator cuff group plus the deltoid, teres major, and latissimus dorsi, are thought to be morphologically related.[18] Their origins appear to be from cervical myotomes.[18]

The trapezius muscle originates from the medial third of the superior nuchal line and the external occipital protuberance of the occipital bone, from the ligamentum nuchae, from the spinous processes of the seventh cervical and all of the thoracic vertebrae, and from the intervening supraspinal ligament (Plate. 4.1).[19,20] Insertion for this muscle is the lateral third of the clavicle, the medial border of the acromion, and the upper border of the crest of the spine of the scapula.[19,20] The trapezius assists in suspending the shoulder girdle, pulling or extension movements of the arm, abduction of the arm, and upward rotation of the scapula.[19,20] With the shoulder fixed, the trapezius may bend the head and neck posterolaterally.[19,20]

The latissimus dorsi muscle originates medially from tendinous fibers that attach to the lower six thoracic spines and through the thoracolumbar fascia to the lumbar and sacral spines, supraspinous ligaments, and the posterior portion of the iliac crest (Plate 4.1).[19,20] It also originates, via muscular attachments, from the outer lip of the iliac crest, the lower three or four ribs, and the inferior angle of the scapula.[19,20] This broad muscle subsequently inserts into the floor of the intertubercular groove of the humerus.[19,20] The latissimus dorsi muscle is active in adduction, extension, and medial rotation of the humerus.[19,20] It is typically active with swimming, pulling movements, coughing, sneezing, and deep inspiration.[19,20]

The levator scapulae muscle originates, via four separate tendons, from the transverse processes of the first three or four cervical vertebrae (Plate 4.1).[19,20] It inserts into the medial border of the scapula from the superior angle to the spine.[19,20]

The rhomboideus minor muscle originates from the lower part of the ligamentum nuchae, the spinous process of the last cervical and first thoracic vertebrae, and the associated segment of the supraspinal ligament (Plate 4.1).[19,20] It inserts into the medial border of the scapula at the root of the scapular spine.[19,20]

The rhomboideus major muscle originates from the spinous processes of the second to the fifth thoracic vertebrae and the corresponding segment of the supraspinous ligament (Plate 4.1).[19,20] It inserts into the medial border of the scapula below its spine.[19,20]

The rhomboideus minor and major muscles work together to draw the scapula upward and medially and assist the serratus anterior muscle in holding it firmly to the chest wall.[19,20] The levator scapulae muscle assists in elevation, support, and rotation of the scapula.[19,20] With the shoulder fixed, it laterally flexes the cervical spine to the same side.[19,20]

The platysma is a broad muscular sheet that spreads from its fascial attachments over the upper parts of the pectoralis major and deltoid muscles and ascends medially across the clavicle to the side of the neck.[20] Attachment sites include the symphysis menti, lower border of the mandibular body, lateral half of the lower lip, and muscles at the modiolus near the buccal angle.[20] The platysma wrinkles the nuchal skin obliquely, may assist in mandibular depression, helps express horror and surprise, is active in

sudden deep inspiration, and is significantly contracted in sudden violent efforts.[20]

The deep cervical fascia, internal to platysma, is fibroareolar tissue between muscles, viscera, and vessels.[20] Its superficial layer is continuous with the ligamentum nuchae and periosteum of the seventh cervical spine.[20] It covers the trapezius and sternocleidomastoid muscles and adheres to the symphysis menti and the body of the hyoid bone.[20] The deep fascia is attached to the acromion, clavicle, and manubrium sterni, fusing with their periostea.[20]

The sternocleidomastoid muscle originates from the lateral aspect of the mastoid process and, by a thin aponeurosis, to the lateral half of the superior nuchal line (Plate 4.2).[20] It inserts into the upper anterior surface of the manubrium sterni and the medial third of the clavicle.[20] The sternocleidomastoid muscle side-bends the head ipsilaterally and rotates it contralaterally.[20] It also assists in flexion of the cervical spine.[20] With the head fixed, the muscles work together to aid thoracic elevation and inspiration.[20]

The suprahyoid muscles (digastric, stylohyoid, mylohyoid, and geniohyoid) are important in that they work in coordination with the infrahyoid muscles (sternohyoid, sternothyroid, thyrohyoid, and omohyoid), which have direct attachments to the shoulder girdle (Plate 4.2).[20] The suprahyoid muscles are active in mandibular depression, hyoid elevation, swallowing, and chewing.[20] The infrahyoid muscles are active in hyoid depression, elevation and depression of the larynx, speech, and mastication.[20]

The omohyoid, one of the infrahyoid muscles, has two bellies that meet at an angle as an intermediate tendon (Plates 4.1 and 4.2). The superior belly originates from the lower border of the hyoid bone and descends into the intermediate tendon.[20] This tendon is ensheathed by a band of deep cervical fascia that descends to the clavicle and first rib.[20] The inferior belly descends from this tendon to attach to the upper scapular border, near the scapular notch, and occasionally to the superior transverse scapular ligament.[20] Its actions include hyoid depression with prolonged inspiratory efforts and tensing of the lower deep cervical fascia.[20]

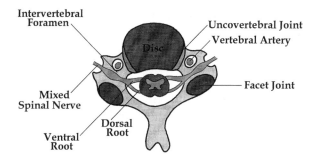

FIGURE 4.1 *Anatomy of the dorsal and ventral nerve roots in a typical cross-section segment of the cervical spine.*

Neurogenic Relationship

The shoulder is tied to the spine neurologically via sensory, motor, sympathetic, reflex, mechanoreceptor, segmental facilitation, and referred pain relationships. Each of these relationships will be examined in greater detail throughout this section and the rest of the chapter.

The spinal cord is surrounded by meninges (dura, arachnoid, and pia mater), which at the level of the foramen magnum are directly continuous with those covering the brain.[21] The spinal cord is a segmented structure, as indicated by the attachments of 31 pairs (8 cervical, 12 thoracic, 5 lumbar, 5 sacral, and 1 coccygeal) of spinal nerves.[21] The cervical spinal nerve, or mixed spinal nerve, is formed by the convergence of the dorsal and ventral spinal nerve roots close to the intervertebral foramina (Fig. 4.1).[21] The ventral root is composed primarily of efferent (80 percent motor, 20 percent sensory) somatic fibers, which are the axons of cell bodies in the ventral horn of the gray matter, that carry motor impulses to the voluntary muscles.[21] The corresponding cervical intervertebral disc and uncovertebral joint are in close proximity to the ventral nerve root (Fig. 4.2).[21] The dorsal nerve root is entirely sensory, and it conveys afferent impulses back to the dorsal horn of the spinal cord from somatic, visceral, and vascular sources.[21] The cell bodies of the afferent fibers are located in the spinal ganglia of the dorsal root.[21] The dorsal root ganglia is oval and usually located between the perforation in the dura mater, by the

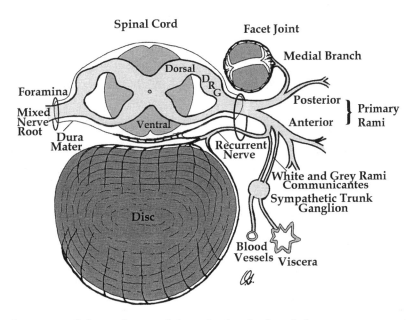

FIGURE 4.2 *Anatomy of the pathway of the mixed spinal and the recurrent meningeal nerve in a typical cross-section of the cervical spine.*

dorsal root, and the intervertebral foramina (Fig. 4.2).[21] The first and second cervical ganglia, however, are on the vertebral arches of the atlas and axis, respectively.[21] The cervical facet joints are in close proximity to the dorsal nerve roots (Fig. 4.1).

As the mixed spinal nerve emerges from the intervertebral foramina it immediately gives off the recurrent meningeal (sinuvertebral) nerve branch (Fig. 4.2).[10,21–23] The recurrent meningeal nerve then receives input from the gray rami communicans.[10,21–23] This nerve, now a mixture of sensory and sympathetic nerves, returns back through the intervertebral foramina to innervate the dura mater, walls of blood vessels, periosteum, ligaments, uncovertebral joints, and intervertebral discs in the ventrolateral region of the spinal canal.[10,21–24] Occasionally, branches of the recurrent meningeal nerve will innervate the dorsal dura, periosteum, and ligaments.[10,21–23]

After leaving the intervertebral foramina, the mixed spinal nerve divides into dorsal (posterior) and ventral (anterior) rami (Fig. 4.2).[21,22] Near its origin, each ventral ramus receives a grey ramus communicans from the corresponding sympathetic ganglion.[21,22] The dorsal rami of the cervical spinal nerves divides, except the first cervical, into medial and lateral branches to supply the muscles and skin of the posterior regions of the neck.[10,21,22] The medial branch is also distributed to the capsules of the cervical facet joints, where it relays afferent input from fibers of type I, II, and III encapsulated mechanoreceptors and the type IV unencapsulated nociceptors back to the dorsal horn of the spinal cord.[10,24,25]

The type I receptors are most abundant in the joint capsules of the cervical facet joints, shoulder, and hip.[26] The actual number of active type I receptors may decline more rapidly in elderly patients or those whom have suffered repeated traumas, due to the superficial location of these mechanoreceptors within the joint capsule. Research has demonstrated a higher density of type II versus type I mechanoreceptors in the cervical spine.[25] The subjects (n = 3) were few, however, and they were either deceased or had suffered traumatic cervical spine injuries

previous to the time of the study.[25] Type I receptors fire impulses for up to 1 minute (slowly adapting) after stimulation, and they are activated by deformation in the beginning or end range of tension for the capsule.[24] The type I receptors produce tonic reflexogenic affects on the neck and limb muscles, postural (low threshold) and kinesthetic sensation, and pain inhibition.[24–27]

The type II receptors are located deep in the joint capsule, fire an impulse for 0.5 seconds (rapidly adapting) after stimulation, and are activated by deformation in the beginning or midrange of tension for the joint capsule.[24] These receptors are most abundant in the ankle and foot, wrist and hand, and temporomandibular joints.[26] Type II receptors are responsible for dynamic (phasic) reflexogenic effects on the muscles of the trunk and limbs.[24–27] They also provide information on joint acceleration and deceleration (low threshold).[26] Type II mechanoreceptors may also be activated to inhibit pain.

Type III receptors are also dynamic mechanoreceptors. Within the facet joint capsules of the cervical spine, these receptors are found at the junction between the dense fibrous capsule and the loose areolar subsynovial tissue.[25] These mechanoreceptors are also found in ligaments and tendons.[25,26] They have a high threshold for activation and are very slow to adapt.[25,26] The type III mechanoreceptors have the lowest density in the facet joint capsules of the cervical spine when compared to types I and II.[25]

The type IV receptors are responsible for transmitting impulses that eventually reach the higher centers of the brain for perception as painful stimuli.[26] These nociceptors may be activated by abnormal neck posture, trauma, disc lesion, or chemical stimulation.[24] In addition, the three encapsulated mechanoreceptors (types I to III) can produce a noxious stimulus in response to excessive joint motion.[25]

The cervical ventral rami supply the anterior and lateral portions of the neck.[21,22] The third cervical ventral ramus appears between the longus capitis and the scalenus medius.[21,22] The ventral rami of the fourth through eighth cervical spinal nerve emerge between the scalenus anterior and scalenus medius.[21,22]

The upper four cervical ventral rami form the cervical plexus (Plate 4.3); the lower four, including the first thoracic ventral ramus, form the brachial plexus (Plate 4.4).[22,28] The cervical plexus supplies some nuchal muscles, the diaphragm, and areas of skin in the head, neck, and chest.[22,28] The formation of the brachial plexus allows for rearrangements of the efferent and afferent somatic and autonomic fibers so that they are redirected through the various trunks, divisions, and cords into the most appropriate channels (terminal branches) for distribution to the muscles, skin, vessels, and glands in the upper limbs.[22,28]

The dorsal scapular nerve (C5) arises from the uppermost root of the brachial plexus.[22,28] It pierces the scalenus medius muscle as it travels to supply the levator scapulae and the rhomboid major and minor muscles (Plates 4.4 and 4.5).[22,28] The suprascapular nerve (C5 and C6) arises from the superior trunk of the brachial plexus (Plate 4.3).[22,28] It supplies the supraspinatus and infraspinatus muscles, glenohumeral and acromioclavicular joints, and suprascapular vessels (Fig. 4.3).[22,28] The axillary nerve (C5 and C6) originates from the posterior cord of the brachial plexus (Plate 4.4).[22,28] It supplies the glenohumeral joint and the deltoid and teres minor muscles (Fig. 4.3).[22,28] The upper subscapular nerve (C5 and C6) arises from the posterior cord and innervates the subscapularis muscle (Plate 4.4).[19,22] The middle subscapular nerve, or thoracodorsal nerve (C7 and C8), arises from the posterior cord and innervates the latissimus dorsi muscle (Plate 4.4).[19,22] The lower subscapular nerve (C5 and C6) also arises from the posterior cord in proximity to the upper subscapular and the thoracodorsal nerves. The former innervates the subscapularis and teres major muscles (Plates 4.4 and 4.5).[19,22]

Biomechanic Relationship

The shoulder girdle is designed to be extremely mobile. One of its primary functions is to allow our hands to be used to their greatest advantage.

All movements of the shoulder girdle involve the direct or indirect participation of the cervical, thoracic, and/or lumbar spine. Most of the movement of the shoulder occurs between the head of the humerus and the glenoid fossa. Suspension and stabilization of the whole girdle are designed to enhance this action. The goal is scapular stability in concert with glenohumeral mobility.

Lifting the arm from the side of the body and up over head, abduction (normal range = 180°), involves all the joints of the shoulder girdle. The primary muscles involved are the trapezius, levator scapulae, serratus anterior, deltoid, and rotator cuff muscles. The rhomboid major and minor muscles simulate the activity of the middle trapezius and are most active in abduction as a stabilizing synergist via eccentric contraction during upward rotation of the scapula.[29] A force couple is formed using the upper trapezius and upper serratus anterior muscles to produce upward rotation and elevation of the scapula.[29] These two muscle segments, in concert with the levator scapulae muscle, will also support the shoulder girdle against the downward pull of gravity.[29] A second force couple, active in the same task, uses the lower trapezius and lower serratus anterior muscles.[29] Besides the activity of muscles originating from the spine, direct involvement of the joints of the spine occurs with end range (usually greater than 150°) of abduction. As the shoulder and arm are abducted beyond approximately 150°, there is a component motion of contralateral sidebending and extension of the thoracic spine.[30] For this reason, thoracic spine segmental mobility should be examined in any patient demonstrating restricted shoulder elevation. When both arms are raised, there is a necessary increase in the lumbar lordosis through activity of the lumbar erector spinae muscles.[30] Lumbar lordosis may also be increased secondary to a tight latissimus dorsi muscle. In order to ensure full functional recovery of motion around the shoulder girdle, it is important to treat all thoracic and lumbar spine segments with limitations in sidebending or extension.[29–31]

In a person with good postural alignment, elevation of the arm is free to proceed through

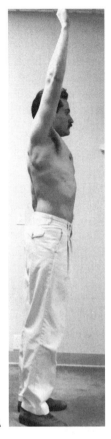
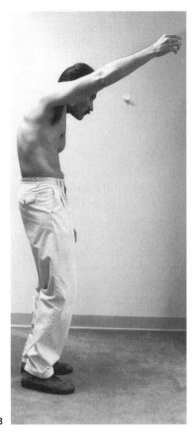

A   B

FIGURE 4.3 *Elevation of the arm.* **(A)** *Person with good postural alignment.* **(B)** *Same person, now demonstrating the effect of poor posture on elevation of the arm.*

Appreciation of the biomechanics of the shoulder requires a study of the sternoclavicular, acromioclavicular, scapulothoracic, and glenohumeral joints; their intrarelationship; and the collective interrelationship of the entire shoulder girdle complex to the spine. In addition, the kinesiology of almost 30 muscles that control motion at the shoulder needs to be understood. There is no room in this chapter for such an extensive undertaking. Please refer to Kapandji[30] or Norkin and Levangie.[29]

Postural Relationship

Poor posture can be a source of neck and shoulder pain.[33-36] Normal postural alignment, starting at the external auditory meatus of the skull, will allow a line of gravity to pass through the odontoid process, anterior to the axis of motion for flexion and extension of the occiput, posterior to the midcervical spine, through the glenohumeral joint, anterior to the thoracic spine, and posterior to the lumbar spine (Fig. 4.4).[37]

Sitting postures with the whole spine flexed will result in high levels of electromyographic (EMG) activity in the neck and shoulder muscles.[38] Standing postures associated with a forward head will demonstrate an increase in the cervical and lumbar lordosis, as well as an increase in thoracic kyphosis. In addition, the forward head posture forces the midcervical spine into hyperextension, with subsequent narrowing of the intervertebral foramina and increased weightbearing of the facet joints, especially at the C4–5 and C5–6 segments (Fig. 4.5).[34,39] This may lead to irritation of the C5 and C6 spinal nerve roots, respectively.[17,34,39] It may also lead to irritation of the dorsal root of C1, vertebral artery symptoms or entrapment of the suprascapular and dorsal scapular nerves.[40] Headaches are a common sequelae of chronic poor posture. One source of these headaches could be the increased stress on the C2–3 facet joints and the associated intervertebral foramen. Headaches originating from the C2–3 facet joints or the C3 dorsal ramus are fairly common in patients with chronic neck pain and headaches.[41,42]

a full 160° to 180° of motion without impingement of soft tissues in the subacromial space (Fig. 4.3). In the patient with the classic forward head, rounded shoulders, and increased thoracic kyphosis, the scapula rotates forward and downward, depressing the acromial process and changing the direction of the glenoid fossa. Now as the patient attempts to elevate the arm, the supraspinatus tendon and/or the subdeltoid bursa may become impinged against the anterior portion of the acromion process (Fig. 4.3). Repeated motions of this nature may accelerate overuse injuries or cumulative trauma disorders and lead to early changes consistent with bursitis and/or tendinitis.[32]

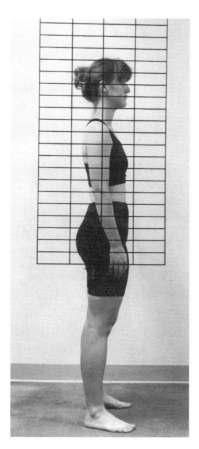

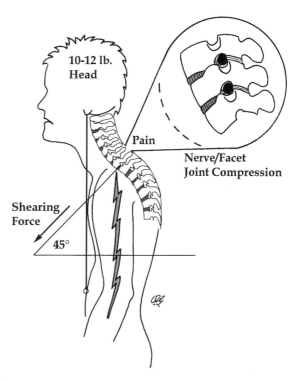

FIGURE 4.5 *Schematic of a forward head posture resulting in nerve and facet joint compression with increased shearing forces at the discs.*

FIGURE 4.4 *Normal postural alignment in standing.*

The cervical facet joints are at risk due to the increased weightbearing stress encountered in the forward head posture. The cartilage and synovial capsule of the facet joint will be exposed to persistent and recurrent trauma.[22] This may lead to arthritic changes and restrictions within the involved joints.[22] Any injury or irritation to these facet joints will contribute, via type I mechanoreceptor damage, to disorders involving the static postural reflexes of the upper extremities.[24,43] Finally, the intervertebral discs are put at risk due to the increase in shearing force as a result of increasing the cervical lordosis (Fig. 4.5). The normal lordosis in the cervical spine allows for an adequate balance of compressive forces with shearing forces. If the spine were to straighten, then there would be greater compres-

sive forces and lesser shearing forces acting on the discs.

When seated at a desk or table, the forward head posture may be secondary to one or more of the following: a seat height that is too high, a table or visual display terminal height that is too low and/or a seat that is too far away from the table (Fig. 4.6).[44] Neck and shoulder muscle activity is lowest in a sitting posture of slight thoracolumbar extension and a vertical cervical spine.[38]

Additional consequences of the forward head posture are a shortening of the sternocleidomastoid, upper trapezius, and levator scapulae, which will elevate the scapula.[40,45] The subsequent increase in thoracic kyphosis will abduct the scapula, allowing for a lengthening of the rhomboids and lower trapezius in association with a shortening of the serratus anterior.[40] Also, the shortening of the latissimus dorsi, teres

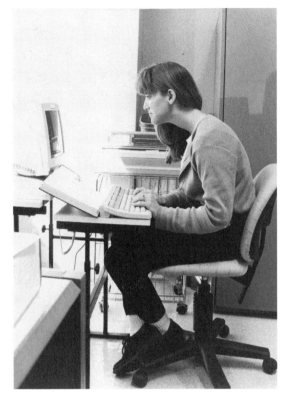

FIGURE 4.6 *Poor sitting posture at a work station.*

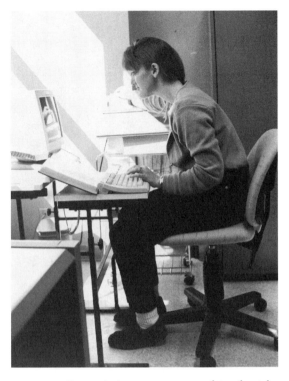

FIGURE 4.7 *Poor sitting posture combined with repetitive elevation of the arm.*

major, subscapularis, and pectoralis major and minor muscles will pull the humerus into a relative internally rotated posture.[40] This posture will alter the normal scapulohumeral rhythm and may precipitate an impingement of soft tissues, subdeltoid bursa, and supraspinatus tendon, in the subacromial space during elevation of the arm (Figs. 4.4 and 4.7).[40] An abducted scapula may have additional sequelae, such as increased acromioclavicular joint compression, shortened conoid ligament with a lengthened trapezoid ligament, and a posterior glide of the proximal clavicle that results in a shortening of the anterior capsule of the sternoclavicular joint.[40] During abduction or flexion of the shoulder girdle in persons with a kyphotic thoracic spine posture (arms abducted and internally rotated), they must keep increased tone in the rotator cuff musculature to compensate for loss of capsular stabilization.

Scoliosis will also affect the postural relationship of the scapula to the spine. The scapula will be elevated on the convex side and depressed on the concave side of the scoliosis.[37] There may also be a slight winging over a rib hump secondary to ipsilateral rotation of the spine at that level.[37]

Occupational Relationship

The cervical spine and the shoulder girdle are inseparable with regard to their coordinated functions in job-related tasks. Holding a prolonged and abnormal posture at the neck and shoulder is a major cause of cumulative trauma disorder (CTD).[46,47] The posture assumed by the neck and shoulder will determine how well the arm, wrist, and hand will tolerate the demands at work.[47] Cumulative trauma disorder involves repetitive microtrauma, to specific musculoskeletal tissues, collected over a period of time at a faster rate than the body can heal itself.[46] If the extent of damage continues to exceed the repair process, then it will eventually lead to pain, decreased work performance and loss of function.[46] The physical work demands that lead to CTD are repetitive motion and holding a sustained posture (Fig. 4.7).[46,47]

The neck and shoulder are dynamic structures that are mobile by design.[46] The neck and shoulder, however, are often required to perform static work as the hands perform a skilled task.[46–48] Maintaining a sustained work posture of the neck, in association with repetitive movements of an elevated shoulder, can restrict circulation to the working tissues of the arm and hand.[48] This can be a major hurdle for persons trying to return to work following a musculoskeletal injury. Patients with chronic neck and shoulder pain, following a whiplash injury in a motor vehicle accident, have shown a decreased ability to achieve a normal increase in blood flow to the upper trapezius muscle during progressive workloads.[49] Myofascial disorders of the trapezius, sternocleidomastoid, or infraspinatus muscles are capable of referred autonomic phenomena, including vasoconstriction.[50] Jobs that require holding a sustained posture for a prolonged period of time can restrict circulation to working tissues, resulting in early fatigue and a slower rate of repair of microtraumas to the musculoskeletal system.[46]

Forward head posture is a major risk factor in CTD.[46] The shifting forward of the weight of the head makes the neck and upper back muscles work harder.[46] This stressful posture can upset nerve control and circulation to the arms.[46] Poor posture is as much a problem in CTD as is repetitive motion.[46] Repetitive motion jobs are usually carried out in prolonged sitting or standing positions.[46,47]

Occupational neck and shoulder disorders are usually the result of prolonged flexion and/or abduction of the shoulders, repetitive arm work, high-speed work, poor head posture, and a maintained static muscle load.[17,35,44,47,51–53] A high level of static muscle activity is one reason for the high incidence of neck and shoulder disorders in persons working with cash registers or computer keyboards.[35,47,51,53] Working in a posture with the shoulder flexed and/or abducted will increase the (EMG) activity levels in the upper trapezius, cervical, and thoracic erector spinae muscles.[38,44,47] One solution is to have the cashier stand rather than sit, which will put less stress on the trapezius, infraspinatus, and thoracic erector spinae muscles.[47] For computer keyboard operators, ergonomically designed chairs and foot and arm rests are available (Fig. 4.8). The top portion of the visual display terminal should be at eye level. Other occupations at risk for neck and shoulder disorders are dentists, meat carriers, miners, heavy laborers and shipyard welders.[51]

Jobs that require sustained elevation of the arms may cause supraspinatus tendinitis, due to

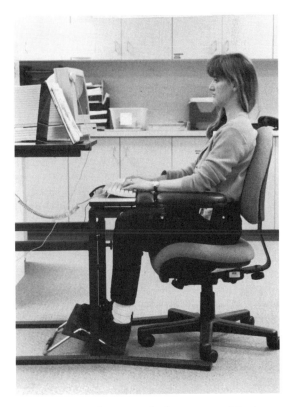

FIGURE 4.8 *Good postural alignment with the appropriate use of ergonomic design for a person seated at a visual display terminal.*

compression of the humeral head against the coracoacromial arch as the head of the humerus migrates cranially due to rotator cuff fatigue, and as a result of sustained tension in the muscle that will inhibit venous circulation.[52] Bicipital tendinitis can occur with similar working postures due to repeated friction between the synovial sheath of the tendon (long head) and the lesser tuberosity of the humerus.[52]

Ergonomic solutions to CTD include correcting both sitting and standing posture (Fig. 4.4); adjusting seat, table, and visual display terminal heights to allow for a supportive posture (Fig. 4.8); brief but frequent rest periods throughout the workday; light exercise during breaks to keep the blood flowing freely to all tissues; balancing repetitive motions of ADL or sports, that simulate job duties, with appropriate periods of rest; and training the worker's body to become fit, like an athlete, through exercise, nutrition, and rest, in order to withstand the stresses on the job.

Syndromes Related to the Neck and Shoulder

OMOHYOID SYNDROME

Neck, shoulder, and/or arm pain may be the presenting complaint of a patient with omohyoid syndrome.[54–58] This syndrome is characterized by the sudden onset of a severe muscle spasm on one lateral side of the neck.[54–57] The symptoms are typically aggravated by swallowing.[54–57] The omohyoid muscle belly may contain myofascial trigger points.[58] The etiology is often a contraction combined with a stretching of the omohyoid muscle.[55] An example would be a yawn combined with an attempt to swallow as the head is sidebent to one side.[54] Forceful motions, such as vomiting, may also cause the omohyoid muscle to go into spasm.[58]

Symptoms

Patients will report the sudden onset of pain and muscle spasm, often during yawning, swallowing, or vomiting.[54–56] Pain will be on one lateral side of the neck and may include the shoulder and arm.[54–58]

Signs

The patients will often present with the head flexed and sidebent ipsilaterally.[54,55] There will be audible breathing and an alteration in the quality of the voice, such as slurred speech.[55] Swallowing will be painful.[54–57] Neck flexion will decrease the symptoms.[55] Pain will be reproduced with stretching (extension, sidebending, or rotation away) or palpation of the omohyoid muscle.[54–56]

LEVATOR SCAPULAE SYNDROME

Another source of neck and shoulder pain is the levator scapulae syndrome.[59,60] This is proposed to be a bursitis involving a bursa associated with the levator scapulae at its attachment to the scapula.[59] It is thought to occur due to friction between the levator scapulae, serratus anterior, and the scapula as the muscles pull in opposite directions during repeated upper extremity tasks with the arm elevated.[59] A sustained head posture in rotation during prolonged typing or telephone calls may also precipitate a problem in the levator scapulae.[60] Additional risk factors include vigorous tennis or swimming.[60]

Symptoms

Patients will complain of pain over the superior medial angle of the scapula. There may be a "heaviness" or "burning" sensation that will radiate to the neck or shoulder.[59]

Signs

There is full active and passive ROM at the neck and shoulder. Symptoms are reproduced through palpation or stretching of the levator scapulae muscle. Thoracic outlet, impingement, and neurologic testing is negative. Plain radiographs of the shoulder will be negative.[59]

DROOPY SHOULDER SYNDROME

The droopy shoulder syndrome, a source of neck and shoulder pain, may be considered a brachial plexus stretch injury due to chronic postural strain. This syndrome is normally exclusive to women.[61,62]

Symptoms

The patient may complain of head, neck, chest, and bilateral shoulder and arm pain. Patients often report paresthesias in the upper extremities, without objective numbness, weakness, or atrophy. The patients may describe their symptoms as "tightness," "electrical," "jabbing" or "pulling."[61,62]

Signs

Postural examination will reveal a swan neck with low-set shoulders and horizontal clavicles. Symptoms are reproduced with stretch or palpation, at the supraclavicular fossa, of the brachial plexus. Passive scapular depression will increase the symptoms, whereas passive elevation will decrease the symptoms. There is no vascular insufficiency, claudication, or Raynaud's phenomenon. Lateral radiographs of the cervical spine will allow visualization of the second thoracic vertebrae. Normally a lateral radiograph of the neck will only allow visual inspection down to the sixth cervical vertebrae due to interference by the shoulder girdle. Electromyographic (EMG) studies are within normal limits.[61,62]

Myofascial Neck and Shoulder Pain

Myofascial pain in the neck and shoulders may be due to tenderness at motor points in muscle, secondary to cervical spine disease (Fig. 4.9).[12,14] Specifically, the early stage of C5 and/or C6 radiculopathy may precipitate these symptoms.[12] Clinically, it may be difficult to detect early radiculopathy referring myofascial pain and tenderness to the shoulder. There are no physical signs

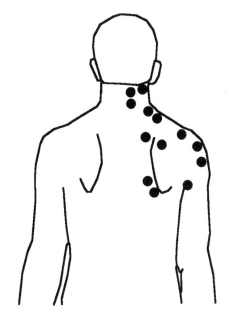

FIGURE 4.9 *Myofascial trigger points of the neck and shoulder. (Adapted from Kirkesola and Schjelderup,[110] with permission.)*

other than tenderness at motor points within the involved muscles.[12] An EMG study will be positive for neuropathy.[12,14] Patients with cervical spondylosis or an intrinsic shoulder problem will not have clinically significant tenderness at their motor points.[12]

A similar perspective on "myofascial" pain in the neck and shoulder states that these symptoms may be due to hyperalgesia from an entrapped peripheral nerve.[63] Entrapment of the suprascapular, dorsal scapular, axillary, or long thoracic nerves may account for the symptoms (Plate 4.5).[63] Peripheral nerve entrapment may occur without neurologic deficit and with normal findings on electrodiagnostic examination.[63]

Facilitated Segment and Mild Reflex Sympathetic Dystrophy

A facilitated segment may be defined as any segment of the spinal cord that has a lower than normal threshold for activation of the interneur-

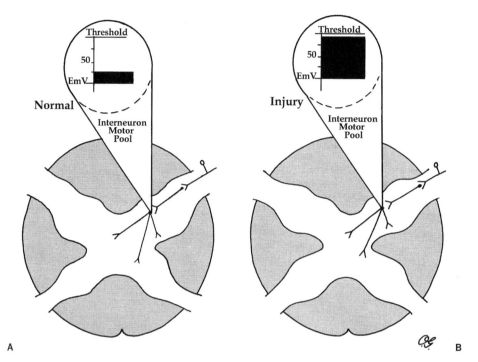

FIGURE 4.10 *A normal and a facilitated segment of the cervical spinal cord.* **(A)** *A normal segment with a low level of electrical activity and a high threshold for activation of the interneurons.* **(B)** *A facilitated segment with a high level of electrical activity and a low threshold for activation of the interneurons.*

ons within the interneuron pool (IP) (Fig. 4.10).[64] A large portion of the neurons are maintained in a state of facilitation due to chronic bombardment by afferent impulses from a segmentally related tissue that is irritated due to macrotrauma, repetitive microtrauma, or disease.[64] Repeated impingement of cervical nerve roots can produce chronic irritation of the dorsal root fibers, which then bombard the IP of the spinal cord with afferent nociceptive impulses.[15] This nerve root impingement may occur secondary to repeated upper extremity motion with the shoulder elevated; or a high-risk occupational activity, which produces repeated muscular pulls on the cervical spine that allows the intervertebral foramina to slightly "pinch" the nerve root.[15] Once these nociceptive impulses reach the IP, a response is elicited that may continue beyond the period of the actual stimulation.[15] This can occur via self-perpetuating chains of neurons within

the pool.[15] The IP is then sensitized by the barrage of afferent impulses cycling around within the pool.[15] This then becomes a segment of the spinal cord that facilitates, through a lowered threshold of activation for interneurons within the IP, the ability of incoming afferent stimuli to reach the critical threshold in order to elicit an efferent response or to travel to the higher centers of the brain to be perceived as pain.

Another way that the spinal cord may get facilitated is through a loss of the almost constant barrage of inhibitory impulses from type I or type II mechanoreceptors.[24] Due to the superficial location of the type I receptors within the facet joint capsules, they are at a greater risk of being damaged. As a result of cervical spondylosis or trauma, there will be a decline in the number of type I mechanoreceptors available to produce inhibitory impulses into the internuncial pool.[24] This will subsequently lead to a lowering of the threshold for activation of the interneurons within that segment of the spinal cord.[24] Remember, however, that each facet joint supplies the medial branch of the dorsal primary rami at its own level, as well as one level above and below.[24] Corpuscular mechanoreceptors in the skin and subcutaneous tissues will also send inhibitory impulses to the spinal cord.[24] The loss of these receptors, via scarring, burns, superficial wounds, or diseases, may lead to the lowering of the threshold and subsequent formation of a facilitated segment.[24]

In this way a normally subliminal afferent stimuli may actually produce a motor or sympathetic efferent impulse, or reach the higher centers of the brain and be perceived as pain, because the interneurons in that segment of the spinal cord have been facilitated; that is, their threshold for activation has been lowered (Fig. 4.10).[15]

The segment of the spinal cord that is facilitated acts as a neurologic magnifying glass (Fig. 4.5). The facilitated segment will focus and exaggerate the effects of the incoming afferent impulses, from multiple sources, upon the tissues innervated from that segment.[65] The individual is then subjected to an exaggerated impact of normal activities of daily living upon tissues that are segmentally related to the site of injury, disease, or dysfunction.[65] Even ordinary innocuous life situations become relatively stressful and taxing to the neuromusculoskeletal system (Fig. 4.11).[65]

The sympathetic nervous system (SNS) can adjust circulatory, metabolic and visceral activity according to postural and musculoskeletal demand.[66] In order for the SNS to perform this role, it must receive direct (via segmental somatic afferents) and indirect (via higher centers of the central nervous system) sensory input from the musculoskeletal system.[66] Sympathetic

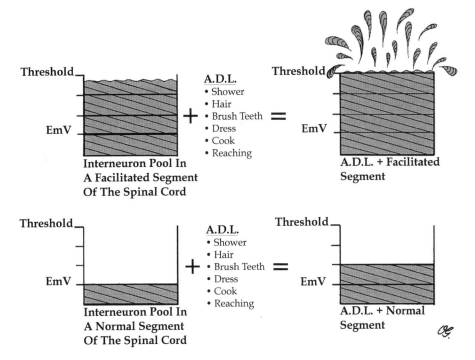

FIGURE 4.11 *Eletrical activity within the interneuron pool and the effect of activities of daily living (ADL). On the bottom is a normal segment with a low level of electrical activity that increases with ADL, but does not reach the threshold. On the top is a facilitated segment with a high level of electrical activity that easily reaches the threshold for activation due to the normal ADL.*

nervous system hyperactivity has been associated with, and segmentally related to, musculoskeletal trauma and dysfunction.[66] Long-term hyperactivity of particular sympathetic pathways is deleterious to the associated tissue.[66] Some of the consequences of prolonged hyperactivity of the SNS are (1) ischemia due to vasoconstriction and (2) shortening of tendons, muscle atrophy, and joint contractures.[66]

The cervical spine is capable of inducing real pathology (adhesive capsulitis, tendinitis, or bursitis) within the shoulder joint.[10,11,14–17,27,67,68] These shoulder pathologies may be precipitated by vasoconstriction to the shoulder joint via cervical sympathetic activity due to cervical nerve root irritation.[15,16,27] Sympathetic cell bodies are found in spinal cord segments C4–8; and the transmission of the preganglionic fibers, in the ventral roots of C5–8, has been demonstrated.[14,69]

Through synapses in the IP with sympathetic neurons, vasoconstrictor impulses can emerge and influence tissues in and around the shoulder joint.[15] The lowest somatic segmental supply to the upper extremity is T3, and the sympathetic supply to the upper extremity may be as low as T8.[69] These impulses may produce inflammation, exudation, fibrosis, adhesions, capsular thickening, degeneration, and calcification within the rotator cuff and joint capsule.[15,27] Cervical nerve root irritation may also give rise to reflex sympathetic dystrophy (RSD) with the changes mentioned to the capsule and tendons associated with the shoulder.[27] A previously asymptomatic event, active motion of the shoulder, may become symptomatic due to (1) cervical spine-initiated vasoconstriction of tissues in and around the shoulder; and (2) the formation of a facilitated segment (C3, C4, C5, or C6) within the spinal cord, via afferent nociceptive impulses, or a loss of type I or type II inhibitory impulses, from a cervical spine disorder (which may involve anything from scarred skin to spondylosis), that results in a lower threshold of activation of interneurons responsible for relaying nociceptive impulses to the higher brain centers for perception of pain.[15,24,49]

Patients who complain of shoulder pain during movement and also report stiffness or tightness, without actual joint contracture, may benefit from treatment exclusive to the cervical spine.[15] An example treatment regime may include a stretch articulation, preferably distraction, of the C2–3, C3–4, C4–5, and/or C5–6 facet joints in the beginning or end range of capsular tension in order to stimulate the type I mechanoreceptors to fire. Another example begins with the premise that chronic spondylosis or repeated cervical traumas have significantly reduced the population of type I mechanoreceptors. Treatment would now focus on stimulating the type II mechanoreceptors via oscillation in the beginning or midrange of capsular tension. This may send an inhibitory impulse to the sensitized IP, resulting in an increase of the threshold needed to elicit a motor or sympathetic response, and an increase in the threshold for activation of neurons within the anterolateral spinothalamic tract that respond to nociceptive stimuli to be relayed to the higher brain centers for perception of pain.[27]

The facilitated segment of the spinal cord, which can produce signs and symptoms identical to a mild RSD, will have the following effects on the nervous system: (1) an increased response, hypersensitivity, to sensory stimuli; (2) an increased motor response leading to muscle guarding; and (3) an increase in the activity of the SNS, resulting in vasoconstriction and the subsequent ischemia of the associated tissues.[65,70] Each cervical-shoulder disorder is progressive.[27] The initial cervical pathology, causing referred pain and sympathetic outflow to the asymptomatic shoulder, will lead to tissue changes in the shoulder girdle.[27] These changes will eventually lead to an intrinsic shoulder pathology that will show up positive on an examination of the shoulder.[27,67] The cervical spine symptoms may then become minimal or nonexistent.[27,67]

Adhesive Capsulitis, Tendinitis, and Bursitis of the Shoulder

Frozen shoulders, or adhesive capsulitis, are known to be associated with a decrease in the glenohumeral joint space.[71] In at least two studies, however, adhesions of the infraglenoid recess were not found in patients who presented with a diagnosis of a frozen shoulder.[72,73] Other causes of frozen shoulder include bicipital tendinitis, myofascial trigger points in the subscapularis muscle, and bursitis of the subscapular bursa (Plate 4.5).[50,72]

A frozen shoulder can be initiated by myofascial trigger points in the shoulder girdle muscles (Fig. 4.9).[50] This is especially true when the subscapularis muscle is involved. Guarding of this muscle will restrict abduction and external rotation.[50] Inflammation of the subscapular bursa, "bursitis," may also cause the subscapularis muscle to go into guarding. An acutely "frozen shoulder" may actually be due to muscle guarding, primarily of the subscapularis muscle, and not from adhesions within the glenohumeral joint capsule.[27] The subscapularis muscle can exert a strong influence on reflex sympathetic vasomotor control, which may result in fibrotic changes in the glenohumeral joint capsule that can eventually lead to an adhesive capsulitis.[50] It is interesting to note that an irritation or entrapment of the lower subscapular nerve (Plate 4.5), which innervates the subscapularis and teres major muscles, will produce muscle guarding at the shoulder that will restrict motion into external rotation, abduction, or flexion.

Pathology within the cervical spine can lead to an "intrinsic" shoulder problem such as adhesive capsulitis, tendinitis, or bursitis.[10,11,14–17,27, 67,68] Muscle guarding of the rotator cuff muscles, due to a lesion at the C5 or C6 segment of the spine, can lead to tendinitis.[27] A frozen shoulder may be caused by cervical disc disease or a C5 or C6 radiculopathy.[16,27,67,68] Cervical spondylosis is found in 40 percent of patients with a frozen shoulder.[9] When examined by thermography, 80 percent of these patients will have hot spots over the cervical spine, with only 20 percent of them demonstrating hot spots over the shoulder.[9]

Even though a patient may have reproduction of symptoms from a mechanical examination of the shoulder, it is important to remember that a cervical disorder can lead to a real shoulder pathology and the patient is then likely to have dual pathology.[10,11,15,17]

Neurologic Diseases Producing Shoulder Dysfunction

Suspect neuropathy and/or myelopathy if a young patient presents with painless and nontraumatic weakness and atrophy, especially if the problem is bilateral.

UPPER MOTOR NEURON DISEASE

- Stroke
- Head injury
- Tumors of brain/spinal cord
- Cerebral palsy
- Multiple sclerosis

LOWER MOTOR NEURON DISEASE

- Idiopathic brachial neuritis
- Infectious or idiopathic neuropathy/myelopathy

  Poliomyelitis

  Guillain Barré syndrome

  Motor neuron disease (progressive muscular atrophy)

  Herpes zoster

  Mononeuritis multiplex (metabolic or other)

  Diffuse peripheral neuropathy

BRACHIAL PLEXUS INJURIES

  Supraclavicular

  Subclavicular

  Infraclavicular

  Open wounds

  Post anesthetic palsy

  Radiation neuropathy

- Cervical radiculopathy
- Spinal cord tumors (extrinsic)
- Compression neuropathy

Suprascapular nerve

Thoracic outlet syndrome

Quadrilateral space syndrome

- Cranial nerve injuries

    Spinal accessory nerve

- Peripheral nerve injuries

    Axillary

    Musculocutaneous

    Long thoracic

    Suprascapular

MYOPATHIES

- Muscular dystrophy

    X-linked (Duchenne, Becker)

    Autosomal recessive (limb girdle, scapulo-humeral; childhood; congenital)

    Autosomal dominant (fascioscapulohumeral)

- Metabolic myopathies
- Inflammatory myopathies

    Polymyositis

    Dermatomyositis

- Endocrine myopathies
- Toxic and drug-induced myopathies

MIXED PATHOLOGY AND MISCELLANEOUS

- Reflex sympathetic dystrophy

    Shoulder–hand syndrome

- Arthrogryposis

Cervical Spine Pathology Causing Shoulder Symptoms

DISC

Cervical disc disease (internal disruption, degeneration, herniation, or prolapse), without nerve root involvement, can be a source of shoulder pain.[7,9,11–14] Degenerative disc disease will produce instability at that segment, that may lead to injury of ligaments or facet joint capsules.[74]

The recurrent meningeal nerve receives afferent impulses from the posterior and posterior lateral regions of the intervertebral disc and posterior longitudinal ligament (Fig. 4.2). This nerve then joins the mixed spinal nerve, which at the C3 to C6 levels is relaying afferent impulses from the shoulder, and sends sensory information into the dorsal horn of the spinal cord.[21–23] In this way, referred pain at the shoulder may be experienced with disc pathology at the same segmental levels that innervate the shoulder; that is, C2–3 to C5–6. In the late stages of this disease, osteophytes, or a prolapsed disc, can induce nerve root irritation.[74]

Symptoms

Pain, usually a dull ache, that can vary in distribution from the neck to the top of the shoulder, posterior shoulder, interscapular region, and scapula, and/or laterally down the arm to the insertion of the deltoid muscle. Pain may be unilateral or bilateral. Pain normally will not travel below the elbow. There are generally no complaints of numbness, pins and needles sensation, or specific muscle weakness. Pain is normally not referred to the anterior shoulder or the area of the biceps brachaii muscle.

Signs

Positive signs include: Valsalva;[75] compression of the cervical spine in neutral, flexed, and extended postures (Figs. 4.12 and 4.13); relief of symptoms with axial distraction; and possible increased segmental shearing (with the translatory shear test) if disc degeneration is present, muscle guarding is minimal, and there are no facet joint restrictions. Neurologic signs are negative including nerve root compression and nerve tension tests. In general, you may find that the symptoms are reproduced with provocation of the cervical spine and not the shoulder. Chronic cervical disc disease, however, may have induced true intrinsic pathology at the shoulder. In this example, the shoulder may respond with pain immediately during provocational testing, whereas the cervical spine may only be symptomatic after prolonged activity.[74]

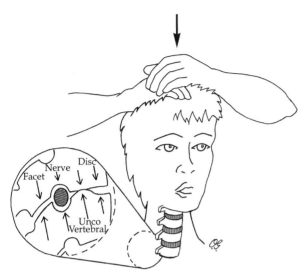

FIGURE 4.12 *Axial compression of the cervical spine in neutral may produce pain from the intervertebral disc, uncovertebral joint, inflamed nerve, or facet joint.*

Physician-Ordered Tests

Plain radiographs are not diagnostic; they may or may not demonstrate decreased disc height or osteophytosis. Myelography can demonstrate spinal cord or nerve root compression, but it cannot tell if it is a disc, osteophyte, or tumor creating the compression. Computed tomography (CT) following a myelogram will allow for the differential diagnosis of the tissue responsible for compression of neurologic tissues, but it cannot tell if a specific disc itself is symptomatic.[76,77] Magnetic resonance imaging (MRI) can identify a degenerated (dark image on a T2-weighted image) or herniated/prolapsed disc, but it cannot tell if the disc is symptomatic.[76–78] Discography can clearly identify a symptomatic disc and internal disc disruption.[7,11,13,78,79] This procedure may be used to provoke or briefly abolish the patient's symptoms.[7,11,13,79]

FACET JOINT

Irritation of a cervical facet (zygapophyseal) joint (C5–6, C6–7) can refer pain to the shoulder

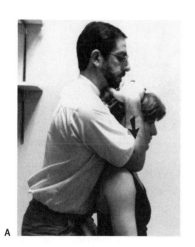
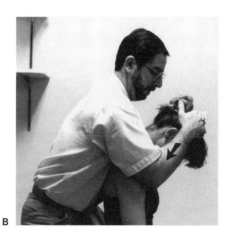
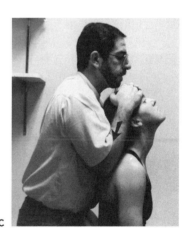

A   B   C

FIGURE 4.13 *Differential diagnosis using compression testing of the cervical spine.* **(A)** *With the cervical spine in neutral, pain may be produced from the intervertebral disc, uncovertebral joint, inflamed nerve, or facet joint.* **(B)** *With the cervical spine in flexion, pain may be produced from the intervertebral disc or the uncovertebral joint. Flexion combined with ipsilateral sidebending will primarily stress the uncovertebral joint.* **(C)** *With the cervical spine in extension, pain may be from the intervertebral disc, inflamed nerve, or facet joint. In the case of an inflamed nerve, you can expect to produce paresthesias that may be accompanied by the distal radiation of pain. Other neurologic tests will also be positive.*

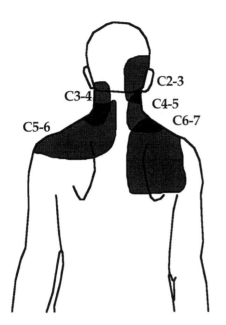

FIGURE 4.14 *Referred pain patterns from specific cervical facet joints. (From Dwyer et al.,[6] with permission.)*

(Fig. 4.14).[4–6,12] Structures of the facet joint that are capable of provoking pain include the joint capsule and the meniscoids within the joint itself.[26,80] It has been suggested that the articular cartilage within the joint, normally considered to be avascular and without nervous innervation, may acquire nociceptive fibers if the tissue is undergoing "remodeling" due to arthritic disease of the cartilage. Research has documented that it is much more likely for a patient to have a symptomatic cervical disc along with a symptomatic facet joint, than it is to have either pathology on its own.[81]

Symptoms

Pain is unilateral and may be felt in the neck, top or posterior portions of the shoulder, scapula, or interscapular region (Fig. 4.14). Pain is generally not referred to the anterior shoulder, biceps brachaii muscle, or below the elbow. There are no complaints of numbness, pins and needles, or specific weakness in the upper extremity.

Signs

Positive signs include Spurling's test (Fig. 4.15); passive cervical spine extension, and often with ipsilateral passive sidebending or rotation; cervical spine compression test, in extension and occasionally in neutral (Fig. 4.13); and facet joint tenderness to palpation. Segmental mobility examination is usually abnormal at the suspected level. Quite often you will find that the symptomatic facet joint is part of a hypermobile segment. This segment, however, may initially test hypomobile due to an acute entrapment of a menis-

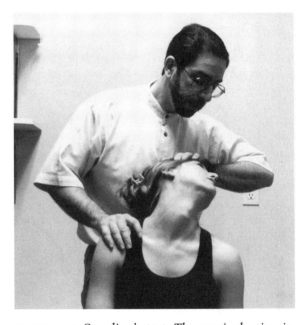

FIGURE 4.15 *Spurling's test. The cervical spine is maximally rotated and then sidebent ipsilaterally. This position maximally stresses the intervertebral foramen as well as applying a compressive stress ipsilateral and a stretching strain contralateral to the facet joints. Pain may be produced from the intervertebral disc (posterolateral compression), inflamed nerve, or facet joint. Holding the position for 10 seconds will help you assess if the initial pain subsides or if neurologic signs and symptoms start to appear. A slight over-pressure may be given if no symptoms occur initially. This position may also stress the vertebral artery.*

coid or from acute muscle guarding. Neurologic examination is negative, including nerve root compression and nerve tension tests. Valsalva is negative.

Physician-Ordered Tests

Plain radiographs are not diagnostic, but may show decreased disc height and/or arthritic changes of the facet joints. MRI and CT scan are not diagnostic, but may show degenerative changes within the disc or facet joints.[82] Myelography is not useful in this instance. Facet joint blocks, anaesthesia of the medial branch of the dorsal ramus, are the most accurate, specific, and sensitive diagnostic examination of the facet joints.[4,5,81]

NERVE

Irritation or compression of an inflamed cervical nerve root (dorsal root, ventral root, or the mixed spinal nerve) by a intervertebral disc, osteophytes from a facet or uncovertebral joint, or tumor or other space-occupying lesion can be a source of neck, shoulder, and arm pain (Fig. 4.13 and 4.16).[2,7–10,27] Compression of a normal, un-

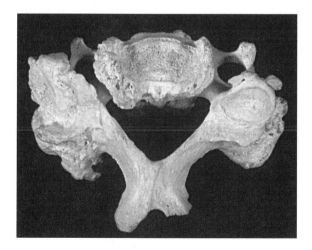

FIGURE 4.16 *Degenerative joint disease and osteophytosis of the left cervical facet and uncovertebral joint. Notice the narrowing of the intervertebral foramen and the bony encroachment towards the transverse foramen (vertebral artery). (From Tillmann,[111] with permission.)*

injured spinal nerve root does not give rise to pain.[8]

Symptoms

Patients often describe the pain as sharp, electrical, or "like a nerve is being pinched." Pain may start in the neck or shoulder and radiate as far as the finger tips. Pain may also be felt in the posterior shoulder, scapula, or interscapular regions. Pain may be felt in a dermatome, myotome, or sclerotome.[27] The patient may complain of numbness, pins and needles, or weakness down the arm. Symptoms may be bilateral to the shoulder, but are unilateral with respect to the upper extremities.

Signs

Patients often get relief of symptoms by resting their involved hand on their heads.[75,83,84] Positive signs include Spurling's test (Fig. 4.15)[14,75,83,84]; pain with passive extension, ipsilateral sidebending, or ipsilateral rotation of the cervical spine; at least one abnormal finding with neurologic testing of motor (Fig. 4.17), sensory, or deep tendon reflexes; and doorbell test[10] (palpation of the vertebral gutter outside the intervertebral foramina). Axial compression in neutral posture of the cervical spine may be positive or negative, whereas compression in a flexed posture will be negative and compression in an extended posture will be positive (Fig. 4.13). Cervical axial distraction or traction in a flexed posture will often bring temporary relief of symptoms,[2,75,83] but symptoms can be aggravated if an inflamed and tethered nerve root is stretched over a bulging disc or osteophyte.

Osteophytes from a cervical facet joint may hit the mixed spinal nerve or the dorsal (sensory) root only (Figs. 4.1 and 4.16). In the latter case, expect to see sensory, but no motor, disturbances. If the ventral (motor) root is spared, then expect EMG testing to be negative.[85] A cervical herniated disc, or osteophytes from the uncovertebral joint (Fig. 4.16), may hit the mixed spinal nerve or the ventral root alone (Fig. 4.1).[85] In this case, expect motor, but not sensory, signs

C1	C2	C3	C4	C5	C6	C7	C8	T1

Sternocleidomastoid-Trapezius

Rectus capitis posterior major
Rectus capitis posterior minor
Obliquus capitis superior
Obliquus capitis inferior
Geniohyoid
Thyrohyoid
Rectus capitis lateralis
Rectus capitis anterior
Sternohyoid
Sternothyroid
Omohyoid
Longus capitis
Semispinalis capitis
Levator scapulae
Longus colli
Anterior intertransversarii
Posterior intertransversarii
Diaphragm
Splenius capitis
Scalenus medius
Interspinales
Multifidus
Scalenus anterior
Semispinalis cervicis
Rhomboids-Major & Minor
Supraspinatus
Infraspinatus
Teres major
Deltoid
Teres minor
Subscapularis
Brachioradalis

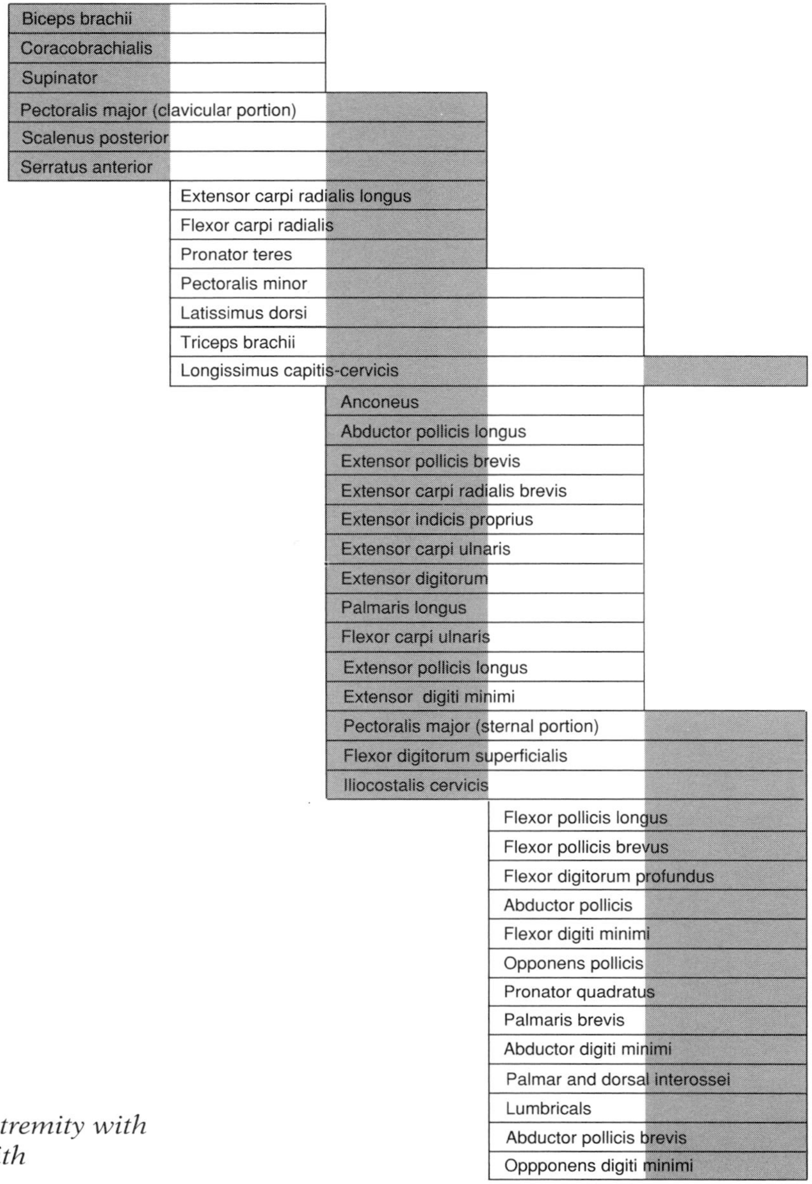

Biceps brachii
Coracobrachialis
Supinator
Pectoralis major (clavicular portion)
Scalenus posterior
Serratus anterior

Extensor carpi radialis longus
Flexor carpi radialis
Pronator teres
Pectoralis minor
Latissimus dorsi
Triceps brachii
Longissimus capitis-cervicis

Anconeus
Abductor pollicis longus
Extensor pollicis brevis
Extensor carpi radialis brevis
Extensor indicis proprius
Extensor carpi ulnaris
Extensor digitorum
Palmaris longus
Flexor carpi ulnaris
Extensor pollicis longus
Extensor digiti minimi
Pectoralis major (sternal portion)
Flexor digitorum superficialis
Iliocostalis cervicis

Flexor pollicis longus
Flexor pollicis brevis
Flexor digitorum profundus
Abductor pollicis
Flexor digiti minimi
Opponens pollicis
Pronator quadratus
Palmaris brevis
Abductor digiti minimi
Palmar and dorsal interossei
Lumbricals
Abductor pollicis brevis
Opponens digiti minimi

FIGURE 4.17 *Muscles of the cervical spine, shoulder, and upper extremity with their corresponding motor nerve innervation. (From Bland,[112] with permission.)*

115

and symptoms. If nerve root pathology is secondary to a disc problem, then the patient may also demonstrate positive signs for disc pathology. If the nerve root pathology is due to an osteophyte on the uncovertebral joint, then the patient may also have positive signs for this joint lesion. If the nerve root pathology is secondary to an osteophyte on the facet joint, then the patient may also demonstrate positive signs of this joint lesion. Signs of specific nerve root compression follow.[67,74,75,84,86,87]

C5 NERVE ROOT

- Weakness of shoulder abduction and external rotation
- Weakness of elbow flexion
- Decreased biceps and brachioradialis DTR
- Decreased sensation in upper arm and proximal forearm

C6 NERVE ROOT

- Tenderness in biceps and pectorals
- Weakness of elbow and finger flexors
- Weakness of shoulder internal rotation
- Weakness of pronation and wrist extension
- Occasionally, weakness in shoulder abduction
- Decreased biceps and brachioradialis DTR
- Decreased pinprick in radial forearm; radial 3 digits

C7 NERVE ROOT

- Weakness of elbow extension and forearm supination
- Weakness in wrist and finger flexion or extension
- Decreased triceps DTR
- Decreased sensation in ulnar forearm; ulnar 2 digits

C8 NERVE ROOT

- Weakness in elbow and wrist extension
- Weakness in wrist flexion and intrinsics of the hand

- Decreased triceps DTR
- Decreased sensation in the ulnar 2 digits
- Mimics a brachial plexus injury or ulnar neuropathy

Note that sensory changes are variable and may not correspond to anatomical dermatomes.

Physician-Ordered Tests

Plain radiographs are not diagnostic, but they may show foraminal stenosis or osteophytes on the uncovertebral or facet joints. MRI (74 to 88 percent accuracy), CT scan (72 to 91 percent accuracy), myelography (67 to 92 percent accuracy), and CT-myelography (75 to 96 percent accuracy) are diagnostic for nerve root irritation and compression.[77] EMG and NCV tests can provide information on the extent of the nerve damage.[79,83]

Brachial Plexus

The brachial plexus supplies motor and sensory innervation to the upper extremities and shoulder girdle structures (Plate 4.4). Lesions to this plexus affect the neurologic integrity, and therefore function, of the whole upper extremity. Autonomic sympathetic nervous system fibers are present throughout the brachial plexus, being mostly postganglionic fibers from the sympathetic ganglion chain.[22] The only preganglionic fibers are at the T1 primary ramus.[22] Because the sympathetic supply to the eye is via the T1 nerve root, Horner's syndrome (constriction of the pupil, ptosis of the eyelid, and a loss of sweating on the skin on the side of the face ipsilateral to the injury) is found in patients with a traction injury and presumed avulsion to that root.

Peripheral Nerve Entrapments

DORSAL SCAPULAR

Dorsal scapular nerve palsy results in rhomboid and levator scapulae weakness (Plates 4.4 and 4.5). This muscle is entirely motor.[88] It can be

Color Plates

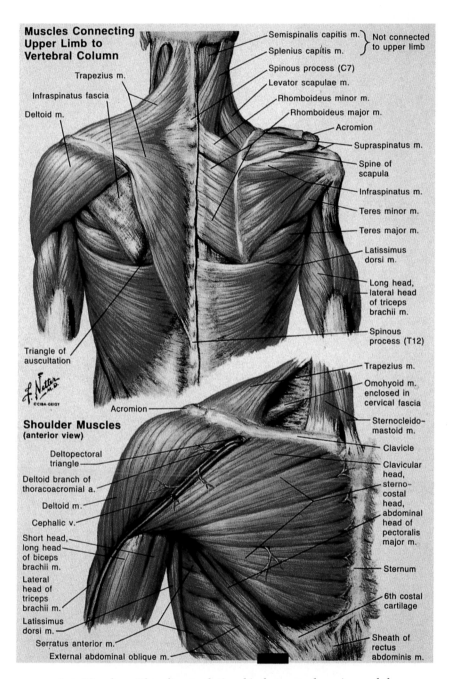

Muscles Connecting Upper Limb to Vertebral Column

- Trapezius m.
- Infraspinatus fascia
- Deltoid m.
- Triangle of auscultation
- Acromion
- Semispinalis capitis m.
- Splenius capitis m.
- Not connected to upper limb
- Spinous process (C7)
- Levator scapulae m.
- Rhomboideus minor m.
- Rhomboideus major m.
- Acromion
- Supraspinatus m.
- Spine of scapula
- Infraspinatus m.
- Teres minor m.
- Teres major m.
- Latissimus dorsi m.
- Long head, lateral head of triceps brachii m.
- Spinous process (T12)

Shoulder Muscles (anterior view)

- Deltopectoral triangle
- Deltoid branch of thoracoacromial a.
- Deltoid m.
- Cephalic v.
- Short head, long head of biceps brachii m.
- Lateral head of triceps brachii m.
- Latissimus dorsi m.
- Serratus anterior m.
- External abdominal oblique m.
- Acromion
- Trapezius m.
- Omohyoid m. enclosed in cervical fascia
- Sternocleido-mastoid m.
- Clavicle
- Clavicular head, sterno-costal head, abdominal head of pectoralis major m.
- Sternum
- 6th costal cartilage
- Sheath of rectus abdominis m.

PLATE 4.1 *Muscles with a direct relationship between the spine and the shoulder girdle. (Copyright 1996. CIBA-GEIGY Corporation. Reprinted with permission from the Ciba Collection of Medical Illustrations, illustrated by Frank Netter, M.D. All rights reserved.)*

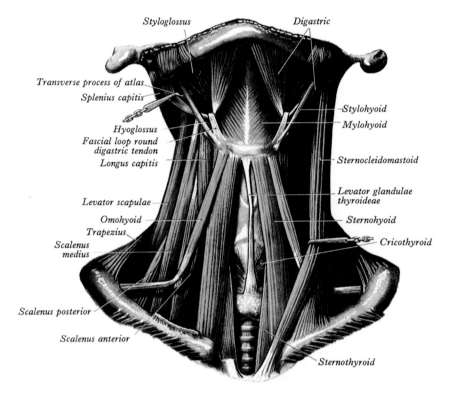

Styloglossus

Digastric

Transverse process of atlas

Splenius capitis

Hyoglossus

Fascial loop round digastric tendon

Longus capitis

Levator scapulae

Omohyoid

Trapezius

Scalenus medius

Scalenus posterior

Scalenus anterior

Stylohyoid

Mylohyoid

Sternocleidomastoid

Levator glandulae thyroideae

Sternohyoid

Cricothyroid

Sternothyroid

PLATE **4.2** *Muscles of the front of the neck. (From Williams PL, Warwick R, Dyson M, Bannister LH (eds): Gray's Anatomy. 37th ed. Churchhill Livingstone, Edinburgh 1989, p. 585.)*

PLATE **4.3** *The cervical plexus. (Copyright 1996. CIBA-GEIGY Corporation. Reprinted with permission from the Ciba Collection of Medical Illustrations, illustrated by Frank Netter, M.D. All rights reserved.)*

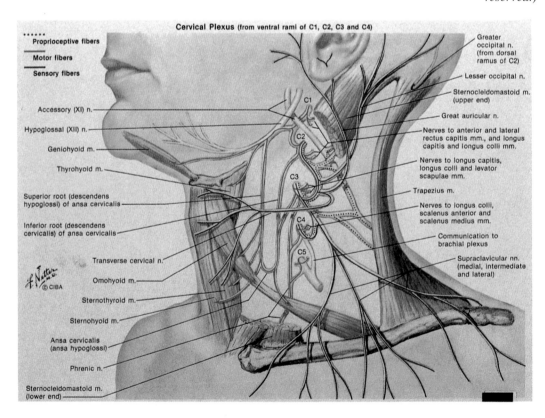

Cervical Plexus (from ventral rami of C1, C2, C3 and C4)

Proprioceptive fibers

Motor fibers

Sensory fibers

Accessory (XI) n.

Hypoglossal (XII) n.

Geniohyoid m.

Thyrohyoid m.

Superior root (descendens hypoglossi) of ansa cervicalis

Inferior root (descendens cervicalis) of ansa cervicalis

Transverse cervical n.

Omohyoid m.

Sternothyroid m.

Sternohyoid m.

Ansa cervicalis (ansa hypoglossi)

Phrenic n.

Sternocleidomastoid m. (lower end)

Greater occipital n. (from dorsal ramus of C2)

Lesser occipital n.

Sternocleidomastoid m. (upper end)

Great auricular n.

Nerves to anterior and lateral rectus capitis mm., and longus capitis and longus colli mm.

Nerves to longus capitis, longus colli and levator scapulae mm.

Trapezius m.

Nerves to longus colli, scalenus anterior and scalenus medius mm.

Communication to brachial plexus

Supraclavicular nn. (medial, intermediate and lateral)

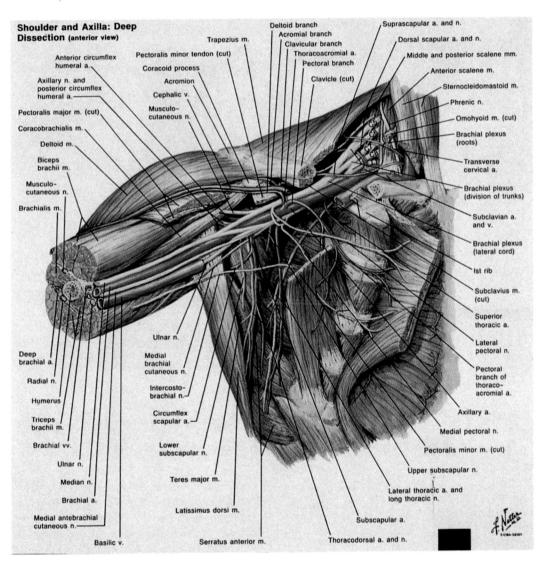

Shoulder and Axilla: Deep Dissection (anterior view)

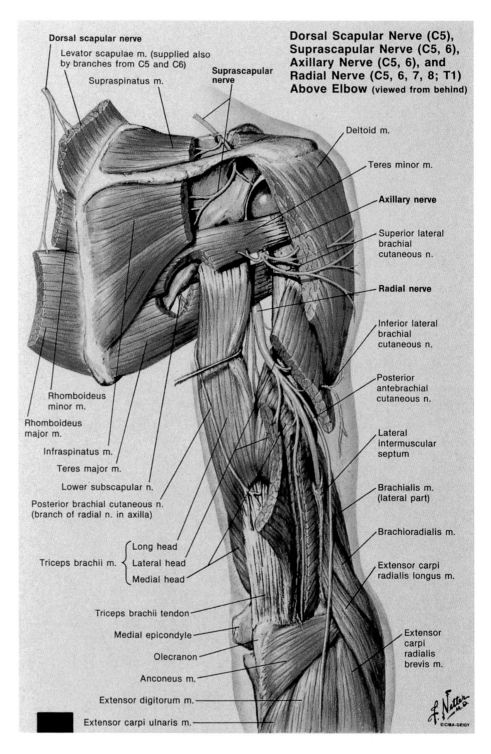

Dorsal scapular nerve

Levator scapulae m. (supplied also by branches from C5 and C6)

Suprascapular m.

Suprascapular nerve

Dorsal Scapular Nerve (C5), Suprascapular Nerve (C5, 6), Axillary Nerve (C5, 6), and Radial Nerve (C5, 6, 7, 8; T1) Above Elbow (viewed from behind)

Deltoid m.

Teres minor m.

Axillary nerve

Superior lateral brachial cutaneous n.

Radial nerve

Inferior lateral brachial cutaneous n.

Posterior antebrachial cutaneous n.

Lateral intermuscular septum

Brachialis m. (lateral part)

Brachioradialis m.

Extensor carpi radialis longus m.

Rhomboideus minor m.

Rhomboideus major m.

Infraspinatus m.

Teres major m.

Lower subscapular n.

Posterior brachial cutaneous n. (branch of radial n. in axilla)

Triceps brachii m. { Long head / Lateral head / Medial head }

Triceps brachii tendon

Medial epicondyle

Olecranon

Anconeus m.

Extensor digitorum m.

Extensor carpi ulnaris m.

Extensor carpi radialis brevis m.

PLATE 4.5 *Peripheral nerves of the shoulder. (Copyright 1996. CIBA-GEIGY Corporation. Reprinted with permission from the Ciba Collection of Medical Illustrations, illustrated by Frank Netter, M.D. All rights reserved.)*

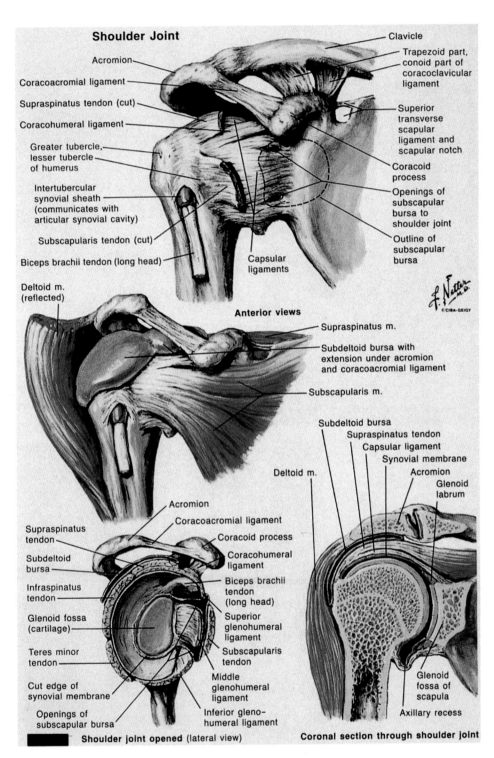

Shoulder Joint

Acromion

Coracoacromial ligament

Supraspinatus tendon (cut)

Coracohumeral ligament

Greater tubercle, lesser tubercle of humerus

Intertubercular synovial sheath (communicates with articular synovial cavity)

Subscapularis tendon (cut)

Biceps brachii tendon (long head)

Capsular ligaments

Clavicle

Trapezoid part, conoid part of coracoclavicular ligament

Superior transverse scapular ligament and scapular notch

Coracoid process

Openings of subscapular bursa to shoulder joint

Outline of subscapular bursa

Anterior views

Deltoid m. (reflected)

Supraspinatus m.

Subdeltoid bursa with extension under acromion and coracoacromial ligament

Subscapularis m.

Supraspinatus tendon

Subdeltoid bursa

Infraspinatus tendon

Glenoid fossa (cartilage)

Teres minor tendon

Cut edge of synovial membrane

Openings of subscapular bursa

Acromion

Coracoacromial ligament

Coracoid process

Coracohumeral ligament

Biceps brachii tendon (long head)

Superior glenohumeral ligament

Subscapularis tendon

Middle glenohumeral ligament

Inferior gleno-humeral ligament

Shoulder joint opened (lateral view)

Deltoid m.

Subdeltoid bursa

Supraspinatus tendon

Capsular ligament

Synovial membrane

Acromion

Glenoid labrum

Glenoid fossa of scapula

Axillary recess

Coronal section through shoulder joint

PLATE 4.6 *Anatomic relationship of the subscapular muscle and bursa. Also note the supraspinatus tendon and the subdeltoid bursa in the subacromial space. (Copyright 1996. CIBA-GEIGY Corporation. Reprinted with permission from the Ciba Collection of Medical Illustrations, illustrated by Frank Netter, M.D. All rights reserved.)*

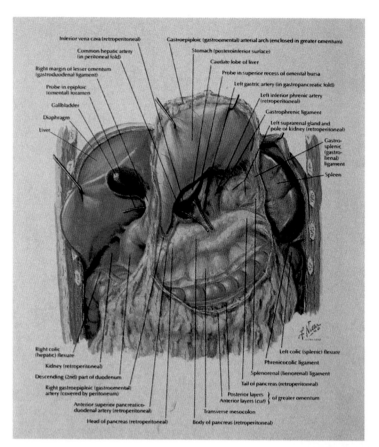

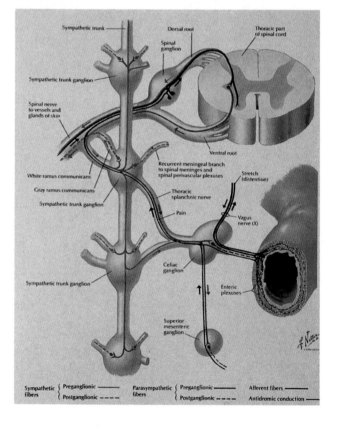

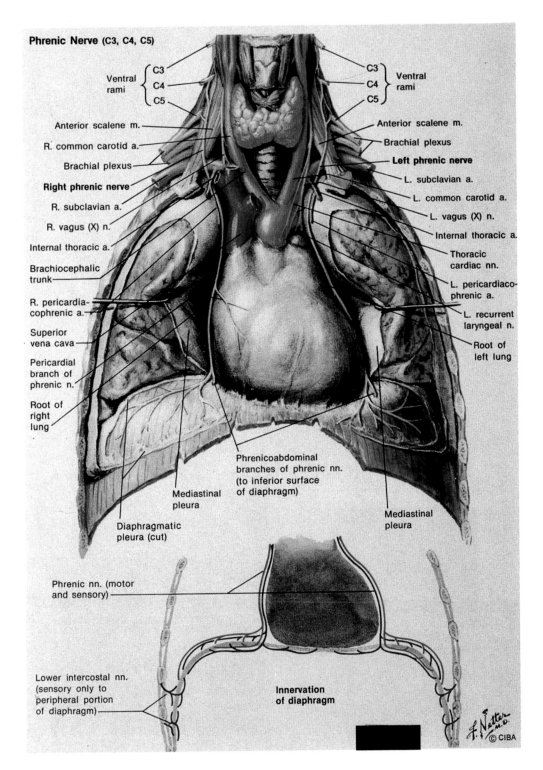

Phrenic Nerve (C3, C4, C5)

Ventral rami — C3, C4, C5

Anterior scalene m.

R. common carotid a.

Brachial plexus

Right phrenic nerve

R. subclavian a.

R. vagus (X) n.

Internal thoracic a.

Brachiocephalic trunk

R. pericardiacophrenic a.

Superior vena cava

Pericardial branch of phrenic n.

Root of right lung

Ventral rami — C3, C4, C5

Anterior scalene m.

Brachial plexus

Left phrenic nerve

L. subclavian a.

L. common carotid a.

L. vagus (X) n.

Internal thoracic a.

Thoracic cardiac nn.

L. pericardiacophrenic a.

L. recurrent laryngeal n.

Root of left lung

Phrenicoabdominal branches of phrenic nn. (to inferior surface of diaphragm)

Mediastinal pleura

Diaphragmatic pleura (cut)

Mediastinal pleura

Phrenic nn. (motor and sensory)

Lower intercostal nn. (sensory only to peripheral portion of diaphragm)

Innervation of diaphragm

PLATE 12.3 *Anatomy of the phrenic nerve and its innervation of the diaphragm. (Copyright 1996. CIBA-GEIGY Corporation. Reprinted with permission from the Ciba Collection of Medical Illustrations, illustrated by Frank Netter, M.D. All rights reserved.)*

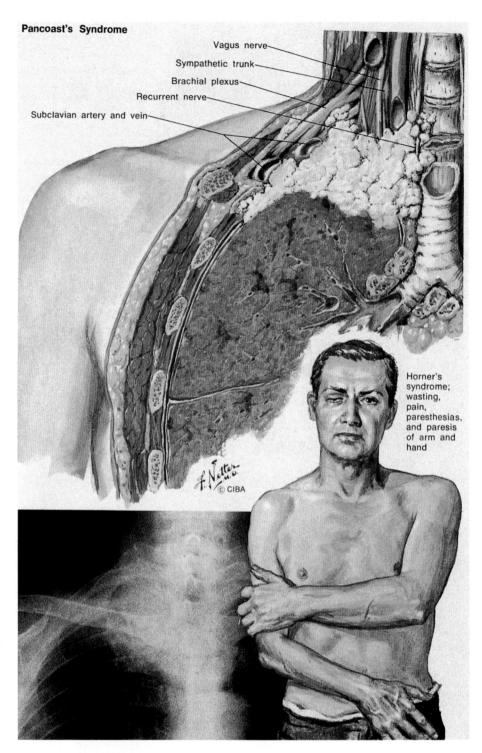

Pancoast's Syndrome

Vagus nerve
Sympathetic trunk
Brachial plexus
Recurrent nerve
Subclavian artery and vein

Horner's syndrome; wasting, pain, paresthesias, and paresis of arm and hand

PLATE **12.4** *Pancoast's tumor. (Copyright 1996. CIBA-GEIGY Corporation. Reprinted with permission from the Ciba Collection of Medical Illustrations, illustrated by Frank Netter, M.D. All rights reserved.)*

impinged through the middle and posterior scalenes or involved in the thoracic outlet syndrome.[88] Postural tension, as noted with a forward head position, or shortening of the scalenes, may induce abnormal tension on the dorsal scapular nerve.[88]

Symptoms

Patient may complain of shoulder weakness and/or pain along the medial border of the scapula.[63,88]

Signs

A forward head posture may be noted. Symptoms are exacerbated by ipsilateral rotation or extension. Palpation of the scalenus muscle will reproduce symptoms. There will be no sensory loss.[88]

Physician-Ordered Tests

Denervation signs will be evident on EMG of the rhomboids.[88] Radiographs and other imaging studies are not diagnostic.

LONG THORACIC

Long thoracic nerve palsy affects scapular stability, as the serratus anterior muscle is weakened. This nerve is derived from the C5 to C7 nerve roots as they exit the intervertebral foramen (Plate 4.4). Isolated long thoracic nerve palsy may be secondary to viral illness, lying motionless for long periods of time, or lying on the operating table under general anesthesia. Traction injury may occur with closed trauma to the shoulder girdle.

SUPRASCAPULAR

Suprascapular nerve palsy results in paralysis or reduced function of the supraspinatus and infraspinatus muscles (Plate 4.4 and 4.5). This nerve is entirely motor.[89] It may be affected by a fracture of the supraclavicular notch or be entrapped in that notch as the transverse suprascapular ligament courses over it.[89,90] Forward-sloped

shoulder postures may also increase tension on the nerve. Suprascapular nerve injury may be iatrogenic secondary to prolonged awkward positioning during unrelated surgery or as a result of surgical repair of a massive rotator cuff tear.[91,92] The nerve is fixed in the suprascapular foramen and is at risk of being stretched during forceful movements of the scapula.[2,93] Persons at risk are those who work above their heads or place their arms in the extremes of abduction or external rotation.[90] It is frequently a problem for baseball pitchers, who injure the nerve through traction in the deceleration phase of throwing. Tennis players, volleyball players, painters, electricians, weightlifters, boxers, and persons who suffer a cervical whiplash or shoulder dislocation injury are also at risk.[90,93]

Symptoms

Patients may complain of shoulder pain or weakness.[63,89,91,93,94]

Signs

There will be weakness of abduction at the shoulder, with atrophy of the supraspinatus and infraspinatus, and tenderness at the suprascapular notch.[90,93,94] There is reproduction of pain with passive horizontal adduction (scapular protraction) of the humerus.[90] There is no sensory loss.

Physician-Ordered Tests

Denervation of the supraspinatus will be apparent on an EMG study.[89,90,93,94] Radiographs and other imaging studies are not diagnostic.

AXILLARY

Axillary nerve palsy results in weakness of the deltoid and teres minor muscles (Plate 4.4 and 4.5). It is derived from the posterior cord, a terminal branch of C5 and C6 nerve roots. It can be directly traumatized through fracture or dislocation. It is also vulnerable with operative procedures at the inferior aspect of the shoulder. Blunt injury to the deltoid from hard falls on the shoulder, or direct trauma, can injure the nerve as it courses rather superficially through the deltoid. Sports that imply risk for the axillary nerve are swimming, baseball, and backpacking.

MUSCULOCUTANEOUS

Musculocutaneous nerve palsy affects the biceps, coracobrachialis, and brachialis muscles. From the C5 and C6 portion of the lateral cord it passes inferior to the pectoralis minor and pierces the coracobrachialis (Plate 4.4). Throwing injuries may affect the nerve.

MEDIAL AND LATERAL PECTORAL

Medial and lateral pectoral nerve palsy affects the pectoralis major and minor muscles (Plate 4.4). Weakness with shoulder adduction, forward flexion, and horizontal adduction are indications of a problem with the pectoralis major muscle. These nerves may be injured during body building exercises, such as horizontal adduction ("flys") for the chest.

Entrapped distal nerves can refer pain back to the shoulder.[2] Shoulder pain is a complaint for 15 percent of patients with median nerve compression at the carpal tunnel.[2]

Differential Diagnosis

The principles of differential diagnosis of cervical and shoulder disorders are as follows.[68]

1. A thorough history is necessary to elucidate information regarding the type or direction of any trauma, gradual onset of symptoms, and a description and location of all symptoms.
2. If the predominant symptom is not pain, then you may be dealing with a neurologic disease.
3. If pain is not reproduced through a mechanical examination, then consider viscera or tumor-referred symptoms (see Ch. 9).
4. The cervical spine may refer symptoms to both shoulders, whereas intrinsic shoulder disorders are usually unilateral.

5. Perform specific stress testing to specific tissues.
6. In the acute stage of healing, an examination of the shoulder will be positive only for a lesion localized to the shoulder. Using the same scenario, an examination of the neck will be positive only for a local cervical spine disorder. Although in the latter case there may be referred pain to the shoulder, an examination of the shoulder will be negative.
7. In the late stages following an injury, there may be dual pathology in the cervical spine and shoulder. The neck may appear asymptomatic.

CASE STUDY

This is a case in which a patient was referred to physical therapy following surgery to her shoulder, yet most of her symptoms were referred from the cervical spine. Evaluation was performed on November 3, 1994.

HISTORY

A 44-year-old right-handed female presented with a prescription for work hardening and the following diagnosis, "S/P left shoulder A-scope with decompression." Surgery was on May 5, 1994 and included bursectomy, acromioplasty, and excision of the distal clavicle. Patient reported that surgery was performed due to chronic shoulder pain. She denied experiencing any trauma to the shoulder. She received 2 months of physical therapy (at another facility) following surgery, but her symptoms progressively worsened. She then went for approximately 2 months without therapy and her symptoms subsided. Three weeks ago the patient started working out on her own by lifting weights up and over her head. Subsequently she experienced a severe exacerbation of neck and left shoulder pain.

SYMPTOMS

The patient complained of periodic severe ($\%_{10}$ to $\%_{10}$) neck and left shoulder pain (Fig. 4.18). She also complained of a periodic "slipping out" of her left shoulder. The patient denied radiation of pain down the upper extremities, headaches, tinnitus, and numbness or paresthesias in either extremity. The patient reported that driving, talking on the telephone, and sitting increased her symptoms. Her symptoms decreased with rest.

PAST MEDICAL HISTORY

1991–1992: Decompression (per patient) surgery, arthroscopically, of the left shoulder due to a work related injury. She received a total of at least 6 months of physical therapy (elsewhere)

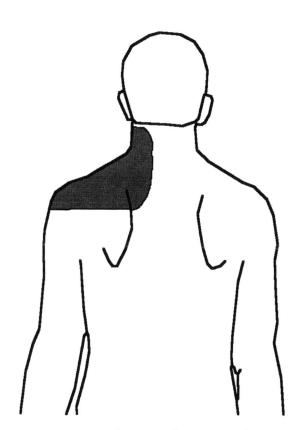

FIGURE 4.18 *Pain diagram of a 44-year-old right-handed female patient following surgery for subacromial decompression of the left shoulder.*

before and after her surgery. Most of her symptoms resolved.

1984–1985: Neck injury at work due to a tray table that hit her on the head. She complained of neck and shoulder pain for 1 year.

OCCUPATION

The patient is a flight attendant (D.O.T. #352.367–010) with a light physical demand level.[95,96] Her job duties include stooping, kneeling, crouching, reaching, lifting overhead up to 20 pounds, and frequent lifting of up to 10 pounds overhead.[96] The patient has been out of work since May 1, 1994.

PREVIOUS LEVEL OF ACTIVITY

Prior to surgery and the onset of her symptoms, the patient's exercise routine included running, stairmaster, step aerobics, and lifting free weights.

CURRENT FUNCTIONAL STATUS

She reported difficulty working, driving more than 30 minutes, sitting more than 45 minutes, and talking on the phone for more than 2 minutes.

PATIENT'S GOALS

"Get rid of the pain."

POSTURE

In standing she presented with a forward head posture with rounded shoulders, protracted scapula, and a slight increase in her thoracic kyphosis. An increase in lumbar lordosis, tibial internal rotation, and pes planus was also noted bilaterally.

CERVICAL SPINE ACTIVE ROM

There were moderate restrictions to cardinal movements of extension, left sidebending, and left rotation. Pain (Fig. 4.18) was reproduced during each of these motions. The patient's head deviated to the left during flexion and to the right during extension. Repeated flexion, right sidebending or right rotation failed to reproduce the patient's primary complaints of pain. Combined motions of flexion-left sidebending-left rotation, flexion-right sidebending-right rotation, and extension-right sidebending-right rotation were all negative. Pain was reproduced with combined extension-left sidebending-left rotation.

CERVICAL SPINE PASSIVE ROM

The same restrictions to movement were found as with active ROM. Pain (Fig. 4.18) was reproduced during the cardinal motions of extension, left sidebending or left rotation. Sustained overpressure into flexion, right sidebending or right rotation failed to reproduce patient's primary complaint of pain. Combined motions of flexion-left sidebending-left rotation, flexion-right sidebending-right rotation, and extension (slight)-right sidebending-left rotation failed to reproduce pain. Pain was reproduced with combined extension (slight)-left sidebending-right rotation. This last combined motion produces the most compression to the facet joints on the left.

CERVICAL SPINE RESISTED TESTING

Each resisted direction (six) is isometrically tested in three different muscle lengths—shortened, mid, and lengthened. The purpose is to differentiate pain arising from contractile tissue (painful in all three muscle lengths tested) versus noncontractile tissue (pain may occur only in a position that allows the contracting muscle to compress or stretch the involved tissue). For example, if resisted left sidebending is positive in the shortened (cervical spine is sidebent left into a painfree range), mid (cervical spine is in neutral), and lengthened (cervical spine is sidebent right into a pain-free range) positions, then it is reasonable to assume the pain is arising from the contractile tissues of the left scaleni muscle group. If, however, resisted left sidebending is painful (on the left side) only in the shortened muscle length, then the pain is probably from compression of noncontractile tissue such as the facet joint, uncovertebral joint, disc or nerve root.

For the above case study, pain (Fig. 4.18) was reproduced in the shortened range of resisted extension, left sidebending or left rotation. These same symptoms were reproduced in the length-

ened range of resisted flexion, right sidebending or right rotation. All of these painful positions are compressive to noncontractile tissues, such as the facet joints, on the left side of the cervical spine. Resisted testing to the cervical spine was negative when the facet joints on the left were not in a closed pack position.

SHOULDER ACTIVE ROM

Pain was reproduced with flexion and horizontal adduction only. There were no limitations to motion.

SHOULDER PASSIVE ROM

Pain was reproduced in all directions except internal rotation. There were no limitations to motion.

SHOULDER RESISTED TESTING

Pain was reproduced during flexion and abduction only with the muscle in the shortened position. External rotation was only painful when the muscle was in the lengthened range. When pain was reported, it occurred at the time resistance was released.

ACTIVE, PASSIVE, AND RESISTED TESTING OF THE SCAPULAE AND ELBOWS

Testing was negative and noncontributory.

PALPATION OF CERVICAL SPINE AND SHOULDER

Pain and discomfort were reported with palpation of the C6–7 facet joint on the left. Tenderness was noted within the left supraspinatus and infraspinatus muscle bellies, left subclavius, C5–6 left and coracoid process.

NEUROLOGIC EXAMINATION

There was no painless-weakness noted in the cervical spine, shoulders, or upper extremities. Sensation, light touch, and pin prick were WNL for the cervical spine, shoulders, and upper extremities. The deep tendon reflexes in the upper extremities were WNL.

SPECIAL TESTS

Cervical spine compression tests were negative in a flexed or neutral-positioned spine. Compression testing of the spine in extension reproduced neck and left shoulder pain (Fig. 4.13). Cervical spine bilateral facet distraction provided relief. Compression of the cervical spine in a flexed and sidebent posture was positive for discomfort on the side being stretched in each case. Spurling's test towards the left was positive for pain (Fig. 4.15). Distraction and compression of the glenohumeral joint was negative. Passive shoulder flexion was positive with the humerus internally or externally rotated. Apprehension test (abduction and external rotation) was negative for anterior dislocation.

SHOULDER GIRDLE MOBILITY EXAMINATION

Glenohumeral: Hypermobile, grade 4, in distraction and inferior glide.
Sternoclavicular: Normal, grade 3, in all directions.
Acromioclavicular: Normal, grade 3, an all directions.
Scapulothoracic: Normal, grade 3, in all directions.

CERVICAL SPINE SEGMENTAL MOBILITY EXAMINATION

Hypomobility, grade 2, at C5–6 in all directions.

THORACIC AND LUMBAR SPINE SEGMENTAL MOBILITY EXAMINATION

Mobility was graded as normal.

RADIOLOGY

There were no cervical or shoulder radiographs taken of this patient in the past 3 years.

ASSESSMENT

Patient's signs and symptoms were consistent with referred pain from the left cervical facet joint at C5–6. Restricted mobility was recorded at the C5–6 segment of the cervical spine. Mild laxity of the left glenohumeral joint capsule was also noted.

TREATMENT PLAN

1. Soft tissue massage to the cervical spine and shoulder muscles in guarding. Minimal amounts of lotion should be used so that there is less sliding on the skin and more motion against the deep muscle fibers. Techniques include massage without joint motion, massage with joint motion, passive pump massage, active pump massage, and massage with a contract-relax component.

2. Joint articulation, also known as passive joint motion or mobilization, to the C5–6 segments in order to inhibit pain and guarding and also to increase joint mobility. This involves stretch articulation (to facilitate mainly type I mechanoreceptors) of the facet joints into distraction. This may be performed with the patient supine, using a technique that distracts the facet joints bilaterally (Fig. 4-19). A stretch articulation is usually held for at least 10 seconds. An alternate technique is performed with the patient seated, using a technique that unilaterally distracts only the involved facet joint (Fig. 4.20). This last technique can also be used to manipulate the facet joint (using a short-amplitude, high-velocity thrust). Manipulation is particularly helpful in patients with an acute meniscoid entrapment. Oscillatory articulations, gliding the facet joint back and forth, are used (1) to maintain newly gained ROM following a stretch articulation, (2) to inhibit pain via activation of type II mechanoreceptors, and (3) to provide nutrition to the cartilage of the facet joint through repeated intermittent compression-decompression and gliding motions.

3. Therapeutic exercises involving the principles of STEP (scientific therapeutic exercise progressions), which originated from MET (medical exercise therapy).[97,98] Initially the patient will be instructed to exercise the muscles at less than 60 percent of their one isometric repetition maximum (usually 25 to 50 repetitions per set), to vascularize the muscles and tissues that have been in guarding, ischemic, and full of lactic acid and

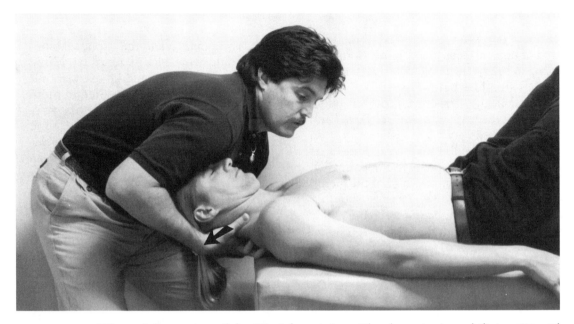

FIGURE 4.19 *Bilateral distraction of the C5–6 facet joints. The therapist is stabilizing C6 with the left hand and firmly grasping C5 with the right hand. The spine is flexed to the involved segment C5–6. At this point a distraction force (arrow) is produced by pressure from the therapist's shoulder pushing downward and from the right hand pulling C5 downward in the direction of the arrow.*

other metabolic waste products. The shoulder muscle most often in guarding, and subsequently responsible for limited abduction and external rotation, is the subscapularis. Therefore, one of the first exercises most shoulder patients should receive is internal rotation (Fig. 4.21). In order to vascularize all the shoulder muscles in guarding, it is helpful to add adduction and extension exercises. Development of muscle coordination usually requires thousands and thousands of repetitions. To achieve this level of repetitions, six to eight different shoulder exercises are often required. As the muscle guarding subsides, additional exercises may include assisted flexion, assisted abduction, scapular elevation (shrugs), scapular retraction (rows), scapular protraction, scapular depression, elbow flexion, elbow extension, and external rotation.

As for the neck, rotation exercise away from the painful injury will allow the mus-

cles on the involved side (sternocleidomastoid, upper trapezius, multifidus, and other transversospinal muscles) to be exercised while the involved facet joint is protected from further provocation or irritation (Fig. 4.22). As pain subsides, rotation in the inner ROM can begin towards the involved segment of the spine. A late progression will incorporate cervical spine extension. Finally, the STEP program will include dynamic coordination and stabilization exercises to the shoulder, followed with coordination of the tonic and phasic muscles of the neck and shoulder in a functional synergy (Fig. 4.23).

4. Nutritional advice for this patient was as follows. Avoid sources of arachidonic acid, which is a precursor to prostaglandin E2.[99] The latter stimulates both the inflammatory response and nociceptors. Sources to avoid include red meats (beef, pork, lamb, organ meats); shellfish (lobster, shrimp, clams);

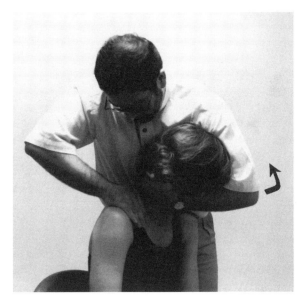

FIGURE 4.20 *Unilateral distraction of the left C5–6 facet joint. The therapist flexes the cervical spine through C4–5 with slight flexion at C5–6. The C5–6 segment is then sidebent right and rotated left. The arrow points in the direction of the rotational force used to produce the unilateral distraction. The thumb of the therapist's right hand is on the right side of the spinous process of C6. The little finger of the left hand is wrapped around the spinous process of C5.*

and dairy fats (milk, cheese). Avoid caffeinatted drinks such as coffee, tea, and soda. The caffeine increases the urinary loss of calcium and magnesium.[100,101] Avoid sodas or drinks that contain phosphoric acid. This also increases the urinary loss of calcium. Avoid drinks that contain alcohol. Alcohol increases the loss of magnesium from the body.[102–104] Supplement the diet with omega-3 fatty acids (EPA, or eicosapentaenoic acid, and DHA, or docosahexaenoic acid), which have been shown to inhibit the metabolism of arachidonic acid and therefore provide an anti-inflammatory effect.[99,105,106] Sources of omega-3 fatty acids include (1) cold-water fish (Atlantic mackerel, Atlantic herring, bluefin tuna, salmon); (2) nuts (butternuts, walnuts);

and (3) oils (flaxseed, soybean, canola, fish oil, cod liver oil, walnut). Supplement the diet with appropriate vitamins and minerals. For muscle, tendon, and collagen injuries these are vitamin C, calcium, magnesium, manganese, and glucosamine sulfate.[107–109]

Summary

Every patient who presents with a history of shoulder pain of gradual onset, even occupational repetitive injuries, should always receive a screening of the cervical and thoracic spine in order to rule out referred symptoms. A previously asymptomatic event, active motion of the shoulder, may become symptomatic due to (1) cervical spine-initiated vasoconstriction of tissues in and around the shoulder and (2) the formation of a facilitated segment (C3, C4, C5 or C6) within the spinal cord, via afferent impulses from a cervical spine disorder, that results in a lower threshold of activation of interneurons responsible for relaying nociceptive impulses to the higher brain centers for perception of pain.

Even in the absence of an identifiable cervical disorder, it may be wise to articulate the joints of the cervical spine in order to achieve pain and muscle guarding reduction in cases where shoulder mobilization is contraindicated; that is, in acute injury, immediately postsurgery, or in cases of patient anxiety. Successful treatment of the shoulder is dependent on eliminating aberrant afferent input to the spinal cord and sympathetic ganglia from an obvious or clinically subliminal cervical spine disorder.

The cervical spine and shoulder are codependent, and as such, inseparable. You cannot just work on the neck of a patient with complaints in the cervical spine. The muscles surrounding the neck, and attaching to the shoulder girdle, need to be massaged and exercised. Also, you cannot simply treat the shoulder of a patient who presents with complaints of shoulder pain. As noted in this chapter, the cervical spine needs to be evaluated and treated appropriately.

FIGURE 4.21 *Resisted internal rotation of the left shoulder using a pulley. The pulley height is adjusted so that the rope is perpendicular to the humerus. The treatment bench is moved to the appropriate angle that will allow the rope to be perpendicular to the forearm at the muscle length at which the patient is the strongest. This normally occurs at 20 percent beyond the resting length of the muscle.*

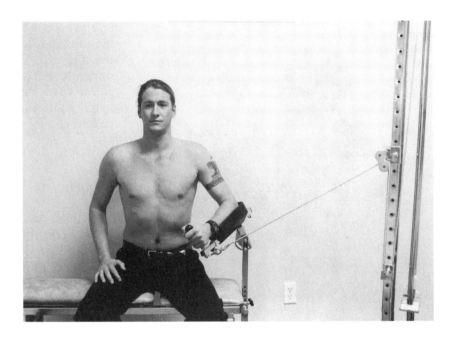

FIGURE 4.22 *Resisted right rotation of the cervical spine in a non-weight-bearing position. The pulley height is adjusted so that the pulley exerts maximum resistance at the point in the ROM that the muscles of the cervical spine are at their strongest. Note the counter-weight (upper left hand corner) that is necessary in order to reduce the resistance below 1.0 kg.*

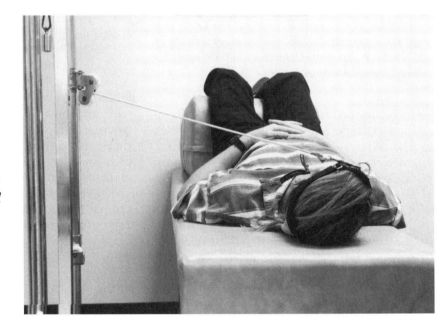

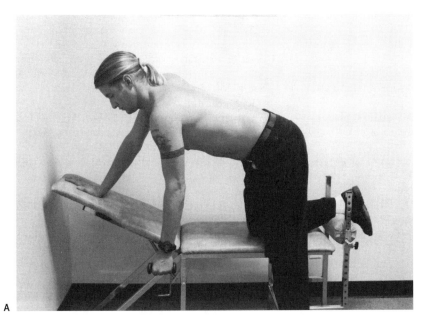

A

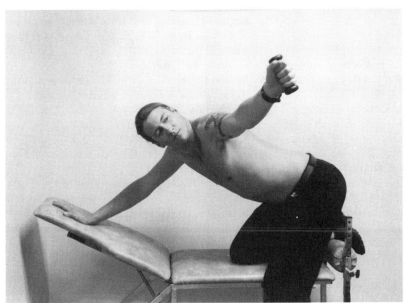

B

FIGURE 4.23 *Coordination of the tonic and phasic muscles of the neck and shoulder into a functional synergy.* **(A)** *Starting position.* **(B)** *Final position. The patient rotates his head to the left while simultaneously raising his left arm into horizontal abduction with scapular retraction.*

Acknowledgement

The authors would like to thank Jim Rivard for his invaluable assistance in preparing the illustrations in this chapter for publication.

References

1. Bateman JE: Lesions producing shoulder pain predominately. p. 195. In Bateman JE (ed): The Shoulder and Neck. WB. Saunders, Philadelphia, 1972

2. Campbell SM: Referred shoulder pain: an elusive diagnosis. Postgrad Med 73:193, 1983

3. Leland JS: Visceral aspects of shoulder pain. Bull Hosp J Dis 14:71, 1953

4. Barnsley L, Lord SM, Wallis BJ: The prevalence of chronic cervical zygapophysial joint pain after whiplash. Spine 20:20, 1995

5. Bogduk N, Marsland A: The cervical zygapophysial joints as a source of neck pain. Spine 13:610, 1988

6. Dwyer A, Aprill C, Bogduk N: Cervical zygapophyseal joint pain patterns, 1. A study in normal volunteers. Spine 15:453, 1990

7. Macnab I: Symptoms in cervical disc degeneration. p. 599. In Sherk HH, Dunn EJ, Eismont FJ et al (eds): The Cervical Spine. JB Lippincott, New York, 1989

8. Chabot MC, Montgomery DM: The pathophysiology of axial and radicular neck pain. Semin Spine Surg 7:2, 1995

9. Middleditch A, Jarman P: An investigation of frozen shoulders using thermography. Physiotherapy 70:433, 1984

10. Heller JG: The syndromes of degenerative cervical disease. Orthop Clin North Am 23:381, 1992

11. Hawkins RJ, Bilco T, Bonutti P: Cervical spine and shoulder pain. Clin Orthop Rel Res 258:142, 1990

12. Gunn CC, Milbrandt WE: Tenderness at motor points: an aid in the diagnosis of pain in the shoulder referred from the cervical spine. JAOA 77:196, 1977

13. Roth DA: Cervical analgesic discography: a new test for the definitive diagnosis of the painful-disk syndrome. JAMA 235:1713, 1976

14. Wells P: Cervical dysfunction and shoulder problems. Physiotherapy 68:66, 1982

15. Cinquegrana OD: Chronic cervical radiculitis and its relationship to "chronic bursitis." Am J Phys Med 47:23, 1968

16. Hargreaves C, Cooper C, Kidd BL et al: Frozen shoulder and cervical spine disease. Br J Rheumatol, letter. 28:78, 1989

17. Coventry MB: Problem of painful shoulder. JAMA 151:177, 1953

18. Kato K: Innervation of the scapular muscles and its morphological significance in man. Anat Anz 168:155, 1989

19. Netter FH: Upper limb. p. 20. In Woodburn RT, Crelin ES, Kaplan FS (eds): The Ciba Collection of Medical Illustrations. Vol. 8. Part 1. Ciba-Geigy, Summit, NJ, 1987

20. Williams PL, Warwick R, Dyson M et al (eds): Myology. p. 545. In: Gray's Anatomy. 37th Ed. Churchill Livingstone, New York, 1989

21. Netter FH: Gross anatomy of brain and spinal cord. p. 23. In Brass A (ed): The Ciba Collection of Medical Illustrations. Vol. 1. Part 1. Ciba-Geigy, Summit, NJ, 1991

22. Williams PL, Warwick R, Dyson M et al (eds): Neurology. p. 859. In: Gray's Anatomy. 37th Ed. Churchill Livingstone, New York, 1989

23. Bogduk N, Windsor M, Inglis A: The innervation of the cervical intervertebral discs. Spine 13:2, 1988

24. Wyke B: Neurology of the cervical spinal joints. Physiotherapy 65:72, 1979

25. McLain RF: Mechanoreceptor endings in human cervical facet joints. Spine 19:495, 1994

26. Wyke B: Articular neurology—a review. Physiotherapy 58:94, 1972

27. Grieve GP: Clinical features. p. 159. In: Common Vertebral Joint Problems. Churchill Livingstone, New York, 1981

28. Netter FH: Nerve plexuses and peripheral nerves. p. 113. In Brass A (ed): The Ciba Collection of Medical Illustrations. Vol. 1. Part 1. Ciba-Geigy, Summit, NJ, 1991

29. Norkin CC, Levangie PK: The shoulder complex. p. 157. In: Joint Structure and Function: A Comprehensive Analysis. FA Davis, Philadelphia, 1983

30. Kapandji IA: The shoulder. p. 2. In: The Physiology of the Joints. 5th Ed. Vol. 1. Churchill Livingstone, New York, 1982

31. Bateman JE: Applied physiology of the shoulder and neck. p. 67. In: The Shoulder and Neck. WB Saunders, Philadelphia, 1972

32. Cailliet R: Posture in shoulder pain. p. 124. In: Shoulder Pain. 3rd Ed. FA Davis, Philadelphia, 1991

33. Pecina MM, Krmpotic-Nemanic J, Markiewitz AD: Scapulocostal syndrome. p. 21. In: Tunnel Syndromes. CRC Press, Boston, 1991

34. Cailliet R: Mechanisms of pain in the neck and from the neck. p. 59. In: Neck and Arm Pain. 3rd Ed. FA Davis, Philadelphia, 1991

35. Cailliet R: Differential diagnosis of neck, arm, and hand pain. p. 194. In: Neck and Arm Pain. 3rd Ed. FA Davis, Philadelphia, 1991

36. Bateman JE: Lesions producing neck plus shoulder pain. p. 173. In: The Shoulder and Neck. WB Saunders, Philadelphia, 1972

37. Norkin CC, Levangie PK: Posture. p. 367. In:

Joint Structure and Function: A Comprehensive Analysis. FA Davis, Philadelphia, 1985

38. Schultz K, Ekholm J, Harms-Ringdahl K et al: Effects of changes in sitting work posture on static neck and shoulder muscle activity. Ergonomics 29:1525, 1986
39. Kendall FP, McCreary EK: Muscle function in relation to posture. p. 269. In: Muscles: Testing and Function. 3rd Ed. Williams & Wilkins, Los Angeles, 1983
40. Ayub E: Posture and the upper quarter. p. 81. In Donatelli RA (ed): Physical Therapy of the Shoulder. 2nd Ed. Churchill Livingstone, New York, 1991
41. Bogduk N, Marsland A: On the concept of third occipital headache. J Neurol Neurosurg Psychiatry 49:775, 1986
42. Lord SM, Barnsley L, Wallis BJ et al: Third occipital nerve headache: a prevalence study. J Neurol Neurosurg Psychiatry 57:1187, 1994
43. Wyke B: Cervical articular contributions to posture and gait: their relation to senile disequilibrium. Age Ageing 8:251, 1979
44. Chaffin DB, Andersson GBJ: Biomechanical considerations in machine control and workplace design. p. 324. In: Occupational Biomechanics. John Wiley & Sons, New York, 1984
45. Travell JG, Simons DG: Sternocleidomastoid muscle. p. 202. In: Myofascial Pain and Dysfunction: The Trigger Point Manual. William & Wilkins, Los Angeles, 1983
46. Hebert LA: The Neck Arm Hand Book: The Master Guide for Eliminating Cumulative Trauma Disorders from the Work Place. Impacc, Bangor, 1989
47. Lannersten L, Harms-Ringdahl K: Neck and shoulder muscle activity during work with different cash register systems. Ergonomics 33:49, 1990
48. Palmer JB, Uematsu S, Jankel WR et al: A cellist with arm pain: thermal asymmetry in scalenus anticus syndrome. Arch Phys Med Rehabil 72:237, 1991
49. Larsson SE, Alund M, Cai H et al: Chronic pain after soft-tissue injury of the cervical spine: trapezius muscle blood flow and electromyography at static loads and fatigue. Pain 57:173, 1994
50. Travell JG, Simons DG: Subscapularis muscle. p. 410. In: Myofascial Pain and Dysfunction: The Trigger Point Manual. William & Wilkins, Los Angeles, 1983
51. Hagberg M, Wegman DH: Prevalence rates and odds ratios of shoulder-neck diseases in different occupational groups. Br J Industrial Med 44:602, 1987
52. Hagberg M: Occupational musculoskeletal stress and disorders of the neck and shoulder: a review of possible pathophysiology. Int Arch Occup Environ Health 53:269, 1984
53. Travell JG, Simons DG: Trapezius muscle. p. 183. In: Myofascial Pain and Dysfunction: The Trigger Point Manual. William & Wilkins, Los Angeles, 1983
54. Caswell HT: The omohyoid syndrome. Lancet 1969:319, 1969
55. Zachary RB, Young A, Hammond JDS: The omohyoid syndrome. Lancet 1969:104, 1969
56. Valtonen EJ: The omohyoid syndrome. Lancet 1969:1073, 1969
57. Wilmot TJ: The omohyoid syndrome. Lancet 1969:1298, 1969
58. Rask MR: The omohyoideus myofascial pain syndrome: report of four patients. J Craniomandibular Pract 2:256, 1984
59. Menachem A, Kaplan O, Dekel S: Levator scapulae syndrome: an anatomic-clinical study. Bull Hosp J Dis 53:21, 1993
60. Travell JG, Simons DG: Levator scapulae muscle. p. 334. In: Myofascial Pain and Dysfunction: The Trigger Point Manual. William & Wilkins, Los Angeles, 1983
61. Swift TR, Nichols FT: The droopy shoulder syndrome. Neurology 34:212, 1984
62. Clein LJ: The droopy shoulder syndrome. CMA J 114:343, 1976
63. Quintner JL, Cohen ML: Referred pain of peripheral nerve origin: an alternative to the "myofascial pain" construct. Clin J Pain 10:243, 1994
64. Denslow JS, Korr IM, Krems AD: Quantitative studies of chronic facilitation in human motoneuron pools. Am J Physiol 150:229, 1947
65. Korr IM: Clinical significance of the facilitated state. J Am Osteopath Assoc 54:277, 1955
66. Korr IM: Sustained sympathicotonia as a factor in disease. p. 229. In: The Neurobiologic Mechanisms in Manipulative Therapy. Plenum, New York, 1978
67. Simeone FA: Cervical disc disease with radiculopathy. p. 553. In Rothman RH, Simeone FA (eds): The Spine. Vol. 1. 3rd Ed. WB Saunders, Philadelphia, 1992
68. Macnab I, McCulloch J: Differential diagnosis of neck ache and shoulder pain. p. 439. In: Neck

Ache and Shoulder Pain. Williams & Wilkins, Philadelphia, 1994

69. Grieve GP: The autonomic nervous system in vertebral pain syndromes. p. 259. In: Modern Manual Therapy of the Vertebral Column. Churchill Livingstone, New York, 1986

70. Korr IM: The concept of facilitation and its origins. J Am Osteopath Assoc 54:265, 1955

71. Neviaser JS: Adhesive capsulitis of the shoulder: a study of the pathological findings in periarthritis of the shoulder. J Bone Joint Surgery 27:211, 1945

72. Wiley AM: Arthroscopic appearance of frozen shoulder. Arthroscopy 7:138, 1991

73. Simmonds FA: Shoulder pain: with particular reference to the "frozen" shoulder. J Bone Joint Surg 31B:426, 1949

74. Macnab I: Cervical spondylosis. Clin Orthop Rel Res 109:69, 1975

75. Foreman SM, Croft AC: Physical examination. p. 73. In: Whiplash Injuries: The Cervical Acceleration/Deceleration Syndrome. Williams & Wilkins, Baltimore, 1988

76. Wesolowski D, Wang A: The radiology of cervical disc disease. Semin Spine Surg 1:209, 1989

77. Bell GR, Ross JS: The accuracy of imaging studies of the degenerative cervical spine: myelography, myelo-computed tomography, and magnetic resonance imaging. Semin Spine Surg 7:9, 1995

78. Schellhas KP, Smith MD, Gundry CR et al: Cervical discogenic pain: prospective correlation of magnetic resonance imaging and discography in asymptomatic subjects and pain sufferers. Spine 21:300, 1996

79. Bateman JE: Neurological and dystrophic disorders. p. 483. In: The Shoulder and Neck. WB Saunders, Philadelphia, 1972

80. Mercer S, Bogduk N: Intra-articular inclusions of the cervical synovial joints. Br J Rheumatol 32:705, 1993

81. Bogduk N, Aprill C: On the nature of neck pain, discography and cervical zygapophysial joint blocks. Pain 54:213, 1993

82. Schwarzer AC, Wang S, O'Driscoll D et al: The ability of computed tomography to identify a painful zygapophysial joint in patients with chronic low back pain. Spine 20:907, 1995

83. Viikari-Juntura E, Porras M, Laasonen EM: Validity of clinical tests in the diagnosis of root compression in cervical disc disease. Spine 14:253, 1989

84. Macnab I, McCulloch J: Cervical disc disease: clinical assessment. p. 54. In: Neck Ache and Shoulder Pain. Williams & Wilkins, Philadelphia, 1994

85. Cailliet R: Spondylosis: degenerative disk disease. p. 165. In: Neck and Arm Pain. 3rd Ed. FA Davis, Philadelphia, 1991

86. Cailliet R: Cervical disk disease in the production of pain and disability. p. 129. In: Neck and Arm Pain. 3rd Ed. FA Davis, Philadelphia, 1991

87. McQueen JD, Khan MI: Neurologic evaluation. p. 199. In Sherk HH, Dunn EJ, Eismont FJ et al (eds): The Cervical Spine. 2nd Ed. JB Lippincott, New York, 1989

88. Plezbert JA, Nicholson CV: Dorsal scapular nerve entrapment neuropathy: a unique clinical syndrome. J Neuromusculo System 2:206, 1994

89. Stewart JD, Aguayo AJ: Compression and entrapment neuropathies. p. 1435. In Dyck PJ, Thomas PK, Lambert EH et al (eds): Peripheral Neuropathy. 2nd Ed. Vol. 2. WB Saunders, Philadelphia, 1984

90. Pecina MM, Krmpotic-Nemanic J, Markiewitz AD: Suprascapular nerve syndrome. p. 23. In: Tunnel Syndromes. CRC Press, Boston, 1991

91. Shaffer JW: Suprascapular nerve injury during spine surgery: a case report. Spine 19:70, 1994

92. Warner JJP, Krushell RJ, Masquelet A et al: Anatomy and relationships of the suprascapular nerve: anatomical constraints to mobilization of the supraspinatus and infraspinatus muscles in the management of massive rotatorcuff tears. J Bone Joint Surg 74-A:36, 1992

93. Yoon TN, Grabois M, Guillen M: Suprascapular nerve injury following trauma to the shoulder. J Trauma 21:652, 1981

94. Vastamaki M, Goransson H: Suprascapular nerve entrapment, abstracted. Acta Orthop Scand, suppl. 65:S28, 1994

95. Marshall R, Green EG: Service occupations. p. 223. In: Dictionary of Occupational Titles. 4th Ed. U.S. Government Printing Office, Washington, D.C., 1977

96. Field JE, Field TF: Worker trait profiles. p. 63. In: Classification of Jobs. 3rd Ed. Vol. 1. Elliott & Fitzpatrick, Athens, Georgia, 1988

97. Jacobsen F: Medical exercise therapy. Sci Phys Ther 3:1, 1992

98. Torstensen TA, Meen HD, Stiris M: The effect of medical exercise therapy on a patient with chronic supraspinatus tendinitis. Diagnostic ul-

trasound—tissue regeneration: a case study. J Orthop Sports Phys Ther 20:319, 1994

99. Siekerka JR: Nutrition and biochemistry of the intervertebral disc: a clinical approach. Chiropractic Technique 3:116, 1991

100. Massey L, Wise K: Effects of dietary caffeine on mineral status. Nutr Res 4:43, 1984

101. Bergman EA, Massey LK, Wise KJ et al: Effects of dietary caffeine on renal handling of minerals in adult women. Life Sci 47:557, 1990

102. Wester PO, Dyckner T: The importance of the magnesium ion: magnesium deficiency-symptomatology and occurrence. Acta Med Scand, suppl. 661:3, 1982

103. Lim P, Jacob E: Magnesium status of alcoholic patients. Metabolism 21:1045, 1972

104. McCollister RJ, Flink EB, Lewis MD: Urinary excretion of magnesium in man following the ingestion of ethanol. Am J Clin Nutr 12:415, 1963

105. Lee TH, Hoover RL, Williams JD et al: Effect of dietary enrichment with eicosapentaenoic and docosahexaenoic acids on in vitro neutrophil and monocyte leukotriene generation and neutrophil function. N Engl J Med 312:1217, 1985

106. Simopoulos AP: Omega-3 fatty acids in health and disease and in growth and development. Am J Clin Nutr 54:438, 1991

107. Brilla LR, Haley TF: Effect of magnesium supplementation on strength training in humans. J Am Coll Nutr 11:326, 1992

108. Hunt AH: The role of vitamin C in wound healing. Br J Surg 28:436, 1941

109. Bucci LR: Glycosaminoglycans. p. 177. In: Nutrition Applied to Injury Rehabilitation and Sports Medicine. CRC Press, Boca Raton, 1994

110. Kirkesola G, Schjelderup J: Pain regions. p. 1. In: Diagnostic Atlas of Myofascial Pain Syndromes. Hoyskole Forlaget, Kristiansand, Norway, 1993

111. Tillmann B: Slides in Human Arthrology. JF Bergman Verlag, Munich, 1985

112. Bland JH: Embryology: practical clinical implications and interpretation. p. 11. In: Disorders of the Cervical Spine: Diagnosis and Medical Management. 2nd Ed. WB Saunders, Philadelphia, 1994

5

Neural Tissue Evaluation and Treatment

ROBERT L. ELVEY

TOBY HALL

Upper quarter pain includes pain perceived in variable regions of the neck, upper back, upper chest, suprascapular area towards the shoulder, shoulder, and arm. Associated headache is a frequent accompaniment. In the absence of any form of neurologic deficit of the peripheral nervous system or in the absence of definitive results from diagnostic tests such as imagery techniques, diagnoses may ensue as a result of individual clinician bias. Although diagnostic bias with respect to upper quarter pain syndromes may be due to trends and areas of clinician specialty, it may frequently relate to inadequate physical examination of the neuromusculoskeletal system.

In this chapter an aspect of clinical practice and physical examination is presented that we have found fundamental to the clinical reasoning process, or the logic, necessary to evaluate upper quarter pain syndromes. Presentation of the topic in this way should not be construed as author bias toward regarding neural tissue as a major tissue of origin of pain, or the tissue of involvement in most upper quarter pain syndromes. A detailed examination and assessment of the findings is required before any clinical hypothesis or diagnosis regarding neural tissue as a pain source can be made. Even then, an open

mind is essential, and continued critical assessment is necessary.

In neuromuscular disorders, identification of the source of pain is essential prior to administration of physical treatment or prescription of patient-generated treatment programs. Among a range of physical evaluation tests to assist in this task are neural tissue provocation tests. Tests for use in upper quarter pain disorders, originally described by Elvey in 1979, [1,2] in recent years have gained popularity in physical therapy literature.[3,4]

The chapter deals with pain disorders unaccompanied by neurologic deficit and without definitive investigative diagnostic results. This type of disorder of the upper quarter is very common in physical therapy and manual therapy practice. The most apt descriptive term is *cervicobrachial pain syndrome* or *cervicobrachial disorder*.

The diagnostic term *radiculopathy*, although technically incorrect for the cervical spine, is frequently and loosely used in upper quarter pain disorders when pain radiates as far as the forearm or hand. Radiculopathy may therefore be considered an appropriate term for communication purposes within the context of neuromusculosketal pain, but it may also be considered incorrect in the absence of evidence of neurologic deficit of the peripheral nervous system.

Incidence in the Community

When measured in terms of lost productivity, medical treatment costs, and disability insurance claims, upper quarter pain in the form of cervicobrachial pain syndrome and cervical radiculopathy represents a substantial problem for society. In the United States there has been an increase of 45 per cent in the rate of hospitalization for cervical spine surgery between 1979 and 1990.[5]

Due to the lack of population-based studies, the precise incidence of cervicobrachial pain is not known.[6] However, several investigators have addressed this problem. Thirty-four percent of responders to a cross-sectional questionnaire of Norwegian adults reported "neck pain" in the previous year. Fourteen percent reported neck pain that lasted more than 1 year.[7] Lawrence,[8] who surveyed 3,950 persons in England, found that 9 percent of men and 12 percent of women complained of cervicobrachial pain. Furthermore, the mean prevalence of neck stiffness and arm pain in Swedish working males aged 25 to 54 years was shown by Hult[9] to be 51 percent. The maximum prevalence was between the ages of 45 and 49 years. An extensive epidemiologic survey of cervical radiculopathy was carried out in Rochester, Minnesota, between 1976 and 1990.[10] This survey of a population of 70,000 people identified 561 subjects with cervical radiculopathy, with a male preponderance. Their ages ranged from 13 to 91 years, with a mean age of 38 years for both males and females. The average annual age-adjusted incidence rates per 100,000 were 83 for the total, 107 for males, and 64 for females. The age-specific annual incidence rate per 100,000 population reached a peak of 203 for the age group between 50 and 54 years.

The onset of cervicobrachial pain or radiculopathy can either be traumatic or insidious. In the older patient with preexisting cervical spon-

dylosis, frequently no single traumatic event is recalled, and the clinical picture develops insidiously.[11] In their review of cervical radiculopathy, Ellenberg et al.[12] reported that 80 to 100% of patients present with neck and arm pain, with or without motor weakness or paresthesia, generally without preceding trauma or other determinable precipitating cause.

In summary, cervicobrachial pain and cervical radiculopathy are relatively common; recurrent episodes of cervicobrachial pain and cervical radiculopathy increase in incidence with age; and there is usually no precipitating trauma. A frequently seen cause of these disorders is motor vehicle accidents involving "whiplash" injuries of the cervical spine.[13]

Upper Quarter Pain

In the evaluation of pain and the various types of "pain patterns" that may accompany disorders of the upper quarter, it is essential for the clinician to keep an open mind with respect to any judgement of the tissue of origin of pain. Although symptoms such as tingling, burning, pins and needles, and numbness are generally accepted as an indication of pathology affecting the nerve root or peripheral nerve trunk, unaccompanied by paraesthesia, pain may be very difficult to analyze in terms of tissue of origin. The pain may be of the following types:

1. Local pain, where it may be an indication of pathology of somatic tissues immediately underlying the cutaneous area of perceived pain
2. Visceral referred pain, where a visceral disorder may cause a perception of pain in cutaneous tissues distant to the viscera involved
3. Somatic referred pain, giving rise to perceived pain in cutaneous tissues distant to the somatic tissue
4. Radicular referred and neuropathic referred pain, where it is again perceived in cuta-

neous tissues that may be distant from pathologic neural tissue

5. Variable combinations of the preceding

Although detailed descriptions of nociception—the physiology of pain and the mechanisms of somatic, visceral, and radicular referral of pain—are beyond the scope of this chapter, a brief outline will be given to help gain an understanding of the topic

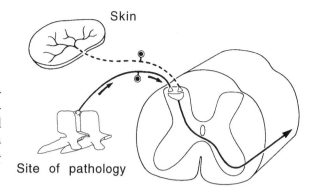

FIGURE 5.1 *A physiologic mechanism for somatic referred pain.*

REFERRED PAIN

The phenomenon of referred pain is well recognized but not well understood. It is a frequent source of difficulty in the identification of symptomatic vertebral segments and soft tissues, and therefore in correctly localizing treatment.[14] The topography and nature of referred pain in any one patient is inadequate as a single factor in differential diagnosis, of both the tissue involved and the segmental level.[15] Two types of referred pain are recognized: somatic referred pain and radicular pain.

SOMATIC REFERRED PAIN

Somatic referred pain is pain perceived in an area adjacent to, or at a distance from, its site of origin, but usually within the same spinal segment.[16] A number of theoretical models have been put forward to explain somatic referred pain.[17] One theory, which is supported by sound experimental evidence, is that the anatomic substrate for somatic referred pain is the convergence of afferent neurons from one body region onto central nervous system neurons that also receive afferents from topographically separate body tissues.[15] Figure 5.1 illustrates one of the physiologic mechanisms thought responsible for somatic referred pain. In this case there is afferent input from an intervertebral disc converging on the same neuron in the dorsal horn as neurons from the skin in a topographically separate area.

Inman and Saunders[18] put forward the con-

cept of myotomes and sclerotomes to explain segmentally referred pain from deep structures, a concept similar to that of the dermatomes for cutaneous sensation mapped by Foerster.[19] Dermatomal, sclerotomal, and myotomal charts published in standard texts should not be taken as patterns to which referred pain must invariably conform. There is known to be wide variation between individuals in the patterns of referred pain.[20,21]

There have been numerous studies of referred pain patterns following noxious stimulation of different tissues in the cervical spine. Landmarks in the study of referred pain are the investigations by Kellgren,[22] Cloward,[23] and Inman and Saunders.[18] Cloward[23] studied pain referral patterns during cervical discography. His findings prompted him to assert that pain radiated almost exclusively into the dorsal aspect of the upper trunk and arm. These findings have subsequently not been supported.[24] Recently pain patterns associated with cervical zygapophyseal joint stimulation have been investigated.[25–27] The results have vindicated the use of pain charts to accurately predict the segmental location of the symptomatic joint(s) in patients with cervical zygapophyseal joint pain.[26]

RADICULAR PAIN

Radicular or projected pain is that pain perceived to be transmitted along the course of a nerve either with a segmental or a peripheral nerve distribution, depending on the site of the lesion.[16] Examples of projected pain with segmental distribution are the pain of radiculopathy caused by herpes zoster or other diseases involving the nerve trunk before it divides into its major peripheral branches. Examples of projected pain with peripheral distribution include trigeminal neuralgia, brachial plexus neuralgia, and meralgia paraesthetica.[16]

Two types of pain following peripheral nerve injury (neuropathic pain) have been recognized: dysesthetic pain and nerve trunk pain.[28] Dysesthetic pain is pain perceived in that part of the body served by the damaged axons (Fig. 5.2). This pain has features that are not found in deep pain arising from either somatic or visceral tissues. These include abnormal or unfamiliar sensations, frequently having a burning or electrical quality; pain felt in the region of sensory deficit; pain with a paroxysmal brief shooting or stabbing component; and the presence of allodynia.[17]

Nerve trunk pain is pain that follows the course of the nerve trunk. It is commonly described as deep and aching, familiar "like a toothache," and made worse with movement, nerve stretch, or palpation.[28]

In an individual patient with nerve injury, dysesthetic pain, nerve trunk pain, or both may be present.[28] For this reason it can sometimes be difficult to distinguish, on subjective grounds,

between referred pain arising from somatic tissues and arising from neural tissues.[29] The pain and paresthesia that occur in cervical radiculopathy are not well localized anatomically, because a number of roots may cause a similar distribution of pain or even paraesthesia. In a series of 841 subjects with cervical radiculopathy, Henderson et al.[30] found only 55 percent presented with pain following a typical discrete dermatomal pattern. The remainder presented with diffuse non dermatomally distributed pain. By contrast, Smyth and Wright[31] stated that lower limb radicular pain is felt along a narrow band "no more than one and a half inches wide."

Evaluation

In disorders evaluated for physical therapy intervention, combinations of local pain of somatic origin, somatic referred pain, and radicular referred pain are commonly encountered. Peripheral referred neuropathic pain is also seen as a discrete symptom or again, in combination with other patterns of pain.

In order to evaluate a disorder for effective manual therapy management, the clinician must carry out a physical examination without presuming the source of symptoms and in a manner that results in a sufficient number of signs correlating and supporting each other in the formulation of a clinical hypothesis or diagnosis.

In the physical examination and evaluation of neural tissue for its possible involvement in a disorder, clinical experience indicates that a number of very specific correlating signs must be present before any suggestion that neural tissue is involved can be made. This is necessary for accurate treatment prescription when considering a manual therapy approach. Physical treatment, in the form of manual therapy, cannot be prescribed from imagery or nerve conduction studies, although it may well be strongly influenced and be guided by such studies even to the degree where results of either may contraindicate manual therapy.

The physical signs of neural tissue involvement include the following:

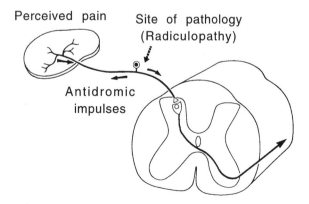

FIGURE 5.2 *Radicular pain.*

Physical Signs of Neural Tissue Involvement

1. Active movement dysfunction.

2. Passive movement dysfunction, which must correlate specifically with 1.

3. Adverse responses to neural tissue provocation tests, which must relate specifically and anatomically to 1 and 2.

4. Hyperalgesic responses to palpation of specific nerve trunks, which must relate specifically and anatomically to 1 to 3.

5. Hyperalgesic responses to palpation of cutaneous tissues, which relate specifically and anatomically to 4 and 6.

6. Evidence in the physical examination of a local area of pathology, which would involve the neural tissue showing the responses in 3 to 5.

The physical therapist involved in treating disorders of the upper quarter must also consider visceral referred pain. Obviously medical referral of patients should overcome this potential problem for the physical therapist; however, not all visceral conditions are readily diagnosed during a routine medical, clinical evaluation. Should a condition of viscera be accompanied by strong shoulder pain and active shoulder movement restriction, there may be some difficulty in making a diagnosis clinically that would involve viscera.

The liver, diaphragm, and heart are viscera requiring particular consideration when the physical therapist is suspicious of the possibility of visceral referred pain. If any suspicion or doubt exists, medical opinion must be sought.

We have seen examples of this need twice in the past year. The first example was a liver disorder in a middle-aged woman who saw her doctor because of increasing severity of pain in the right lower chest and upper right abdominal quadrant, which she said radiated from her midback region. She had right neck pain, right shoulder pain, upper arm pain, and difficulty elevating her arm above shoulder level. She was very tender on palpation of the right upper abdominal quadrant and the midthoracic spine. Her doctor referred her for investigations, including ultrasonography of the liver and plain radiographs of the thoracic spine.

The ultrasonography was reported as normal, and the plain radiographs indicated mild degenerative changes evident in the midthroacic levels. She was referred for physical therapy for treatment with the thought that her chest pain was either somatic or radicular referred. We were not happy with the situation and contacted the referring doctor, who investigated the patient further. The result culminated in a diagnosis of liver disease.

Of concern to us was the paucity of physical evaluation findings to suggest a muscular or neuromusculoskeletal disorder. In addition, we were concerned by reproduction of right lower chest pain on palpation of the anterior surface of the right scalenus anterior muscle, which the phrenic nerve travels over; reproduction of shoulder pain on palpation of the upper trunk of the brachial plexus in the right posterior triangle of the neck; and reproduction of both shoulder and chest pain on provocation tests of the right upper limb when involving the upper trunk. In addition, although palpation of the right upper abdominal quadrant was extremely painful locally, it also caused pain to be perceived in the right neck.

In the absence of other physical findings, in particular any spinal dysfunction, in keeping with the severity of the pain, we postulated a liver disorder with resultant diaphragm irritation, phrenic nerve sensitization, and subsequent facilitation of the related cervical dorsal horn neurones resulting in perceived shoulder and arm pain and sensitization of the upper trunk of the right brachial plexus. These findings excluded physical therapy as a treatment option and she was treated by a physician.

A second example was a middle-aged man who had received physical therapy in the past for neck and bilateral shoulder pain upon referral by his doctor. On this occasion he was not referred but had seen his doctor. He complained of neck stiffness and a heavy feeling with some pain in both upper arms, which was said to extend from his neck. Because of his previous history of neck-related shoulder symptoms he sought physical therapy. The symptoms on all occasions were activity related.

As in the first example, physical evaluation did not reveal any dysfunction of the neuromusculoskeletal system in keeping with his complaint. He was then referred back to his doctor, who referred him for cardiac stress testing. This revealed coronary artery insufficiency and he underwent medical management.

Of note were the right upper limb symptoms, which would relate again to spinal dorsal horn sensitization including a mechanism of contralateral sensitization resulting in the bilateral referred pain of visceral origin.

These cases, together with three cases of thoracic outlet area tumors also seen in our practice and referred for treatment for "stiff painful shoulder" syndrome, highlight the need for careful evaluation of presenting signs resulting from accurate differential physical tests. With respect to neural tissue involvement, the signs were listed earlier and will be discussed further.

In order to understand the structured scheme of examination as listed for the presence of specific signs, it is necessary to consider the sensory innervation of the connective tissues by the peripheral nervous system and the relative dynamics of peripheral nerves. Due to an inherent sensory innervation[28] nerves and nerve tissue, when sensitized by pathologic events, can become a source of pain. When pathologic, nerve tissue may cause a projection of pain to be perceived along the course of anatomically related peripheral nerve trunks. The peripheral nerve trunks in turn become sensitized and thus hyperalgesic. The target cutaneous tissues of the affected neural tissues become sensitized and tender.[20] Herpes zoster (shingles) and causalgia are good examples of these signs attribual to pathologic neural tissue, nerve as a pain source, and peripheral nerve trunks that can become hyperalgesic.

Peripheral nerve trunks are dynamic, relative to the associated movement of anatomically surrounding tissue and structures. This means that nerve trunks have to adapt to positional changes of posture with movement of both the trunk and limbs; in other words, they have to be compliant to movement. Therefore nerve trunks can be physically tested in a selective manner.

Should nerve tissue become pathologic and therefore tender and hyperalgesic, the outcome would be pain associated with any trunk or limb movement with which the trunks of that nerve tissue had to adapt. Due to pain, the nerve trunks would become noncompliant to movement. This non compliance would be demonstrated by painful limitation of movement, where the limitation is due to muscle tone and activity in groups of muscles antagonistic to the direction of movement. In other words, muscles would be recruited via central nervous system processing to prevent pain by preventing movement. (See the section on EMG responses later in the chapter.)

In more severe cases of pain of neural tissue origin, the increased tone of muscles becomes widespread and may involve muscles quite distant to the source of pain. In addition, a type of dystonia may be present, whereby an upper quarter pain syndrome of neural tissue origin may appear as "painful stiff shoulder" or "frozen shoulder." Hence the common clinical presentation of tumors of the thoracic outlet region (e.g., Pancoast tumor), when the tumor cells invade the nerve trunks resulting in nerve trunk pain, is one of "stiff painful shoulder" or "frozen shoulder."

The signs associated with neural tissue pathology listed above required very careful and precise evaluation, an open mind as to the significance of each sign, and an open mind with respect to the formulation of a clinical hypothesis.

ACTIVE MOVEMENT DYSFUNCTION

Previous studies[1] have shown that a position of shoulder girdle depression, shoulder abduction/lateral rotation, elbow extension, and wrist/finger extension with the cervical spine in contralateral lateral flexion has the effect of placing the neural tissues of the brachial plexus and related cervical neural tissues and peripheral nerve trunks in the upper limb in a maximum anatomic lengthened state.

It has also been demonstrated that any movement of the upper quarter to attain this position will influence the same neural tissues to variable degrees. Neural tissues as a structure slide within the anatomic surrounding tissues; or the surrounding anatomic tissues glide over the neural tissues; or both occur, as in functional movement. Hence, in causalgia conditions where a nerve is painful, a patient will display active movement dysfunction, as will a patient with shingles when the herpes zoster virus affects a doral root ganglion of the brachial plexus. In the same manner, a patient with a Pancoast tumor affecting the lower trunk of the brachial plexus will present with a "painful stiff shoulder."

With applied anatomy it becomes clearly evident that different anatomic positions of the shoulder, elbow, and wrist will influence the peripheral trunks of the brachial plexus in different ways. The median nerve will be in its most lengthened state in the position described at the start of this section. The radial nerve will be in its most lengthened position with abduction/medial rotation of the shoulder, elbow extension, wrist/finger flexion in the position of the shoulder girdle depression, and cervical spine contralateral lateral flexion. The ulnar nerve will be in its most lengthened position with abduction/lateral rotation of the shoulder, elbow flexion, wrist/finger extension, and again with the same common position of the shoulder girdle and cervical spine.

Should any neural tissue tract of the upper quarter become involved in a painful disorder, various active movements will be affected, depending on the particular tract involved. Obviously active shoulder abduction, with shoulder girdle depression and contralateral flexion of the cervical spine, will affect all tracts of neural tissue from C5 to T1.

In testing a disorder to determine the possibility of neural tissue involvement, active shoulder abduction should be examined in or behind the coronal plane. If pain is provoked or the range of movement is limited, the clinician can differentiate between shoulder joint pathology

and neural tissue by gently resisting the concurrent shoulder girdle elevation occurring with active abduction and at the same time positioning the patient's head and neck in a position of contralateral lateral flexion. Should neural tissue be involved, the response to active abduction would be more painful and the range of movement further limited.

This is a basic approach to analysis of active movement in the physical evaluation of neural tissue. With some thought to applied anatomy, the clinician can examine active movements in different directions and in various ways to support a clinical hypothesis formed at this early stage of evaluation. For example, a disorder of the C4–5 motion segment may involve the C5 nerve roots or spinal nerve, which may cause an observable dysfunction of shoulder abduction and movement of the hand behind the back, due to the increased tension that these movements place on the suprascapular and axillary nerve trunks. Contralateral lateral flexion of the head and neck would increase the dysfunction.

PASSIVE MOVEMENT DYSFUNCTION

Neural tissue tracts must comply to passive movement as they do with active movement. If there is a specific painful active movement dysfunction due to a disorder involving neural tissues, passive movement in the same directions must also be affected by pain, and as a consequence, limitation of range.

As with active movement, the clinician works through a differential evaluation process for a determination of possible neural tissue involvement where there is a painful limitation of range. Should passive abduction be painfully limited in range, it would correlate with a painful active limitation of range. In addition, the pain would increase and the range decrease, should passive shoulder abduction be performed with the shoulder girdle fixed in depression or the head and neck be positioned in contralateral lateral flexion.

This clinical approach applies to applicable passive movements in different directions correlating always with active movement dysfunction. The quadrant position of shoulder joint exami-

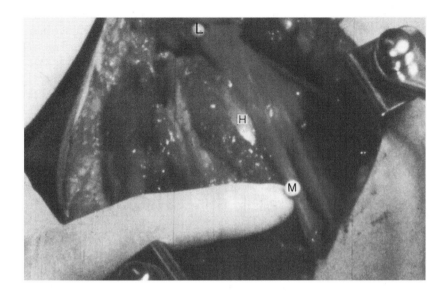

FIGURE 5.3 *Cadaver study at autopsy demonstrating the fulcrum affect of the humeral head on neural tissue at the level of the shoulder with abduction/lateral rotation. This indicates how shoulder motion may be affected by sensitized neural tissue, as may be the case in radiculopathy. L, lateral cord of the brachial plexus; H, head of the humerus; M, median nerve streched over a finger.*

nation described by Maitland[32] is of particular interest in passive movement examination. In the quadrant position the humeral head has an upward fulcrum affect on the overlying neurovascular bundle in the region of the axilla (Fig. 5.3).[1] Therefore it is conceivable to use this test not only as a test of the shoulder but also the compliance of the neurovascular tissues, and in the context of this chapter the neural tissues of the brachial plexus and its proximal and distal extensions. To do this, the quadrant test is performed as described by Maitland,[32] and in addition with the shoulder girdle in elevation and depression and with the head and neck in ipsilateral and contralateral lateral flexion.

These additional positions subtract or add distance over which the neural tissues travel, thereby affording the clinician the ability to differentiate the test responses as to whether they may represent neural tissue or shoulder joint signs.

ADVERSE RESPONSES TO NEURAL TISSUE PROVOCATION TESTS

Provocation tests are passive tests that are applied in a manner of selectivity for the examination of compliance of different neural tissues to functional positions. This means that identifying a specific type of functional position noncompli-

ance enables the clinician to form a hypothesis not only on the possible involvement of neural tissue in a disorder but also, importantly, on the possible site of involvement. Validity with respect to the clinical implications of such tests as described by Elvey[1,2] has been demonstrated by Selvaratnam et al.[4]

Provocation tests can only be carried out within the available ranges of passive movement, which are governed by the severity of pain associated with the disorder being evaluated. These passive movements are those that would lengthen the course over which the neural tissue extends to reach its maximum length capacity. In more severe painful conditions involving neural tissue, it is obvious that passive movements and positions, well short of its maximum length capacity, would result in a pain response sufficient to cause limitation of range or inability to gain a functional position due to the pain and protective muscle.

Therefore it really is unrealistic to document a standard form of provocation test technique. The clinician in practice is required to formulate a methodology of test technique according to the presentation of each patient with a unique presentation of symptoms and signs.

There is a necessary requirement for functional anatomic knowledge, an appreciation of the affects of evoked pain and associated muscle activity, and a methodological approach taking into account these considerations in the physical examination of neural tissues. However, in order to introduce the physical examination of neural tissues by provocation tests, a written formula is necessary as a baseline starting point.

Test Technique From Distal to Proximal

Subject in supine; clinicians hands positioned to control shoulder girdle elevation and elbow and wrist/finger flexion/extension, and also to be able to alter shoulder rotation, head/neck lateral flexion, and forearm pronation/supination.

1. *Via median nerve.* Shoulder abduction/lateral rotation, forearm supinated, head/neck neutral, shoulder girdle neutral; extend elbow. Increase effect of the test with incremental, wrist/finger extension, shoulder girdle depression, and head/neck contralateral lateral flexion.

2. *Via radial nerve.* Shoulder abduction/medial rotation, forearm pronation, head/neck neutral, shoulder girdle neutral; extend elbow. Increase effect with incremental wrist finger (including thumb) flexion, shoulder girdle depression, and head/neck contralateral lateral flexion.

3. *Via ulnar nerve.* Shoulder abduction/lateral rotation, forearm pronation, head/neck neutral, shoulder girdle depression (due to the different inclination of the lower trunk of the brachial plexus to the upper and middle trunks, which form the major part of the median and radial nerves); elbow flexion. Increase the effect with incremental wrist/finger flexion and head/neck contralateral lateral flexion.

TEST TECHNIQUE FROM PROXIMAL TO DISTAL

Subject in supine; clinician's hands in a position to control head/neck lateral flexion, shoulder girdle elevation and depression, and shoulder abduction and rotation.

1. *Via median nerve.* Shoulder abduction lateral rotation, with the arm comfortably in a position of elbow extension, slight wrist extension (positions naturally occurring as a result of the placement of the arm); head/neck contralateral lateral flexion. Increase the effect with shoulder girdle depression.

2. *Via radial nerve.* Shoulder abduction medial rotation, with the arm in a position of elbow extension, slight wrist flexion (positions naturally occurring as a result of the placement of the arm); head/neck contralateral lateral flexion. Increase the effect with shoulder girdle depression.

3. *Via ulnar nerve.* Shoulder abduction lateral rotation, elbow and wrist/finger extension, forearm pronation, shoulder girdle depression; head/neck contralateral lateral flexion. Increase the effect with increased shoulder girdle depression. As the name implies, with passive neural tissue provocation tests a response to the test is the clinicians goal. This response should be threefold in the presence of sensitization of the neural tissue being examined.

   a. Clinician appreciation of increase in muscle tone in muscles that are in a position to prevent further movement in the direction of the test movement — that is, the antagonists to the movement. This increase in tone should coincide with the first experience of the onset of pain.

   b. The identification of the increased muscle tone amounts to a first limitation of range of the passive test movement. This is not a lack of range as might be related to tethering or any other form of physical prevention of movement, but one directly related to an evoked pain response and resultant muscle activity to prevent further pain via the provoking movement.

   c. Having produced an initial adverse response, the test movement should be carefully taken further into range in order to attempt to reproduce the pain of complaint. Reproduction of symptoms is always a requirement in manual therapy evaluation in order to assume a condition is suited to a physical treatment.

HYPERALGESIC RESPONSES TO NERVE TRUNK PALPATION

If neural tissue sensitized due to some form of pathologic process responds with a painful reaction to a stimulus applied through its length in a longitudinal manner, such as with active or passive movement, it must also follow that there would be a painful reaction or response to a stimulus applied directly over or to the nerve trunk. This stimulus in the physical evaluation is a result of nerve trunk palpation, and the response when adverse or abnormal is one of hyperalgesia.

Nerve trunks are selectively palpated. The nerve trunks or neural tissues of the uninvolved upper quarter, or the upper quarter of least severity, is palpated first in order to allow the patient to make a comparison and in order for a correct interpretation of a perception of hyperalgesia to be made.

Nerve trunks are palpated through cutaneous, subcutaneous, and in some regions muscle tissues, gently and precisely, gradually applying increasing pressure until deamed sufficient to complete the examination. Palpation of neural tissue of the upper quarter is done in the following way.

Nerve Trunk Palpation in Supine Lying Position

1. The trunks of the brachial plexus in the posterior triangle of the neck. Selectively examining from cranial to caudal and from the lateral margins of scalenus anterior and medius towards the mid third of the clavicle and hence the first rib.
2. The neurovascular bundle of the brachial plexus as it travels beneath the coracoid process.
3. The three major peripheral nerve trunks of the arm at their commencement in the axilla, where they may not be identifiable individually, but where they can certainly be identified as nerve trunks.
4. The median nerve, in the lower third of the medial upper arm, where it can be identified as a structure, and anterior at the level of the wrist, where it cannot be identified as a structure.
5. The radial nerve, in the posterolateral aspect of the upper arm, where in some individuals it can be identified as a structure, at the lower third of the lateral aspect of the upper arm, where it crosses into the anterior compartment, at the lateral aspect of the forearm below the elbow, and over the posterolateral region of the wrist. The nerve cannot be identified as a structure at the latter sites.
6. The ulnar nerve, at the posteromedial aspect of the elbow, where it is readily identifiable, and at the anteromedial aspect of the wrist.

Nerve Trunk Palpation in Prone Lying Position

1. The suprascapular nerve, through trapezius on the superior border of the scapular, where it cannot be identified as a structure.
2. The axillary nerve, through the posterior aspect of the deltoid and on the upper lateral border of the scapula as it enters teres minor. The nerve is unidentifiable as a structure at either site.
3. The dorsal scapular nerve, through the rhomboids and medial to the scapula, where it cannot be identified.

HYPERALGESIC RESPONSES TO PALPATION OF CUTANEOUS TISSUES

In disorders of pain involving neural tissue it becomes readily apparent that palpation of tissue in regions anatomically related to the involved neural tissue will reveal marked tenderness to the point of being hyperalgesic. These tender points will be predictably found in areas that appear to be target tissues of the involved nerve or its spinal anatomical segments of origin.

There is a suggestion that the tender points may represent ectopic pacemaker sites,[38] perhaps terminating cutaneous or subcutaneous branches of the nerve in question. The most common area found in disorders of the upper quarter such as cervicobrachial syndrome is medial to the medial border of the scapula.

EVALUATION FOR SIGNS OF A LOCAL AREA OF PATHOLOGY

In pathologic conditions of nerve tissue, all of the features discussed may readily be found or determined during a physical evaluation. However, this does not mean the condition is one suited to manual therapy management. It is quite possible for a painful diabetic neuropathy, a painful neuropathy caused by a tumor infiltration, or carpal tunnel syndrome to cause all of the features discussed thus far, including limitation of active and passive movement. Therefore the clinician must determine a cause for the neural involvement.

As an example in the upper quarter, disc disease will often result in radicular arm pain and a specific cervical spine motion segment dysfunction. This would be manifested by passive spinal segmental motion palpation for aberrant movement, and by accessory spinal segmental motion palpation where an association between an abnormal pain response and aberrant motion can be made. An example of this would be evident where a radiculopathy of C6 resulted in all of the features discussed and there was a well-defined motion segment dysfunction consisting of a painful restriction of passive movement at the C5–6 motion segment.

EMG Responses to Non-Noxious Mechanical Stimulation of Nerve Trunks in Cervical Radiculopathy.

The concept of neural tissue provocation testing[1,2] has been investigated for clinical relevance,[4] as have the mechanisms of muscle responses in positive tests.[33] The concept of neural tissue provocation testing[1,2] has been investigated for clinical relevance,[4] as have the mechanisms of muscle responses in positive tests.[33] EMG activity indicates a mechanosensitivity of the peripheral nerve trunks that bear anatomic relationships to the anatomic levels of spinal radiculopathy,[33] and also presents a logical reason for the clinical signs previously outlined before a clinical diagnosis of cervicobrachial syndrome or radiculopathy can be made. This indicates a mechanosensitivity of the peripheral nerve trunks that bears an anatomic relationship to the anatomic level of spinal radiculopathy, and also presents a logical reason for the clinical signs previously outlined that must be present before a clinical diagnoses of cervicobrachial syndrome or radiculopathy can be made.

Manual Therapy Treatment of Neural Tissue

The treatment of neural tissue in manual therapy involves passive movement techniques, where the anatomic tissues or structures surrounding the affected neural tissue are gently mobilized with controlled and gentle oscillatory movement. Treatment can be more progressive by using mobilizing techniques in a similar manner but involving movement of the surrounding anatomic tissues or structures and the affected neural tissue together in the oscillatory movement.[34]

Passive movement of the pathologic neural tissue without movement of its surrounding anatomic tissues should be avoided, and any stretching of affected neural tissue is absolutely contraindicated.

With clinician experimentation in treatment of neural tissue disorders, it becomes readily apparent that the disorder may show acute exacerbation if the guidelines outlined are not followed. Clinicians report that due to frequent exacerbations of conditions they tend to avoid the use of such techniques. It becomes obvious that the clinician in these circumstances is not prescribing treatment according to the physical signs demonstrated on evaluation, is treating too strongly, or commonly is mobilizing neural tissue solely, rather than with the surrounding anatomic tissues, and therefore producing a stretch effect. It stands to reason that if neural tissue is sensitized, undue stimulation of it will cause further sensitization and exacerbate the condition. This is the fundamental reason for the muscle activity that results from provoking manouevers—to prevent further and undue stimulation of already sensitized neural tissue. The clinician must be guided at all times by an appreciation of protective muscle activity.

In general manual therapy terms, treatment of neural tissue is indicated when the physical evaluation demonstrates that neural tissue is the tissue of origin of the subjective complaint of pain; or in the more commonly seen presentations, where it is the dominant tissue of origin.

To meet this requirement, it is essential that all the signs previously listed are present in the physical evaluation of the disorder to be treated. If they are not present, another form of treatment, directed to tissue other than neural, would have to be considered. In addition, these signs must dominate over signs of other tissue or structure involvement.

The authors have used passive movement techniques in the treatment of neural tissue disorders for many years with excellent results when a disorder has not developed on a pathologic basis to one of a more severe neuropathic type, particularly where there are central nervous system mechanisms of pain and sympathetically maintained pain syndromes. Although to date, support for such treatment outcome is ancedotal, a study presently being conducted gives support in its early results and therefore is demonstrating the validation of treating appropriate disorders involving neural tissue with passive movement techniques.[35]

With regard to treatment of the upper quarter, two treatment techniques, which have been found to be the most useful, will be described: cervical lateral glide and shoulder girdle oscillation.

Cervical Lateral Glide

Patient supine, shoulder slightly abducted with a few degrees of medial rotation, elbow flexion to about 90° such that the hand rests on the chest or abdomen. The clinician gently supports the shoulder over the acromial region with one hand while comfortably holding and supporting the head and neck. *Technique*: Gentle controlled lateral glide to the contralateral side in a slow oscillating manner up to a point in range where the first resistance in the form of antagonistic muscle activity occurs.

The first resistance represents the treatment barrier. Should this barrier not be reached, the patient's arm position should be changed. This would involve more abduction or possibly extending the elbow with the shoulder position maintained. The arm must be fully supported on the treatment couch at all times, and in more acute conditions additional support should be given with the use of a pillow.

The technique progresses on subsequent treatment days, but only when indicated by a demonstrable improvement, by performing the lateral glide with the shoulder in gradually increased amounts of abduction. The most obvious indicator of successful treatment using this technique would be an improvement of active shoulder abduction.

Shoulder Girdle Oscillation

Patient prone, forehead resting on the palm of the hand of the uninvolved side, the involved arm supported by the clinician in a position of comfort towards a position of hand behind the back. The clinician places the other hand over the acromial area. *Technique:* Gentle oscillation of the shoulder girdle in a caudad cephalad direction. The range of oscillation is governed by the onset of first resistance in the caudad direction. This represents the treatment barrier and is the commencement of increased muscle tone.

The technique progresses on subsequent treatment sessions and when indicated by performing the oscillation in gradually increased amounts of hand behind the back position. The most obvious indicator of successful treatment would be an improvement of active hand behind the back function.

The amount of time the techniques are performed is variable, depending largely on the experience of the clinician, but as in any disorder also on symptom severity and irritability. The composure of the patient is a prime consideration with regard to the amount of time devoted to a technique. Should the patient shown any signs of the beginnings of lack of total relaxation, the technique should be temporarily ceased and methods of soft tissue mobilization should be employed until composure is regained.

With experience, a clinician will learn to use different techniques; however, the two just described will serve very well when applied appropriately and correctly. In general, in conditions that are more acute, the anatomic tissues surrounding the neural tissue should be mobilized. In the less acute conditions, or where progression is required, the neural tissues together with the surrounding anatomic tissues should be mobilized.

As in so many disorders managed by manual therapy techniques, it is necessary to consider treatment of tissues affected secondarily and as a consequence of the primary neural tissue pathology. Treatment would commonly be given for adaptive shortening that inevitably follows neuropathy. This shortening mostly involves muscles that have been facilitated and involved in tonic reflex activity to prevent movement, which if it occurred, would cause pain. In addition, long-term lack of movement affects articular and periarticular tissue mobility, and therefore joint treatment may well be a requirement. The treatment for these associated dysfunctions must be chosen at a time when the neural tissue signs are resolving, and the treatment must be carried out without any disturbance by stretch of the neural tissue.

Commonly in upper quarter conditions involving neural tissue, a time will come in the treatment program to treat the scalenii and the shoulder abductors/medial rotators for loss of extensibility and to facilitate the shoulder abductors/lateral rotators. In addition, the cervical spine and the shoulder joint may require mobilizing treatment. The extent of the treatment to other tissues and structures would be dependent on the chronicity of the disorder and its severity.

Self-treatment and management is most important. For neural tissue of the upper quarter, this can be performed in a variety of ways. A relatively simple treatment can be carried out by placing the hand of the involved side against a wall in a comfortable position with a degree of elbow flexion, followed by very gentle and controlled contralateral flexion. This should not cause pain, but a feeling of a pulling sensation in the shoulder and upper arm region would be acceptable.

The movement is repeated three times once daily. This may appear insubstantial, but it is essential to regard the movement as self-treatment and not exercise. It becomes very evident to the inexperienced that in regarding this technique as an exercise rather than a treatment, a condition can readily be exacerbated, or a condition that has settled to chronicity can readily become acute. Functional training in the form of exercise at a time deemed appropriate by the clinician also becomes essential to the self-management program.

CASE STUDY

HISTORY

Mrs. F.O. was sitting in her stationary motor vehicle when it was struck from behind in February 1991. She sustained a "whiplash" defined injury to her neck. Her immediate complaint was one of left-sided neck pain extending into her upper back. Treatment and management consisted of rest, medication, and physical therapy. Mrs. F.O. continued her work in a nursing home, but due to steady deterioration of symptoms she was forced to cease work some months after the accident. Bilateral upper arm pain developed and deteriorated to the degree where the left arm pain radiated to the hand into the thumb and index finger and was accompanied by a sensation of "pins and needles." Plain radiographs identified ossification of the anterior longitudinal ligament at the C4 and C5 levels and prominent ossification adjacent to the C6–7 disc. Active left shoulder mobility become so painfully limited that she was said to have developed a "frozen shoulder."

Her symptoms slowly improved through 1993 to 1994, but remained significant. Right shoulder mobility was full range, but left shoulder mobility and neck mobility remained limited. All litigation was completed in 1994.

In early 1995 there was a gradual increase in pain, culminating in a severe exacerbation of left upper quarter symptoms without reason. In particular she complained of severe left shoulder pain radiating down the arm to the hand accompanied again by a pins and needles sensation of in the thumb and index finger. Marked restriction of shoulder mobility by pain once again mimicked a frozen shoulder. CT scan of the cervical spine in March 1995 identified degenerative facet changes and at the C5–6 level disc degeneration with anterior and posterior osteophytic spurring.

In May 1995, Mrs. F.O. was referred to us by a consultant physician specializing in assessment for pain management for evaluation and for treatment if we felt it indicated, The working diagnosis at that time was left C6 radiculopathy. The referring physician's next option of treatment was to be a C6 nerve root sleeve block.

PHYSICAL EVALUATION

At initial evaluation, the left shoulder girdle was elevated with the arm held in a protective position. Left shoulder function was recorded as flexion 80° and abduction 40° (Fig. 5.4).

Although cervical range of motion was limited in all directions, particular note was made of greater limitation of right lateral flexion than left lateral flexion. Of further interest was the fact that active shoulder mobility was more painful and more limited in range when performed with head and neck positions in contralateral lateral flexion. Passive left shoulder mobility was limited in range by pain to the same degree as active mobility. Retesting passive mobility with the head and neck positioned in contralateral lateral flexion demonstrated a further decrease in range and increased pain.

Neural tissue provocation tests could only be carried out in the available range of shoulder abduction of 40°. Consequently, there was a need to compensate for an inability to reach a sufficient anatomic length of neural tissue in test positions by making maximum use of maximum shoulder girdle depression and contralateral lateral flexion of the cervical spine (Figs. 5.4 and 5.5). Although wrist extension in shoulder girdle depression reproduced symptoms, the shoulder girdle elevated wrist extension did not reproduce the shoulder and arm pain.

Neural tissue provocation tests via the median and radian nerves reproduced symptoms, but testing via the the ulnar nerve did not, thus indicating a spinal level of involvement from C5 to C7. In testing from proximal to distal, the shoulder could again only be positioned in a small available range of abduction, and the shoulder girdle therefore had to be fixed in cauded depression to compensate for the lack of ability to be able to place the neural tissue in a more maximal length position.

Palpation of particular peripheral nerve trunks of the left upper quarter produced hyperalgesic responses. These responses were not produced on palpation of all peripheral nerve trunks. Hyperalgesic responses were obtained in the left posterior triangle; with respect to the upper trunks of the brachial plexus, immediately inferior to the left coracoid process; with respect to the neurovascular bundle, the axilla; and with respect to the neurovascular bundle and the upper arm with respect to the median and radial nerves. Palpation over the suprascapular and axillary nerves also produced hyperalgesic responses.

Palpation of cutaneous and subcutaneous tissues in regions that had a neuroanatomic relationship to the hyperalgesic upper trunk of the left brachial plexus also indicated hyperalgesic responses. These areas were particularly evident medial to the medial border of the scapula, the upper chest, shoulder, and upper arm. Responses of a similar nature were not found in corresponding tissues on the right.

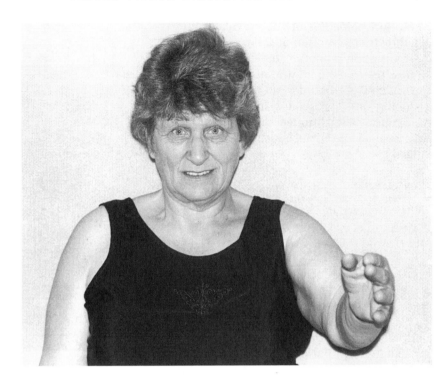

FIGURE 5.4 *Mrs. F.O., demonstration of gross limitation of active range shoulder motion due to sensitization of neural tissues.*

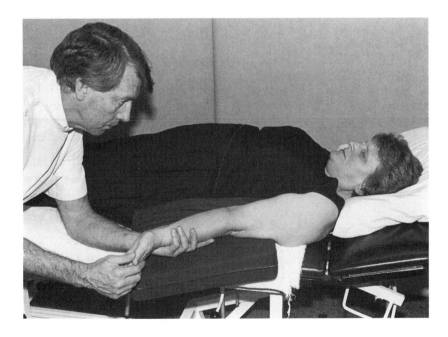

FIGURE 5.5 *Neural tissue provocation test. Wrist extension performed in maximum available range of shoulder abduction, influencing the median nerve, brachial plexus, and ultimately the cervical nerve roots. Note should be made of the small pillow elevating the arm from the couch. At the time of initial evaluation due to shoulder and arm pain, the patient was unable to lie supine with the arm resting on the couch by her side.*

Motion palpation of the cervical spine revealed restricted motion at C5–6 and C6–7. Accessory motion palpation indicated a pain and stiffness relationship at the same levels. In spite of palpation of shoulder subcutaneous tissues producing painful responses and active and passive motion being limited in range, accessory movement of the articular surfaces was freely available.

EMG RESPONSES

For the subject in this case history, EMG responses to upper limb nerve trunk palpation were recorded using the protocol described by Hall and Quintner.[33] EMG responses were recorded from the ipsilateral biceps, triceps, deltoid, and upper trapezius muscles on the side of the arm being tested. EMG activity in the four muscles was simultaneously recorded during gentle deep palpation over the anatomic site of the ipsilateral radial and median nerve trunks in the upper arm, and of the ulnar nerve trunk behind the medial epicondyle. Recordings were also made during gentle palpation of the skin and subcutaneous tissues overlying each presumed tender nerve trunk; and also, in the case of the median and radial nerve trunks, during palpation of the bellies of the adjacent biceps and triceps brachii muscles.

A burst of activity was recorded in left biceps, triceps, and upper trapezius muscles sampled on the painful side when the radial and median nerve trunks were palpated (Fig. 5.6). The other stimuli, including palpation of the ulnar nerve, had no effect upon EMG activity, nor were they painful. On the opposite (asymptomatic side), there were no EMG responses to nerve trunk palpation (Fig. 5.7).

ASSESSMENT

The physical findings and the EMG analysis correlated accurately with the subjective complaint and supported a disorder categorization of cervicobrachial pain syndrome, in which there was strong evidence of neural tissue involvement and of it being the major pain source. In view of the pins and needles sensation felt in the thumb and

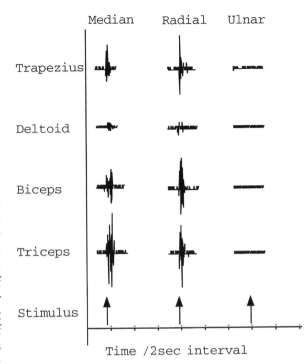

FIGURE 5.6 *EMG responses in this subject with cervical radiculopathy are similar to those documented by Hall and Quintner[33] in a similar case. They found painful responses to gentle palpation over the radial and median nerve trunks in the symptomatic arm of their patient, and recorded widespread (multisegmental) EMG responses on palpation of these putatively tender nerve trunks. Neither pain nor EMG responses were noted during palpation, in turn, of the skin and the subcutaneous tissues overlying these nerve trunks, and of the adjacent muscle bellies of biceps and triceps brachii.*

index finger and the CT results, a diagnosis of C6 radiculopathy was also loosely supported. Treatment of choice, with respect to physical treatment, was therefore using a technique that indirectly had a postulated physiologic effect, and hence a therapeutic affect, on neural tissue.

TREATMENT

Treatment commenced with therapist intervention only. Severity of pain prevented any patient-generated management at that time. Treatment

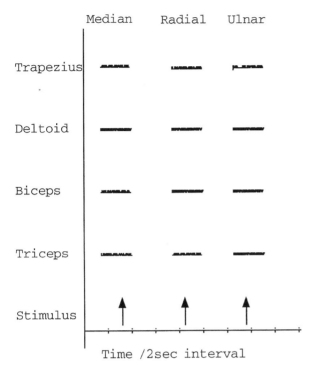

Median   Radial   Ulnar

Trapezius

Deltoid

Biceps

Triceps

Stimulus

Time /2sec interval

FIGURE 5.7 *EMG activity of the right biceps, triceps, deltoid, and upper trapezius muscles during palpation of the radial, median, and ulnar nerves in the upper arm/elbow of the asymptomatic side.*

to overcome the provocation affect of the drag on sensitized neural tissue by the weight of the shoulder girdle. Medications and medical advice remained unchanged.

Mrs. F.O. was given a complete understanding of the disorder, and it was explained to her and accepted that improvement would be extremely slow and that it would be at least 2 months before the true value of the treatment approach would be known. This was also acceptable to her referring physician.

With some subjective improvement occurring after 2 weeks and a knowledge that the disorder was stabilizing, as judged by maintenance of improved function, treatment was stepped up to involve techniques to facilitate the shoulder abductors and lateral rotators, the function of which appeared inhibited, presumably due to pain; and to inhibit the abnormal excessive influence of the adductors and medial rotators, which appeared facilitated presumably as a protective measure to prevent pain.

This was done in supine lying with controlled isometric hold relax techniques supplemented as time went on with proprioceptive neuromuscular facilitation PNF patterning techniques stimulating the abductors and lateral rotators. These techniques were performed in painless positions.

Mrs. F.O. commenced her own treatment program involving neural tissue after 4 weeks. This consisted of the method described earlier. As the condition improved and the symptoms became more stable, a program of left shoulder abductor and lateral rotation was begun. This involved sitting sideways at a table with the left arm supported on a pillow to give 90° abduction. An active abduction was then performed to take the weight of the arm only, held for 2 seconds, and then relaxed back onto the pillow. At the same time the shoulder girdle was not elevating. This was repeated six times, and followed by lifting the forearm from the pillow without lifting the elbow as a maneuver of lateral rotation of the shoulder. This was repeated six times with the same relaxation between lifts. The aim of these techniques was to stimulate the abductors

consisted of gentle, controlled oscillation of the neck from the midline towards the right by performing a right lateral glide of C5 on C6. The left arm was supported in the position shown in Figure 5.8. Assessment of treatment was carried out by reevaluation of active left shoulder mobility. Due to the severity of the condition, small fractional improvements of range were deemed acceptable. Treatment initially was carried out three times per week. Mrs. F.O. was instructed to use a thin pillow but firm under the axilla to support the shoulder girdle in a degree of elevation when sitting. She was asked to refrain from anything causing depression or caudad stress to the shoulder girdle, and while walking, to place her hand in the waistband of her clothing. These measures were taken to shorten the course over which the brachial plexus traveled and therefore

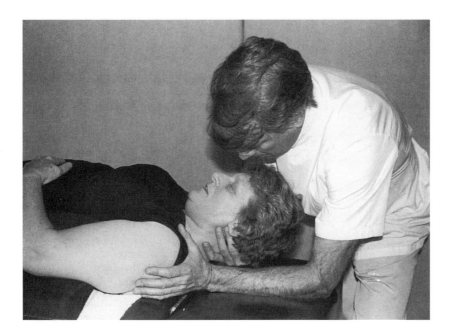

FIGURE 5.8 *Neural tissue treatment technique. The arm is in a position to shorten the course over which neural tissue travels in the upper quarter. Note again the pillow under the arm. The shoulder girdle is supported lightly by the therapist's left hand, while the right index finger is at C5 with the head and neck fully supported. The technique is one of a passive lateral glide to the right in an oscillatory manner.*

and lateral rotators and to regain normal muscle recruitment patterns of arm elevation.

Treatment was successful at the time of writing this report. The severity of pain was reduced and the range of left shoulder mobility was increased in unison, as treatment proceeded. The improvement of both variables was on the order of 50 percent, a level of improvement acceptable to all parties concerned when considering the history and severity of the disorder. The same medications were continued but decreased in quantity, and a nerve root sleeve block was not carried out. Prior to the treatment intervention symptomatic deterioration was reported.

It is anticipated Mrs. F.O. will continue to improve, and with more time progress to an active functional training program.

DISCUSSION

Many disorders encountered in physical therapy practice have multiple possibilities as to the tissue of origin of pain. A ready example is the patient referred for treatment for shoulder arm pain, when there are numerous possible sources of the pain, from lateral epicondylitis, to im-

pingement syndrome, to degenerative disease of the cervical spine. In such cases, the physical evaluation by necessity has to be very precise, with the clinician being skilled enough to perform a competent and detailed analytical evaluation not only to determine the source(s). The depth of such an examination must be of a type that will thoroughly evaluate all structures capable of referring pain. Only then can a working diagnostic hypothesis be formed and tested with a technique of treatment prescribed from the examination findings.

This perspective is quite different from treatment in the form of anti-inflammatory medication or management of pain with analgesic medication, transcutaneous electrical nerve stimulation (TENS), or other forms of modalities. In these approaches the physical examination needs only to be of sufficient extent to determine the existence of an organic musculoskeletal disorder. The examination in that case does not need to be so detailed, and as a result the tissues of origin of pain need only be presumed.

This approach obviously has its success. In Mrs. F.O.'s case, unfortunately, this approach was not successful. A great deal of thought is needed to understand why it was not, but it may be that the tissues causing the symptoms were not receiving any therapeutic form of stimulus to promote a decrease in peripheral afferent neural discharge. To speculate on the reason for improvement from a therapist's intervention in the form of passive movement, some consideration needs to be given to the physical signs, the tissues those signs related to, the mode of possible involvement of the same tissues at the time of the rear-end collision in 1991, and the evolving pathologic events thereafter.

The physical evaluation findings clearly indicated neural tissue at the major pain source. The physical evaluation also showed that there was a direct relationship, as a result of pain caused through movement and relative dynamics associated with function, between those same neural tissues and the active movement dysfunction demonstrated. If this was the case, some explanation for the possible cause of neural tissue pathology, or at the least sensitization, can be offered. It is known that extension of the cervical spine reduces the lumen or diameter of the intervertebral foramen.[36] It is also known that this reduction in lumen has an associated affect of increased pressure within the intervertebral foramen. Should a high-velocity decrease in the diameter of the intervertebral foramen occur, as appears to happen in whiplash injuries, there may well be a concussion affect involving tissues within the confines of the intervertebral foramen resulting in injury and bleeding. Studies by Taylor and Twomey (personal communication, 1999) have demonstrated this very possibility. Figure 5.9 from their cadaver dissection studies shows both intraneural and extraneural bleeding within the intervertebral foramen.

In addition to many additional possible sources of pain, it could be speculated that bleeding of this nature may indicate neural tissue sensitization either directly in the case of the intraneural pathology or indirectly in the case of the extraneural pathology. It could further be speculated that this sensitization would result in pain of a radicular type and associated neuromusculoskeletal dysfunction. This dysfunction might have resulted in active and passive move-

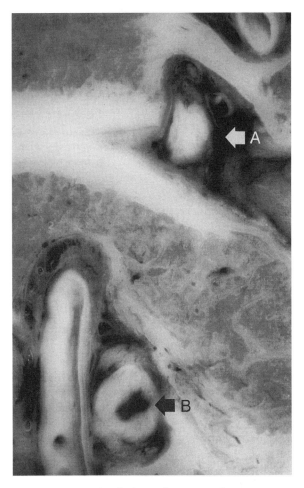

FIGURE 5.9 *Saggital slice of a cervical spine showing bleeding within the intervertebral foramen* **(A)** *and intraneurally* **(B)** *as a result of a motor vehicle accident. This indicates pathology that may result in neural tissue sensitization and hence painful limitation of shoulder motion. (Courtesy of Professor James Taylor, Perth Pain Management Centre.)*

ment limitation when movement affected the neural tissue in question, by positive neural tissue provocation tests, by hyperalgesic responses to palpation, and by the demonstration of spinal motion segment dysfunction.

Further speculation can be made based on the known facts of active movement dysfunction that the condition resolves with great difficulty simply because the normal physiologic effects associated with movement of tissues in and around the intervertebral foramen do not occur. Due to pain and muscle reflex activity directly resulting from movement transferred to the pathologic neural tissue, the patient is unable to perform any movement that would influence the pathologic tissue favorably in terms of having a therapeutic affect. In other words, stasis within the intervertebral segment and motion segment of involvement would not only exist but persist.

In this context, the patient told to exercise would be unable to do so with any therapeutic influence on the pathology, and would in fact reinforce movement patterns that prevented physiologic movement of the pathologic neural tissue, thus denying the tissue the beneficial effects of movement.

The value of therapist intervention as seen in the case study again can be answered in terms of the physiologic benefit of movement. The patient position during treatment is such that movement can be promoted within the intervertebral foramen and motion segment of the pathologic level without evoking pain. In this way, reflex muscle activity is avoided, and the therapeutic effects of movement can therefore be gained. Salter[39] has outlined the effects of passive movement on pathologic tissues, and with respect to the tissues occupying the intervertebral foramen it could be postulated that the same premises apply.

The advancement from direct therapist intervention to patient intervention and eventually functional training therefore lies in the response to passive movement with respect to its presumed physiologic influence on the pathologic tissue, the therapeutic effects of this influence, and with time a resulting decreased severity of pain. With decreased pain, the patient is able to move without prompting reflex muscle activity, and therefore in a manner more in keeping with an ability to have a physiologic and remedial influence on the improving pathologic neural tissues. At this stage, patient self-treatment techniques can be prescribed, and with further time and the regaining of normal physiologic ranges

of movement, functional training programs can be implemented.

Summary

As extensive an outline as possible of neural tissue in upper quarter disorders has been given, although the extent has been governed by the constraints of a chapter in a clinical text. It is up to the individual clinician to challenge the content of the chapter in order to gain a full understanding of the role that neural tissue may play in the painful dysfunctions seen daily in the physical therapy clinic. It is also up to the individual to maintain an open mind with respect to implicating neural tissue in a painful disorder and a very thoughtful approach to techniques of treatment when neural tissue is involved.

An understanding of neural tissue relative dynamics, sensitization, and nociception including physiologic pain and clinical pain, is essential, and readers are encouraged to study these topics in detail. An understanding of pain mechanisms will lead to understanding of the movement dysfunctions of pathologies such as reflex sympathetic dystrophy, herpes zoster, Pancoast tumor, and other pathologies such as those mentioned at the start of the chapter that may result in "frozen shoulder."

Many physical signs must be present in order to imply that neural tissue is involved. The reasons why dysfunction of movement will be apparent when neural tissue is sensitized and therefore a source of pain have been outlined, and postulations have been offered as to why nonpainful passive movement techniques of treatment may be beneficial. It must be readily apparent that pain is of the utmost significance in guiding both the examination and treatment. Should this be overlooked, it will become very obvious why a patient's condition deteriorates during examination and treatment of neural tissue.

The greatest single example of poor technique, as a result of lack of understanding, is the use of stretch, either in examination or treatment. The credibility of the profession rests with the individual.

References

1. Elvey RL: Brachial plexus tension tests and the pathoanatomical origin of arm pain. p. 105. In Idczak RM ed: Proceedings. Aspects of Manipulative Therapy, Lincoln Institute of Health Sciences, Melbourne, 1979
2. Elvey RL: The investigation of arm pain. In Grieve GP (ed): Modern Manual Therapy. Churchill Livingstone, Edinburgh, 1986
3. Butler DS: Mobilisation of the nervous system. Churchill Livingstone, Melbourne, 1991
4. Selvaratnam PJ, Matyas TA, Glasgow EF: Noninvasive discrimination of brachial plexus involvement in upper limb pain. Spine 19:26, 1994
5. Davis H: Increasing rate of cervical and lumbar spine surgery in the United States 1979–1990. Spine 19:1117, 1994
6. Loeser JD: Cervicobrachial neuralgia. p. 868. In Bonica JJ (ed): The Management of Pain. 2nd Ed. Lea & Febiger, Philadelphia, 1990
7. Bovim G, Schrader H, Sand T: Neck pain in the general population. Spine 19:1307, 1994
8. Lawrence JS: Disc degeneration. Its frequency and relationship to symptoms. Ann Rheum Dis 28:121, 1969
9. Hult L: Frequency of symptoms for different age groups and professions. p.17. In Hirsch C, Zotterman Y (eds): Cervical Pain. Proceedings of the international symposium held in Wenner-Gren Centre, Stockholm. Pergamon Press, Oxford, 1971
10. Radhakrishnan K, Litch WJ, O'Fallon WM, Kurland LT: Epidemiology of cervical radiculopathy: a population-based study from Rochester, Minnesota, through 1990. Brain 117:325, 1994
11. Connell MD, Wiesel SW: Natural history and pathogenesis of cervical disc disease. Orth Clin North Am 23:369, 1992
12. Ellenberg MR, Honet JC, Treanor WJ: Cervical radiculopathy. Arch Phys Med Rehab 75:342, 1994
13. Spitzer WO et al: Scientific monograph of the Quebec Task Force on Whiplash-associated Disorders. Spine 20:9, 1995
14. Grieve GP: Common Vertebral Joint Problems. 2nd Ed. Churchill Livingstone, Edinburgh, 1988
15. Grieve GP: Referred pain and other clinical features. p. 271. In Boyling JD, Palstanga N (eds): Grieves Modern Manual Therapy. 2nd Ed. Churchill Livinstone, Edinburgh, 1994
16. Bonica JJ, Procacci P: General considerations of acute pain. p. 159. In Bonica JJ (ed): The Management of Pain. 2nd Ed. Vol. 1. Lea & Febiger, Philadelphia, 1990
17. Fields HL: Pain. McGraw-Hill, New York, 1987
18. Inman VT, Saunders JB: Referred pain from skeletal structures. J Nerv Ment Dis 99:660, 1994
19. Foerster O: The dermatomes in man. Brain 56:1, 1933
20. Elliot FA: Tender muscles in sciatica: EMG studies. Lancet 1:47, 1994
21. Brodal A: Neurological Anatomy in Relation to Clinical Medicine. 3rd Ed. Oxford University Press, Oxford, 1981
22. Kellgren JH: On the distribution of pain arising from deep somatic structures with charts of segmental pain. Clin Science 4:35, 1939
23. Cloward RB: Cervical diskography. A contribution to the etiology and mechanism of neck, shoulder and arm pain. Ann Surg 150:1053, 1959
24. Klafta LA, Collis JS: The diagnostic inaccurancy of the pain response in cervical discography. Clev Clin Quart 36:35, 1969
25. Dwyer A, Aprill C, Bogduk N: Cervical zygapophyseal joint pain patterns, 1: a study of normal volunteers. Spine 15:453, 1990
26. Dwyer A, Aprill C, Bogduk N: Cervical zygapophyseal joint pain patterns 2: a clinical evaluation. Spine 15:458, 1990
27. Dreyfuss P, Michaelson M, Fletcher D: Atlanto-occipital and lateral atlanto-axial joint pain patterns, Spine 19:1125, 1993
28. Asbury AK, Fields HL: Pain due to peripheral nerve damage: an hypothesis. Neurology 34:1587, 1984
29. Dalton PA, Jull GA: The distribution and characteristics of neck-arm pain in patients with and without a neurological deficit. Aust J Physiother 35:3, 1989
30. Henderson CM, Hennessy R, Shuey H: Posterior lateral foraminotomy for an exclusive operative technique for cervical radiculopathy: a review of 846 consecutively operated cases. J Neurosurg 13:504, 1983
31. Smyth MJ, Wright V: Sciatica and the intervertebral disc. An experimental study. JBJS 40A:1401, 1958

32. Maitland GD: Vertebral Manipulation. 5th Ed. Butterworths, London, 1986

33. Hall TM, Quintner JL: Mechanically evoked electromyographic responses in peripheral neuropathic pain: a single case study. In: Abstracts of the Australian and New Zealand Reheumatology Associations Annual Scientific Meeting. Auckland, 1995

34. Elvey RL: Treatment of arm pain associated with abnormal brachial plexus tension. Aust J Physiother 32:224, 1986

35. Vicenzino B: An investigation of the effects of spinal manual therapy on forequarter pressure and thermal pain thresholds and sympathetic nervous system activity in asymptomatic subjects. p.

185. In Shacklock M (ed): Moving in on Pain. Butterworth-Heineman, Australia, 1995

36. Yoo JU, Zou D, Edwards WT et al: Effects of cervical spine motion on neuroforaminal dimension of the human cervical spine. Spine 17:1131, 1992

37. Farmer JC, Wisneski RJ: Cervical spine nerve root compression: an analysis of neuroforaminal pressures with varying head and arm positions. Spine 19:1850, 1994

38. Devor M: Neuropathic pain and injured nerve: peripheral mechanisms. BMJ 47:619, 1991

39. Salter RB: Motion versus rest: Why immobilise joints? pp. 1–11. In : Proceedings of the Manipulative Therapists Association of Australia, Brisbane, 1985

6

Neurovascular Consequences of Cumulative Trauma Disorders Affecting the Thoracic Outlet: A Patient-Centered Treatment Approach

PETER   I.   EDGELOW

Neurovascular compression syndromes of the upper quarter involve a complex and bewildering set of problems when seen as separate diagnoses, but interrelationships must be considered. Issues related to the cumulative trauma disorder of thoracic outlet syndrome will be presented.

Thoracic outlet syndrome (TOS) as a diagnostic entity is receiving increased attention; yet one must not fall into the trap of ignoring other anatomic sites of neurovascular entrapment. Therefore, although issues will be presented that focus on the thoracic outlet and symptoms that can derive from this region, one must consider the potential for multiple entrapment sites.

In the past four years in an outpatient orthopedic clinic, over 500 patients with the diagnosis of TOS received physical therapy treatment. One of the common findings was that patients often exhibited signs and symptoms in multiple areas. These patients presented with severe, chronic pain problems that failed all conservative treatments and, in some instances, failed multiple surgeries. The patients all had 2 or more years of symptoms before being ultimately diagnosed as having TOS. An evaluative procedure and treatment protocol has been the result of this clinical experience.

A clear understanding of the neural consequences of cumulative trauma disorders (CTDs) affecting the thoracic outlet will help the practicing physical therapist comprehend the etiology of these disorders. Also, it is necessary to think of CTDs as multifactoral rather than having a single cause, as the basis for evaluating and developing an effective treatment program.

The guiding principles for effective treatment of neurovascular entrapment build on the fundamental idea that neurovascular entrapments occur as a result of trauma to the nervous system or vascular system. Such trauma may occur in an individual with few or many preexisting risk factors.

Three concepts have been developed based on clinical experience: findings from surgery, hypotheses derived from the basic sciences, and logical common sense.

The first concept is that patients must be in control of their own care in order for treatment to be effective and lasting. In the current medical climate, issues that cannot be controlled by the patient include the interaction between the health care practitioner, the patient's employer, and the patient's insurance provider. Therefore, factors that can be controlled—such as individual risk factors, health habits, daily living demands, and belief systems—take on an increasing importance in the treatment process.

The second concept is that neurovascular entrapments are a problem of stenosis. Stenosis should not be thought of as a rigid narrowing of an anatomic part, but rather a series of events or circumstances, some of which may result in an irreversible narrowing and others of which are reversible. For example, the stenosis caused by the presence of a cervical rib or scalenus minimus may be irreversible, but the stenosis due to postural changes or paradoxical breathing patterns is reversible.

The third concept is that an understanding of fluid dynamics must complement investigations of structural changes. This concept is based on research concerning fluid dynamics in the carpal tunnel and appears to be equally relevant for the thoracic outlet. As structural and fluid changes cause restriction in the size of the outlet, these changes could contribute to disruption of the pressure gradient and effect both the local neural circulation as well as the venous return from the whole upper extremity.

Relevant signs and symptoms will be introduced that are important indicators leading to an understanding of the pathology as well as treatment goals and objectives. This information is essential when treating either a single-tunnel thoracic outlet problem or a multiple-tunnel problem when one of the tunnel problems is in the anatomic region called the thoracic outlet.

A case history of a patient with early signs of a cumulative trauma disorder illustrates the use of the knowledge presented in this chapter in evaluation and treatment. It is my contention that if adequately addressed at the time the symptoms and signs first presented themselves, problems can be prevented from developing into the kind of unremitting condition being discussed.

Importance of Treating the Whole Person

Patient empowerment is an essential ingredient in treatment. It is based on the theory that a successful outcome involves engaging the whole person in treatment. Although TOS is a physical problem, it affects the whole person. Simplistically stated, the impact is to change the person from being in control of their life to being out of control. This feeling state of being out of control negatively affects the body/mind connection. Restoring the feeling of being in control is one method to have a positive impact on this connection.

In order to be empowered, patients must be ready to take control of their own care. Once patients are committed to this process, the physical therapist acts as a coach to guide them through recovery as they learn to monitor daily activities and the home treatment program.

There are two key issues that facilitate the feeling of being in control: Understanding "what is wrong" and "what is the solution." Patients need to understand why they have the problem and how their actions can help resolve it. This requires that the therapist is able to translate the pathoanatomic knowledge inherent in the diagnosis into a language that empowers the patient. This can be done in a number of ways. One method is to give a story that is simple, using analogies to guide rather than using medical terminology. The problem with medical terminology is that it may have a negative connotation based in the patient's belief system. It is this belief system that can increase or decrease the patient's feeling of control. For example, the belief that nothing can be done to correct a problem will have a negative impact on everything that is done to help. If there was a quick fix to this issue then the therapist could overpower this negative belief by fixing the problem. However, it is my experience that there is no quick fix for severe neurovascular entrapments.

Therefore the understanding and commitment on the part of the patient to arrive at a satisfactory outcome involves a significant, sustained change. The first step in resolution can take 3 months before enough stability and positive results have been obtained for the patient to feel in control. For this reason, a negative belief system can sabotage initial treatment efforts if not addressed. This idea can be expressed to the patient by using the analogy of the orthodontist. If you went to the orthodontist with crooked teeth, and he said that he could fix them immediately and took out a pair of pliers, one could understand that you might look for another practitioner. Common sense and experience has taught us that there is no quick fix for crooked teeth. Even if you don't wish to wear braces for 2 years to have a beautiful smile, at least you know that it is the best available answer.

Learning to listen to the language of the body is a critical concept. Pain and muscle tension can be thought of as *words* to listen and respond to. If one thought of symptoms as body language, then one might consider the following translation.

1. Tension = excited awareness.
2. Pain that comes and goes = whining.

3. Pain/numbness and tingling that is constant but does not stop you from doing what you have to do = crying.
4. Pain/numbness and tingling that is severe, constant, and interferes with thought and action, and cannot be relieved = hysteria.

The body speaks to us by symptom change. In the hysterical state it is unable to change, and therefore it cannot "talk." If we ignore tension, then it becomes pain/whine. If we ignore pain/whine, then it becomes constant/crying. If we ignore constant/crying, then it will become so severe that change is not readily apparent and we have no easy way to be lead along the path of healing. Patients who fit the profile of this topic have usually failed other treatment approaches. They may have tried to understand the significance of their symptoms, but not enough to be able to resolve the problem. Therefore in treatment it is important to realize that the progression of treatment will be to reverse the process and go from a stage of hysteria to crying to whining to tension. This process will offer the patient an opportunity to understand the significance of symptoms and cause and effect.

It is important for the patient to understand the risks and rewards of paying close attention to symptoms—not to become a hypochondriac but not to deny the problem, either. Awareness is the first step to solving a problem. This means understanding the problem, understanding the solution, and doing what it takes for the rest of one's life to minimize the problem. Not to the extent of dominating one's life with treatment, but learning how much is necessary to support the body in stressful situations. The statement "pay attention to tension and blow it away" is an example of the use of words that are descriptive of both the problem and the solution.

The common statement of "no pain, no gain" has no place in the treatment of patients, and they must be cautioned that treatment will not be successful if the pain response is not "listened to" and used as a guide to treatment. This is particularly important with injuries to the nervous system as well as the musculoskeletal system, because the body's pain response will be to protect

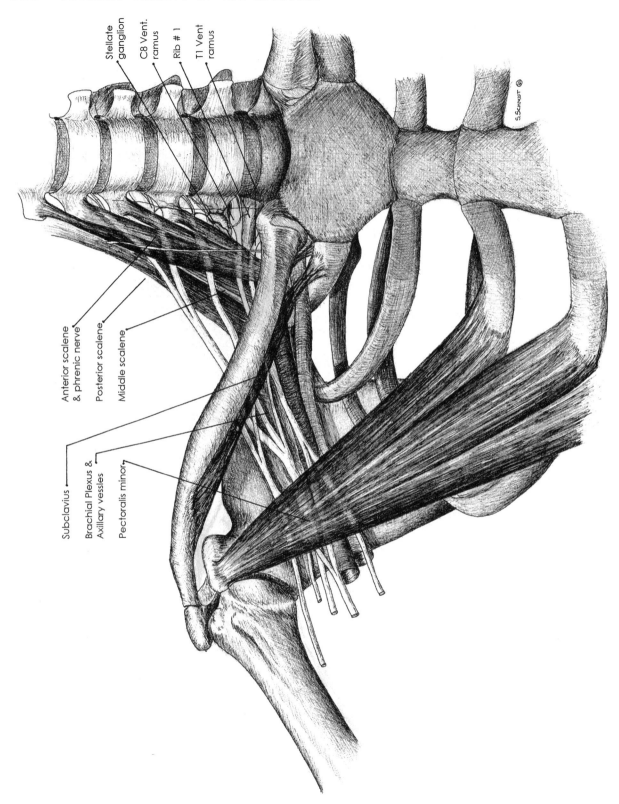

Stellate ganglion

C8 Vent. ramus

Rib # 1

T1 Vent ramus

Anterior scalene & phrenic nerve

Posterior scalene

Middle scalene

Subclavius

Brachial Plexus & Axillary vessels

Pectoralis minor

the neurovascular structures. This protective response has an adverse affect on healing when the muscle tension reaction is prolonged by overuse, overtreatment, or recurrent injury.

Anatomy

A review of the anatomy and potential risk factors will focus on the thoracic outlet. This area is a source of symptoms secondary to congenital factors and/or trauma and is the primary region that exhibits dysfunction as a result of pathologic reflexes secondary to other sites of entrapment. Early evidence points to the fact that neglect in addressing dysfunction in the thoracic outlet may be a contributor to the high incidence of failure in conservative management of patients with CTDs of the upper extremity.

The anatomy of the thoracic outlet might be considered as tunnels made up of bones and muscles. The nerves and blood vessels may become compromised within one or more of these tunnels (Fig. 6.1). The concept of tunnels is an essential perspective to understand the problem associated with TOS and the proposed solutions. Figure 6.2 shows a diagrammatic representation of the major tunnels of the spine and upper extremity, and Figure 6.3 shows an overlay of the tunnels on the anatomy. The author has found these diagrams to be of assistance in explaining the problem to the patient.

The basic anatomic structures will briefly be discussed together with the potential risk factors within these structures.

BONES

The bony tunnel comprises a floor consisting of the first through fifth ribs. The anterior wall is formed by the clavicle. The posterior wall is the scapula, with the medial border made up of the cervical vertebrae and discs with the external opening of the intervertebral foramina, and a lateral border formed by the glenohumeral joint (Fig. 6.1). Potential risk factors within these structures are as follows.

1. Structures that can affect the pathway the lower roots of the brachial plexus must traverse to reach the extremity (the breadth of the first rib).

2. Structures that can affect the diameter of the tunnel based on congenital factors, which might include the size of the transverse process of C7, the length of the clavicle, and the presence of a cervical rib. Although present in less than 1 percent of the population, a cervical rib occurs in 5 percent of TOS patients.[1]

3. Factors that can affect the diameter of the tunnel based on trauma in the past or from the injury that immediately preceded the onset of symptoms. These include callus formation following fracture of the clavicle or first rib; and degenerative hypertrophy of an arthritic glenohumeral joint, which can contribute to trauma of the neurovascular bundle during arm movements.[1]

4. Functional changes such as the mobility of the sternoclavicular, acromioclavicular joints and the first rib occur as a result of postural changes or dysfunctional breathing patterns. These changes affect the course of the lower roots of the plexus by increasing the distance traveled to pass from the intervertebral foramina of T1 up and over the first rib to then join C8 and pass into the arm. The relationship of the clavicle can affect the costoclavicular space and therefore the potential for changing the vascular flow through that space.

FIGURE 6.1 *Anatomy of the thoracic outlet. The clavicular head of the sternocleidomastoid muscle has been removed to view the anterior scalene muscle with the phrenic nerve crossing it. The C5, C6, C7, C8, T1 ventral roots of the plexus are visible as they pass in front of the middle scalene muscle. (© Peter Edgelow. Used with permission.)*

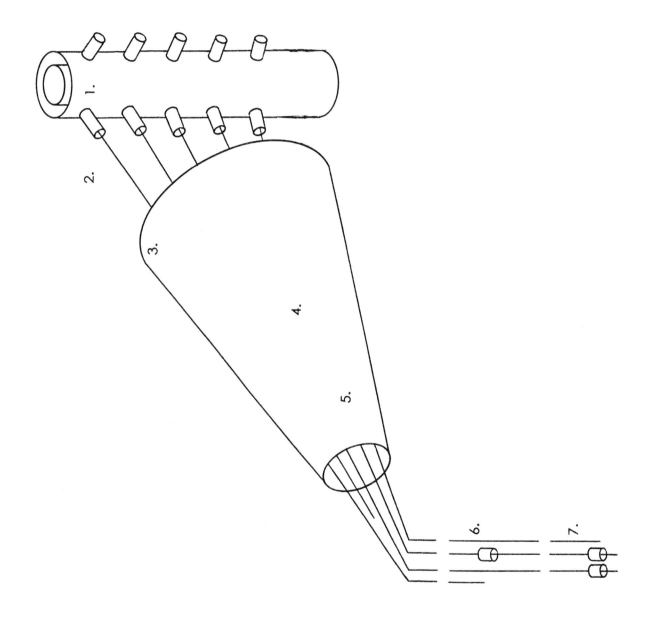

1.

2.

3.

4.

5.

6.

7.

MUSCLES

The muscular components separate this bony tunnel into two additional "soft-tissue" tunnels. A medial tunnel is formed by the anterior and middle scalenes as they pass from their origins to their insertions. The scalenus anterior arises from the anterior knob of the transverse process of each vertebra to insert on the anterior superior surface of the first rib, and the scalenus medius arises from the posterior knob of the transverse process and inserts to the posterior superior surface of the first rib. A lateral muscular tunnel is formed by the pectoralis minor muscle as it passes from its origin on the third, fourth, and fifth ribs to the coracoid process of the scapula (Fig. 6.1). The anterior bony wall of the tunnel is further reinforced by the presence of a muscular component (subclavius), which passes from its point of origin along the lateral one third of the undersurface of the clavicle to its insertion at the medial superior surface of the first rib.

Potential risk factors within these structures are as follows.

1. Narrowing of the scalene triangle and pectoralis minor contractile tunnels as a result of abnormal breathing and overused accessory breathing muscles, in conditions such as asthma or COPD. Paradoxical breathing patterns in which the scalenes and pectorals are used as the initiators of each breath, rather than assisting the diaphragm and lower intercostals during a deep inspiration, could be considered as a reason why the scalenes alter their physiology (see #3).

2. Anatomic variations of the anterior and middle scalene muscles, such as unusual proximity, wide distal attachments of the first rib, distal interdigitations, and the presence of a scalene minimus muscle.[2,3] Fibrous bands that attach lower cervical transverse processes or a cervical rib to the first rib are present in half of the normal population, and fewer than 1 percent develop TOS; so these are not considered a primary risk factor but can certainly provide a predisposition for development of symptoms.[2]

3. Shortening in the muscular elements secondary to poor posture and traumatic scarring. Scalene muscle trauma from injury with resultant inflammation, fibrosis, and contracture as verified by histologic studies.[4] The scalene muscles of patients with traumatic TOS have shown consistent abnormalities in fiber type, size distribution, and amount of connective tissue. Normal scalene muscle fibers comprise 50 percent of type I and 50 percent of type II. Type I fibers contract and relax slowly, develop tension over a narrow range, and are very resistant to fatigue, making these fibers specialized for the long-term contraction necessary in the maintenance of posture. Type II fibers are characterized by rapid contraction and relaxation, develop a wide range of tensions, and often fatigue quite rapidly. They are suited for high-intensity, short-duration muscular activity.[5] The TOS samples showed a predominance of type I (slow) fibers over type II (quick) fibers. TOS samples averaged 77 percent type I to 33 percent type II. These studies also showed a significant increase in connective tissue. The normal average amount of connective tissue in a healthy muscle is 14.5 percent, and the average amount in TOS samples was 36.6 percent. This suggests that fibrosis of the scalene muscles secondary to trauma, such as whiplash, may be an important contributor to the cause of TOS.[4]

4. Post-traumatic scarring along the deep cervical fascia could be another source of dys-

---

FIGURE 6.2 *Diagrammatic representation of tunnels within the upper quarter that may be compromised by acquired, congenital, or postural stenotic lesions. 1., vertebral canal; 2., intervertebral foramina; 3., scalenes; 4., infraclavicular; 5., pectoralis minor; 6., cubital tunnel; 7., carpal tunnel and canal of Guyon. (© Peter Edgelow. Used with permission.)*

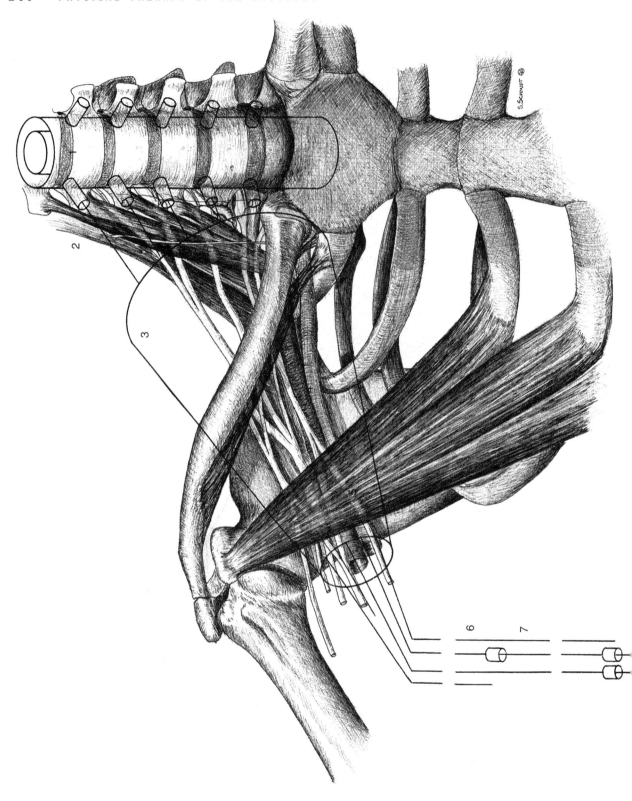

function. The deep cervical fascia is continuous with the axillary sheath that encases the neurovascular bundle.[6] Scarring in one area could lead to decreased mobility throughout the length of the tissue.

NERVES

The brachial plexus comprises the C5 through T1 nerve roots with a contribution from C4 and T2. However, it is the ventral rami of C8 and T1, as they anastomose to form the lower trunk of the brachial plexus, which is of particular importance with TOS, because it is their relationship with the floor of the tunnel (first rib) that places them in jeopardy. The sympathetic supply to the upper extremity comes from the stellate ganglion which lies on the neck of the first rib.(figure 1) Potential risk factors within these structures are as follows.

1. The possibility of an abnormally large contribution of T2 fibers to the T1 root, termed a postfixed plexus. The affect on available neural mobility is to lower the exiting T1 root, resulting in a longer course to get over the first rib and into the arm.
2. Any change in mobility of the plexus or a segment of the plexus as a result of scarring of the extraneural elements with further changes central to the scarring. Such change will affect the segment. That is, slumped posture increases the length of the spinal cord, thereby changing the distance the roots have to traverse to get into the arm.

BLOOD VESSELS

The subclavian vessels enter and exit the chest in this region, together with the nerves. The subclavian artery courses through the scalene trian-gle, which is formed by the anterior and middle scalene muscles and the first rib. There they are joined by the subclavian vein, which passes in front of the anterior scalene muscle. Distal to the first rib, the subclavian vessels are renamed the axillary artery and vein. Normally, there is "harmonious coexistence" among these structures.[7] However, if the delicate balance is disturbed, the osseous or fibromuscular components can cause compression on the neurovascular structures, giving neurogenic or vascular symptoms (Fig. 6.1).[7–10]

Potential risk factors within these structures are as follows. Due to the relationship of the artery and vein to adjacent structures, the vein is more susceptible to compromise than the artery. The first rib, anterior scalene, subclavius, and clavicle form a tunnel with a variable diameter. Narrowing of this space would affect the venous flow more than arterial flow and may be a significant factor in fluid dynamics not only in the thoracic outlet but also in the carpal tunnel. Based on normal pressure gradients, any increase in vascular congestion would have an immediate effect on the pressure within a tunnel, and this would then initiate a sequence of events that could ultimately produce nerve damage.

The nerves and blood vessels are required to traverse both the bony tunnel and the two soft tissue tunnels as the nerves pass from the intervertebral canal to the arm and the blood vessels from the thorax to the arm.

Further Issues in Understanding the Pathophysiology of Cumulative Trauma Disorders

As can be seen, the thoracic outlet tunnel diameters can be narrowed by a combination of bony, soft tissue, neurologic, and traumatic abnormal-

FIGURE 6.3 *This overlay of the tunnels upon the anatomy emphasizes the close proximity of the intervertebral foramina, (2) the space between the anterior and middle scalene, (3) the course of the subclavian vein passing over the first rib and beneath the clavicle between the muscular attachments of the anterior scalene (posteriorly) and the subclavius (anteriorly), (4) and the space posterior to pectoralis minor (5). (© Peter Edgelow. Used with permission.)*

ities. In addition, dysfunctional reflexes, fluid system dynamics, and postural, ergonomic, and gender factors can further affect the scalene first rib triangle and interfere with the course of the neurovascular structures, causing vascular compression.

DYSFUNCTIONAL REFLEXES THAT CAN AFFECT TUNNEL DIAMETER

There are three reflexes that can affect the diameter of the thoracic outlet and the blood flow to the upper extremity. In severe neurovascular entrapments, these reflexes are all pathologic and may worsen if the reflex activity is not normalized.

An abnormal or paradoxical breathing pattern is the most common and frequently overlooked dysfunctional reflex. The common dysfunctional pattern is the tendency to breathe with the upper thorax with an absence of abdominal movement. This could be viewed as a protective response adversely affecting the breathing pattern (e.g., gasping and breath holding). This protective response acts to elevate the first rib, thereby narrowing the tunnel. Changing the breathing pattern to relaxed, diaphragmatic breathing would assist in opening the tunnel and releasing the resultant muscle tension. The normal breathing reflex is to breathe in the quiet mode with the diaphragm and only use the scalene muscles as accessory muscles of breathing when the inspiration deepens. In paradoxical breathing, the scalenes are used even when breathing quietly. The resultant change in the normal reflex pattern of breathing then becomes conditioned into a "new normal" or pathologic breathing. In treatment it is essential to decondition this conditioned reflex, because it perpetuates a vicious cycle of pain/spasm and congestion.

In patients with paradoxical breathing the involved scalene begins to contract with the initiation of inspiration and contracts through the full inspiratory phase. This pattern of contraction can be palpated, and note should be made of the difference in size, time of contraction, and sensitivity to pressure as compared to the unin-

volved side. As the first rib elevates due to the abnormal breathing pattern it approaches the clavicle and affects the available space for the subclavian vein.

Further clinical observation with these patients reveals the issue of increased tone in the muscles of the upper quarter and a decrease in hand temperature and blood flow. This clinical observation and its relevance to the perpetuation of the problem has led to a hypothesis to try to explain this phenomenon and how to restore the system to normal.

The somatic nervous system has a normal protective reflex, which is called the flexion withdrawal reflex. Under normal circumstances, when the extremity experiences a noxious stimulus (such as touching a hot stove), the reflex pulls the extremity away from the stimulus towards the center of the body. Following this reflex, relaxed repeated movements of the extremity will result in a relaxation response of the muscles that produced the withdrawal.[11]

The autonomic nervous system also has a normal protective response: vasoconstriction. If there is a traumatic event such as a cut, the autonomic nervous system causes a vasoconstriction, which results in a decrease in blood flow allowing time for the blood to clot. Following the clotting, there is a reflex vasodilatation, which then increases blood flow to promote more rapid healing. This vasodilatation response can be stimulated by relaxed repeated movements of the injured part. The effect of the relaxed repeated movements is felt as a warming of the extremity.

In patients with cumulative trauma disorders, these reflexes become dysfunctional. The somatic nervous system's flexion withdrawal reflex becomes hyperactive, so that relaxed, repeated movements of the extremity cause an increase in muscle tension of the flexor muscles rather than a softening or release of tension. The autonomic system in the dysfunctional state results in a decrease rather than an increase in blood flow with relaxed, repeated movements. The breathing reflex in the dysfunctional state is paradoxical. These reflexes (flexion withdrawal, vasoconstriction, and paradoxical breathing) become conditioned by repeated noxious stimuli to respond with persistent cooling, with increased muscle tension in the extremity, and with increased tension in the scalenes. An important component in treatment is to decondition these abnormal reflexes by training the patient to perform relaxed, repeated movements in a range that does not elicit the tension/cooling response, but does elicit the relaxation/warming response while maintaining relaxed scalenes during quiet diaphragmatic breathing.

FLUID DYNAMICS, TISSUE REPAIR AND NEURAL MOBILITY

The traditional paradigm in considering the musculoskeletal consequences of an injury is to see the consequences as a loss of flexibility, coordination, endurance, and strength. This paradigm then directs treatment for musculoskeletal injury to restoring losses in flexibility, coordination, endurance, and strength. This paradigm needs to be expanded to include circulation (fluid systems), particularly when considering the cumulative trauma patient population. The problem in these patients is that the nervous system becomes affected in the injury, and the ensuing pain has a negative impact on both the circulation and the healing process.

There are six separate fluid systems within the upper quarter. These fluid systems must be working at their best to maximize healing from trauma to this area. Table 6.1 briefly summarizes

TABLE 6.1 *Fluid systems within the upper quarter*

CIRCULATORY SYSTEM	STRUCTURES SUPPLIED	PUMP
Arteries and veins	Muscles, ligaments, bone	Heart
Lymph	Fascia	Movement
Synovial fluid	Joints	Movement
Cerebral spinal fluid	Dura, meninges, nerve roots	Breathing
Intervertebral disc fluid	Disc	Walking
Intraneuronal transport system	Nerve	Movement

these systems, the structures they supply, and the pumps that maximize the flow necessary for adequate repair and health. Because the key ingredients for adequate circulation of all of the systems involve both movement and diaphragmatic breathing, both the problem and the solution become obvious.

An additional issue is that of pressure and its impact on circulation. The blood supply within a peripheral nerve relies on a pressure gradient system for adequate nutrition. In research on pressure gradients within the carpal tunnel, the pressure in the nutrient arteriole was found to be greater than the pressure in the capillary, which was greater than the pressure in the nerve fascicle, which was greater than the pressure in the vein, which was greater than the pressure in the tunnel (Fig. 6.4). Imbalance in the pressure gradient due to an increase in the tunnel pressure caused the vein to collapse, creating venous stasis and hypoxia. If nothing was done to reverse this problem then the hypoxia continues, leading to edema, which ultimately leads to fibroblastic activity and scar formation within the nerve fascicle.[1,12] From this evolves a hypothesis. Initial trauma around the nerve could lead to extraneural scarring without affecting the intraneural function of the nerve. However, once the pressure gradient changes lead to intraneural fibrosis, then permanent neural change would occur.

Although the pressure gradient research has been described for the median nerve in the carpal tunnel, the model could be generalized to the entire nervous system, as it is continually housed within tunnels of varying structure throughout the body.[12] This is of importance in the thoracic outlet because, as previously mentioned, structural and dynamic changes cause restriction in the size of the outlet, which could contribute to disrupting the pressure gradient and affecting the neural circulation. A useful analogy to describe this situation is to consider a river flowing into a lake and a river flowing out of the lake, in which the inflow equals the outflow. In this state, the volume of the lake is constant, the oxygen content is high, and the pollution content is low. Should there be an obstruction affecting the out-

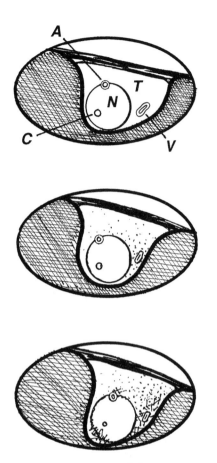

FIGURE 6.4 *Representation of the pressure gradients in the carpal tunnel and the stages that follow alteration of the pressure gradients. For simplicity, one nerve fiber in a fascicle is represented.* **(A)** *Normal tunnel pressure gradient: artery ⟩ capillary ⟩ nerve ⟩ venule ⟩ tunnel.* **(B)** *Hypoxic and edematous tunnel and nerve: increased tunnel pressure ⟩ venule = collapse = venous stasis and hypoxia.* **(C)** *Neural and tunnel fibroblastic response: further increase in tunnel pressure and hypoxia, scar tissue. (A, arteriole; C, capillary; N, nerve; T, tunnel; V, venule.) (Adapted from the work of Sunderland, 1976; © Peter Edgelow. Used with permission.)*

flow, then the volume of the lake would increase, the oxygen content would decrease, and the pollution would increase. This condition would be called a swamp (Fig. 6.5).[13] Because the blood flow to and from the upper extremity passes through the tunnel of the thoracic outlet, the concept of narrowing of the tunnel can be a mechanical explanation for the circulation problem.

A further issue following injury involves the repair process itself. For maximum repair and restoration of function, microstresses are required to stimulate both structural strength and flexibility. An awareness of this issue helps to understand how normal injury and repair can be interfered with in the thoracic outlet region and upper quarter. Normal repair requires an adequate amount of circulation and stress. Circulation feeds the healing tissues, and stress stimulates adequate remodeling so that the repaired tissue can be as close to the pre-injured state as possible. This idea can be expressed to the patient by using the analogy of the orthodontist and how he is able to remodel crooked teeth with the use of braces and small forces in the form of elastic bands. The forces must be small enough not to elicit significant pain, but sustained enough to allow for the tissues to accommodate to the stress. The major factor in this step is a function of time. With post-traumatic cumulative trauma patients, the factor of time taken to remodel the extraneural components of the nerve and the application of small forces are also important considerations in the healing process.

OCCUPATIONAL AND ACTIVITIES OF DAILY LIVING ISSUES

Certain occupations that involve constant turning or sustained flexion of the neck (keyboard jobs), repetitive use of arms (assembly line work), lifting or holding the arms above the shoulders (painters, electricians), and working with vibrating tools seem to predispose people to develop symptoms.[7] Studies have compared occupations of heavy industry work (packers and assembly workers), office work, and cash register work for incidence of TOS symptoms. In one

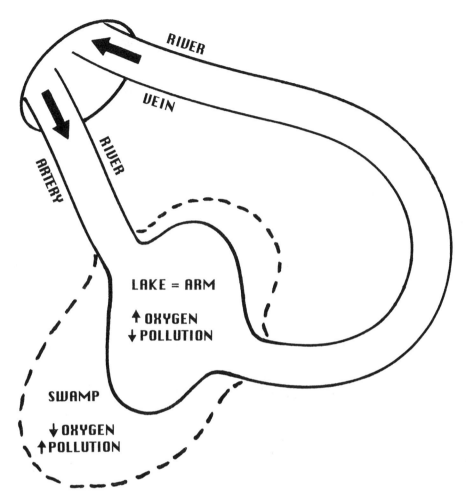

FIGURE 6.5 *An analogy of a healthy lake to describe to the patient the possible scenario of venous stasis leading to congestion (swamp) within the tunnel(s), and hence the need to decongest the tunnel (drain the swamp!) before proceeding to other treatments. (© Peter Edgelow. Used with permission.)*

study, it was found that the awkward work posture and continuous muscle tension of the cash register work produced the highest percentage of TOS symptoms (32% of cash register workers).[5] Some of these symptoms may be due to postural stresses, such as the carrying of heavy packs or weights by those unaccustomed to heavy work, or by debilitation and poor posture.[7,14–16] Recent clinical experience has shown that musicians are another occupational group in which there is a significant incidence of CTDs because of periods of intense sustained highly repetitive physical activity with high cognitive demand.

Another possible cause of symptoms related to the thoracic outlet is the narrowing of the costoclavicular space by a hypomobile, elevated first rib.[16] It is suggested that patients with emphysema are predisposed to TOS because the first rib is chronically elevated.[8] Also, a high thoracic lordosis lifts the upper ribs towards the clavicle, approximating these structures and causing impingement of the neurovascular contents.[17] It is important to remember that anything that affects the circulation through the thoracic outlet could then compromise the nutrition of the nerve at a distal site.

Sleeping postures are often affected, and patients may awaken with their arm having fallen asleep and it may even be momentarily flail and require some passive movements with the aid of the uninvolved arm to restore circulation and mobility.

An important fact to appreciate is that the nervous system is a continuous tissue tract. As the effect of specific trauma and age affects the mobility of the nervous system, certain postures that place the nervous system in its extreme of range can be potentially injurious or irritating, particularly if they are sustained. For example, the common position of many seated office workers is slumped. Slump sitting with the coccyx/sacrum in a flexed position and a loss of lumbar lordosis when accompanied by a thoracic kyphosis has a very profound affect on the mobility of the spinal cord caudal to the cervicothoracic junction. The spinal cord is approaching its end range of motion. Add to this the use of the arms in an extended position, such as working with a mouse on the computer, and you selectively stress the upper roots of the brachial plexus compared to the lower roots. The functional position of holding a phone to the ear would selectively stress the lower roots of the plexus. The information upon which this analysis is based is the pioneering work of Bob Elvey on the upper limb tension test.[18] This knowledge is important in analyzing the stresses of ADL as well as in examination and treatment, as is mentioned later in this chapter.

GENDER ISSUES

It is not known why the incidence of TOS in women is twice that of men. It is speculated that the increased incidence may be due to less developed muscles, more horizontal clavicles, or a greater tendency for drooping shoulders; or it may be due to more prevalent congenital anomalies in the thoracic outlet in women.[19]

It has been suggested that a narrowed thoracic outlet may be due to the lower position of the female sternum, which decreases the angle between the scalene muscles.[20] Another factor not to overlook is the biomechanical consequences of the anatomic fact that women have breasts. Perhaps instead of drooping shoulder girdles, the problem is chronically contracted pectoral muscles or undue tightness of the scalene muscle group.[6]

Differential Diagnosis

Patients are remarkable for lack of objective evidence of neurologic injury or radiological findings, and it is the subtle soft-tissue signs of neural irritability, vascular abnormalities, changes in breathing patterns, changes in first rib and thoracic mobility, and in the quality of muscle contraction that contribute to the clinical diagnosis.

A complete clinical evaluation should always consider conditions that may simulate or coexist with TOS, such as cervical disc disease or spondylosis, angina pectoris, spinal cord neoplasm, Pancoast tumor, multiple sclerosis, carpal tunnel syndrome, ulnar nerve compression at the elbow, orthopedic problems of the shoulder and spine, and inflammatory conditions of the joints and soft tissues.[2,21]

In addition, the T4 syndrome presents symptoms of dull pain, aching, and discomfort or paraesthesia in the arm, which do not follow any dermatomal pattern and often have a vague feeling of tightness or pressure in the posterior midthoracic region. The signs on palpation of the T4 syndrome are located between T3 and T6 as differentiated from the supraclavicular tenderness associated with TOS.[6,22]

Many patients have multiple tunnel issues involving more than one "tunnel" (termed multiple crush). Sorting out the contribution of each is challenging. A major contribution to the clarification of cervical involvement comes from the work of Dr. Herman Kabat.[23] He has devised a simple clinical test to clarify the quality of muscle contraction in two distal arm muscles innervated by the C7 nerve root. These muscles are adductor pollicis and flexor carpi ulnaris. A positive test incriminates the C7 root as a potential source of irritation, and a significant number of patients with TOS also exhibit weakness in adductor pollicis and flexor carpi ulnaris that is reversed by self cervical traction. It is of interest to observe that sometimes the motor root problem is in one arm while the TOS problem is in the other.

Another challenging diagnostic problem concerns carpal tunnel syndrome (CTS). True CTS involves the median nerve only and is often associated with a Tinel and/or Phalen sign. CTS is associated with TOS in 21 to 30 percent of TOS cases. Ulnar nerve compression at the elbow is associated with TOS in 6 to 10 percent of cases.[24,25] The double crush syndrome indicates the existence of more than one area of nerve compression in an extremity.[26] The presence of a more proximal lesion does seem to make the more distal nerve more vulnerable to compression.[27]

It is believed that in some cases there can be a multiple crush syndrome involving any combination of cervical spinal nerves, trunks and cords of the brachial plexus, ulnar nerve compression at the elbow, and carpal tunnel syndrome.[24] In severe cases of TOS, the author's experience is that the lower extremity neural tension signs, such as straight leg raising (SLR) and cord mobility, can also be affected.

Examination Findings

SUBJECTIVE SYMPTOMS

Symptom Patterns for Patients With TOS

Complaints may include paresthesia (numbness and tingling), pain (aching or sharp), and sensory and motor loss. Aching pain is noted as the most common symptom.[19,21] Pain is frequently felt in the lateral aspect of the neck, supraclavicular area, shoulder area, and the area of the arm corresponding to the dermatome(s)

affected, frequently in the hypothenar area and fourth and fifth digits. The pain may radiate to the chest wall.[6,28,29]

Arterial obstruction produces coolness, cold sensitivity, numbness in the hand, and exertional fatigue. Venous obstruction may cause cyanotic discoloration, arm edema, finger stiffness, and a feeling of heaviness.[19,30–32] Venous symptoms are more common than arterial ones. Peripheral embolization can cause gangrene of fingertips and is an arterial complication of TOS.[7,33]

Functional Profile for Patients With TOS

Symptoms are aggravated by dependency of the arm and any use of the arm in lifting, pushing, pulling, reaching over the head, or repetitive activity such as writing, data entry, or playing a musical instrument. Fine coordination may be affected, with patients complaining of symptoms with sustained upper extremity activity, such as combing hair, reaching, holding a newspaper, telephone or steering wheel, or carrying a heavy bag. Pain is often worse after rather than during use, and is referred to as latency. The pain may be particularly disturbing at night,[30] and symptoms can be bilateral or unilateral.[7]

Symptoms are eased by avoiding aggravating activity and through support of the involved extremity, such as wearing a sling or keeping the hand in a pocket.

Present History for Patients With TOS

In the TOS patients referred to the author, there was a high incidence of trauma. The trauma could be sudden or insidious. The most common traumatic event was a motor vehicle accident, often followed by the passage of time and/or a job involving large amounts of static use of the upper extremity, with repetitive use of the hands.[7,34] Insidious onset occurred following prolonged stress to the hand in occupations requiring sustained hand activity under high cognitive demand and with either poor work station design or poor hand/arm/neck use.[35]

Past History for Patients With TOS

There may be a history of traumas to the head or neck or upper extremity that subsequently resolved, leaving the patient apparently asymptomatic or with minor residuals that did not compromise normal function. If this trauma affected the diameter of the canal(s) or the flexibility of the nervous system as it traverses the canals, or caused trauma to the vascular system, then the trauma may have contributed to the onset of symptoms.

TESTS AND MEASURES FOR PATIENTS WITH TOS

Specific diagnosis for TOS can be made by radiograph and computed-tomography (CT) scan. Radiologic studies identify any bony abnormalities, degenerative changes, Pancoast tumors, or other pulmonary diseases.[2] Previous history of clavicular fracture picked up on radiography is important, because it can predispose toward embolization of the subclavian artery.[28] CT and magnetic resonance imaging (MRI) are often necessary to rule out frank cervical disc disease, spinal stenosis and fibrous bands.[7]

An important finding whose significance is often not appreciated is the presence of an elongated transverse process of C7 seen on plain films. It is the experience of a prominent vascular surgeon who has performed over 250 thoracic outlet decompression surgeries that the presence of an elongated transverse process is a marker for other anomalies within the thoracic outlet, such as soft-tissue changes within the scalene triangle and fibrous bands (R. Stoney, personal communication).

Diagnosis for vascular TOS is made by duplex scanning (ultrasound combined with Doppler velocity waveforms), angiography, or venography.[7,36,37] The infraclavicular area should be auscultated for the presence of a bruit with the arm in various positions.[19,20,33] A bruit indicates an arterial lumen narrowing.[7]

Electrodiagnostic tests include electromyography (EMG), late F-wave responses, nerve conduction velocities (NCV), and somatosensory evoked potentials (SSEP). Positive electrodiagnostic studies can reveal chronic, severe lower trunk brachial plexopathy. Such tests may indicate an abnormality in nerve function, but do not give the specific cause. Low-amplitude ulnar sensory responses are the most widely accepted of these studies, but there is disagreement over the reliability of the results. There is a wide range of conduction times found in asymptomatic individuals, which may be the result of inaccurate placement of the proximal electrode at Erb's point.[6,7,24,37,38] Many TOS patients have normal electrodiagnostic studies. This may be due to the intermittent nature of the symptoms, which are dependent on certain positions. Instead of testing these patients in the anatomic position, they should be tested in the symptom-provoking position.[39] Most agree that these studies are helpful in ruling out carpal tunnel syndrome and ulnar nerve entrapment at the elbow.[7,24,32,37]

Thermography has been used by some practitioners as an aid in diagnosis of TOS.[40] Thermography indicates either an increase or decrease in heat emission secondary to blood flow. Alterations in heat emission can be measured by an increased blood flow, as in venous occlusion, or a decreased flow, as in arterial compression or nerve fiber irritation from neurogenic compression. Because pathologies such as cervical radiculopathy, ulnar nerve injury, and reflex sympathetic dystrophy can produce similar patterns, the lack of specificity can make interpretation of thermography difficult.[37]

A muscle block is another technique used as a diagnostic aid. Relief of symptoms after scalene muscle block with lidocaine into the muscle belly can implicate the anterior scalene muscle as the source of pathology. Improvement after the block correlates with good response to surgery.[7]

OBJECTIVE EXAMINATION BY PHYSICAL THERAPIST FOR PATIENTS WITH TOS

The objective examination is limited in the traditional scope and range of motion examined, due to respect for the irritability of the condition. Active movements of the cervical spine are examined to the point of onset or increase of symptoms only. When examining the upper limb tension test, it is essential to examine to the initial barrier or point at which involuntary muscle guarding comes into play. This is before the range in which symptoms are elicited. If this precaution is not adhered to, the risk of a latent flair of symptoms is heightened. It is the irritability of the nervous system which is at the physiologic core of the problem, and because all movements of the spine and extremities have a biomechanical effect on the nervous system, all movements need to be examined to the initial point of muscle tension.

Observation

Typical postural deviations to look for in these patients involve protective positioning of the upper quarter to reduce stress on the neural and vascular structures. This can manifest in subtle protraction and elevation of the shoulder girdle. In more extreme cases the patient may hold the extremity in a fully flexed posture much like the posture seen in hemiplegia. The evaluator should also look for forward head posture, particularly for prominence in the cervical thoracic junction, as well as soft-tissue fullness in the supraclavicular area.

Active Movements

Full active motion testing is not performed initially. The cervical ranges of flexion, extension, and bilateral rotation are assessed to the point of onset of symptoms. This is the point at which tension is felt. The common restriction is to have tension in the left scalene region when rotation is performed to the right, and tension in the right scalene region when rotation is performed to the left.

Neurodynamic Testing

The nervous system is examined both functionally and specifically. Functional examination is to have the patient elevate the arm with the elbow extended and with the elbow flexed.

The patient is asked to move the extremity to the point of increase in tension only. This difference in range between elbow flexion and extension range is compared with the specific examination of the brachial plexus or upper limb tension test.

In my experience, the upper limb tension tests (ULTTs) to evaluate and treat abnormal neural dynamics in the brachial plexus are the most valuable tests for the neurogenic tissues. These tests are discussed in detail in Chapter 5, and so only a brief description will be given here to highlight their importance.

There are four tests designed to test the extensibility of the neural structures. Each one biases a different aspect of the cervical roots, trunks, and peripheral nerves. With TOS, compression of the neural structures provides a site of tensile stress concentration and limits the normal mobility and extensibility necessary to accommodate to the stresses of neck and arm movement. The resulting abnormal amount of tension will produce a positive ULTT.[41]

The first of these tests, ULTT 1, is a general base test for the brachial plexus with a slight bias towards the median nerve and nerve root levels C5, C6. ULTT 2 has two variations that more selectively bias the medial and radial nerves and the C5, C6, and C7 nerve roots. ULTT 3 is biased for the ulnar nerve and nerve root levels C8–T1.[12] (See Ch. 5 for a description of these tests.) In the author's experience the ULTT 1 is positive and symptomatic on all patients. An important feature of these patients is the irritability of the neural structures. For this reason, when examining the neural mobility, one must examine it to the point of muscle tension or muscle guarding. Otherwise the pathologic withdrawal reflex will be elicited. To examine them into the range in which symptoms such as numbness, tingling, or pain are produced is to *over*examine them. Once this has been done it is too late to back up. There will most commonly be a latent flare, which may take hours or days to subside. In less irritable conditions or when the patient has progressed to the stage that the ULTT 1 is improved and no longer irritable, then ULTT 2 or 3 may be used as a refinement in the examination or progression in treatment. This decision is based on clinical judgment.

Palpation

In patients with neurogenic TOS there may be pain with direct pressure over the scalene muscles and also on the brachial plexus. There may also be a positive Tinel sign over the supraclavicular area at the insertion of the anterior scalene muscle.[7,20,24,30] Tenderness in the region of the subclavius muscle as it inserts into the first rib is also common.

Strength Testing

Muscle weakness, if present, is mild and involves most commonly the thenar, hypothenar, and interosseous muscles innervated by the ulnar nerve. Reflexes usually remain intact. Hypesthesia may occur in the C8–T1 dermatomes.[20]

In the case of a specific C7 motor root weakness (adductor pollicis and/or flexor carpi ulnaris), the Kabat protocol is used to determine its significance. If the strength tests are found to demonstrate weakness and this weakness is reversed with self cervical traction (Fig. 6.6), then this technique of self-treatment is incorporated into the treatment protocol.[23] Based on this protocol the identified path of least resistance is used to guide the patient in modifying activities of daily living.[23]

Breathing Pattern

Relaxed breathing is always paradoxical, with the scalene muscle active on inspiration from the initiation of inspiration through the full inspiratory excursion. The patients often have difficulty breathing with the diaphragm, and even when they can, it is the inability to quieten the scalenes that is the dysfunctional pattern.

More Traditional Objective Tests for Thoracic Outlet Syndrome

The standard clinical tests to implicate particular areas that could be responsible for causing compression to the neurovascular structures

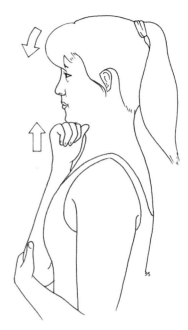

FIGURE 6.6 *Dr. Kabat's method of performing self cervicle traction as a method of reversing identified weakness in adductor pollicis and/or flexor carpi ulnaris. The traction force is sustained for 15 seconds and then slowly released. Retesting of the weak muscles should demonstrate immediate increase in motor power.[23] (© Peter Edgelow. Used with permission.)*

are sometimes equivocal. Among the more common diagnostic tests are the following:

1. Adson's test. This has been used to implicate the anterior scalene muscle's role in obliterating the pulse when the muscle is put on stretch.

2. The exaggerated military position. This purports to test the costoclavicular component of the thoracic outlet by lowering the clavicle onto the first rib, causing compression there.

3. Hyperabduction of the arms (arms overhead with elbows flexed, as assumed in sleep). This produces a pulley effect of the neurovascular structures under the pector-

alis minor tendon and coracoid process, causing compromise at that site. This position can also narrow the costoclavicular space. Both pulse obliteration and typical symptom reproduction are considered positive for these tests.[10,20]

4. The abduction external rotation test (AER), commonly called the hands-up test. This has the reputation of being the most reliable of the TOS tests. This postural maneuver involves shoulder abduction and external rotation to 90°, producing a scissors-like compression of the neurovascular structures by the clavicle on the first rib. It can be considered positive by reproduction of the patient's symptoms or pulse change.[2,7,19] Positive response for pulse obliteration is only 5 to 10 percent in normals.[3]

5. An additional claudication test added to the AER position, during which a patient opens and closes the hands for up to 3 minutes. This is called the elevated arm stress test (EAST). This test will evaluate all three types of TOS due to compression by the position and the added stress of exercise.[2]

The problem with these traditional tests is that when pulse obliteration is used as the critical sign, the tests have shown too many false-positive results to be reliable, because the majority of asymptomatic individuals have pulse changes with the maneuvers.[3] Reproduction of the patient's symptoms using these test positions is a more reliable sign of thoracic outlet syndrome.[20] The hyperabduction and costoclavicular maneuvers are positive if there is simultaneously an obliteration of the arm pulses and reproduction of neurologic symptoms.

Each of these standard TOS tests has components of the ULTT within them. Depression of the shoulder girdle or the exaggerated military position causes a "drag on the nerve roots."[3] Abduction and external rotation of the arm, or the AER test, places a traction force on the brachial plexus and is further exaggerated by the hyperabduction maneuver.[8] Adson's test involves lateral flexion of the head to the contralateral side.

Compared to the ULTT, these tests involve only partial tension of the neuromeningeal system. However, with the more mild cases, progressively adding tension up to the limit of the neuromeningeal system may be required. This may explain why many times the results of these classic tests are negative, and why performing the ULTT is a better test of the limit to which the compromised system can be taken. No single test of the more traditional tests is specific enough to eliminate other potential sources of pathology.

Treatment

GOALS

There are many outcomes that influence a treatment program for patients with thoracic outlet syndrome. They can reflect the education and experience of the therapist, the risks and benefits as viewed by the patients, and the cost and benefits as determined by insurers and employers, to mention a few of the influencing factors. With these factors acknowledged as ongoing parameters, the general goals of the treatment program are to teach the patient to control the problem and prevent recurrence by taking control of selected and individualized therapeutic procedures. This is achieved through training and monitoring of the physical problems; the emotional response to the disabling and painful problem; and an intellectual understanding of the issues related to causes, methods for preventing, and curing the disorder, and the personal role in each. It is the basic premise of this approach that the patient learns through the ability to feel the change that occurs while performing the exercises to both understand the problem and to be guided, by the change in relevant symptoms, towards the solution.

THE EDGELOW PROTOCOL

• Identify physical, intellectual, and emotional issues that contribute to the problem and recognize when treatment is effective.

- Recognize the interdependence of the whole person, physically, intellectually, and emotionally. Appreciate that by training the patient to recognize (pay attention to the tension) and reverse the dysfunctional reflexes, they are gaining the control that will guide them to a state of maximum function.
- Recognize and reverse dysfunctional reflexes.
- Identify variance in normal quiet breathing and decondition the acquired dysfunctional pattern.
- Identify variance in relaxation response to repeated movements of the hand, and use this abnormal tension response for guidance in deconditioning the acquired dysfunctional pattern.
- Identify variance in warming response to repeated movements of the hand, and use this abnormal cooling response for guidance in deconditioning the acquired dysfunctional pattern.
- Develop personal control under the guidance of a professional physical therapist, through monitoring, and teach the patient how to use specific active and passive exercises and certain assistive devices to effectively (1) open the tunnel(s) that are narrowed and (2) assist normalization of the fluid systems through the pumping actions of breathing and movement. Both outcomes must be achieved without increasing pain that the patient perceives as harmful. From a clinical perspective, pain is perceived of as harmful if one of two responses occurs. Either a tension response results in the muscles being used when a relaxation is the intended result, or a cooling response occurs in the involved extremity when a warming response is the intended response.

TREATMENT METHODS TO "OPEN THE TUNNELS"

Breathing

Relaxed diaphragmatic breathing is taught with the patient lying supine with hips and knees bent (Fig. 6.7). The inhalation phase is coordi-

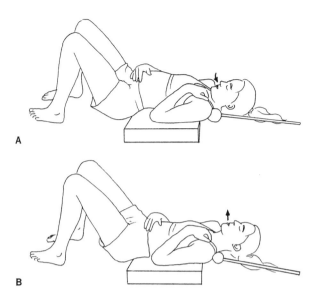

FIGURE 6.7 *Relaxed diaphragmatic breathing.* **(A)** *Patient lying supine, knees flexed with foam wedge positioned to stabilize the shoulder girdle on the affected side. The ball-on-a-stick is positioned superior to the scapula and close to the spine to press against the first rib. Inhale and arch the lumbar spine allowing the chin to nod down as the body shortens relative to the pelvis.* **(B)** *Exhale and flatten the lumbar spine, contracting the abdominal muscles so as to pull the ribs down towards the pelvis and the first rib gently pushes against the ball-on-the-stick, chin nodding up. (© Peter Edgelow. Used with permission.)*

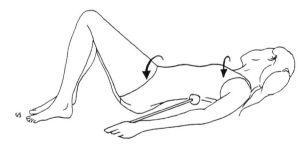

FIGURE 6.8 *Use of the ball-on-a-stick to apply self mobilization to each rib articulation while lying supine. (© Peter Edgelow. Used with permission.)*

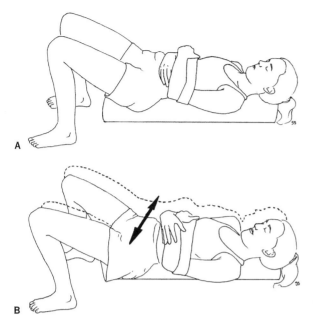

FIGURE 6.9 (A & B) *Patient lying supine on the 6-inch Ethafoam roll. Arms relaxed and supported by belt. Breathe in as balanced in the center and breathe out as rolling from side to side. May perform in standing if supine is too painful. (© Peter Edgelow. Used with permission.)*

contraction of the hip rotators facilitates hip flexor relaxation and scalene relaxation as well.

Rib Mobilizer

The ball on the stick is used to mobilize each rib articulation (Fig. 6.8). Rolling to the side, and placing the ball paraspinally and rolling back onto it while exhaling, assists rib depression.

Ethafoam Rollers

Six-inch and 3-inch Ethafoam rollers are used to mobilize the spine and rib cage with the emphasis on increasing spinal extension, depressing the rib cage, facilitating spinal stabilization and coordination with controlled breathing patterns. A belt is used to assist relaxation of the pectoralis minor muscle (Fig. 6.9). Once patients have achieved increased mobility with the 6-inch

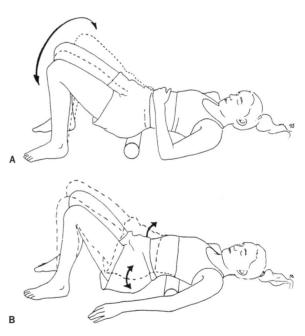

FIGURE 6.10 *Patient mobilizing the pelvis, lumbar spine and thoracic spine with three inch Ethafoam roll. (A) Spinal extension with inhale to pain only. Move up spine to include all segments increasing range as tolerated. (B) Spinal flexion with exhale. (© Peter Edgelow. Used with permission.)*

nated with spinal extension, and the exhalation phase is coordinated with spinal flexion. In this way, relaxation of the abdomen that occurs with lumbar extension allows for full diaphragmatic excursion. Conversely, contraction of the abdomen that occurs with spinal flexion reinforces exhalation while depressing the sternum and rib cage. A further modification is to place a ball on a stick up against the posterior aspect of the elevated first rib. The spinal motion affects a movement of the rib away from the ball during inhalation and a movement towards the ball with exhalation. With the end of the stick stabilized against a wall this provides a very simple assist to first rib depression during active exhalation.[11] Training of this breathing pattern can be progressed by doing it with the legs extended and relaxed and with the legs extended and relaxed during inhalation but with active internal rotation of the hips during exhalation. This active

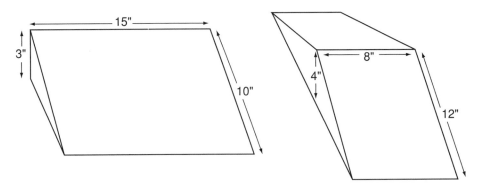

FIGURE 6.11 *Dimensions of foam wedges to assist in relaxed, repeated movements of the cervical spine. (© Peter Edgelow. Used with permission.)*

roller, they progress to the 3-inch roller (Fig. 6.10). A word of caution: these exercises must be able to be performed without significant increase in spinal pain during the exercise. Any increase in spinal pain must not be accompanied by any arm pain. The other issue that must be

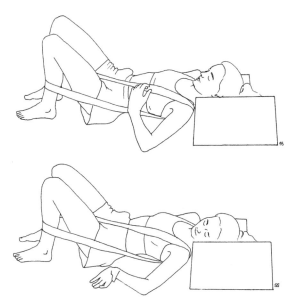

FIGURE 6.12 *The stabilization belt is used to assist patients in checking their own brachial plexus tension. The exercise involves performing relaxed repeated movements of the neck, elbow, and wrist to obtain a relaxation/warming response. (© Peter Edgelow. Used with permission.)*

addressed is the skill necessary to perform the exercise and control the breathing pattern at the same time. If the patient cannot quieten the scalenes during the exercise on the roller, then the patient is not ready to do it. It takes time to decondition a conditioned response.

METHODS TO "DRAIN THE SWAMP"

Relaxed Repeated Movements

I have designed two pillows that allow relaxed, repeated movements of the cervical spine (Fig. 6.11). The patient lies supine with the head on one slope of the double-ended pillow and slowly relaxes the neck and lets it roll downhill. The other pillow is placed on the slope to act as a stop to prevent movement into a range that results in tension or pain. Patients are taught to assess their own neural tension and then perform relaxed repeated movements of the neck, elbow, and wrist. Each movement is performed 10 times and then the neural tension is reassessed. If there is a relaxation response, then the patient repeats the movements (Fig. 6.12). They are also taught to use a handheld thermometer to assess change in hand temperature.

CASE STUDY

HISTORY

A 25-year-old, right-handed billing clerk developed right wrist pain on 10/26/95 while doing computer entry. Over the next 2 days the symptoms spread from the wrist up the forearm to the elbow and down into the hand. Despite rest for 2 days the pain remained constant and did not subside.

SIGNIFICANT PAST HISTORY

The patient had been working overtime 6 days a week, packing records in preparation for a move. Her normal work commute was 45 minutes twice a day. She worked out at the gym for the prior 6 weeks, lifting weight up to 60 pounds. She had two auto accidents, one in 1989 and one in 1991. She reported no prior arm symptoms but occasional neck pain that responded to massage, self-mobilization, and rest. She has had mild asthma since age 16. She wears glasses and has to "peer at the screen" when tired. She uses roller blades for fun, and 6 weeks ago fell on outstretched hands with sprain of the left wrist, but was "OK" within 2 days.

PAIN PATTERN (BY REPORT)

1. Her greatest pain is in the area of the right wrist, which she describes as a constant pain rated at 7/10, 50 percent of the time at worst and 3/10, 25 percent of the time at best
2. The second area of symptoms in decreasing order of intensity is the right forearm/elbow, which is intermittent and rated as 6/10 at worst.
3. The third area of symptoms is intermittent pain in the right thumb, thenar eminence, and fifth digit.
4. The fourth area of pain is a soreness in the right upper arm and tender points to palpation in the neck on the right.
5. She denies any symptoms in the left upper extremity.

FUNCTIONAL PROFILE (BY REPORT)

1. Aggravated by data entry repetition and slight slowness in finger dexterity noted when switches from 10 key entry to key-board and vise versa for the first few seconds. "The hand feels as if it doesn't want to work."
2. Lifting weights at the gym or boxes at work increases her neck pain.
3. Driving to and from work is uncomfortable in the neck and shoulder blade and she feels tight in the right supraclavicular region.

OBJECTIVE

Tested to initial point of pain/increase only. For ease of reading the case study, the following abbreviations will be used:

- C, cervical
- (R), right
- (L), left
- ULTT, upper limb tension test
- wnl, within normal limits

In addition, the recording of the sequence of motions involved in the ULTT is as follows.

1. Shoulder girdle depression
2. Glenohumeral abduction
3. Glenohumeral external rotation
4. Forearm supination (90° = full supination)
5. Wrist extension (85 to 90° = full wrist extension)
6. Elbow extension (180° = full elbow extension)

OBSERVATION

Posture forward, head with loss of normal postural alignment. Apparent "step off" at C7/T1, shoulders level. Height: 5'9"; weight: 150 pounds.

CERVICAL

Flexion: 3" chin from sternum, pulls cervical spine R > L.
Extension: Full range. Pulls anterior cervical spine.

Rotation: (R): Full range. Pulls L supraclavicular region.
Rotation: (L): 80°. Pulls right cervical spine and pain left trap.

SHOULDER FLEXION

(R) (with elbow extension): 135° pulling whole arm to thumb.
(R) (with elbow flexion): 180°.
(L) (with elbow extension): 110° pulling whole arm to thumb.
(L) (with elbow flexion): 135° pulling into the upper arm.

UPPER LIMB TENSION TEST

Recorded in sequence of examination to tension point.
(R): 1/wnl; 2/80°; 3/45°; 4/wnl; 5/wnl; 6/120° with pull in right thumb.
(L): 1/wnl; 2/60°; 3/30°; 4/wnl; 5/wnl; 6/150° with pull in left arm.

BREATHING PATTERN

Paradoxical with early scalene contraction on quiet inspiration, right more than left.

PALPATION

Sensitive scalenes on right compared to the left.

STRENGTH

Flexor carpi ulnaris: (R) 4/5, (L) 5/5. Adductor pollicis: (R) 4/5, (L) 5/5.

EFFECT OF TRIAL SELF CERVICAL TRACTION (KABAT)

Results in increase strength of right thumb and ulnar wrist flexion. Testing reveals that the mechanical sensitivity is from compression through the top of the head.[22]
Thoracic spine, cervical spine, and rib cage: Postural dysfunction in flexion with elevated first rib bilateral.

ASSESSMENT

1. C37 motor root irritability on the right.
2. Findings suggestive of plexus irritability bilaterally, right greater than left, with elevated first rib on the right and left and paradoxical breathing pattern.
3. Postural factors influencing the problem.
4. Cervical and upper thoracic dysfunction in flexion.

TREATMENT PLAN

1. Instruct in "what is wrong" and use home kit for treating upper quarter neurovascular entrapments.
2. Progress through the home program approach to dealing with these dysfunctions beginning with the Kabat protocol and progressing through the diaphragmatic breathing, thoracic and rib mobilization.
3. Restoration of the relaxation and warming response during repeated movements of the upper extremity.
4. Train in protective body mechanics to minimize stress from work.
5. Initial modification of work schedule; no overtime; no lifting; awareness of posture; no sitting with legs crossed; feet flat on floor. Posture instruction.

RESULTS AND DISCUSSION

This case history was chosen to illustrate that findings present in severe cases of neurovascular entrapment are evident early in the history. The problem is that if they are not looked for they will often be missed. If addressed early, they disappear rapidly, and one has a clear picture of the relevance of these findings. When the patient can also see the relationship between the findings and their ability to change those findings, this reinforces the issues they need to address to get well and stay well. There is much yet to learn with these problems. For example:

• Was this an example of a progression of a problem that clearly involved the cervical spine following the auto accidents but now was involving other tunnels as well?

- The initial treatment involved self cervical traction (Fig. 6.6) and breathing. The result in 24 hours was to abolish the right wrist pain, but now she complained of left wrist pain due to using the left wrist and hand for self-traction. Examination of the left wrist uncovered slight carpal dysfunction secondary to the recent rollerblade fall on the wrists. Self-mobilization of the left wrist cleared that complaint in 24 hours and it did not return.

- Progression of treatment through the foam rollers and self-mobilization of the neural tissues cleared all symptoms, and she has remained free of any arm symptoms for 6 months.

- Slight ongoing neck discomfort associated with stress from data entry is relieved with the home program.

Summary

Even though diagnostic procedures are more thorough and treatment is growing more sophisticated, much additional research is needed to aid in devising improved evaluation and treatment procedures for the TOS patient. The ability to change symptoms and signs early in the course of the condition needs to be followed over time to see if early intervention will have a long-term affect on the course of the pathology.

References

1. Sunderland S: Sixth biennial conference proceedings, Manipulative Therapists Association of Australia, Adelaide, 1989
2. Roos DB: New concepts of thoracic outlet syndrome that explain etiology, symptoms, diagnosis and treatment. Vasc Surg 13:313, 1979
3. Telford ED, Mottershead S: The "costoclavicular syndrome." 1:325, 1947
4. Sanders RJ, Ratzin Jackson CG, Banchero N, Pearce WH: Scalene muscle abnormalities in traumatic thoracic outlet syndrome. 159:231, 1990
5. Kandel ER, Schwartz JH: Principles of Neural Science, Edward Arnold, London, 1981
6. Phillips H, Grieve GP: The thoracic outlet syndrome. p. 359. In Grieve G (ed): Modern Manual Therapy of the Vertebral Column. Churchill Livingstone, New York, 1986
7. Sanders J, Haug CE: Thoracic Outlet Syndrome. Philadelphia, JB Lippincott, 1991
8. Pratt NE: Neurovascular entrapment in the regions of the shoulder and posterior triangle of the neck. Phys Ther 48:1894, 1986
9. Karas S: Thoracic outlet syndrome. Clin Sports Med 9:297, 1990
10. Lord JW, Rosati LM: Thoracic-outlet syndromes. Clinical Symposia, CIBA Pharmaceutical Company, Summit, N, 1971
11. Edgelow PI: Thoracic outlet syndrome: a patient centered treatment approach. p. 132. In Shackloch MO (ed): Moving in on Pain. Butterworth-Heinemann, Sydney, 1995
12. Butler D: Mobilisation of the Nervous System, Churchill Livingstone, London, 1991
13. Gifford L: Fluid movement may partially account for the behavior of symptoms associated with nociception in disc injury and disease. In Shacklock M (ed): Moving in on Pain. Butterworth-Heineman, Sydney, 1995
14. Nichols HM: Anatomic structures of the thoracic outlet. Clin Orthop 207:13, 1986
15. Peet RM, Henriksen JD, Anderson TP, Martin GM: Thoracic outlet syndrome. Mayo Clinic Proc 31:281, 1956
16. Lindgren KA, Leino E: Subluxation of the first rib: A possible thoracic outlet syndrome mechanism. Arch Phys Med Rehabil 68:692, 1988
17. Celegin Z: Thoracic outlet syndrome: What does it mean for physiotherapists? p. 825. In Proceedings of IXth Congress World Confederation for Physical Therapy, Stockholm, 1982
18. Elvey RL: The investigation of arm pain. p. 530. In Grieve G (ed): Modern Manual Therapy of the Vertebral Column. Churchill Livingstone, New York, 1986
19. Sallstrom J, Schmidt H: Cervicobrachial disorders in certain occupations with special reference to compression in the thoracic outlet. Am J Ind Med 6:45, 1984
20. Hursh LF, Thanki A: The thoracic outlet syndrome. Postgrad Med 77:197, 1985

21. Crawford FA: Thoracic outlet syndrome. Surg Clin North Am 60:947, 1980

22. Kabat H: Low Back and Leg Pain from Herniated Cervical Disc. St. Louis, Warren H. Green, 1980

23. Adson AW: Surgical treatment for symptoms produced by cervical ribs and the scalenus anticus muscle. Surg Gynecol 85:687, 1947 Reprinted in Clin Orthop 207:3, 1986

24. Wood VE, Twito R, Verska JM: Thoracic outlet syndrome. The results of first rib resection in 100 patients. Orthop Clin North Am 19:131, 1988

25. Narakas A, Bonnard C, Egloff DV: The ceravico thoracic outlet compression syndrome. Analysis of surgical treatment. Ann Chir Main 5:195, 1986

26. Upton ARM, McComas AJ: The double crush in nerve entrapment syndromes. Lancet 2:359, 1973

27. Osterman AL: The double crush syndrome. Orthop Clin North Am 19:147, 1988

28. Liebenson CS: Thoracic outlet syndrome: Diagnosis and conservative management. J Manipulative Physiol Ther 11:493, 1988

29. Young HA, Hardy DG: Thoracic outlet syndrome. Br J Hosp Med 29:457, 1983

30. Roos DB, Owens JC: Thoracic outlet syndrome. Arch Surg 93:71, 1966

31. Etheredge S, Wilbur B, Stoney RJ: Thoracic outlet syndrome. Am J Surg 138:175, 1979

32. Karas S: Thoracic outlet syndrome. Clin Sports Med 9:297, 1990

33. Riddell DH, Smith BM: Thoracic and vascular aspects of thoracic outlet syndrome. Clin Orthop 207:31, 1986

34. Machleder HI: Thoracic outlet syndromes: New concepts from a century of discovery. Cardiovasc Surg 2:137, 1994

35. Pascarelli E, Quilter D: Repetitive Strain Injury: A Computer User's Guide. John Wiley & Sons, New York, 1994

36. Baxter BT, Blackburn D, Payne K, Pearche WH, Yao JST: Noninvasive evaluation of the upper extremity. Surg Clin North Am 70:87, 1990

37. Sucher BM: Thoracic outlet syndrome—A myofascial variant, 1. Pathology and diagnosis. JAOA 90:686, 1990

38. Dawson DM, Hallett M, Millender LH: Thoracic outlet syndromes in Entrapment Neuropathies. Little, Brown, Boston, 1983

39. Chodoroff G, Dong WLG, Honet JC: Dynamic approach in the diagnosis of thoracic outlet syndrome using somatosensory evoked responses. Arch Phys Med Rehabil 66:3, 1985

40. Pavot AP, Ignacio DR: Value of infrared imaging in the diagnosis of thoracic outlet syndrome. Thermology 1:142, 1986

41. McNair JFS, Maitland GD: Manipulative therapy technique in the management of some thoracic syndromes. In Grant R (ed). Physical Therapy of the Cervical and Thoracic Spine. Churchill Livingstone, New York, 1988

7

Evaluation and Treatment of Brachial Plexus Lesions

BRUCE H. GREENFIELD

DORIE B. SYEN

The brachial plexus supplies both motor and sensory innervation to the upper extremities and related shoulder girdle structures. Lesions to the brachial plexus compromise the neurologic integrity, and hence the function, of the shoulder and related upper extremity. Evaluation of shoulder dysfunction should include an assessment of the integrity and functional status of the brachial plexus. The complex structure of the brachial plexus requires a thorough understanding of the multiple innervation patterns to the various muscles. An understanding of the mechanisms of injuries to the brachial plexus, pathophysiologic changes of nerve fibers and nerve roots, and potential for recovery is essential for proper and effective clinical management. Therefore, this chapter provides a review of the anatomy of the brachial plexus, classification of brachial plexus injuries, description of pathomechanical and pathologic changes to the specific nerve fibers and nerve roots, and a review of a clarifying evaluation to assess the nature and extent of brachial plexus lesions. Clinical case studies offer a combined physical and occupational therapy management of a patient with a brachial plexus injury.

Anatomy of the Brachial Plexus

The anatomy of the brachial plexus is divided into a review of the gross anatomy of the plexus and its relationship to surrounding structures, as well as a review of the microscopic anatomy of the nerve and nerve trunks.

SUPERFICIAL ANATOMY

The brachial plexus comprises the anterior primary divisions of spinal segments C5, C6, C7, C8, and T1, as shown in Figure 7.1. The components of the brachial plexus include the following:

1. Undivided anterior primary rami
2. Trunks—upper, middle, lower
3. Divisions of the trunks—anterior and posterior
4. Cords—lateral, posterior, and medial
5. Branches—peripheral nerves derived from the cords

The segmental motor innervation of the brachial plexus to the muscles of the shoulder is shown in Figure 7.2. The anatomy of the plexus has been previously described.[1] The fourth cervical nerve usually gives a branch to the fifth cervical, and the first thoracic nerve frequently receives one from the second thoracic. When the branch from C4 is large, the branch from T2 is frequently absent and the branch from T1 is reduced in size. This constitutes the prefixed type of plexus. Conversely, when the branch from C4 is small or ab-

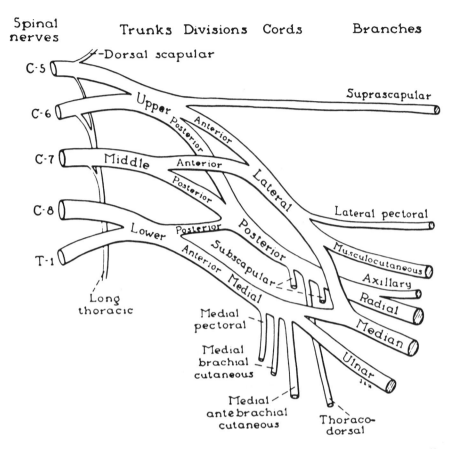

FIGURE 7.1 *Segmental motor innervation of the muscles of the shoulder. (From Hollinshead,[53] with permission.)*

sent, the contribution of C5 is reduced in size, that of T1 is larger, and the branch from T2 is always present. This arrangement constitutes the post fixed type of plexus.

The most typical arrangement of the brachial plexus is as follows. The fifth and sixth cervical nerves unite at the lateral border of the scalenus medius muscles to form the upper trunk of the plexus. The eighth cervical and first thoracic nerves unite behind the scalenus anterior to form the lower trunk of the plexus, while the seventh cervical nerve itself constitutes the middle trunk. These three trunks travel downward and laterally and just above or behind the clavicle, each splitting into an anterior and a posterior divi-

sion. The anterior division of the upper and middle trunks unite to form a cord, which is situated on the lateral side of the axillary artery and is called the lateral cord. The anterior division of the lower trunk passes downward, first behind and then on the medial side of the axillary artery, and forms the medial cord; this cord frequently receives fibers from the seventh cervical nerve. The posterior divisions of all three trunks unite to form the posterior cord, which is situated at first above and then behind the axillary artery.[1]

Autonomic sympathetic nerve fibers are present in all parts of the brachial plexus, consisting mostly of postganglionic fibers derived from the sympathetic ganglionated chain. The

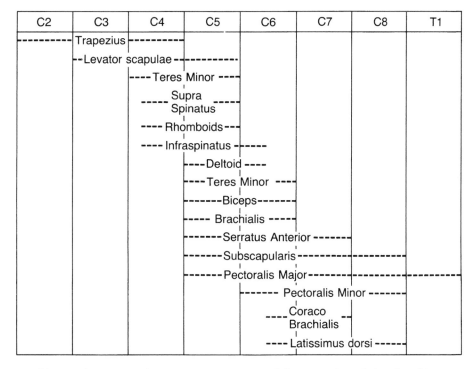

FIGURE 7.2 *Additional segmental motor innervation of the muscles of the shoulder.*

only preganglionic fibers in the brachial plexus are those of primary ramus T1.[1] Because the sympathetic supply to the eye travels through the T1 nerve root, the occurrence of Horner's syndrome, characterized by constriction of the pupil and ptosis of the eyelid on the involved side, in a patient who has sustained a traction injury is presumptive evidence of avulsion to that root.[2]

ANATOMIC RELATIONSHIPS TO THE BRACHIAL PLEXUS

The clinician should understand the relationship of the brachial plexus to the anatomic structures about the neck, shoulder girdle, and arms. To effectively isolate a plexus lesion, especially in the presence of open trauma, the clinician must identify the plexus and its relationship to the anatomic structures. For example, knowledge of the portion of plexus that lies between the clavicle and the first rib, in the presence of clavicular fracture, can help the clinician isolate the af-

fected nerve and predict the affected muscles. Topographic relationships of the plexus are delineated in *Gray's Anatomy.*[1]

In the neck, the brachial plexus is situated in the posterior triangle, which is the angle between the clavicle and the lower posterior border of the sternocleidomastoid muscle. The plexus in this area is covered by skin, platysma, and deep fascia.

The plexus emerges between the scalenus anterior and scalenus medius muscles, passes behind the anterior convexity of the medial two-thirds of the clavicle, and lies on the first digitation of the serratus anterior and subscapularis muscles. In the axilla, the lateral and posterior cords of the plexus are on the lateral side of the axillary artery and the medial cord is behind the axillary artery. The cords surround the middle part of the axillary artery on three sides, the medial cord lying on the medial side, the posterior cord behind, and the lateral cord on the lateral side of the axillary artery. In the lower part of the axilla, the cord split into the nerves for the upper limb.

ANATOMY OF THE NERVE TRUNKS

The nerve trunks and their branches are composed of parallel bundles of nerve fibers comprising the efferent and afferent axons and their ensheathing Schwann cells, which in some cases contain myelin sheaths.[1] The fibers are grouped together within trunks in a number of fasciculi, each of which contains from a few to many hundreds of nerve fibers. The architecture of the nerve trunk is shown in Figure 7.3. A dense irregular connective tissue sheath, the epineurium, surrounds the whole trunk, and a similar but less fibrous perineurium encloses each fasciculus of nerve fibers. The spaces between nerve fibers are penetrated by a loose delicate connective tissue network, the endoneurium. These connective tissue sheaths serve as planes of access for the vasculature of peripheral nerves, as well as protective cushions for the nerve fibers.

Features of Nerve Trunks Providing Protection from Physical Deformation

Several factors protect the brachial plexus and related nerve trunks from both traction and deformation injuries. First, with two notable exceptions, the ulnar nerve at the elbow and the sciatic nerve at the hip, the nerve trunks cross the flexor aspect of joints. Because extension is more limited in range than flexion, the nerves are subjected to less tension during limb movements.

Second, the nerve trunk runs an undulating course in its bed, the funiculi run an undulating course in the epineurium, and the nerve fibers run an undulating course inside the funiculi, as shown in Figure 7.4. This means that the length of nerve fibers between any two fixed points on the limb is considerably greater than the distance between those points.

Third, during traction, the perineurium, by virtue of a relatively large amount of elastic fibers compared with the endoneurium and epi-

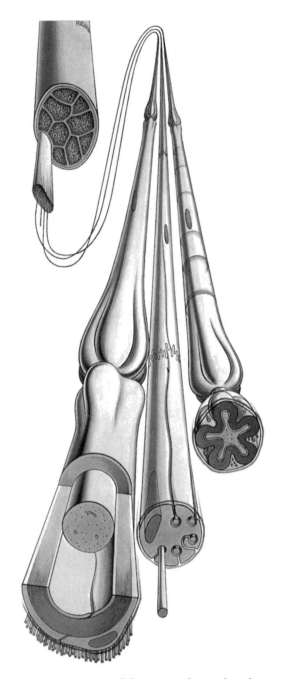

FIGURE 7.3 *Structural features of peripheral nerve fibers and a nerve trunk cut away, showing a large number of fasciculi, which each contain a large number of nerve fibers. (From Williams and Warwick,[1] with permission.)*

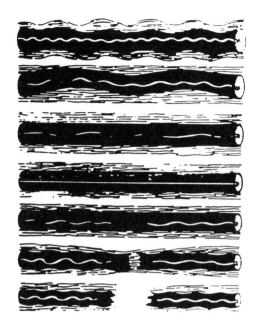

FIGURE 7.4 *Example of the undulating structure of the funiculi, which contains nerve fibers of a nerve trunk to the point of failure. (From Sunderland,*[3] *with permission.)*

neurium, imparts a degree of elasticity in the nerve trunk. Fourth, each peripheral nerve contains, within the nerve trunk, a large amount of epineurial connective tissue that separates the fasciculi. According to Sunderland,[3] values of epineurial connective tissue of various peripheral nerves range in the body from 30 to 75 percent of the cross-sectional area of the total number of nerve fibers contained in each nerve trunk. Therefore, the epineurium, by providing a loose matrix for the contained fasciculi, cushions the nerve fibers against deforming forces.

Features of the Nerve Roots Providing Protection from Injury

The nerve roots at the intervertebral foramen possess several mechanisms that protect them from traction injury.[3] Repetitive strains are placed on the nerve roots forming the brachial plexus during normal cervical spine, shoulder girdle, and shoulder motions. Overstretching of

nerve roots by transmitted forces generated in this manner is normally prevented by the following factors.

First, the dura is adherent to and part of the nerve complex at the level of the intervertebral foramen, so that when traction pulls the entire system outward, a dural funnel is drawn laterally into the foramen. The dura, at a junction of the intervertebral foramen, being cone-shaped, plugs the foramen in such a way as to resist further displacement of the nerve (Fig. 7.5). Second, the fourth, fifth, sixth, and seventh cervical nerve roots are securely attached to the vertebral column. Each nerve root, on leaving the foramen, is lodged into the gutter of the corresponding transverse process, bound securely by reflections of the prevertebral fascia and by slips from the dura attachment to the transverse processess (Fig. 7.5). Sunderland suggests that the significance of this attachment emerges on examination of the relative susceptibility to avulsion injury of the several nerve roots contributing to the brachial plexus. Traction injuries, which do not avulse nerve roots, more commonly involve the spinal nerves where these attachments exist, whereas the incidence of avulsion injuries is much higher in the case of the nerve roots, which do not have these soft tissue attachments to the transverse processes.

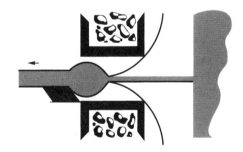

FIGURE 7.5 *Displacement of the nerve complex laterally through the foramen is resisted by plugging the funnel-shaped dura, as well as the dural attachment to the transverse process. (From Sunderland,*[3] *with permission.)*

Classification of Brachial Plexus Injuries

Numerous types of classifications of brachial plexus injuries have been proposed (Table 7.1). The majority of brachial plexus lesions result from trauma, either direct, as if struck by an instrument, or indirect, as in a traction lesion to the cervical spine or upper extremity.[5–12] Lesions may be described as preganglionic or postganglionic. Preganglionic avulsion injuries indicate that the nerve root has been torn from the spinal cord and preclude the possibility of recovery. Post ganglionic lesions may be either in continu-

TABLE 7.1. *Etiologic classification of brachial plexus injuries as related to the shoulder and cervical spine*

Traumatic
    Open injuries
        Fractures
    Closed injuries
        Fractures
        Obstetric
        Postnatal exogenous
    Sports injuries (e.g. 'burner' syndrome, shoulder dislocations)
Compression
    Exogenous (sometimes isolated branches)
    Anatomic predisposition (sometimes isolated branches)
    Genetically determined (sometimes isolated branches)
    Posture (muscle imbalances/spasms)
Tumors
    Primary tumors of brachial plexus
    Secondary involvement of plexus by tumors of surrounding tissues
Vascular
    Local vascular processes or lesions
    Participation in generalized vasculopathies (e.g., polyarteritis nodosa and lupus erythematosus)
Physical factors
    Radiotherapy
    Electric shock
Infectious, inflammatory, and toxic processes
    Involvement of local sepsis
    Viral or infectious
Cryptogenic (neuralgic amyotrophy)
    Parainfectious
    Related to serum therapy
    Genetic predisposition
    Cryptogenic

(Modified from Mumenthaler et al,[9] with permission.)

ity (root and sheath intact) or ruptured (root intact and nerve sheath ruptured).[4] Spontaneous recovery may occur with the first injury; but without surgical repair of the rupture, no recovery will occur in the second lesion.

Finally, the postganglionic avulsion is classified as either supraclavicular, which involves the trunks and divisions of the plexus, or infraclavicular, which involves the cords and branches.[5] In a series of 420 brachial plexus cases that underwent operations, Alnot reported that 75 percent were supraclavicular lesions and 25 percent were infraclavicular lesions.[5]

SUPRACLAVICULAR LESION

Isolated supraclavicular lesions affect the upper, middle, or lower trunks of the brachial plexus. However, according to Alnot, in his series of patients, 15 percent of the supraclavicular lesions were double level, affecting two trunks, or combined supraclavicular and infraclavicular lesions. These lesions occur when the arm is forced violently into abduction and the middle part of the plexus is blocked temporarily in the coracoid region. Terminal branches are torn away and concomitant supraclavicular lesions occur when the head is jerked violently to the opposite side. Lower down in the plexus, the musculocutaneous nerve (which is tightly attached near the origin of the coracobrachialis muscle), the axillary nerve in the quadrilateral space behind the shoulder, or the suprascapular nerve in the suprascapular notch of the scapula is entrapped and torn.[5–6]

UPPER TRUNK LESION

Palsy of the C5 and C6 roots of the brachial plexus is known as Erb's palsy or Duchenne-Erb paralysis.[7] The muscles affected include the deltoid, biceps, brachialis, infraspinatus, supraspinatus, and serratus anterior. Also usually involved are the rhomboids, levator scapula, and supinator muscles. Therefore, this injury causes severe restriction of movement at the shoulder and elbow joints. The patient is unable to abduct or externally rotate the shoulder. The patient cannot supinate the forearm because of weakness of the supinator muscle. Sensory involvement is usually confined along the deltoid muscle and along the distribution of the musculocutaneous nerve. According to Comtet et al.[7] partial or total spontaneous recovery of traumatic Duchenne-Erb paralysis is a frequent occurrence. The delay between the injury and reinnervation of the corresponding muscle varies from 3 to 24 months. Therefore, long-term rehabilitation with periods of reevaluations is imperative.

MIDDLE TRUNK LESION

The middle trunk receives innervation from the C7 nerve root and courses distally to form a major portion of the posterior cord.[7] The middle trunk offers a major neural contribution to the radial nerve. Therefore, a lesion affecting the middle trunk of the brachial plexus weakens the extensor muscles of the arm and forearm, excluding the brachioradialis, which receives primary innervation from the C6 nerve root. Sensory deficit occurs along the radial distribution of the posterior arm and forearm and along the dorsal radial aspect of the hand. Brunelli and Brunelli found 11 percent of a total series of brachial plexus injuries were isolated lesions to the middle trunk.[8] Middle trunk lesions were produced by trauma to the shoulder in an anteroposterior direction.

LOWER TRUNK LESION

The lower trunk of the brachial plexus receives innervation from nerve roots C7 and T1. Therefore, injury to the lower trunk known as Dejerine Klumpke, affects motor control in the fingers and wrist. The extent of disability is determined by whether the plexus is prefixed or postfixed. The intrinsic muscles of the hand are only slightly affected in a lesion involving a prefixed plexus, whereas paralysis of the flexors of the hand and forearm occur in a lesion to a postfixed plexus.[9] Sensory deficit is present along the ulnar border of the arm, forearm, and hand. Horner's syndrome occurs if the sympathetic fibers contained within the anterior primary ramus of T1 are injured.[2] The sympathetic fibers of T1 provide motor control to the eye.

INFRACLAVICULAR LESION

Infraclavicular lesions include injuries to the cords or the individual peripheral nerves of the brachial plexus. In Alnot's series of 105 patients with infraclavicular brachial plexus injuries, 90 percent of the cases were seen in young people (15 to 30 years of age) after car or motorcycle accidents.[5] The causes included (1) anteromedial shoulder dislocation, which caused most of the isolated lesions of the axillary nerve and the posterior cord; (2) violent downward and backward movement of the shoulder, which caused stretching of the plexus; and (3) complex trauma with multiple fractures of the clavicle, scapula, or upper extremity of the humerus, which caused more diffused lesions affecting multiple cords and terminal branches.

LATERAL CORD LESION

According to Alnot,[5] injury to the lateral cord is rare. Because the musculocutaneous nerve and the lateral head of the median nerve are affected, motor deficit consists of palsy of elbow flexion, associated with a deficit of muscle pronators of the forearm and wrist and finger flexors. When the lesion is proximal, the lateral pectoral nerve is injured, resulting in partial or total palsy of the upper portion of the pectoralis major muscle. Sensory deficit is localized at the forearm and at the thumb level.

MEDIAL CORD LESION

Isolated injury to the medial cord is also rare. Upper medio-ulnar palsy results in injury that is total in the distribution of the ulnar nerve and only partial in the distribution of the median nerve, the flexor pollicis longus muscle, and the flexor digitorum profundus muscle of the index finger. Partial palsy of the lower portion of the pectoralis muscle results in injury to the medial pectoral nerve.[5]

POSTERIOR CORD LESION

A posterior cord lesion involves the areas of distribution of the radial, axillary, subscapular, and thoracodorsal nerves. The lesion results in weakness of the extensors in the arm, with impairment of medial rotation and elevation of the arm at the shoulder.

PERIPHERAL NERVE LESION

Common peripheral nerve or branch injuries include, but are not limited to, lesions of the long thoracic nerve, axillary nerve, dorsal scapular nerve, and suprascapular nerve. Injuries to the dorsal scapular and suprascapular nerves are reviewed in Chapter 4

LONG THORACIC NERVE LESION

The long thoracic nerve originates from the anterior primary rami of C5, C6, and C7 nerve roots after these nerves emerge from their respective intervertebral foramen. The nerve reaches the serratus anterior muscle by traversing the neck behind the brachial plexus cords, entering the medial aspect of the axilla, and continuing downward along the lateral wall of the thorax.[1] Although isolated injuries to the long thoracic nerve are rare, traumatic wounds or traction injuries to the neck that result in isolated weakness of the serratus anterior muscle with winging of the medial border of the scapula are presumptive evidence of a long thoracic nerve lesion.[2] Normal shoulder abduction and flexion results from a synchronized pattern of movements between scapula rotation and humeral bone elevation. Variations in the scapulohumeral rhythm in the literature have been reported.[13–16] For every 15° of abduction of the arm, 10° occurs at the glenohumeral joint and 5° occurs from rotation of the scapula along the posterior thoracic wall.[13] The rotation of the scapula results from a force couple mechanism combining the upward pull of the upper trapezius muscle, the downward pull of the lower trapezius muscle, and the outward pull of the serratus anterior muscle.[16] Therefore, palsy of the serratus anterior muscle in the presence of a long thoracic nerve injury, during abduction or flexion of the arm, results in partial loss of scapular rotation. The ability of the upper and lower trapezius muscles to temporarily compensate the loss of the serratus anterior muscle to externally rotate the scapula allows for close to full range (180°) flexion and abduction of the arm.[17] However, these muscles quickly fatigue after four or five repetitions, resulting in significant loss of full active shoulder flexion and abduction range of motion.

AXILLARY NERVE LESION

The axillary nerve originates from spinal segments C5 and C6, travels to the distal aspect of the posterior cord of the brachial plexus, and advances laterally through the axilla.[1] The nerve bends around the posterior aspect of the surgical neck of the humerus to innervate the deltoid muscle and the overlying skin, as well as the teres minor muscle.

The most frequent cause of isolated axillary nerve lesion is anteromedial shoulder dislocation.[5,7] In 80 percent of cases, anteromedial dislocation results in a neuropraxia of the axillary nerve, with total recovery in 4 to 6 months.[5]

Complete lesion to the axillary nerve results in loss of active shoulder abduction. Sensory changes include an area of anesthesia along the deltoid muscle. However, even in the presence of a total axillary nerve lesion, some active shoulder abduction and external rotation is possible. Residual shoulder abduction results from the actions of the supraspinatus and infraspinatus muscles, as well as the biceps muscle. The stabilization of the humeral head by the supraspinatus muscle combined with the action of the long head of the biceps muscle allows, in some cases, full overhead abduction. Specifically, by externally rotating the arm, the patient places the long head of the biceps muscle in the line of abduction pull. However, the strength of abduction under these conditions is poor, and loss of muscle power occurs quickly with repetitive movements.

Pathomechanics of Traumatic Injuries to the Nerves

According to Stevens, the majority of traumatic injuries to the brachial plexus results in traction or tensile strains.[18] The brachial plexus is stretched between two firm points of attachment, the transverse processes proximally and the clavopectoral fascial junction distally, in the upper axilla. Stevens compares the cords of the plexus as a traction apparatus with a neutral axis at the C7 vertebra, when the arm is at the horizontal position. Specifically, he compares the brachial plexus as a single cord with five separate points of attachment firmly snubbed at the transverse processes, as shown in Figure 7.6. According to Stevens, a traction apparatus must have a neutral axis and a line of resistance. When the force of traction falls through this neutral center of axis at the C7 vertebra, the traction is equally borne by all parts of the apparatus, represented by nerve roots C5 through T1. A slight deviation from this neutral axis creates an unequal pull to one side or the other of the apparatus. That is, if the line of traction falls outside the neutral axis of C7, the entire force is transmitted from the neutral axis and all tension is released on the cords on the other side. Therefore, if tension is imparted to an arm elevated above the horizontal, stress is increased to the lower roots of the brachial plexus. Conversely, if tension is imparted to an arm depressed below the horizontal, stress is increased to the upper roots of the brachial plexus (Fig. 7.6)[18] Therefore, the relative position of the shoulder and neck at the time of injury, as well as the magnitude of the forces, dictates the area and extent of injury to the brachial plexus.

Musculoskeletal Injuries

As previously mentioned, a majority of brachial plexus injuries result from trauma, and occur as a complication of musculoskeletal injuries. Examples of these injuries include the so-called "burner syndrome," shoulder dislocations, and fractures.

"BURNER" SYNDROME

The "burner" or "stinger" syndrome is one of the most common type of sports injuries that occur to the upper trunk of the brachial plexus.[6,10-12] This injury often has been thought to occur secondary to traction to the brachial plexus when an athlete sustains a lateral flexion injury to the neck. Specifically, the syndrome is an abrupt change in the neck and shoulder angle, as experienced by football players making a tackle, with depression of the shoulder and rotation of the neck to the contralateral shoulder.[6,10-11] Markey et al reported another common mechanism of injury due to compression of the fixed brachial plexus between the shoulder pad and the superior medial scapula when the pad is pushed into the area of Erb's point.[10] Regardless of the mechanism of injury, at the time of injury the athlete

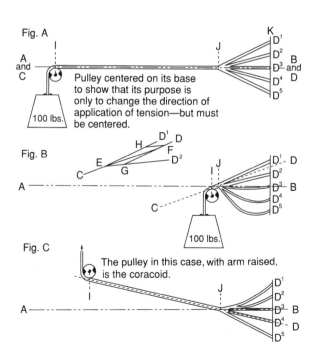

FIGURE 7.6 *Traction apparatus representing brachial plexus. (From Stevens,*[18] *with permission.)*

relates a stinging or burning pain, radiating from the shoulder into the arm.[10-12] Location of the lesion varies, and cervical root avulsion has been seen in severe cases.

Most "burner" injuries are self-limiting and resolve within minutes of insult. Potential problems include persistent neck tenderness and upper extremity weakness. If these problems persist, electromyography should be performed at 3 to 4 weeks to assess for serious nerve damage.[10-12]

DISLOCATIONS

Injuries to the brachial plexus can occur as a result of shoulder dislocation. The incidence of secondary brachial plexus injury after shoulder dislocation ranges from 2 to 35 percent in the literature. Guven et al. reported the "unhappy triad" at the shoulder that included concomitant shoulder dislocation, rotator cuff tear, and brachial plexus injury.[19] Axillary nerve injury sometimes occurs with acute anterior dislocation of the humeral head. Wang et al. presented a case with concomitant mixed brachial plexus injury in the presence of inferior dislocation of the glenohumeral joint.[20] Travlos et al. classified brachial plexus lexions due to shoulder dislocation into diffuse infraclavicular, posterior cord, lateral cord, and medial cord injuries.[21] The type of injury partly depends on the mechanism of injury and the direction of dislocation of the humeral head.

FRACTURES

Traumatic injuries associated with fractures in the shoulder girdle and humerus bones have been associated with brachial plexus injuries. Della Santa et al. found sixteen cases of costoclavicular syndrome related to compression of the subclavian artery and brachial plexus were due to callous and scar formation as a result of fractures of the clavicle.[22] Stromquist et al. reported three cases of injury to the axillary artery and brachial plexus complicating a displaced proximal fracture of the humerus.[23] Blom and Dahlback found two cases in a series of 31 cases of

proximal humeral fractures with associates brachial plexus injuries.[24] Silliman and Dean report that an associated complication of scapular fractures around the scapular spine is suprascapular nerve injury.[6]

Pathophysiology of Injury

The extent of injury to the nerve trunk, ranging from a nondegenerative neuropraxia to a severance of the nerve or plexus (neurotmesis), will dictate the course of treatment (surgical versus nonsurgical) and the prognosis and relative time frames for full recovery.

Five major degrees of injury are described by Sunderland[25]:

1. *First-degree nerve injury*. This injury is characterized by interruption of conduction at the site of injury with preservation of the anatomic continuity of all components comprising the nerve trunk, including the axon. Clinical features include temporary loss of motor function to the affected muscles, but the presence of electric potential due to axonal continuity is retained. Cutaneous sensory loss may occur, but will recover in advance of motor function. Most patients recover spontaneously within 6 weeks after injury.

2. *Second-degree nerve injury*. In this injury, the axon is severed and fails to survive below the level of injury and, for a variable but short distance, the axon degenerates proximal to the point of the lesion. However, the endoneurium is preserved within the endoneurial tube. Histologic changes to the nerve include breakdown of the myelin sheath, Schwann cell degeneration, and phagocytic activity with eventual fibrosis. Clinical features include temporary complete loss of motor, sensory, and sympathetic functions in the autonomous distribution of the injured nerve. Several months will pass before recovery begins, with proxi-

mal reinnervation occurring before distal re-innervation to the involved muscles.

3. *Third-degree nerve injury.* This condition is characterized by axonal disintegration, Wallerian degeneration both distal and proximal to the site of the lesion, and disorganization of the internal structure of the endoneural fasciculi. The general fascicular pattern of the nerve trunk is retained with minimal damage to both the perineurium and epineurium. Because the endoneural tube is destroyed, intrafascicular fibrosis may obviate axonal regeneration. Many axons fail to reach their original or functionally related endoneurial tubes, and are instead misdirected into foreign endoneurial tubes. Clinically, motor, sensory, and sympathetic functions of the related nerves are lost. The recovery is long, up to 2 to 3 years, with a chance of significant residual dysfunction.

4. *Fourth-degree nerve injury.* This type of injury is similar to third-degree nerve injury, but the perineurium is disrupted. Therefore, the chance for a residual dysfunction due to fibrosis and mixing of regenerating fibers at the site of injury, which may distort the normal pattern of innervation, is high.

5. *Fifth-degree nerve injury.* In this injury, the entire nerve trunk is severed, with resultant complete loss of function to the affected structures. Obviously, without surgical grafting, recovery is negligible.

Clarifying Evaluation

A thorough and systematic clarifying evaluation is essential for the clinician to accurately assess the nature and extent of the brachial plexus lesion and to develop an appropriate and effective treatment plan. Because most brachial plexus lesions slowly improve over a long period of time, the clinician must maintain and update accurate records concerning the progress of the patient.

The clinician should use any one of a number of charts for recording results of the physical examination, as shown in Figure 7.7. Evaluation and treatment is a conjoint effort by a physical and an occupational therapist who specializes in the treatment of hand and upper extremity injuries. Knowledge of hand management and rehabilitation is particularly important in lower trunk injuries to the brachial plexus. Additionally, in the presence of fourth-and fifth-degree nerve injuries to the brachial plexus, occupational therapy offers strategies for splinting as well as equipment modification or assurance to assist permanently dysfunctional individuals.

History

MECHANISMS OF INJURY

Because most brachial plexus injuries result from trauma, a thorough history should include questions concerning the nature and mechanisms of injury. According to Stevens, the different varieties of stress, and the relative position of the arm and head at the time of the stress, make tremendous differences in the kinds of lesions suffered, in the locality of the lesion, and in prognosis.[18] The magnitude of forces, that is, high-speed versus slow-speed injuries, is important to ascertain. According to Frampton, high-speed, large-impact accidents are commonly associated with preganglionic plexus injuries, while slow-speed, small-impact accidents are commonly associated with postganglionic injuries.[4] Examples of high-velocity injuries are those resulting from falls from speeding motorcycles, while examples of low-velocity injuries are those resulting from a fall down a stairway.

PAIN

The area and nature of pain should be documented. Pain, described as a constant burning, crushing pain with sudden shoots of paroxysms of pain, is central in nature. This pain occurs as a result of deafferentation of the spinal cord

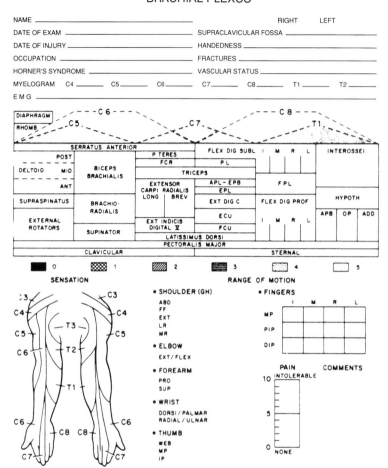

FIGURE 7.7 *Chart for recording results of physical examination for brachial plexus injury. (From Leffert[2], with permission.)*

at the damaged root level, leading to undampened excitation of the cells in the dorsal horn of the spinal cord. The confused barrage of abnormal firings is received and interpreted centrally as pain and is eventually felt in the dermatomes of the nerve root that is avulsed.[26] In a series of 188 patients with post-traumatic brachial plexus lesions, Bruxelle et al found that 91 percent experienced pain at least 3 years after injury.[26] Pain may also result from secondary injuries to bones or related soft tissues. The report of any anesthesias or paresthesias should be noted and documented. The presence of Horner's syndrome, which is characterized by en-

ophthalmos, myosis, and ptosis, along with a deficit of facial sweating on the affected side, reflects damage to the T1 nerve root. Questions concerning the course of events since injury or a change in the severity of the symptoms establish an indication of an improving or worsening lesion. A condition that is resolving spontaneously may indicate first- or second-degree nerve injuries, while a condition that has not changed across the course of 6 weeks may indicate at least a third-degree nerve injury, according to Sunderland's classification.

Finally, the clinician should document the patient's occupation, handedness, and previous state of health to assist in establishing feasible goals for return to the patient's premorbid activity level.

Physical Evaluation

The components of the physical evaluation include: (1) posture; (2) passive range of motion of the cervical spine, shoulder, and upper extremity; (3) motor strength; (4) sensation; (5) palpation; and (6) special tests. The occupational therapy evaluation includes assessment for (1) edema; (2) coordination; (3) activities of daily living; and (4) vocational and avocational pursuits. The physical evaluation should be repeated frequently during the process of rehabilitation to carefully assess subtle signs of nerve reinnervation.

POSTURE

The patient is observed from the front, side, and behind. From behind, the clinician observes for muscle atrophy as well as winging of the scapula. Winging of the scapula signifies weakness of the serratus anterior muscle, which may indicate a lesion of the long thoracic nerve. Ipsilateral atrophy of the supraspinatus or infraspinatus muscles can signify suprascapular nerve entrapment. Atrophy of the deltoid muscle, in addition to the supraspinatus and infraspinatus muscles, can indicate an upper trunk plexus lesion, such as Duchenne-Erb Paralysis of the C5 and C6 nerve trunks. Isolated atrophy of the deltoid muscle indicates an isolated axillary nerve lesion. From the side, the clinician should observe for changes consistent with a forward head posture: accentuated upper thoracic spine kyphosis, protraction and elevation of the scapulae, increased cervical spine inclination, and backward bending at the atlanto-occipital junction. The forward head posture results in muscle imbalances that can further result in entrapment of various nerves of the brachial plexus in the area of the thoracic outlet.[27] Thoracic outlet syndrome is discussed in detail in Chapter 16. From the front, the clini-

cian should observe the attitude or position of the upper extremity and hand. An arm position of adduction and internal rotation can result from Duchenne-Erb paralysis. Pronation of the forearm with flexion at the wrist and metacarpophalangeal and proximal interphalangeal joints can result from injury to the lower trunk of the brachial plexus.[7] External deformities along the clavicle, which may indicate fracture, should be noted. Both nonunions and malunions of the clavicle can result in significant compression of the brachial plexus. The supraclavicular fossa is inspected for the presence of swelling or ecchymosis in those patients with recent injury and for nodularity and induration in the brachial plexus where the injury is old.[4] The eyes are observed for constriction of the pupils or ptosis of the eyelids, which can indicate the presence of Horner's syndrome.[2]

PASSIVE RANGE OF MOTION

The passive range of motion of all joints of the shoulder girdle and upper limb must be assessed and recorded using a standard goniometer. Deficits of joint motion from immobility result in contractures of joint capsule, adhesions in the joints, and shortening of both muscle and tendons above the affected joints. The classic studies of Akeson et al demonstrated the deleterious effects of 9 weeks of immobilization on periarticular structures, including the loss of water and glycoaminoglycans, randomization and abnormal cross-linking of newly synthesized collagen, and infiltration in the joint spaces of fatty fibrous materials.[28]

MOTOR STRENGTH

Several manuals are available that review proper isolation, stabilization, and grading procedures for manual muscle testing.[29,30] Most grading systems grade muscle for 0 to 5, with 0 being a flaccid muscle and 5 representing normal muscle strength.[29] A complete upper extremity test should be performed initially to provide the clinician a data base from which to measure improvement. Therefore, retests should be performed periodically. A thorough manual muscle test assists the clinician in pinpointing the site and extent of the plexus lesion. Establishing an appropriate strengthening program is based on isolating and grading involved muscles. Isokinetic testing can also assist clinicians in measuring muscle strength deficits, usually for peak torque, power, and work, compared with the uninvolved upper extremity. Refer to Chapter 16 for a review of isokinetic testing protocols in the shoulder.

SENSATION

Assessment of sensory loss assists in the diagnosis of the level and extent of the plexus lesion. Total avulsion of the plexus results in total anesthesia of the related areas. However, in a mixed lesion, and when recovery is occurring, the sensory pattern may vary in the arm. The sensory evaluation may include deep pressure, light touch, temperature, stereognosis, and two-point discrimination, depending on the patient's status.[4] Sensory changes are documented along dermatomes, as illustrated in Figure 7.7.

COORDINATION

Loss of sensation and muscle control in the presence of a brachial plexus injury results in a loss of gross and fine motor coordination in the affected upper extremity. There are numerous tests on the market designed to assess an individual's coordination. Each requires varying amounts of fine and/or gross motor coordination. The Purdue pegboard (Lafayette Instructional Co.. Lafayette, IN), for example, assists the clinician in assessing the patient's manual dexterity. Patients are requested to place pegs with both the right and left hands, singularly and in tandem, and to perform a specific assembly task using pins, collars and washers. These tests are timed and compared with normative values.[31] The therapist should determine the most appropriate tests based on the patient's level of functioning.

VASCULAR

In the presence of severe brachial plexus injuries, particularly with associated fractures of the clavicle, disruption of the subclavian or axillary arteries may occur. Additionally, all patients who have had a significant nerve injury will have evidence of vasomotor changes.[2] Assessment of the brachial and radial pulses and inspection for dusky, cool skin indicating venous insufficiency should be performed by the clinician.

EDEMA

Edema must be assessed and treated to prevent stiffness in the joints. The concept of volumetrics to measure upper extremity edema is well established. The patient's hand is submerged in a lucite container (Volumeter, Volumeters Unlimited, Idyllwild, CA), and the amount of water displaced is measured using a 500-ml graduated cylinder. Both extremities should be measured and the results recorded. Circumferential measurements of the hand and forearm are another method of measuring edema. However, this technique is best suited for individual digit swelling or in the case of open wounds, which may preclude the patient getting the extremity wet. Manual palpation is also used to measure edema. The severity of the edema is usually rated from 1 to 3, with 1 being minimal and 3 being severe or pitting edema.

PALPATION

Manual palpation is used to assess for myofascial trigger points about the affected shoulder girdle and upper extremity musculature. Trigger points result from tight and contracted muscles or from partially denervated muscles exhibiting poor muscle control and altered movement patterns. Active trigger points refer pain into the affected upper extremity, as well as the shoulder girdle, neck, and head.[32,33]

SPECIAL TESTS

The presence of Tinel's sign, demonstrated by tapping over the brachial plexus above the clavicle, can be quite useful in distinguishing rupture from a lesion in continuity.[2,4] A distal Tinel's sign indicates a lesion in continuity where the axonal connections within the nerve trunk are intact.

This may correspond to a first-degree nerve injury or a regenerating second- or third-degree nerve injury, as described by Sunderland. Conversely, the presence of a localized tenderness to tapping above the clavicle indicates a possible neuroma resulting from disruption of part of the plexus. This type of injury would correspond to a fourth- or fifth-degree nerve injury.

ACTIVITIES OF DAILY LIVING

The patient is questioned regarding all aspects of self-care to identify those specific tasks he or she is not able to perform owing to the extent of the brachial plexus injury. Such areas include self-care skills such as feeding, bathing, grooming, and dressing, Based on the specific limitations of the patient, the occupational therapist then determines whether to provide the patient with specific adaptive equipment or to instruct the patient in one-handed techniques.

ASSESSMENT FOR SPLINTING

In the case of a complete brachial plexus injury, the patient is fitted with a flail arm splint that allows the patient to use the extremity at home and at work. The splint is fitted early, to prevent the patient from relying on one-handed methods as a means of performing specific activities.[4] In the case of a C5–7 injury, the patient might require a long wrist and finger extension assist splint (Fig. 7.8). The patient may also be fitted with a resting hand splint (Fig. 7.9) to wear at night to help maintain the wrist and fingers in a balanced position.

VOCATIONAL

A detailed job description is obtained to assess the patient's potential to return to work. In addition, a functional capacity evaluation can be performed later in the rehabilitation process to assess the patient's physical demand level.

AVOCATIONAL

Because the brachial plexus-injured patient is unable to work, avocational pursuits are often an important source of much-needed diversional activity. The occupational therapist questions the patient closely as to premorbid hobbies or potential areas of interests. Activities of interest are developed that encourage use of the affected extremity.

Laboratory Evaluations of Brachial Plexus Lesions

Also included in the overall evaluation of a patient with a brachial plexus injury are laboratory evaluations involving electrodiagnostic testing, myelography, and radiographic assessment. These evaluations help the clinician diagnose the area and extent of the lesion and provide baseline measurements to help evaluate progress.

RADIOGRAPHIC ASSESSMENT

Every patient who has sustained a significant injury to the brachial plexus should have a complete radiographic series done of the cervical spine and involved shoulder gridle, including the clavicle.[2] Fractures of the clavicle with callus, which can impinge on the nerve trunks along the costoclavicular juncture, or fractures of the cervical transverse processes, which can indicate a root avulsion, must be ruled out.[2,4]

Magnetic resonance imaging (MRI) has been used to detect injuries to the brachial plexus. Bilbey et al evaluated 64 consecutive patients with suspected brahial plexus abnormalities of diverse causes with MRI.[34] MRI was found to be 63 percent sensitive, 100 percent specific, and 73 percent accurate in demonstrating the abnormality in a diverse patient population with multiple etiologies of brachial plexus injuries.

MYELOGRAPHY

Myelography is used to indicate the status of the nerve roots in the presence of traction injuries to the brachial plexus. According to Leffert, root avulsion can occur in the presence of a normal myelogram.[2] However, a well-documented study by Yeoman indicates the efficacy of myelography as a valuable adjunct to the diagnosis of brachial plexus root lesions.[35]

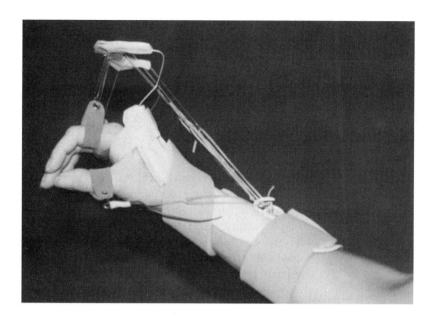

FIGURE 7.8 *A long metacarpophalangeal extension splint used with a patient who has weak wrist extension and trace finger extension.*

ELECTROMYOGRAPHY

Because the loss of axonal continuity results in predictable, time-related electric charges, knowledge and assessment of these electric charges can be used to provide information concerning muscle denervation and reinnervation.[2]

For example, while normally innervated muscle exhibits no spontaneous electric activity at rest when examined with needle electrodes, denervated muscle produces readily recognizable small potentials (fibrillations) or large potentials (sharp waves), which are the hallmark of denervation. These electric discharges usually appear 3 weeks following injury to the plexus and signal the onset of Wallerian degeneration of a

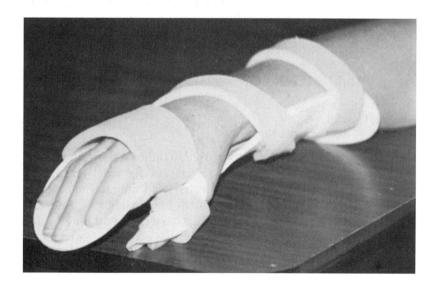

FIGURE 7.9 *A resting hand splint used following a brachial plexus lesion to prevent overstretching of weak and finger extensor muscles by maintaining the wrist in approximately 20° of dorsiflexion.*

specific nerve. The clinician is able to localize the lesion by sampling muscles innervated by different nerves and root levels.

Additionally, when a root avulsion is suspected in a patient who has sustained a traction injury of the brachial plexus, the clinician should also peform an electromyographic evaluation of the posterior cervical musculature. The posterior cervical muscles are segmentally innervated by the posterior primary rami of the spinal nerves that provide the anterior primary rami to form the plexus. Denervation of the deep posterior cervical muscles is highly correlated with root avulsion. Conversely, if the electromyogram is positive for the muscles innervated by the anterior primary rami but not for the posterior cervical muscles, whatever possible damage exists is presumed to be infraganglionic in nature.[36]

Nerve Conduction Studies

Nerve conduction velocity tests may be used to help distinguish muscular weakness in the affected upper extremity from cervical intervertebral disc protrusion, anterior horn cell disease, or a brachial plexus lesion. Because anterior horn cell diseases and intervertebral disc protrusions do not influence nerve conduction latency, the clinician can be certain that a proximal nerve conduction delay is a result of a brachial plexus lesion.[37]

Another type of electrodiagnostic testing is the F response, an outgrowth of the measurement of velocity of conduction; this is a late reaction that potentially results from the backfiring of antidromically activated anterior horn cells. Electrical stimulation of motor points assesses the strength–duration curves of affected muscles.[38] A denervated or partially denervated muscle requires more time and current than a normally innervated muscle. Serial strength–duration testing therefore allows the clinician to assess neuromuscular recovery.[38]

Rehabilitation Goals and Treatment

The approach to rehabilitation for brachial plexus lesions is directed at maintaining or improving soft tissue mobility, muscle strength and function within the constraint of the nerve injury, and function. Because regeneration is excruciatingly slow, rehabilitation in severe cases is a long-term process, lasting as long as 3 years. Therefore, patient and family education, as well as home exercise programs, are an integral component of treatment.

Surgical grafting in the presence of fourth- and fifth-degree nerve injuries necessitates, on the part of the therapist, knowledge of soft tissue healing constraints. The relatively high chance of residual upper extremity dysfunction in some cases requires vocational and avocational retraining, as well as occupational therapy intervention for assistance-providing devices and splints.

According to Framptom,[4] rehabilitation falls into three stages: the early stage, consisting of diagnosis, neurovascular repair, and education concerning passive movement and self-care of the affected extremity; the middle stage, when recovery is occurring and intensive reeducation may be indicated; and the late stage, when no future recovery is expected and assessment for reconstructive surgery can take place. The time frames and extent of each phase are predicted based on the extent of the lesion and the individual's own motivation and recuperative capabilities. Goals, treatments, and rationales for the treatments for each stage of rehabilitation are exemplified in the case study presented below.

CASE STUDY 1

This case study presents a typical brachial plexus injury affecting the shoulder and upper extremity function. Initial findings are delineated in the clarifying evaluation. The goals and phases of treatment are presented as a combined physical and occupational therapy approach. Rationales for specific treatments are presented, when relevant.

HISTORY

A 25-year-old right-handed man was involved in a motor vehicle accident and suffered a traction lesion to his brachial plexus. Electrodiagnostic testing indicated an infraganglionic lesion to his left brachial plexus at Erb's joint, that portion of the brachial plexus where C5 and C6 unite to join the upper trunk. Radiologic studies indicated no fractures at the cervical spine or clavicle. The patient was referred to physical and occupational therapy 4 weeks after the initial injury.

The patient reported numbness and tingling along the lateral aspect of his left shoulder, in the area of the deltoid muscle, and weakness in his left shoulder, elbow, wrist, and hand. He reports intermittent pain in his left shoulder and neck made worse with attempted elevation of his left arm. He reported less numbness and increased strength in his left arm since the initial injury.

VOCATION

The patient works as a carpenter.

POSTURAL/VISUAL INSPECTION

Atrophy was observed in the deltoid, supraspinatus, and infraspinatus muscles on the left compared with the right side. His left arm was held in internal rotation along his lateral trunk, with his forearm pronated and his wrist and fingers in slight flexion.

PASSIVE RANGE OF MOTION

Elevation in the plane of scapula measured 120°, external rotation in adduction measured 30°, external rotation in 45° abduction measured 60°, and external rotation in 90° abduction measured 70°. His elbow, forearm, wrist, and hand passive range of motion were all within normal limits.

ACTIVE RANGE OF MOTION

Elevation in the plane of scapula measured 60°, external rotation in adduction from full internal rotation measured 20°, elbow flexion measured 30°, and supination measured 50°. The patient had full pronation and wrist and finger flexion and extension.

MOTOR STRENGTH

Motor strength was graded as follows:

- Grade 0 = no contraction
- Grade 1 = trace
- Grade 2 = poor
- Grade 3 = fair
- Grade 4 = good
- Grade 5 = normal

The patient's muscles were graded as follows: deltoid = 2, supraspinatus = 3, infraspinatus = 3, teres minor = 2, biceps brachii = 2, brachialis = 2, serratus anterior = 5, subscapularis = 3, extensor carpi radialis longus and brevis = 3, and supinator = 3. His grip strength was 88 lb on the right and 10 lb on the left.

SENSATION

Sensation was impaired to light touch and to sharp/dull along the lateral aspect of the left shoulder, in the area of the deltoid muscle, and along the radial side of the forearm.

COORDINATION

Coordination was assessed using the Purdue pegboard and rated as follows: right hand, 14; left hand, 2; both hands, 4; assembly task, 6.

EDEMA

The patient had 2 + edema palpated along the dorsum of the left fingers at the proximal interphalangeal joints and metacarpal joints and along the dorsum of the left hand. His volumetric measurements were 482 cc on the right and 525 cc on the left.

PALPATION

Trigger points were palpated in muscle bellies of the left upper trapezius, left rhomboid, and left subscapularis muscles.

ACTIVITIES OF DAILY LIVING (ADL)

The patient was unable to perform the following self-care activities:

- *Feeding*—unable to cut his food.
- *Bathing*—unable to wash his right shoulder and upper arm.
- *Grooming*—unable to apply deodorant to his right underarm.
- *Dressing*—unable to tie shoes, button shirt, zip pants or jacket, or buckle belt.

ASSESSMENT

This is a patient whose history revealed a traction injury to the upper trunk of the brachial plexus involving nerve trunks C5 and C6. Because he demonstrated at least poor muscle control of the affected muscles, which is spontaneously improving since the initial injury, the extent of the injury is classified as between a first- and second-degree injury, according to Sunderland's classification.[25] Therefore, one can expect combined resolution of nerve function, with full return of function of the left upper extremity.

Passive range of motion is moderately limited in the affected shoulder with restrictions of the related joint capsule, fascia, tendon, and muscle. Soft tissue limitations are consistent with the findings of Akeson et al.,[28] Tabary et al.,[39] and Cooper,[40] who studied the affects of immobilization on periarticular capsule, tendon, and muscle, respectively. The loss of motor control results in altered scapulohumeral rhythm. The rotator cuff muscles, particularly the supraspinatus, infraspinatus, and teres minor muscles, are unable to adequately control gliding of the humeral head during elevation of the shoulder. The resultant weakness, even in the presence of a weak deltoid muscle, results in impingement of the suprahumeral soft tissues underneath the unyielding corocoacromial ligament. Chronic impingement results in inflammation and degeneration of the rotator cuff tendons.

Compensation of the scapula muscles to elevate the arm in the presence of weakness of the rotator cuff and deltoid muscles results in irritation and trigger points in both the left upper trapezius and left rhomboid muscles. A trigger point palpated in the subscapularis muscle is the result of the shoulder and arm positioned in internal rotation and along the lateral trunk wall, which maintained the subscapularis muscle in a shortened position. The contracted subscapularis muscle resulted in the greater limitation of passive external rotation with the arm adducted along the lateral trunk wall, as opposed to external rotation with the arm abducted to 45° or 90°. (R. Donatelli, personal communication.)

The weakness in the left upper extremity and hand result in a loss of normal muscle pumping activity to remove interstitial fluid. In addition, the patient tended to keep his arm down at his side. These two factors result in increased edema in the left upper extremity, especially the left fingers and hand, compared with the right. The weakness in the left upper extremity, as well as the patient's decreased manual dexterity, interfered with some self-care activities. Fortunately, the patient is right-handed, which will expedite his return to employment as a carpenter.

REHABILITATION GOALS AND TREATMENT

EARLY STAGE

FIRST GOAL

The first goal is to reduce pain.

TREATMENT. Heat, low-voltage surge stimulation, and spray and stretch (see Ch. 12) were applied to the active trigger points in the left upper trapezius and left rhomboid muscles in our patient. Transcutaneous neuromuscular stimulation, using a high-rate, low-intensity conventional setting with dual channels and four electrodes, was applied around the left shoulder. The transcutaneous neuromuscular stimulation device was worn 8 hours per day.

RATIONALE. According to Travell and Simons, myofascial trigger points in the shoulder girdle muscles refer pain into the left shoulder and arm in a consistent pattern.[32] Therefore, reduction of trigger point tenderness in the left upper trapezius and left rhomboid muscles will alleviate part of this patient's pain. The conventional transcutaneous neuromuscular stimulation setting stimulates large A-beta sensory fibers that modulate impulses from the small A-delta and C fibers in the dorsal horn of the spinal cord.[41,42] Pain impulses along the A-delta and C fibers in this patient resulted from irritation of nociceptor endings in the connective tissue sheaths surrounding the nerve fibers and trunks, due to the traction injury.[42]

SECOND GOAL

The second goal is to restore full passive range of motion and soft tissue mobility.

TREATMENT. In our patient, low-voltage surge stimulation followed by spray and stretch techniques were applied to the active trigger points in the muscle belly of the subscapularis. Mobilization techniques, in the grades III and IV range according to Maitland's classification, were applied to the various joints in the left upper extremity.[43] Special attention was directed at manual distraction of the specific details concerning mobilization techniques at the shoulder complex.

Patients with this condition are given a program of range of motion self-exercises in order to preserve the range of motion at those joints where there is no, or only limited, active range of motion. Each patient is given an active range of motion exercise program for the uninvolved joints so that these joints do not become restricted due to disuse of the extremity in general. The patient's family should be familiar with the exercise program so that they can encourage the patient to follow through and become active participants in the patient's rehabilitation.

RATIONALE. In our patient, the painful limitation of external rotation with the shoulder adducted along the lateral trunk wall results from a contracted subscapularis muscle. Therefore, spray and stretch, followed by distraction of the medial scapula border, elongates the subscapularis muscle and improves external rotation with the shoulder in the adducted position. Mobilization techniques at the shoulder are directed at the inferior and anterior capsules, respectively, to promote abduction and external rotation move-

ments, respectively. The scientific literature indicates no optimum time frames for applying grade IV manual stretching to the periarticular capsule. Clinically, we use three sets of 1-minute grade IV oscillations into the restricted tissue preceded by heat and followed by ice.

THIRD GOAL

The third goal is to avoid neural dissociation to the reinnervating muscles.

TREATMENT. High-frequency low-volt muscle stimulation with a pulse duration of 30 msec was applied to the partially denervated muscles. The preferred duty cycle was 10 seconds on and 20 seconds off, for a period of 30 minutes. The patient was instructed to use a home stimulator three to four times daily.

RATIONALE. According to strength-duration studies, muscle stimulation to a partially denervated muscle requires a higher current and longer pulse duration than does stimulation to a normally innervated muscle.[38] In addition to maintaining reinnervating muscle tissue viability, electrically induced muscle contractions facilitate normal circulation, decrease edema, and present potential nutritional or tropic skin changes.[44,45]

FOURTH GOAL

Reducing edema is the fourth goal.

TREATMENT. Retrograde massage was applied to the hand from a distal to proximal direction, with the patient's hand and forearm elevated above his heart.[46] In addition, the patient and his wife were provided with written instructions regarding elevation of the arm, retrograde massage, and first pumping to activate muscle pumping action in the hand and forearm.

Coban (3M Medical-Surgical, St Paul, MN) is a gentle elastic wrap used for edema control. It is wrapped diagonally from the fingertips proximally and should overlap approximately $\frac{1}{2}$ in. The advantages of Coban are that it is reusable (thus reducing costs), may be worn for prolonged periods, and allows for full range of motion.[47]

RATIONALE. Retrograde massage, in a gravity-assisted position, facilitates the reabsorption of interstitial fluids into the lymphatic system. Fist pumping, resulting in alternate contraction and relaxation of the musculature in the hand and forearm, promotes venous blood return to the heart.

FIFTH GOAL

The fifth goal is to increase the patient's ADL independence.

TREATMENT. The patient was issued adaptive equipment to increase his self-care independence until he exhibited a greater degree of motor control. For example, he was issued a rocker knife to help him cut his meat and a button hook to help him button his shirt. In addition, he was instructed in specific one-handed methods of performing certain tasks, such as tying his shoe laces.

SIXTH GOAL

Providing emotional support education is the sixth goal.

TREATMENT. Patient and family education and psychological referral were used to accomplish the sixth goal.

In certain instances, the therapist must help the patient through the initial stages of denial, anger, and depression associated with a severe brachial plexus injury. A patient's emotional state will affect his or her performance in therapy. The therapist should be an active listener and recognize the normal process of emotional recovery in patients with severe disability. Fear is a major component and compounds a patient's anxiety. This anxiety can often be reduced if the patient is educated as to the nature and extent of the injury, the course of recovery, the course of therapy, and the prognosis for recovery. One cannot stress enough the importance of involving the patient's family in the rehabilitation process. Family relationships often become strained as a result of serious injury. Financial issues may become a source of worry and concern for all involved. The family members may need as much support as the patient and will also benefit from the education process.

MIDDLE STAGE

FIRST GOAL

The first goal in the middle stage is to reeducate reinnervating muscles.

TREATMENT. Manual proprioceptive neuromuscular facilitation techniques emphasizing diagonal patterns, with the patient supine, were begun at approximately 3 weeks after the initial evaluation. Light-weight isotonic strengthening was added to the program, using adjustable-weight cuffs. Initial isotonic strengthening emphasized external rotation movement patterns at the shoulder as well as flexion and extension movements at the elbow and pronation and supination at the forearm. As strength improved, the patient was progressed to isokinetic strengthening at slow speeds of approximately 60°/s, emphasizing rotational movement patterns in the shoulder. The patient was progressed to isokinetic diagonal movement patterns in the supine position when isokinetic testing indicated a difference of left to right external rotation strength, as measured in peak torque, and power was within 20 percent. Refer to Chapter 3 for isokinetic testing and strengthening strategies for the shoulder.

Modalities such as vibration and tapping are used while the patient is exercising or performing functional activities. Appropriate sensory stimuli can evoke desired muscular responses, and this stimulation must be followed by purposeful activities if motor learning is to take place.[48] Biofeedback and neuromuscular electrical stimulation are used on selected weak muscles to facilitate muscle reeducational strength.

RATIONALE. Manual proprioceptive neuromuscular facilitation diagonals allow the clinician to assess early subtle strength changes across treatments. Early isotonic strengthening is directed at restoring strength in the shoulder rotator cuff muscles, specifically the supraspinatus, infraspinatus, and teres minor muscles. The goal is to restore, during elevation of the shoulder, the dynamic steering mechanism of the rotator cuff muscles on the humeral head.[49] The restoration of rotator cuff muscle strength reestablishes the normal balance between these muscles and the upward pull of the deltoid muscle. Isokinetic strengthening is instituted as soon as the patient is actively exercising with 1- or 2-lb weights. Isokinetic contraction offers the advantage of accommodating resistance to maximally load a contracting muscle throughout the range of motion.[50] The patient exercises at preselected speeds, beginning with slower speeds, so that he or she can consistently "catch" and maintain the speed of the dynamometer. External rotational strengthening is emphasized early, as previously mentioned, to restore the dynamic glide of the humeral head along the glenoid fossa by reestablishing strength in the supraspinatus, infraspinatus, and teres minor muscles. Isokinetic testing is performed every 2 to 3 weeks to assess peak torque and power values of the involved compared with the uninvolved upper extremity. Isokinetic diagonal strengthening patterns are performed initially supine, to eliminate the affect of the muscles working directly against gravity. Diagonal patterns are eventually performed with the patient sitting or standing, after bilateral strength deficits between the left and right shoulder rotators are within 20 percent. Although not scientifically substantiated, we have observed that when bilateral shoulder rotational strength deficits are greater than 20 percent, impingement of the suprahumeral soft tissues and pain, during active shoulder elevation, occurs.

OCCUPATIONAL THERAPY. In occupational therapy, our patient worked on tabletop activities with his left upper extremity supported. The activities were directed toward strengthening his elbow, forearm, and wrist musculature. For example, he transferred pegs from one bucket placed in front of him to a bucket placed to his far left. This activity required active elbow flexion and extension in a gravity-eliminated position. As his shoulder strength improved, he was able to perform this same activity unsupported. Additionally, he was able to stack cones, which required active shoulder abduction against gravity. He used light weights to strengthen wrist flexion and extension, supination, and pronation. Elastic rubber tubing, such as Theraband (Hygenic, Akron, OH), was used at home to improve elbow

and wrist strength. He was issued therapeutic putty and instructed in hand-strengthening exercises.

SECOND GOAL

The second goal is to continue mobilization to the restricted joints.

TREATMENT. Low-load prolonged stretching using surgical tubing was applied to the restricted periarticular capsules, especially the anterior aspect of the glenohumeral capsule, to promote external rotation. The patient was positioned with his shoulder in 45° of abduction and his elbow in 90° flexion. Surgical tubing attached to his wrist provided a 30-minute low-load stretch into external rotation.

RATIONALE. Using rat tail tendons, Lehman et al demonstrated that the optimum method to stretch pericapsular tissue is to use low-load prolonged stretch.[51] According to Lehman et al the prolonged stretching allows the viscoelastic material in the capsular tissue, including the water and glycoaminoglycans, to creep or to elongate with the tissue.

THIRD GOAL

If necessary, continue the third goal for edema control.

FOURTH GOAL

The fourth goal is to reevaluate the use of assistance-providing devices and to modify the use of these devices.

FIFTH GOAL

Increasing coordination is the fifth goal.

TREATMENT. As our patient's motor performance improved, coordination activities became an integral part of his treatment program. Initially, the activities focus on such gross motor skills as placing large pegs into a bucket while being timed and, later, placing those same pegs into a pegboard. As he continued to improve, the activities required more fine motor skills, such as manipulating nuts and bolts (graded from large to small), practicing on an ADL board, turning coins and so forth. All activities were timed to document progress. Trombly and Scott state that in order to increase coordination, activities should be graded along a continuum from gross to fine and that as the patient's coordination improves, the activities should require faster speeds and more accuracy.[52]

LATE STAGE

FIRST GOAL

The first goal in the late stage is to optimize muscle strengthening within the constraints of reinnervation.

TREATMENT. Isokinetic strengthening is continued to all major affected muscle groups in the left upper extremity. Rotational and diagonal strengthening at the shoulder is continued. Fast-speed training, at 180°/s, is added when bilateral slow-speed deficits, at 60°/s, are within 20 percent. The patient is instructed in an aggressive home strengthening program using adjustable cuff weights. Functional training, including lifting, carrying various-size weights, hammering, and sawing activities, is instituted.

RATIONALE. Strengthening in the clinic is continued if the patient continues to exhibit strength gains with periodic isokinetic strength retests. Fast-speed training is instituted to improve muscular endurance. Fast-speed training is not instituted until slow-speed bilateral deficits are within 20 percent. We have observed clinically that, in the presence of slow-speed, bilateral deficits greater than 20 percent, the patient cannot consistently "catch" and maintain the faster speeds of the dynamometer. Functional training for this particular patient is designed to simulate the working conditions and motor requirements of carpentry.

SECOND GOAL

Optimizing joint and soft tissue mobility is the second goal.

THIRD GOAL

The third goal is to help the patient return to work.

TREATMENT. At 1 year postinjury, a job analysis was done to identify those tasks the patient would need to perform in order to be able to safely and accurately perform his job. At that time, the patient started on woodworking projects that required minimal fine motor tasks sanding, staining. At 15 months, he progressed to working on more intricate projects and, at 18 months, he returned to work.

CASE STUDY 2

The second case study presents a pattern of injury that occured to the lower portion of the brachial plexus Klumpke. Initial findings are delineated in the clarifying evaluation and should be compared and contrasted to the findings in Case Study 1. Goals, phases of treatment, and principles of treatment are similar to Case Study 1 and have been omitted to avoid redundancy.

HISTORY *A*

42-year-old male construction worker was working on a scaffold, slipped, and grabbed a railing with his right hand. The result was a forceful upward pull of the arm. This injury occured approximately 7 weeks ago. The patient reports numbness and tingling along the ulnar border of his right arm into the fourth and fifth fingers. He reports occasional burning pain along the same distribution as well as along the lower portion of his right neck. He reports weakness in his right grip. He also has slight "drooping" of his right eyelid. A neurologist performed an EMG last week that indicated increased insertional activity within the medial finger and wrist flexors and intrinsic hand muscles. A diagnosis of a second-degree/third-degree lower trunk brachial plexus injury was made. The patient was given nonsteriodal anti-inflammatory medication and referred to a program of physical and occupational therapy.

VOCATION

The patient is a construction worker and is right-hand dominant.

POSTURAL/VISUAL INSPECTION

Mild atrophy was observed in the intrinsic muscles of the right hand. A mild clawhand deformity was observed and characterized by hyperextension of the fourth and fifth digits at the metatarsal-phalangeal joints and flexion of the interphalangeal joints.

ACTIVE AND PASSIVE RANGE OF MOTION

Mild to moderate restriction in flexion of fourth and fifth metatarsal-phalangeal joints and extension of fourth and fifth interphalangeal joints.

MOTOR STRENGTH

The patient's muscles were graded as follows: flexor carpi ulnaris = 3+, medial half of flexor digitorum profundus = 3, opponens digiti minimi = 3, abductor digiti minimi = 3, flexor digiti minimi = 3, interossei muscles = 3, medial lumbricales (fourth and fifth digits) = 3, flexor pollicis brevis = 3+, and adductor pollicis brevis = 3.

SENSATION

Sensation was impaired to light touch and sharp/dull along the ulnar side of the arm, forearm, and hand. Special tests: Froment's sign was equivocal; the patient was asked to grasp a piece of paper between the thumb and index finger. With full paralysis of the adductor pollicis brevis, the thumb would flex; however, only slight flexion was produced when the paper was pulled away.

EDEMA

1+ edema along the dorsum of right hand; the hand was slightly cool to palpation, but no trophic changes were noted.

The Purdue peg board indicated coordination deficits in the right hand; ADL assessment indicated difficulties in self-care similar to those outlined in Case Study 1.

ASSESSMENT

The pathomechanics of injury involved an upward traction injury of the right limb that affected the lower portion of the brachial plexus, as described by Stevens. Lower plexus injuries affect nerve roots C8 and T1. Ptosis of the right eyelid indicated a potential sympathetic component (Horner's syndrome) and the physical/occupational therapist should monitor the condition carefully for sympathetic dystrophy in the right hand. Fibrillation potentials with EMG examination combined with clinical testing that produced a minimum strength grade of 3 in all affected muscle groups indicated a probable partial denervation of muscles affected by C8 and T1 nerve roots. The extent of the injury was therefore diagnosed as a second degree (rule out third degree) [axonotmesis] with Wallerian degeneration of some muscle fibers but probable preservation of the endoneurial tube. Spontaneous recovery will occur in case of axonotmesis, but axonal outgrowth takes a long time in these cases (at least a year) due to the limited growth rate and the long distance to their target muscles. A comprehensive program of both physical and occupational therapy based on a phased approach outlined in the initial case is indicated; as with all lower trunk brachial plexus injuries, a comprehensive hand therapy program should be designed by a certified hand therapist. Periodic electromyographic evaluations should be performed to check for reinneravation characterized by polphasic action potentials. If signs of recovery fail to appear after 1 year, surgical exploration should be performed.

Summary

The case studies illustrate the problem-solving approach to patient treatment. Signs and symptoms evaluated during the clarifying evaluation are prioritized in order of their clinical significance. Treatment is divided into three phases to allow the clinician to establish appropriate goals within the constraints of nerve reinnervation. The patient is progressed through each phase based on continued re-evaluation of signs and symptoms. The patient is discharged when clinical tests and evaluation indicate no further improvement in motor capabilities. The patient is discharged on a home program and is periodically reevaluated. Treatment is resumed if reevaluation confirms additional signs of motor re-innervation. A combined physical and occupational therapy approach recognizes the potential of significant long-term dysfunction of the patient's upper extremity.

References

1. Williams PL, Warwick R: Gray's Anatomy. 36th British Ed. Churchill Livingstone, Edinburgh, 1980
2. Leffert RD: Clinical diagnosis, testing, and electromyographic study in brachial plexus traction injuries. Clin Orthop Rel Res 237:24, 1988
3. Sunderland S: Traumatized nerves, roots and ganglia: musculoskeletal factors and neuropathological consequences. p. 137. In Korr IM (ed): The Neurobiologic Mechanisms in Manipulative Therapy. Plenum, New York, 1978
4. Framptom VM: Management of brachial plexus lesions. J Hand Ther 115:120, 1988
5. Alnot JY: Traumatic brachial plexus palsy in the adult: retro- and infraclavicular lesions. Clin Orthop Rel Res 237:9, 1988
6. Silliman JT, Dean MT: Neurovascular injuries to the shoulder complex. J Orthop Sports Phys Ther 18:442, 1993
7. Comtet JJ, Sedel L, Fredenucci JF: Duchenne-Erb palsy: experience with direct surgery. Clin Orthop Rel Res 237:17, 1988
8. Brunelli GA, Brunelli GR: A fourth type of brachial plexus injury: middle lesions (C7). Ital J Orthop Traumatol (Austria) 18:389, 1992
9. Mumenthaler M, Narakas A, Gilliat RW: Brachial plexus disorders. p. 1325. In Dyck PJ, Thomas PK, Lambert EH, Bunge R (eds): Peripheral Neuropathy. Vol. 2. WB Saunders, Philadelphia, 1984
10. Markey KL, DiBendetto M, Curl WW: Upper trunk brachial plexopathy. The stinger syndrome. Am J Sports Med 21:650, 1993
11. Hershman EB, Wilbourn AJ, Bergfeld JA: Acute brachial neuropathy in athletes. Am J Sports Med 17:655, 1989
12. Speer KP, Bassett FH III: The prolonged burner syndrome. Am J Sports Med 18:591, 1990
13. Inman VT, Saunders M, Abbot LC: Observations on the function of the shoulder joint. J Bone Joint Surg 26A:1, 1944
14. Freedman L, Munro RR: Abduction of the arm in the scapular plane: scapular and glenohumeral movements. A roentgenographic study. J Bone Joint Surg 48A:1503, 1966
15. Poppen NK, Walker PS: Normal and abnormal motion of the shoulder. J Bone Joint Surg 58A:195, 1976
16. Inman VT, Ralston HJ, Saunders JB et al: Relation of human electromyograms to muscular tension. Electroencephalogr Clin Neurophysiol 4:187, 1952
17. Kendall HO, Kendall FP, Wadsworth GE: Muscles: Testing and Function. 2nd Ed. Williams & Wilkins, Baltimore, 1971
18. Stevens JH: Brachial plexus paralysis. p. 344. In Codman EA (ed): The Shoulder. Krieger Publishing, Melbourne, 1937
19. Guven O, Akbar Z, Yalcin S, Gundes H: Concomitant rotator cuff tear and brachial plexus injury in association with anterior shoulder dislocation: unhappy triad of the shoulder. J Orthop Trauma 8:429, 1994
20. Wang KC, Hsa KY, Shik CH: Brachial plexus injury with erect dislocation of the shoulder. Orthop Rev 21:1345, 1992
21. Travlos J, Goldberg I, Boome RS: Brachial plexus lesions associated with dislocated shoulder. J Bone Joint Surg 72B: 68, 1990
22. Della Santa D, Narakos A, Bonnard C: Late lesions of the brachial plexus after fracture of the clavicle. Ann Chir Main Memb Super (France) 10:531, 1991
23. Stromquist Lidgren L, Norgren L, Odenberg S: Neurovascular injury complicating displaced proximal fractures of the humerus. Injury 18:423, 1989
24. Blom S, Dahlback LO: Nerve injuries in dislocation of the shoulder joint and fractures of the neck of the humerus. Acta Chir Scand 136:461, 1970
25. Sunderland S: Nerves and Nerve Injuries. 2nd Ed. Churchill Livingstone, Edinburgh, 1978
26. Bruxelle J, Travers V, Thiebaut JB: Occurrence and treatment of pain after brachial plexus injury. Clin Orthop Rel Res 237:87, 1988
27. Janda V: Muscles, central nervous motor regulation and back problems. p. 29. In Korr IM (ed): The Neurobiologic Mechanisms in Manipulative Therapy. Plenum, New York, 1978
28. Akeson WH, Amiel D, Mechanis GI et al: Collagen cross-linking alterations in joint contractures: changes in the reducible cross-links in periarticular connective tissue collagen after nine weeks of immobilization. Connect Tissue Res 5:15, 1977
29. Highet WB: Grading of motor and sensory recov-

ery in nerve injuries. p. 356. In Seddon HJ (ed): Peripheral Nerve Injuries. Medical Research Council Report Series T2 282. Her Majesty's Stationary Office, London, 1954

30. Daniels L, Worthingham C: Muscle Testing. Techniques of Manual Examination. 4th Ed. WB Saunders, Philadelphia, 1980

31. Hamm NH, Curtis D: Normative data for the Purdue pegboard on a sample of adult candidates for vocational rehabilitation. Percept Mot Skills 50: 309, 1980

32. Travell JG, Simons DG: Myofascial Pain and Dysfunction. The Trigger Point Manual. Williams & Wilkins, Baltimore, 1984

33. Janda V: Some aspects of extracranial causes of facial pain. J Prosthet Dent 56:4, 1986

34. Bilbey JH, Lamond RG, Mattrey RF: MR imaging of disorders of the brachial plexus. J Magn Reson Imaging 4:13, 1994

35. Yeoman PM: Cervical myelography in traction injuries of the brachial plexus. J Bone Joint Surg 50B:25, 1968

36. Bufalini C, Pesatori G: Posterior cervical electromyography in the diagnosis and prognosis of brachial plexus injuries. J Bone Joint Surg 51B:627, 1969

37. Bonney G, Gilliat RW: Sensory nerve conduction after traction lesion of the brachial plexus. Proc R Soc Med 51:365, 1958

38. Scott PM: Clayton's Electrotherapy and Actinotherapy. 7th Ed. Balliere Tindall, London, 1975

39. Tabary JC, Tardieu C, Tardieu G, Tabary C: Experimental rapid sarcomere loss with concomitant hypoextensibility. Muscle Nerve 4:198, 1981

40. Cooper RR: Alterations during immobilization and regeneration of skeletal muscles in cats. J Bone Joint Surg 54:919, 1972

41. Lampe GN, Mannheimer JS: Stimulation Characteristics of T.E.N.S. FA Davis, Philadelphia, 1984

42. Guyton AC: Organ Physiology: Structure and Function of the Nervous System. 2nd Ed. WB Saunders, Philadelphia, 1976

43. Maitland GD: Peripheral Manipulation. 2nd Ed. Butterworths, London, 1977

44. Gutman E, Guttman L: Effects of electrotherapy on denervated muscles in rabbits. Lancet 1:169, 1942

45. Hatano E et al: Electrical stimulation on denervated skeletal muscles. p. 469. In Goria A (ed): Posttraumatic Peripheral Nerve Regeneration: Experimental Basis and Clinical Implications. Raven Press, New York, 1981

46. Reynold C: The stiff hand. p. 95. In Malick H, Kasch M (eds): Manual on Management of Specific Hand Problems. AREN Publication, Pittsburgh, 1984

47. Enos L, Lane K, MacDougal B: Brief or new: the use of self-adherent wrap in hand rehabilitation. Am J Occup Ther 38:265, 1984

48. Trombly C, Scott A: Occupational Therapy for Physical Dysfunction. Williams & Wilkins, Baltimore, 1977, p. 71

49. Saha AK: Dynamic stability of the glenohumeral joint. Acta Orthop Scand 42:491, 1971

50. Hislop HJ, Perrine JJ: The isokinetic concept of exercise. Phys Ther 47:114, 1967

51. Lehman JF, Masock AJ, Warren CG, Koblanski JN: Effect of therapeutic temperature on tendon extensibility. Arch Phys Med Rehabil 51:48, 1970

52. Trombly C, Scott A: Occupational Therapy for Physical Dysfunction. Williams & Wilkins, Baltimore, 1984

53. Hollinshead W: Functional Anatomy of the Limbs and Back. 4th Ed. WB Saunders, Philadelphia, 1976.

8

The Shoulder in Hemiplegia

SUSAN RYERSON

KATHRYN LEVIT

Hemiplegia, a paralysis of one side of the body, occurs with strokes or cerebrovascular accidents involving the cerebral hemisphere or brain stem. Although hemiplegia is the classic and most obvious sign of neurovascular disease of the brain, it can also occur as a result of cerebral tumor or trauma.[1]

One of the most worrisome physical problems for clients with hemiplegia is the shoulder.[2] Shoulder pain, subluxation, loss of muscular activity, and loss of functional use are the most common complaints. These problems can be avoided with proper assessment and treatment and can be ameliorated if they already exist. This chapter reviews biomechanical and motor control impairments and presents a framework for the clinical management of these shoulder problems in hemiplegia.

Normal Shoulder Girdle Mechanics

Before beginning a study of the shoulder girdle in hemiplegia, it is important to review the normal mechanics of the shoulder (see Ch. 1). Three areas of normal shoulder mechanics should be emphasized: (1) the mobility of the scapula on the thorax,[3] (2) scapulohumeral rhythm and the

factors influencing both humeral mobility and humeral stability in the glenoid fossa,[4,5] and (3) the muscular attachments of the shoulder–girdle complex.[3,6] Because muscles that move the scapula and humerus have attachments to the cervical, thoracic, and lumbar spine, and to the rib cage, a loss of motor control and alignment will have multiple effects on the shoulder girdle.

Abnormal Biomechanics

The loss of motor control of the shoulder in patients with a hemiplegia affects the operation of normal biomechanical principles. In hemiplegia, three factors prevent normal shoulder biomechanical patterns from occurring: loss of muscular control and the development of abnormal movement patterns; secondary soft tissue changes that block motion; and glenohumeral joint subluxations. These three factors combine to allow at least three distinct types of shoulder and arm dysfunction.

LOSS OF MUSCULAR CONTROL AND DEVELOPMENT OF ABNORMAL MOVEMENT

Following the onset of a cerebrovascular accident with hemiplegia, a low tone or flaccid state is present. The length of the lower tone state varies from a short period of hours or days to a period of weeks or months. This state is characterized by a decrease in active postural tone and a loss of motor control in the musculature of the head, neck, trunk, and extremities. Initially, no movement is possible. As motor return occurs, individual muscles gradually become stronger.

In other patients, as motor return occurs, the pattern of control is imbalanced; not all muscles around a joint return at the same strength. Spinal extensor control becomes more evident than spinal flexor control. Early patterns of motor return pull the scapula and arm into abnormal postures. When the scapula and humerus are pulled severely out of alignment, certain muscle groups are positioned in shortened ranges. This results in lengthening or mechanical disadvantage in opposing muscle groups. Because the shortened muscles are available to the patient to use actively, muscle activity in these shortened groups is reinforced cortically with the attempt to move the arm. Muscle firing in these groups may also be reinforced by associated movements.[7] Thus, "functional spasticity" can develop when muscles of the upper extremity are maintained in an almost constant state of excitation.

A third pattern of motor dysfunction in patients is characterized by abnormal coactivation of limb or trunk muscles. These patients get return in both flexor and extensor muscle groups, but have difficulty integrating the firing patterns to produce lateral or rotational movement patterns. These patients also have the ability to recruit distal muscle groups. However, these distal muscle groups are recruited abnormally in what appears to be an attempt to substitute for proximal weakness. As an example, the biceps and wrist flexors may be recruited to help lift the weight of the arm during shoulder flexion while no contraction of the deltoid can be palpated (Fig. 8.1). Over time, a more constant state of excitation develops in the biceps and wrist flexor muscles, leading to muscle shortening. The constant muscle firing in these shortened groups can quickly pull the carpal bones out of alignment, leading to deformities in the forearm, wrist, and hand. The emergence of spasticity will perpetu-

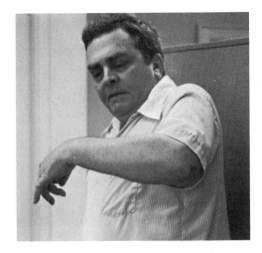

FIGURE 8.1 *Left hemiplegia: biceps and wrist flexors recruited to help move shoulder.*

ate abnormal alignment. However, inhibition of spasticity alone will not produce a functional arm. Motor reeducation must be directed toward both the recruitment or strengthening of absent or weak muscle groups and the retraining of available muscles to fire appropriately. Thus, treatment must address the abnormal tonal state, abnormal movement components, and abnormal joint alignment to restore normal movement. To restore the normal mechanical relationships of the bones, soft tissue stretching may be necessary.

Soft Tissue Blocks to Motion

Soft tissue blocks to motion can be categorized as loss of scapular mobility, loss of glenohumeral mobility, and loss of the ability to dissociate the scapula and humerus. The loss of scapular stability on the thorax occurs in all but the most minor strokes, and is influenced initially by such factors as the pull of the arm into gravity, the development of postural asymmetry, and the influence of patterns of motor return and treatment. As the scapula assumes a position that combines elements of elevation, downward rotation, and abduction, the position of the scapula prevents forward flexion of the arm past 60° to 80°. Because upward rotation is not available for the scapula, glenohumeral movement greater than 60° is not possible.

Without treatment, the scapula loses its mobility on the thorax and becomes fixed, thus eliminating the scapular component of scapulohumeral rhythm. The loss of this scapular component, consisting of scapular abduction and upward rotation, results in the substitution of scapula elevation. The loss of scapula upward rotation and protraction is important functionally because it is necessary for reach and pain-free elevation of the arm. However, loss of scapular adduction and depression has equal functional importance for resistive tasks such as lifting, pushing, carrying, and upper extremity weight-bearing. The goal in treatment is to restore the normal resting position of the scapula on the thorax and to regain mobility and motor control in all planes of motion.

Changes in scapula position will alter the ori-

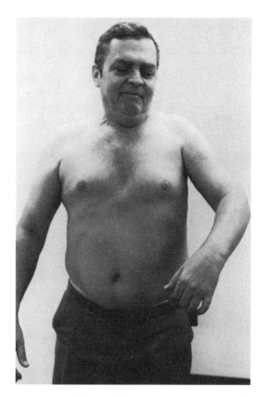

FIGURE 8.3 *Left hemiplegia: impingement of humeral greater tuberosity beneath acromion.*

entation of the glenoid fossa and affect the resting position of the humerus. In cases of chronic hemiplegia, the humerus is always positioned in some degree of internal rotation, but its position relative to the glenoid fossa will depend on the alignment of the scapula. With a downward-rotated and depressed scapula, inferior subluxation and internal rotation result (Fig. 8.2). In patients with an elevated, abducted scapula and a hyperextended humerus, the humeral head will be positioned anteriorly in the fossa. In patients with an elevated, abducted scapula and a humerus that postures in abduction and internal rotation, the humeral greater tubercle will impinge under the coracoid process (Fig. 8.3).

Loss of dissociation of the humerus from the scapula is the third block to normal movement. In this case, the scapula has mobility on the thorax and the humerus retains mobility in the glenoid fossa, but any movement of the humerus

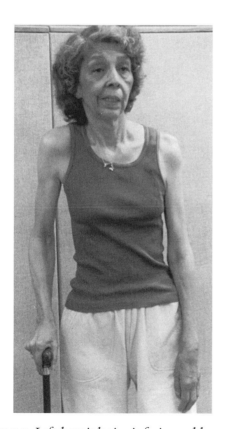

FIGURE 8.2 *Left hemiplegia: inferior subluxation.*

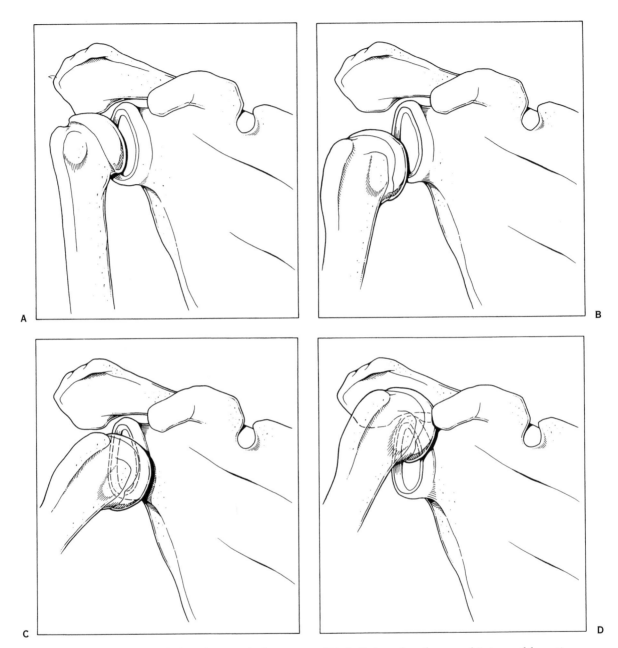

FIGURE 8.4 (A) *Normal glenohumeral alignment.* **(B)** *Inferior glenohumeral joint subluxation.* **(C)** *Anterior glenohumeral joint subluxation.* **(D)** *Superior glenohumeral joint subluxation.*

into flexion or abduction results in simultaneous scapular abduction.

SHOULDER SUBLUXATION

Shoulder subluxation occurs in hemiplegia when any of the biomechanical factors contributing to glenohumeral stability are disturbed. The most important factor is the position of the scapula on the thorax. The scapula is normally held on the thorax at an angle 30° from the frontal plane.[3] When the slope of the glenoid fossa becomes less oblique and no longer faces upward, the humerus "slides down" the slope of the fossa, and inferior subluxation, the subluxation most frequently mentioned, occurs.[4,6]

Two other forms of subluxation exist in the hemiplegic shoulder: anterior and superior subluxation. Each of these subluxations have downward-rotated scapulae, as does the inferior subluxation, but the other scapula and humeral planes of movement vary (Fig. 8.4). These subluxations are discussed in detail in the next section.

Subluxation is not painful as long as the scapula is mobile.[7] However, the subluxed shoulder should not be allowed to progress into a painful shoulder with loss of passive range of motion (ROM).

Type I Arm

With a severe loss of muscular activity, head and trunk control are virtually absent. This loss of trunk control results in increased lateral trunk flexion on the hemiplegia side.

The scapula in these patients is downwardly rotated for one or more of the following reasons. First, the loss of scapular muscle activity allows the scapula to lose its normal orientation on the thorax and rotate downward (the superolateral angle moves inferiorly). Second, loss of trunk control results in increased lateral trunk flexion. The scapula, moving on this laterally flexed trunk, becomes relatively downward rotated, and the glenoid fossa faces inferiorly.[3,4] Third, the weight of the arm, if not supported, will pull the weakened scapula downward and place the

humerus in relative abduction. With humeral abduction, the shoulder capsule is lax superiorly, and the head of the humerus can slide down the glenoid fossa.[4]

With scapular downward rotation, the glenoid fossa orients downward and the passive locking mechanism of the shoulder joint, as described by Basmajian,[6] is lost. The loss of this mechanism, the loss of postural tone, and the loss of tension of the shoulder capsule result in an inferior humeral subluxation of the hemiplegic shoulder.

When the body is in an upright position, the weight of the paretic arm and upper trunk will cause the spine to curve with the concavity to the hemiplegic side or to flex forward (Fig. 8.5). This laterally flexed position of the spine places the scapula lower on the thorax, with inferior angle winging. As motion return occurs and the upper trapezius and levator scapular become active, an inferior subluxation may be found with an elevated scapula. In either case, the humerus

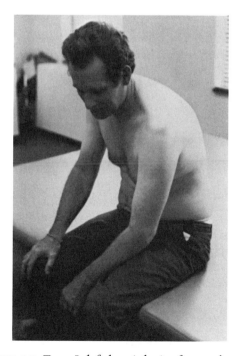

FIGURE 8.5 *Type I, left hemiplegia: forward flexion of trunk with flaccid arm influencing scapula position.*

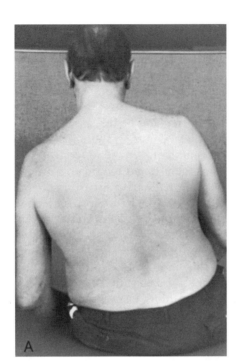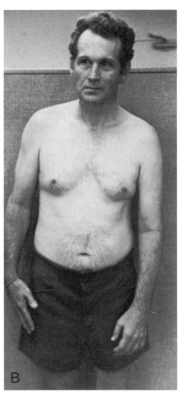

FIGURE 8.6 **(A)** *Type I, left hemiplegia: left side of body falling laterally into gravity, scapula lower on thorax.* **(B)** *Type I, left hemiplegia: humerus hangs by the side in internal rotation, elbow extension, and forearm pronation.*

will hang by the side in internal rotation, the elbow will extend passively, and the forearm will pronate (Fig. 8.6).

With an inferior subluxation, the humeral head is located below the inferior lip of the glenoid fossa. As subluxation occurs, the shoulder capsule is vulnerable to stretch, especially when the humerus is hanging by the side of the body. In this position, the superior portion of the capsule is taut.[4] The weight of the dependent humerus will place an immediate stretch on the taut capsule. Over time, the superior portion of the capsule will become permanently lax.[8]

When subluxation occurs, the movement possibilities are limited owing to the mechanical position of the humeral head. Any movement that occurs will not follow the rules of scapulohumeral rhythm. With an inferior subluxation of

long standing, scapular elevation with humeral internal rotation may be the only movement available.

Soft tissue tightness is found in both sections of the pectoral muscles, and posteriorly in the rotator cuff and the insertion of the latissimus dorsi muscle.

REDUCTION OF INFERIOR SUBLUXATION. To reduce an inferior subluxation, the scapula must first be upwardly rotated to neutral and moved to its normal position in the frontal plane (elevated if low on the rib cage and depressed if high on the rib cage). The humerus is then moved to neutral from internal rotation and lifted up into the fossa. Care must be given to keep the spine aligned vertically during the subluxation reduction.

Biochemical shoulder problems resulting from this type of arm include

1. Downward rotation of the scapula
2. Vertebral border and/or inferior angle winging of the scapula
3. Inferior glenohumeral joint subluxation
4. Humeral internal rotation

Type II Arm

The second pattern develops as the trunk gains more extension control than flexion control. An increase in cervical and lumbar extension is evident. The head and neck assume a position of ipsilateral flexion and contralateral rotation. At the thoracic level, this imbalance results in a unilateral loss of control of the abdominals. Therefore, the rib cage loses its abdominal "anchor" and will flare laterally and/or rotate (Fig. 8.7). The scapula and humerus are strongly

influenced mechanically by this rib cage deviation. The downward-rotated scapula begins to move superiorly on the thorax, and the humerus hyperextends with internal rotation. The glenohumeral joint will sublux anteriorly. With an anterior subluxation, the humerus is internally rotated and positioned inferior to and forward of the glenoid fossa (Fig. 8.4B). The humeral head appears aligned with the acromion in the sagittal plane, resulting in an apparent shortening of the length of the clavicle. As the humeral head moves forward out of the socket, the distal end of the humerus moves into hyperextension. Inferior angle or vertebral border winging of the scapula will occur.

This combination of rib cage rotation and humeral hyperextension allows the elbow to flex and the forearm to pronate (Fig. 8.8). As the scapula continues to elevate on the thorax, and the subluxed, internally rotated humerus moves into stronger hyperextension, the humeral head protrudes forward against the proximal end of the

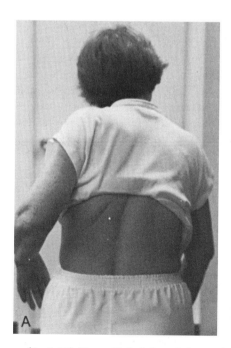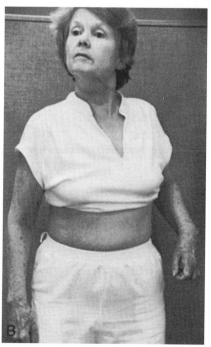

FIGURE 8.7 (A & B) *Type II, left hemiplegia: loss of rib cage anchor with rib cage rotated backward and humeral hyperextension with internal rotation.*

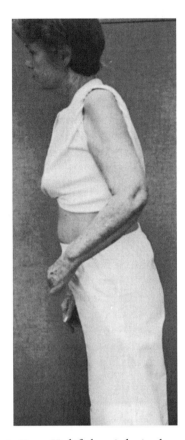

FIGURE 8.8 *Type II, left hemiplegia: humeral hyperextension with forearm pronation.*

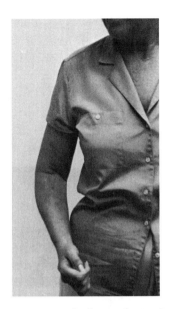

FIGURE 8.9 *Type II, right hemiplegia: humeral hyperextension with forearm supination.*

biceps tendon. This forward pressure of the humerus against the already shortened biceps tendon will mechanically move the forearm into a supinated position (Fig. 8.9). The wrist may appear to be less flexed as the carpals move dorso-laterally.

This anterior subluxation will limit movements that require the humerus and hand to be in front of the body. If the patient is asked to lift the arm, shoulder elevation with humeral internal rotation, hyperextension, and elbow flexion will be the movement pattern available.

Soft tissue tightness will be present in the pectoral muscle groups, rotator cuff, biceps, forearm, and hand.

REDUCTION OF ANTERIOR SUBLUXATION. To correct this subluxation, the rib cage is derotated and spinal alignment is corrected; the scapula can then be realigned on the rib cage. To realign the scapula on the rib cage, it must be moved down from its elevated position and upwardly rotated to neutral. While stabilizing the scapula in its corrected position, the humerus is moved from internal rotation to neutral. The humeral head can then be moved back as the distal end of the humerus is brought forward out of hyperextension, and then lifted up into the fossa.

Biomechanical shoulder problems resulting from this type of arm include

1. Downward rotation and elevation of the scapula
2. Scapular inferior angle and/or vertebral border winging
3. Anterior subluxation
4. Humeral internal rotation

In chronic cases of anterior subluxation, elbow flexion becomes more dominant and the forearm adducts across the abdomen. Shortening and spasticity in pectoral and biceps groups may develop, and the scapula loses mobility in the direction of depression and upward rotation.

Type III Arm

The third type of arm pattern is characterized by abnormal coactivation of the limb muscles. This gives an appearance of "mass" flexion in the hemiplegic upper extremity. The neck and trunk control in clients with this upper extremity pattern contain elements of both flexion and extension. The control patterns are not sufficiently integrated to allow selective combinations of movement, and rib cage flairing accompanies active movement of the hemiplegic arm. The scapula is usually elevated and abducted on the thorax. The scapula moves superiorly and tilts anteriorly, causing the humerus to lie under the coracoid process in a superior subluxation. The humerus is tightly held in internal rotation and abduction, so that the elbow joint lies directly below the shoulder in the frontal plane but is abducted away from the rib cage.

Passive motion of the glenohumeral joint is severely limited because the humeral head is lodged under the coracoid process. Although the deltoid and biceps attempt to initiate humeral motion, no dissociation occurs between the humerus and scapula. During attempts to move, these patients typically "fire" strongly in this elevation–abduction–internal rotation pattern, with elbow and wrist flexion (Fig. 8.10). By increasing humeral internal rotation, patients can "lock" their elbows into elbow extension. When distal movement exists, it is used to reinforce the active shoulder pattern. The wrist assumes a flexed and radially deviated position. This moves the forearm from pronation in the direction of supination.

Soft tissue tightness in the deltoids, pectorals, and rotator cuff are frequent secondary complications. Soft tissue tightness in these groups is often mistaken for atrophy from brachial plexus injury.

REDUCTION OF SUPERIOR SUBLUXATION. The superior subluxation is the most difficult to reduce. The scapula is returned to a neutral posi-

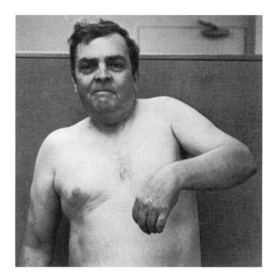

FIGURE 8.10 *Type III, left hemiplegia: active motion available in shoulder elevation, humeral abduction, internal rotation, and elbow flexion.*

tion; it must be lowered, rotated upward, and adducted. The humerus is externally rotated to neutral, using slight traction if necessary. External rotation of the humerus is then combined with horizontal adduction of the distal humerus as the humeral head is brought back into the fossa.

Biomechanical shoulder problems resulting from this type of arm include

1. Scapula elevation and abduction with vertebral border winging
2. Superior subluxation
3. Humeral internal rotation
4. Lack of dissociation between scapula and humerus, and between scapula and rib cage

Relationship of Subluxation to Control

The type of shoulder subluxation and the motor control available affect the hemiplegic patient's ability to move the arm functionally in three ways. First, the loss of antigravity postural tone and the subsequent patterns of motion return will change the relationship of the scapula to the trunk and the relationship of the distal arm to the scapula. This change in position will alter the anatomic relationship of the joints. Second, the changes in bony alignment will change the resting length and direction of pull of the major muscle groups of the shoulder and arm. Biomechanically, this will lead to muscle imbalance and problems of motor control. Third, changes in muscle excitation and recruitment patterns may occur in these muscles, in which resting lengths have been altered. Patterns of spasticity or abnormal coactivation of muscles may result in problems in any or all of these areas and will contribute to the abnormal and inefficient motor patterns associated with hemiplegia. Clinically, it is necessary to analyze the patient's motor patterns to identify the segments of abnormal motion. This will facilitate more effective treatment.

ance or improper movement patterns. When the joint is improperly aligned, passive or active motion either with or without weight-bearing will result in joint pain. This pain is sharp and stabbing in nature. It is relieved immediately when joint alignment is corrected. At the shoulder, joint pain occurs when glenohumeral alignment and rhythm is not maintained. The most frequent reasons for poor alignment are (1) lack of appropriate humeral rotation during forward flexion and (2) improper placement of the humeral head in the glenoid fossa.

Treatment for this type of pain begins with immediate cessation of the movement pattern. Forced motion with pain must *never* be allowed. The movement should STOP; the limb should be lowered, and the bones must be correctly realigned before treatment begins again. If soft tissue or joint tightness exists, realignment may not be possible unless soft tissue or joint mobility is improved or increased.

Musculoskeletal Considerations

SHOULDER PAIN

Shoulder pain is one of the major problem areas in hemiplegia.[2] Pain occurs in the hemiplegic shoulder as a result of muscle imbalance with loss of joint range, impingement of the shoulder capsule during improper ROM, improper muscle stretching, tendinitis, hypersensitivity, or hyposensitivity; pain also is caused by sympathetic changes.

To plan a treatment program, the nature of the pain, the precise anatomic location of the pain, the duration of the pain, and the body position during the movement that causes the pain must be assessed. Four categories of shoulder pain can be identified: joint pain, muscle pain, pain from altered sensitivity, and shoulder–hand pain syndrome.

Joint Pain

Joint pain in hemiplegia occurs when a joint is placed in a biomechanically compromised position as a result of either shoulder muscle imbal-

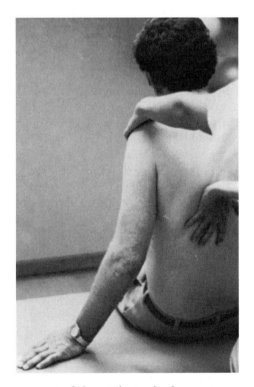

FIGURE 8.11 *Left hemiplegia: body moving on weight-bearing upper extremity.*

Muscle Pain

Muscle pain occurs as a shortened or spastic muscle is lengthened too fast or lengthened beyond the range to which the shortened muscle is "accustomed." Often, this type of pain occurs when the upper extremity is in a weight-bearing position and the patient is asked to move the body on the limb (Fig. 8.11). Muscle pain is perceived as a "pulling" sensation and is localized to the region of the muscle belly that is being stretched. The pain is immediately relieved if the amount of severe stretch is decreased a few degrees. Because lengthening shortened muscles is a goal of treatment, the muscle is not allowed to move back to the shortened range, but is allowed to shorten until the pain is relieved. Treatment can proceed with careful attention given to speed and progression of movement.

The pain that accompanies tendinitis is related to muscle pain, for it is caused by the same mechanisms. Overstretching of a limb muscle followed by overaggressive weight-bearing with poor joint alignment results in tendinitis. The pain is described as aching or sharp, remains after the weight-bearing is stopped, and is referred to other locations. In the hemiplegic upper extremity, the two most common types are bicipital groove tendinitis with pain referred down into the muscle belly, and bicipital tendinitis across the elbow with pain referred down the volar aspect of the forearm. The inappropriate weight-bearing pattern that leads to tendinitis in these cases is severe humeral internal rotation with forced elbow extension, along with an inactive trunk and "leaning" on a weak scapula (Fig. 8.12).

The weight-bearing extended arm activity should be stopped until the pain subsides. When weight-bearing treatment is resumed, particular care should be given to proper joint alignment and active trunk scapular pattern (Fig. 8.13).

Altered Sensitivity

The pain that occurs because of altered sensitivity of the central nervous system (CNS) to sensory input is found at the acute stage of recovery following an insult.

This pain occurs in the upper extremity, and is described as both diffuse and aching and localized to the shoulder and sharp. It typically occurs during the middle of a treatment session that has included tactile, sensory, kinesthetic, and propri-

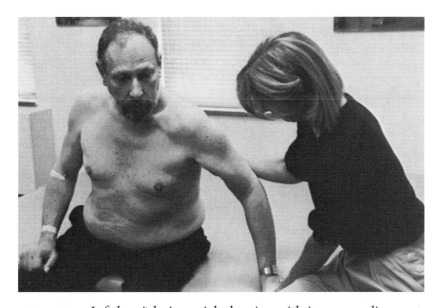

FIGURE 8.12 *Left hemiplegia: weight-bearing with improper alignment.*

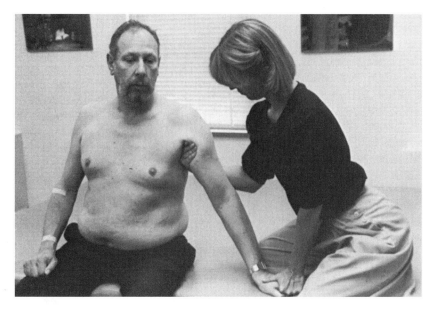

FIGURE 8.13 *Left hemiplegia: weight-bearing with proper alignment.*

oceptive stimuli. One explanation for its occurrence is that the levels of "tolerance" of the impaired CNS have been reached. The treatment should stop for that session, and the duration of treatment and the nature of the treatment should be noted. Subsequent treatment should be graded to allow movement to continue but not to exceed the patient's sensory tolerance. If treatment is stopped completely, these patients may proceed to shoulder–hand syndrome.

Shoulder–Hand Syndrome

Shoulder–hand syndrome begins with diffuse "aching pain" in the shoulder and entire arm. Because this pain interferes with the desire to move the arm, the hand soon becomes swollen and tender. If passive motion is forced on a swollen wrist and hand, the joints will become sharply painful.

The second stage is characterized by decreased ROM of the shoulder girdle, hand, and fingers. Skin changes are also present because of the lack of motion and loss of tactile input.

The syndrome culminates with presence of atrophied bone and severe soft tissue deformity

and joint contractures. Shoulder–hand syndrome can be prevented by a program that

1. Grades the motor program in stages with increasing sensitivity to movement
2. Gradually but consistently uses weight-bearing activities for the entire shoulder girdle and upper extremity
3. Reeducates open-ended activities (non-weight-bearing) with appropriate scapulo-humeral rhythm
4. Prevents edema
5. Teaches patients how to care for their arm

Treatment Planning

The treatment of the deficits in motor control in the patient with hemiplegia focuses on the improvement of function and the prevention of further disability from secondary complications. In this section, treatment objectives for the hemiplegic shoulder will be presented in three major categories. The first category of objectives is designed to help the patient relearn basic postural control. The second set of objectives focuses on the neuromuscular deficits of hemiplegia: loss of extremity motor control and function. In the third category, the objectives for the secondary complications of hemiplegia—subluxation, pain, loss of motion, and spasticity—will be discussed.

REESTABLISHMENT OF POSTURAL CONTROL

The objectives for establishing postural control include (1) facilitating righting reactions, equilibrium reactions, and protective reactions; and (2) providing normal tactile, proprioceptive, and kinesthetic input. Before specific retraining of the shoulder in patients with hemiplegia can begin, postural control of the head, neck, and trunk must be present. This postural trunk control provides the body with the ability to shift weight. The ability of the body to shift and bear weight to one side frees the opposite extremity for the functions of reaching, grasping, and releasing. Along with sensory feedback (tactile, proprioceptive, kinesthetic, visual, and vestibular), movement requires a base of stability or base of support, a point of mobility, and a weight shift. Weight shift, either anterior, posterior, lateral, or diagonal, is followed by one or more of the following: righting reactions, equilibrium reactions, protective reactions, or falling. The establishment of head and neck control allows the shoulder girdle to dissociate or move freely from the thorax and the humerus to dissociate from the scapula. To establish good motor control, the body (trunk) must be able to adjust posture automatically so that an upper extremity movement may achieve its purpose.

NEUROMUSCULAR DEFICITS

Objectives for reestablishing motor control and function of the hemiplegic arm include (1) reestablishing normal alignment, (2) establishing normal weight-bearing patterns in the upper extremity, (3) initiating and "holding" proximal non-weight-bearing patterns, and (4) reeducating distal movement for functional skills.

Reestablishing Normal Alignment

It is necessary to reestablish normal alignment before attempting to reeducate motor control. The shoulder girdle must be properly aligned either by lengthening shortened or spastic muscles or by supporting body parts that do not have sufficient muscular activity.

Establishing Weight-Bearing

The ability to accept and bear weight on the affected arm following a stroke is one of the most important goals of a therapeutic program. Active weight-bearing on either a partially flexed or extended upper extremity is used as a means of increasing mobility; increasing postural control of the trunk; improving motor control of the affected arm; introducing and grading tactile proprioceptive, and kinesthetic stimulation; and preventing edema and pain. Positions that provide weight-bearing for a hemiplegia shoulder and arm include (1) rolling onto the affected side in preparation for getting out of bed (Fig. 8.14A and B), (2) supporting the forearm on a pillow placed in the lap or on a lap board or on a table when sitting (Fig. 8.14C), and (3) extending the weight-bearing arm down onto a countertop while standing.

An active weight-bearing program for the paretic arm stresses "active" patterns in the trunk and does not allow the patient to lean or "hang" on the ligaments of the affected extremity (Fig. 8.15A and B). This active participation of the trunk is accomplished by placing the upper extremity in an aligned weight-bearing position and asking the trunk or "body" to move on the stable arm in anterioposterior, lateral, and rotational directions (Fig. 8–15C to H).

In the acute stage of hemiplegia, when very little postural control is present, upper extremity weight-bearing is used to facilitate proximal motor control. When the upper extremities are "fixed" onto the supporting surface through forearm weight-bearing activities, the arm becomes

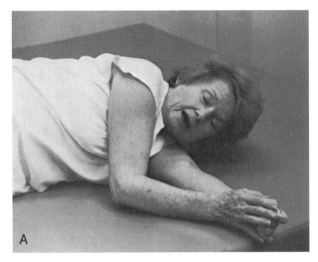

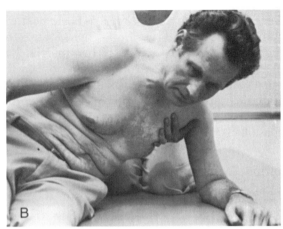

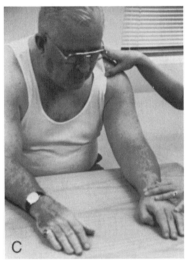

FIGURE 8.14 *Weight-bearing positions for the upper extremity.* **(A)** *Left hemiplegia: rolling onto affected side.* **(B)** *Left hemiplegia: moving onto affected forearm.* **(C)** *Left hemiplegia: supporting forearm on table.*

a point of stability for movements of the trunk and pelvis. As the body moves away from the arm, scapular protraction and upward rotation, humeral flexion, and upper trunk flexion are encouraged (Fig. 8.16A). As the body moves toward the arm, scapular adduction and trunk extension are encouraged as the humerus moves into more extension (Fig. 8.16B). When the pelvis and trunk move laterally, the scapulae move in opposite directions, one into more abduction and one into more adduction. The humerus on the side of the lateral weight shift becomes more externally rotated, while the other humerus becomes more internally rotated (Fig. 8.17).

For patients with available but synergistic movement patterns, upper extremity weight-bearing can be used to lengthen or inhibit tight or spastic muscles while simultaneously facilitating muscles that are not active. When the person sits with hands down and open, a rotational movement of the body toward the affected upper extremity will lengthen tight shoulder depressors and downward rotators, tight humeral internal rotators, and elbow flexors, while simultaneously activating the opposing groups (Fig. 8.18A & B).

*Initiating and "Holding" Proximal
Non-Weight-Bearing Patterns*

When the hand or arm is placed in a position of weight-bearing, the motions of the shoulder girdle occur as a reaction to the body's movement over the fixed extremity. When the arm is taken out of weight-bearing and is asked to move in space, the demands on the shoulder girdle are different from weight-bearing demands. The motor demands on the shoulder for non-weight-bearing (open-ended) activities can be divided into (1) the ability to hold the weight of the limb against gravity; (2) the ability to initiate antigravity movement patterns, including the ability to switch from glenohumeral to scapulohumeral movement as needed; and (3) the ability to recip-

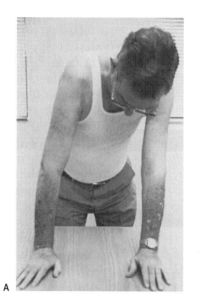

A

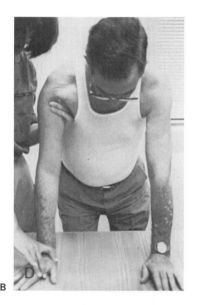

B

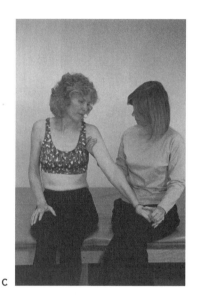

C

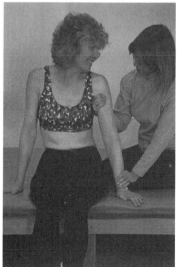

D

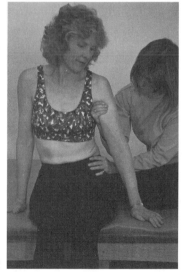

E

FIGURE 8.15 **(A)** *Right hemiplegia: improper weight-bearing on extended arm—"hanging" on shoulder and mechanically locking elbow.* **(B)** *Right hemiplegia: extended arm weight-bearing.* **(C–H)** *Establishing extended-arm weight-bearing in sitting. Therapist aligns patients left shoulder while she practices combining trunk and arm movements. (Figure continues)*

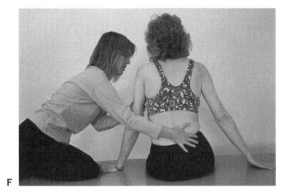

F

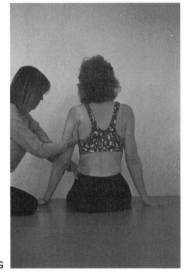

G

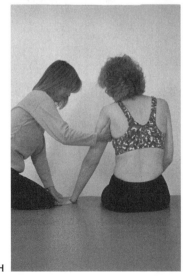

H

FIGURE 8.15 *(Continued)*

rocate and coordinate the combinations of mobility and stability needed for reaching, grasping, carrying, and releasing.

Motor reeducation aimed at training the hemiplegic arm to move against gravity will vary according to the patterns of return present and variables such as pain, spasticity, or malalignment. Techniques for managing pain and spasticity are discussed under "Treatment of Secondary Complications" later in the chapter and should be used before treatment of motor control proceeds. Orthopedic changes, particularly those that are long standing, represent a particular treatment challenge because although orthopaedic malalignment at the shoulder will necessitate compensation or abnormal movement, it is frequently impossible within a treatment session to reposition the scapula or humerus in normal alignment before proceeding with movement reeducation. In these cases, the goal is to gain some increase in mobility in the direction of normal alignment, followed immediately by a movement pattern that uses this new mobility. Over successive treatments, as soft tissue mobility is increased and passive resting positions become closer to normal alignment, the types and combinations of movement can be increased.

When pain, spasticity, and malalignment of the shoulder joints are not problems, treatment can be directed immediately to improving motor control. In the acute stage, in which muscle tone is low and little motion is present, teaching the patient to manage the weight of the arm against gravity is the first stage of motor control to be introduced. This is done by teaching the patient to "hold" the scapula and humerus in an antigravity position (Fig. 8.19A).[7,9] "Place and hold" activities are practiced in supine and, later, in sitting positions until the patient develops control of the arm in various combinations of scapula and humeral patterns (Fig. 8.19B and C).

The patient is then taught to move actively within his or her range of control. When the concept of holding has been achieved, the patient is asked to initiate patterns at the shoulder. This is done by moving the hemiplegic arm in many functional patterns combined with strong sensory stimulation during each treatment session.

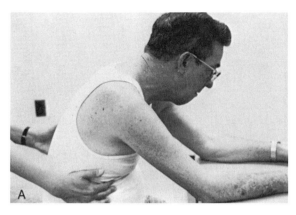 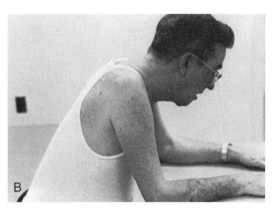

FIGURE 8.16 *Right hemiplegia:* **(A)** *moving body away from weight-bearing arm;* **(B)** *moving body toward weight-bearing arm.*

Muscle groups that are unable to contract after the joint has been realigned need to be stimulated. The techniques of stimulation have been described by Bobath and others. The techniques are the same, although they have been ascribed different names, including joint compression (pressure tapping, joint approximation); resistance with proper alignment maintained; quick stretch (inhibitory tapping, "pull-push"); sweep tapping (brushing, icing); and repetition.

When the patient has movement available,

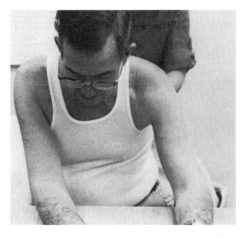

FIGURE 8.17 *Right hemiplegia: weight shifting to right moves right humerus into more external rotation while left humerus begins to move into the direction of internal rotation.*

but efforts to move the arm produce abnormal patterns, treatment is directed toward establishing more normal coordination. This may involve both inhibiting the abnormal way in which muscles are recruited and retraining in the correct pattern of motor recruitment. Problems in motor recruitment can best be addressed by teaching the patient to identify and quiet muscles that are firing inappropriately through techniques of inhibition or biofeedback. The patient is then taught to allow passive motion of the arm without firing muscles inappropriately or allowing muscle tone in the arm to increase. The patient is then encouraged to try to "follow" the movement and finally to perform it actively with less assistance from the therapist. Place and hold exercises are useful in helping the patient use the correct muscles at the shoulder girdle without inappropriately firing distal muscle groups. While new recruitment patterns are being established, the patient is also taught appropriate control of the previously "overused" muscles. Thus, the patient learns to inhibit biceps activity when reaching, but to use the biceps appropriately to bring the hand to the mouth.

Patients who have less spasticity or more complete motor return have fewer problems with abnormal recruitment but more problems with motor control. This category of patients has missing components of motor activity. Compensatory motions resembling an abnormal pattern result. For example, lack of active external rota-

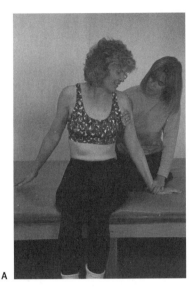
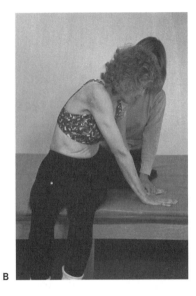

FIGURE 8.18 **(A & B)** *Left hemiplegia: rotational body movements over a weight-bearing upper extremity.*

tion of the humerus will lead to a substitution pattern of abduction, internal rotation of the humerus, and scapula elevation (Fig. 8.20). If this motor pattern is being used because the patient cannot actively externally rotate the humerus, the goal of treatment must be to make external rotation available during active shoulder movement and to establish the ability to hold the humerus in external rotation while moving distally. Similarly, other patients may have difficulties with protraction and upward rotation of the scapula. In this case, the therapist must control the motion of the scapula proximally to facilitate the correct motion of the scapula while the patient works on upper extremity placing or movement sequences.

Reeducating Distal Movements

Distal motor control, to be accurate, must be based on normal patterns of mobility and stability in the scapula and glenohumeral joint. Once the patient can initiate normal motion at the glenohumeral and scapulothoracic joints and can maintain the shoulder in positions against gravity, the patient must learn to add combinations of elbow position and forearm rotation to the control established at the shoulder. To use the hand functionally for grasping, carrying, and releasing, the hemiplegic patient must be able to

position the hand appropriately for grasp by selecting appropriate forearm and wrist positions, hold the hand in position while the fingers move, and sustain grasp while moving proximally. Problems in any of these areas may interfere with adaptive grasp.

As shoulder girdle control builds, the positions and movements of the distal segments must be added in treatment so that various distal positions are available to the patient to use functionally. As new combinations of motor behavior are learned, the patient should be taught a functional task using this pattern to ensure carry-over from exercise into everyday life.

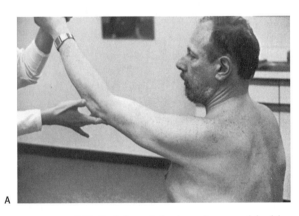

FIGURE 8.19 **(A)** *Left hemiplegia: place and hold position. (Figure continues.)*

Different grasp patterns require varying wrist and forearm positions. In addition, the transition from grasp to manipulation involves the addition of complex fine motor patterns that are often task specific. Improving the level of hand function is thus a separate treatment process that requires good motor control of the shoulder, elbow, forearm, and wrist as a precursor of success.

When the hemiplegic patient has biomechanical shoulder girdle problems, accurate positioning of the hand for function is difficult as the patient attempts to hold the shoulder against gravity and initiate appropriate antigravity movement patterns.[10]

TREATMENT OF SECONDARY COMPLICATIONS

The objectives for each of the secondary complications—subluxation pain, loss of motion, and spasticity—are discussed separately.

Subluxation

Acutely, if subluxation is not present, treatment follows the objectives listed earlier under "Treatment Planning." If subluxation has occurred, treatment must be preceded by careful assessment, reduction of subluxation, and proper support.

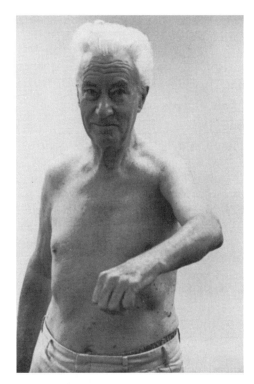

FIGURE 8.20 *Left hemiplegia: lack of active external rotation results in compensation pattern of humeral abduction and internal rotation.*

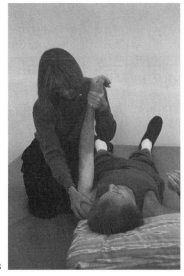

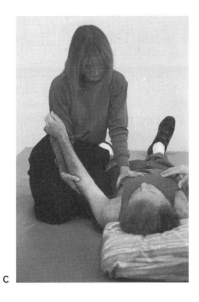

B   C

FIGURE 8.19 *(Continued)* **(B & C)** *Therapist corrects alignment and helps patient learn to move his left arm in a variety of patterns.*

Proper assessment of subluxation includes determination of

1. The exact position of the humeral head, scapula, rib cage, and spine
2. Mobility or passive range of motion
3. Tone
4. Amount and location of motor control

The assessment will reveal the cause of the subluxation (loss of motor control of scapula and/or humerus, soft tissue tightness, and hypotonus or hypertonus). Appropriate treatment can then begin. Treatment of subluxation includes the following goals:

1. Manual alignment and support of scapula on the thorax and humerus in the glenoid fossa during treatment
2. Increase in motor control in shoulder girdle muscle groups
3. Inhibition of spasticity or stretching of soft tissue tightness
4. Maintenance of pain-free ROM with proper glenohumeral rhythm
5. Prevention of stretching of shoulder capsule through proper positioning and/or shoulder supports

Proper positioning can be achieved through the use of lapboards, tables, armrests, or pillows when sitting; self-assisted motion during functional activities; and weight-bearing on the forearm or hand.

SHOULDER SUBLUXATION SUPPORTS. The shoulder should be supported in the acute stage of hemiplegia to prevent stretch on the capsule or to eliminate pain. In the 1950s and 1960s, orthopedic slings were given to patients with hemiplegia (Fig. 8.21A). These slings held the humerus against the body in internal rotation and kept the elbow in flexion. The arm was immobilized and the patient was unable to see the arm or try to use the arm even for support. In the 1970s and 1980s, alternative slings were produced: the Rolyan hemi arm sling, the shoulder saddle sling, and variations on the axillary support as described by Bobath.[7]

- *Rolyan hemi arm sling* (Rolyan Smith and Nephew, Inc., Menomonee Falls, WI): This sling has a humeral cuff and a figure eight suspension. It will provide moderate support to the humerus and allows the elbow to be extended. The arm is free to be moved and used for support (Fig. 8.21B).
- *Shoulder saddle sling* (Fred Sammons, Inc., Brookfield, IL): This sling has a forearm cuff and a shoulder saddle suspension. It provides maximum support to the entire arm and prevents the arm from "banging" around during functional activities. This sling is excellent for the flaccid limb with pain. It allows moderate humeral and elbow movement (Fig. 8.21C).
- *Axillary support* (All Orthopedic Appliances, Inc., Miami, FL): This support elevates the scapula and provides minimal inferior support for the humerus. It should not be used in patients with elevated scapulae. It has been criticized for placing pressure on the brachial plexus when inappropriately donned (Fig. 8.21D).

Because no device is available that upwardly rotates the scapula, no shoulder support will correct glenohumeral joint subluxation. Shoulder supports will help support and/or maintain position on the rib cage once the correction has been made. Shoulder supports will also prevent the flaccid arm from banging against the body during functional activities, thus decreasing shoulder joint pain. They also help to relieve downward traction on the shoulder capsule caused by the weight of the arm.

Therapy clinics should have different types of shoulder supports available and evaluate which support provides the best protection for each patient.

Pain

The causes of shoulder pain have been described in detail. Treatment of the painful shoulder and arm should include

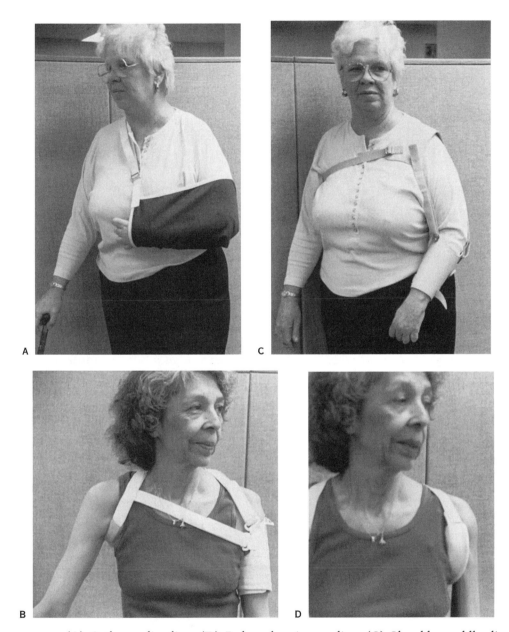

FIGURE 8.21 **(A)** *Orthopaedic sling.* **(B)** *Rolyan hemi arm sling.* **(C)** *Shoulder saddle sling.* **(D)** *Axillary support.*

1. Immediate cessation of any movement or activity that causes or increases the pain
2. Removal of edema, if present
3. Realignment of the shoulder girdle/trunk complex either by the therapist manually

(passively) or by the client actively (this includes lengthening or inhibition of the shortened or spastic muscle groups and realignment of malaligned joints)

4. Reeducation of the inactive muscle groups

5. A graded program of weight-bearing through the shoulder, forearm, and hand

Loss of Range

Loss of ROM at the shoulder can lead to decreased arm function and impaired balance in patients with hemiplegia. Although classic stretching procedures (non-weight-bearing) are often used for loss of shoulder motion in hemiplegia, slow maintained stretching or elongation through weight-bearing (functional stretching in conjunction with retraining motor control) is more effective.

Spasticity

The importance of spasticity in the treatment of hemiplegia is a controversial subject.[11,12] Spasticity is one of the positive symptoms of hemiplegia along with clonus and disinhibition of primitive reflexes. Although spasticity must be dealt with during the treatment of the hemiplegic shoulder, the negative symptoms, paresis, loss of force production, delayed initiation of movement, and pathologic cocontraction of muscles must also be addressed.[13]

Although inhibition of spasticity alone will not result in a functional upper extremity, persistent muscle activity or muscle shortening will block normal movements from occurring. It is only when tone is inhibited that a true assessment of the patient's motor abilities can be performed. The presence and distribution of spasticity in the upper extremity is often influenced by the patient's ability to control the trunk and lower extremity in transitional movements and in standing and walking.

Campbell[11] hypothesizes that by preventing the development of abnormal compensatory motor patterns through activation of normal motor control, the rapists may decrease or even prevent the development of spasticity. From a movement point of view, existing spasticity in the upper extremity can be inhibited by (1) maintained elongation or lengthening in the pattern of shortened muscle groups, (2) activation of the trunk musculature through upper extremity weight-bearing, or (3) reeducation of the pelvis and lower extremity. We believe that in stroke patients who have not developed spasticity, effective treatment can guide motor return and prevent the development of abnormal motor patterns.

Summary

The importance of identifying the exact location and nature of shoulder girdle dysfunction in hemiplegia has been stressed in this chapter. Because the abnormal motor patterns of hemiplegia can arise from a combination of abnormal alignment, unbalanced motor return, and abnormal patterns of muscle recitation and recruitment, treatment strategies must be based on a thorough understanding of the interrelationships between orthopedic and neurologic factors. The presence of subluxation and pain are additional problems that must be addressed before neuromuscular reeducation can begin. The positive results of any treatment regimen will ultimately depend on the clinician's systematic evaluation and skill in implementing appropriate treatment of the shoulder girdle complex.

References

1. Adams RD, Victor M: Principles of Neurology. McGraw-Hill, New York, 1981
2. Davis PM: Steps to Follow. Springer-Verlag, Berlin, 1985
3. Kapandji IA: The Physiology of the Joints: Upper Limb. Churchill Livingstone, Edinburgh, 1970
4. Cailliet R: The Shoulder in Hemiplegia. FA Davis, Philadelphia, 1980
5. Codman EA: The Shoulder. Thomas Todd, Boston, 1934
6. Basmajian JV: Muscles Alive. Williams & Wilkins, Baltimore, 1979
7. Bobath B: Adult Hemiplegia: Evaluation and

Treatment. 2nd Ed. William Heinneman, London, 1979

8. Jensen M: The hemiplegic shoulder. Scand J Rehabil Med, suppl. 7:113, 1980

9. Carr JH, Shepherd R: A Motor Relearning Programme for Stroke. Aspen Systems, London, 1983

10. Rubiana R: Examination of the Hand and Upper Limb. WB Saunders, Philadelphia, 1984

11. Campbell S: Pediatric Neurologic Physical Therapy. Churchill Livingstone, New York, 1984

12. Sahrmann S, Norton BJ: The relationship of voluntary movement to spasticity in the upper motor neuron syndrome. Ann Neurol 2:460, 1977

13. Lance JW: The control of muscle tone, reflexes and movement: Robert Wartenberg lecture. Neurology 30:1303, 1980

9

Impingement Syndrome and Impingement-Related Instability

LORI   A.   THEIN

BRUCE   H.   GREENFIELD

Impingement syndrome has historically been considered to be a continuum of a single pathology, involving the subacromial soft tissues.[1] As our understanding of this complex problem has developed, the simple continuum model has become less effective in guiding appropriate treatment. The purpose of this chapter is to provide the reader with more precise classifications of impingement syndrome and the impingement-instability complex in order to provide more efficient and effective treatment procedures that address the primary pathology.

Compressive Cuff Disease

Impingement syndrome or compressive cuff disease was originally described by Neer[1] as mechanical impingement of the supraspinatus and the long head of the biceps tendon underneath the acromial arch.[1,2] The primary pathology involves a bursal surface lesion. The condition is often classified as primary impingement syndrome, in contrast to secondary impingement, which involves primary instability and will be discussed later. Because primary impingement involves a spectrum of lesions of tissues in the suprahumeral space, a working knowledge of its structural interrelationships will facilitate an understanding of the factors that result in pathology.

SUPRAHUMERAL SPACE

The suprahumeral space, also known as the subacromial space or supraspinatus outlet, is formed by the superior aspect of the humeral head below, and the inferior surface of the acromion, the acromioclavicular joint, and the coracoacromial ligament above (Fig. 9.1). Within the subacromial space are the rotator cuff tendons (supraspinatus, infraspinatus, and teres minor), long head of the biceps, and the subacromial/subdeltoid bursa. The subacromial distance is quite small and has been measured on radiograph and used as an indicator for proximal or superior humeral subluxation due to rotator cuff pathology. The distance was found to be between 9 and 10 mm in 175 asymptomatic shoulders. A distance of less than 6 mm was considered pathologic of rotator cuff disease.[4,5]

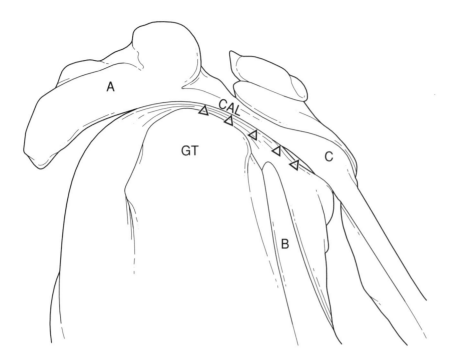

FIGURE 9.1 *The subacromial space. (A, acromion; GT, greater tuberosity; CAL, coracoacromial ligament; B, (long head) biceps; C, coracoid process.)*

A second space for potential primary impingement has been identified by Patte[6] as the so-called coracohumeral compartment. The coracohumeral space is the space between the tuberosity and the lesser tubercle of the humerus. Within the confines of this space are situated the subscapularis bursa, subscapularis tendon, and subcoracoid bursa. In the resting position with the arm in medial rotation, the distance between the tip of the coracoid and the most prominent part of the lesser tuberosity has been measured to be approximately 8.7 mm in healthy shoulders and decreased to 6.8 mm in the presence of subcoracoid impingement.[7] A decrease in the size of the subcoracoid space, caused by a fracture trauma to the tip of the coracoid process, has been implicated in primary subcoracoid impingement.[6] The clinician should be aware of this diagnosis as a potential differential of primary impingement, and in those patients who have not responded to conservative treatment, particularly after acromioplasty.

Because of the narrow confines of the subacromial space, a small margin of error in effect exists to allow for normal excursion of the supra-

humeral tissues to pass safely under acromial process. Several factors have been implicated in pathologic narrowing of the subacromial space and the resulting primary impingement syndrome.[8–15]

Factors Related to Pathology

For purposes of description, factors related to pathology can be divided into intrinsic and extrinsic factors. Intrinsic factors directly involve the subacromial space and include changes in vascularity of the rotator cuff, degeneration, and anatomic or bony anomalies. Extrinsic factors include muscle imbalances and motor control problems of the rotator cuff and parascapular muscles, functional arc of movement, postural changes, and precipitating factors including training errors and occupational or environmental hazards.[15–23] Because several of these problems can coexist with primary impingement, isolating a specific factor as a cause is difficult; more likely, the cause of primary impingement is multifactorial. All factors may be important, and the key factor in any case depends on the individual circumstances.

EXTRINSIC FACTORS

According to Neer,[1] the anteroinferior one-third of the acromion is thought to be the causative factor in mechanical wear of the rotator cuff through a process called impingement. Neer believes that the supraspinatus and long head of the biceps are subjected to repeated compression when the arm is raised in forward flexion. Neer called this the functional arc of elevation of the arm (Fig. 9.2). Arthrokinematic movement dictates that forward flexion of the humerus results in concomitant internal rotation of the humeral head.[24] The result is that the suprahumeral tissues are effectively driven directly under the anteroinferior one-third of the acromion. The coracoacromial ligament and acromioclavicular joint can also be involved in impingement during this functional movement. The Neer Impingement test involves forced forward flexion with internal rotation of the humerus to simulate movement in the functional arc and to provoke pain in symptomatic individuals (Fig. 9.3). By focusing on the anterior acromion as the source of impingement rather than the entire acromion, Neer helped refine the technique and approach to acromial decompression to the area of the anteroinferior acromion, thus avoiding excision

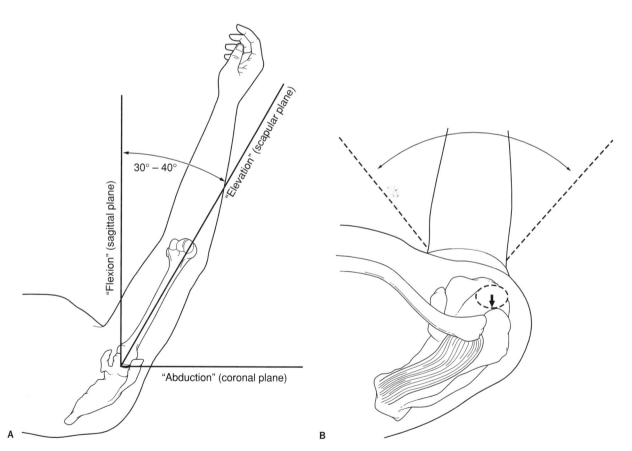

FIGURE 9.2 *Functional arc.* **(A)** *The functional arc of elevation occurs from the sagittal to the plane of the scapula.* **(B)** *Superior view of anterior acromion. Elevation in the functional arc internally rotates the humerus under the anteroinferior one third of the acromion.*

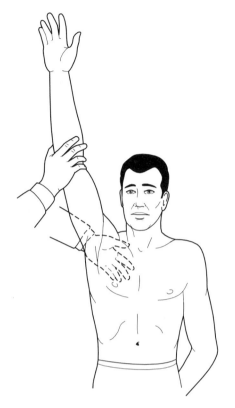

FIGURE 9.3 *Neer Impingement test. Forceful elevation of the humerus with internal rotation results in impingement of the rotator cuff tendons and long head of the biceps underneath the anteroinferior acromion. A positive result is provocation of subacromial pain.*

of the lateral acromion and significant deltoid muscle morbidity. The overall result after acromial decompression or anterior acromioplasty is an accelerated and aggressive rehabilitation program.

MUSCLE IMBALANCES

Control of the scapular and humerus are primarily dictated be a series of muscle force couples.[25] A force couple is defined as two forces of equal magnitude but in opposite direction, that produce rotation on a body.[26] The scapula force couple is formed by the upper fibers of the trapezius muscle, the levator scapula muscle, and the

upper fibers of the serratus anterior muscle. The lower portion of the force couple is formed by the lower fibers of the trapezius muscle and the lower fibers of the serratus anterior muscle.[3] Simultaneous contraction of these muscles produces a smooth rhythmic motion to rotate and protract the scapula along the posterior thorax during elevation of the arm. The scapula functions to provide a stable base of support for the rotating humerus to allow the humeral head to maintain its normal pathway or rotation along the glenoid.[27] Parascapular weakness can result in an unstable base of support for the humerus and may result in inefficient action of the rotator cuff muscles. In addition, the acromion may not sufficiently elevate to provide adequate clearance of the greater tuberosity of the humerus. The coordinated action of the scapula muscles is therefore believed by most clinicians to be indispensable to overall normal shoulder function, and current treatment programs are designed to restore normal parascapular muscle control. However, objective data in assessing changes in parascapular muscle control and position at best are limited, and in some cases equivocal.[16,20,21] The best known test, developed by Kibler, is known as the lateral scapula slide test, which measures the ability of the scapular stabilizers to control the medial border of the scapula during three positions of the limb.[20] Kibler found an increase of 1 cm or more in two of the three positions correlated with shoulder impingement and instability in baseball players.

The inferior and horizontal directed rotator cuff muscle force vectors maintain the humeral head within the shallow glenoid, thereby resisting the upward shear force of the deltoid generated during active elevation of the arm.[25] The result is that the rotator cuff muscles in effect "steer" the humeral head along the glenoid during movement the humerus.[28] The combination of the resultant contractions of the rotator cuff muscles and the deltoid produce the glenohumeral joint force couple (Fig. 9.4). With an intact and normally functioning rotator cuff muscle group, the center of the humeral head is restrained in a very small arc of motion (within 3 mm) along the glenoid fossa. Poppen and

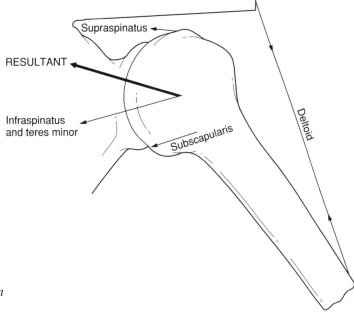

FIGURE 9.4 *Glenohumeral force couple. The resultant force of the rotator cuff muscles results in compression and inferior glide of the humeral head during elevation of the arm.*

Walker[24] and Weiner and MacNab[5] found that in the presence of rotator cuff disease, the center of rotation of the humeral head migrates 6 mm or greater in superior direction during elevation of the arm. The loss of the rotator cuff force couple, therefore, can result in repetitive impingement of the suprahumeral soft tissues. The result is an inflammatory cascade and rotator cuff pathology.

POSTURAL CHANGES

Changes in posture in the upper quarter or quadrant of the body has been implicated as a predisposing factor in primary impingement syndrome.[15,17,19] A common postural change associated with shoulder problems is the forward head and rounded shoulder posture.[17,19] Components of this posture include an increased thoracic kyphosis, protracted and downwardly rotated scapulae, internal rotation of the glenohumeral joints, increased anterior cervical spine inclination, and backward bending at the atlanto-occipital joint. Kendall et al.,[18] Kendall and McCreary,[19] and Janda[17] indicated a sequela of

changes that accompany this posture that result in muscles imbalances, putatively altering the force couple mechanisms about the shoulder with potential pathomechanical changes. Biochemical and clinical studies by Diveta et al.,[21] Culham and Peat,[29] Greenfield et al.,[16] Griegel-Morris et al.,[15] and Kibler[20] have examined postural variables in shoulder patients and found mixed results in correlating postural changes with muscle imbalances and shoulder dysfunction. Differences in methodologies and different operational definitions of postural variables may account for the equivocal results correlating posture with injury. Continued examination of posture and function is important to determine the relevance of posture in the overall evaluation and treatment of shoulder dysfunction.

PRECIPITATING FACTORS

Precipitating factors to injury are any activities that involve repetitive use of the arm, usually overhead or above shoulder level, that results in subacromial impingement.[22,23] The baseball pitcher who pitches a nine inning game early in the season, the retiree who decides to spend the weekend painting her house, and the stock clerk who works two 12-hour shifts to stock inventory, are examples of individuals with precipitating factors that result in overuse to the shoulder. A caveat to practicing clinicians is to identify these factors early and to modify activities appropriate to the stage of pathology of impingement and degree of clinical reactivity.

INTRINSIC FACTORS

The primary intrinsic factors can be divided into vascular, degenerative, and anatomic. The original significance of rotator cuff tendon vascularity was described by Codman.[12] Codman re-

ferred to a critical zone in which rupture of the supraspinatus occurred. This zone was located approximately 1 cm medially to the insertion of the tendon. Moseley and Goldie[30] noted that the anastomosis of the osseous and tendinous vessels in the supraspinatus occurred at this site. Rothman and Parke[10] believed that this location was relatively avascular, a condition intensified by aging. Microinjection studies of normal shoulders in cadavers have shown an area of decreased vascularity within the tendinous portion of the supraspinatus tendon. Rathbun and Macnab[9] noted that the critical zone of the rotator cuff had an adequate blood supply when the vessels were injected with the arm in the abducted position, but this area was hypovascular when

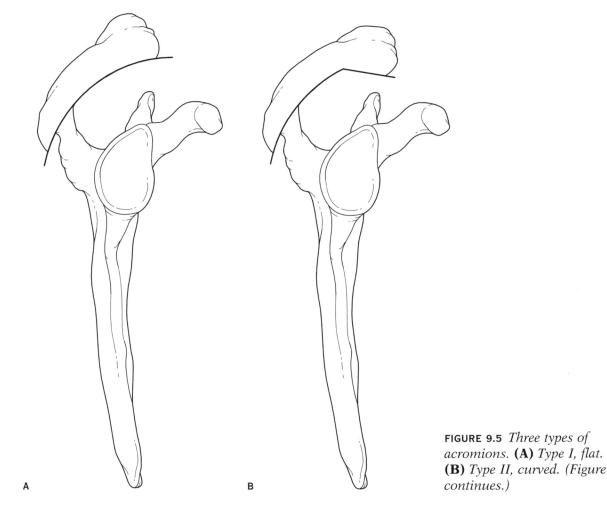

A   B

FIGURE 9.5 *Three types of acromions.* **(A)** *Type I, flat.* **(B)** *Type II, curved. (Figure continues.)*

the injection was given with the arm in the adducted position. The authors propose a hypothesis of transient hypovascularity in the critical zone as a result of vessels being "wrung out" when the arm was in the adducted position. The authors indicated that within this zone most degenerative rotator cuff tears occur, suggesting that hypovascularity of the supraspinatus tendon may play a role in the pathogenesis of rotator cuff tears. Lohr and Uhthoff[31] found that the area of hypovascularity in the critical zone was more pronounced along the articular than the bursal surface of the supraspinatus tendon, and within the site of early degeneration. Although there is not yet any definitive scientific evidence

of a direct cause-and-effect relationship, the finding seem to indicate a vascular predisposition to the pathogenesis of rotator cuff disease and impingement.

DEGENERATION

Evidence indicates a natural age-related degeneration of the rotator cuff tendons. Codman[12] noted that rotator cuff tendon rupture in older patients normally occurred bilaterally and in the presence of preexisting tendon degeneration. Uhthoff et al.[13] and Ozaki et al.[14] found insertional tendinopathy or preexisting tendon degeneration in human specimens. These changes included histologic changes in the arrangement of tendon fibers, fiber disruption at their insertion site, and microcysts and osteopenia along the insertion site. These changes found along the articular side (humeral side) were not usually associated with changes in the acromial process.

ANATOMIC ANOMALIES

Morrison and Bigliani[8] studied the shape of the anteroinferior acromion in anatomic specimens and in patients. The authors identified three types of acromions: type I (flat), type II (curved), and type III (hooked), (Fig. 9.5). In their anatomic specimens studies, 70 percent of rotator cuff tears were associated with type II or III acromions. None had type I acromions. Although no causal relationship between the shape of the acromion and rotator cuff tears or impingement can be concluded, the clinical findings support Neer's theory of impingement occurring primarily along the anteroinferior acromion.

Stages of Pathology and Principles of Treatment

Program design for conservative management of primary impingement syndrome is predicated on a problem-solving approach. This approach necessitates a thorough evaluation to clarify the nature and extent of the pathology, the stage of

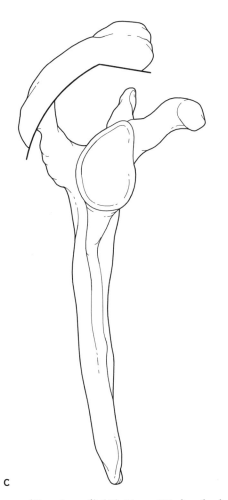

C

FIGURE 9.5 *(Continued).***(C)** *Type III, hooked.*

TABLE 9.1 *Neer stages of impingement*

STAGES	CLINICAL PRESENTATION	TREATMENT PRINCIPLES
Stage I	Subacromial pain/tenderness	Reduce and eliminate inflammation
Age: Less than 25 years	Painful/arc	Patient education
Pathology: Edema and hemorrhage	Positive impingement/Neer test	Restore proximal control
	Strong and painful for resisted abduction and external rotation	(parascapular muscular control)
Stage II	Add: Capsular pattern of limitation at glenohumeral joint	Reestablish glenohumeral capsular mobility
Age: 25 to 40 years		
Pathology: Tendinitis/bursitis and fibrosis		
Stage III	Add: Weakness abduction and external rotation, "squaring" of acromion	Based on size of tear
Age: over 40 years		
Pathology: Bone spurs and tendon disruption		

reactivity, underlying dysfunctions including extrinsic problems to formulate a physical therapy diagnosis, and other factors that may affect treatment planning and outcome (age of patient, motivation, underlying disease). Classifying the pathology based on the progression described by Neer can be correlated to clinical signs and symptoms and can provide a basic framework for preliminary treatment planning and progression. All program designs should be divided into treatment phases that include specific goals and criteria for progression, and include continual reevaluation of both subjective and objective findings.

Table 9.1 presents a summary of the stages of pathology described by Neer. The stages are presented separately but represent a continuum of pathology that in some cases will overlap in a particular patient.

STAGE I IMPINGEMENT

Stage I of impingement is characterized by edema and hemorrhage (inflammation) of the rotator cuff and suprahumeral tissues. The patient is usually less than 25 years of age, and normally there is a precipitating factor of overuse of the shoulder. The clinical symptoms include pain along the anterior and lateral aspect of the shoulder, which when acute or reactive will extend below the elbow. The pain is usually described as a deep dull ache, with sharp subacro-

mial pain with elevation of the limb. The patient presents with full active and passive range of motion (ROM), a painful arc (pain between 60 to 90 and 120 degrees of elevation of the limb), and a positive impingement sign. Muscle strength is usually normal for the abductors, and external rotators of the glenohumeral joint but can be painful and weak in an acute state. Palpation elicits subacromial tenderness usually along the greater tubercle and bicipital groove. Muscle spasms are often present along the ipsilateral upper trapezius, levator scapula, and subscapularis muscles.

Principles of Treatment

Principles of treatment for stage I are based on the stage of clinical reactivity and associated dysfunctions. For an acute presentation, goals of treatment are to reduce and eliminate inflammation, increase the patient's awareness of impingement syndrome, improve proximal (parascapular) muscle control, and prevent muscle atrophy or weakness due to disuse at the glenohumeral joint. The patient should be instructed to rest from activity but not function, and to perform all activities in front of the shoulder and below shoulder level. Forceful active elevation above shoulder level can produce a painful arc and impingement and perpetuate the inflammatory response. The patient would do well to take an oral anti-inflammatory medicine (nonsteroi-

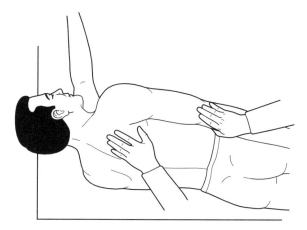

FIGURE 9.6 *Manual technique illustrating resisted posterior scapular depression to facilitate early recruitment of parascapular muscles.*

TABLE 9.2 *Shoulder-strengthening exercises*

MUSCLE	EXERCISE
Supraspinatus	Prone horizontal abduction
	Scaption in internal rotation
Infraspinatus	Prone horizontal abduction in external rotation
Teres minor	Prone horizontal abduction in external rotation
Subscapularis	Scaption in internal rotation
	Military press with dumbbell
Anterior deltoid	Scaption in internal/external rotation
Posterior deltoid	Prone extension
Upper trapezius	Rowing (prone with dumbbell)
	Shrug
Middle trapezius	Prone horizontal abduction in neutral position
Lower trapezius	Prone horizontal abduction in external rotation
Rhomboids	Rowing (prone with dumbbell)
	Prone horizontal abduction in neutral position
Serratus anterior	Push-up with a plus

dal), in conjunction with anti-inflammatory modalities including ice, interferential stimulation, or pulsed or low-intensity ultrasound.[32] Soft tissue work and stretching should be used to alleviate muscle spasms. Exercise including manual resistance can be used early to facilitate scapular parascapular muscle control without further irritation to the suprahumeral tissues (Fig. 9.6).

As reactivity reduces with elimination of rest pain and pain below the elbow, and elimination of painful arc and subacromial tenderness, the patient is progressed into a dynamic strengthening program that emphasizes reestablishment of the force couple mechanisms at both the scapulothoracic junction and glenohumeral joint. Table 9.2 lists exercises that are normally effective at this stage. Emphasis should include high repetitions (3 to 5 sets of 15 repetitions for each exercise), multiple sessions of 3 to 4 daily, working initially in a pain-free range, and using both concentric an eccentric muscle contraction. Exercises are slowly increased to 7 to 10 different movement patterns to isolate different muscle groups. Neer suggests that a patient should continue this conservative approach for several months before surgical treatment is considered. If the patient is an athlete, as signs and symptoms permit, an additional program of sport-spe-

cific exercises and functional training should be incorporated into the program.

STAGE II IMPINGEMENT

Stage II impingement is characterized by fibrosis of the glenohumeral capsule and subacromial bursa and tendinitis of the involved tendons. The condition is normally seen in patients between 20 and 40 years. The clinical presentation can be similar to that of stage I, except that the patient presents with loss of active and passive ROM due to the capsular fibrosis. The loss of ROM normally presents in the so-called capsular pattern described by Cyriax,[33] as significant loss of external rotation and abduction, with less loss of internal rotation.

Principles of Treatment

The principles of treatment are similar to those of stage I with the exception that a major goal is to restore full active and passive ROM to

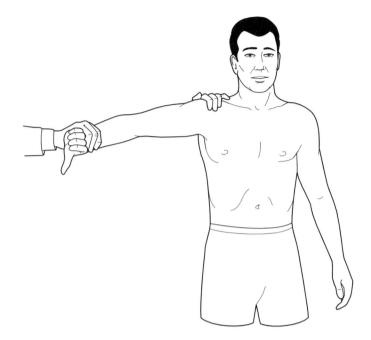

FIGURE 9.7 *Supraspinatus test. The arm is abducted with internal rotation (thumb down) in the plane of the scapula. The patient is asked to resist downward pressure on the abducted arm. A test is considered positive if the patient is unable to hold the arm against resistance.*

avoid further impingement and tissue damage. Cofield and Simonet[34] described how patients with adhesive capsulitis of the glenohumeral joint resulted in subacromial impingement. Specifically, posterior capsule tightness caused the humeral head to roll forward and superiorly into the subacromial arch and anteroinferior acromion. Subsequent treatment should be directed at restoring capsular extensibility to allow the humeral head to attain its normal center of rotation. Several manual techniques described in Chapter 13 in this text are effective for mobilizing the glenohumeral joint capsule. The force and direction of the mobilizing force should be based on the stage of reactivity and clinical mobility testing. Treatment time in patients with a stage II pathology is longer than with stage I, and the prognosis and functional outcome may be more limited.

STAGE III IMPINGEMENT

Stage III impingement is the most difficult to treat conservatively and is characterized by disruption of the rotator cuff tendons. The patient is normally older than 40 years. Clinically, muscle

testing yields weakness, usually for external rotation and abduction. Visual observation indicates a "squaring" of the acromion, which indicates atrophy of both the rotator cuff and deltoid muscles. In significant tendon disruption, a positive "drop-arm" or supraspinatus test will be present (Fig. 9.7).

Principles of Treatment

Treatment principles are based partly on the size and location of the tear (Table 9.3). Tears are classified by size, diameter, location, or topography of the tear.[35,36] The small and moderate-size tears can do relatively well with limited functional goals; the patient is progressed simi-

TABLE 9.3 *Classification of rotator cuff tear based on diameter*

SIZE	TREATMENT PRINCIPLES
≥1 cm	Conservative
1–3 cm	Conservative/acromioplasty/debridement/ mini-open repair
3–5 cm	Mini-open repair
≤5 cm	Open repair

lar to the previous treatment principles. If treatment is ineffective and the patient continues to have pain and inability to raise the arm overhead, surgical options include rotator cuff debridement and anterior acromioplasty, or an mini-open repair. For those with large and massive tears, surgery is usually the most effective option followed by an extensive rehabilitation program incorporating the basic treatment principles of impingement syndrome, and adhering to soft tissue healing guidelines.

CASE STUDY 1: PRIMARY IMPINGEMENT

This case represent a typical progression for a patient who presently clinically with primary impingement syndrome. Goals and treatment are based on some of the principles of treatment discussed in the previous sections.

HISTORY

The patient is a 22-year-old male. He works as a construction worker and enjoys lifting weights. He had an overzealous workout the previous week and attempted to perform maximum resistance during all his exercises. Since that time the patient has reported right anterior and lateral shoulder pain extending to his elbow. The pain is described as a dull ache and sharp during shoulder elevation. He has difficulty sleeping on the right shoulder at night. He is right hand dominant. His family physician prescribed Motrin, and referred him for a trial of physical therapy with a diagnosis of right shoulder muscle strain.

PHYSICAL THERAPY EVALUATION

Visual Inspection: Muscular young male; no external deformities, signs of swelling, or ecchymosis.
AROM: Scapulohumeral elevation in the scapular plane produced a painful arc between 90° and 120°; bilateral scapular winging was noted.
PROM: Full and pain-free in all planes of motion.
Accessory motion testing of the glenohumeral joint: Normal mobility and symmetrical with the uninvolved side.

Resisted testing: Painful and strong for resisted shoulder abduction and external rotation.
Special tests: Positive Neer impingement test.
Palpation: Tender greater tubercle.

ASSESSMENT

Based on presenting signs and symptoms, onset, and patient's age, the physical therapist classified a stage I primary impingement. The stage of clinical reactivity was acute; the patient had pain to the elbow, was unable to sleep on the involved side, had a painful arc, pain with manual resistance, and a positive impingement sign. Resisted testing and palpation seem to indicated primary involvement of the supraspinatus muscle tendon.

TREATMENT PLAN

Initial treatment goals were to reduce and eliminate inflammation of the supraspinatus tendon, to educate the patient concerning his condition and helpful and harmful positions of the arm, and to improve parascapular muscle control (due to scapular winging and possible weakness of the serratus anterior muscle). The patient was instructed to maintain his arm below shoulder level and in front of the shoulder to avoid impingement and stretching of the tendon. He was also instructed not to lift weights. He was instructed to try to maintain his arm in partial abduction and in the scapular plane to promote perfusion to the supraspinatus tendon. Early scapular exercises included manual resistance and simple shoulder shrugs and scapular retraction exercises (Fig. 9.6), and were used to promote parascapular muscle control and coordination. Ice and pulsed ultrasound was applied along the greater tubercle to reduce inflammation and facilitate healing. Pulse ultrasound maintained a low intensity, and produced an acoustical streaming effect for protein synthesis and cellular migration. The frequency of application was 3 MHz because of the superficial penetration that was required for the sound waves.

The patient was seen for five sessions and improved considerably; reevaluation indicated subjective reduction in both the intensity and area of pain, the ability to sleep on the right shoulder at night, elimination of painful arc, and pain with resisted abduction and external rotation.

Treatment goals were updated to facilitate dynamic humeral head control and muscle endurance, and to optimize parascapular muscle control. The patient was instructed in a program of exercises (Table 9.2) to be performed with 2 lbs for 3 sets of 8 repetitions. He was instructed to exercise initially twice daily and in pain-free range. Every two sessions, he was to increase one repetition per set to 20 repetitions for 3 sets. Ice was to be used after exercises. He was instructed to not perform other resistance exercises until he was completely pain-free.

SUMMARY OF CASE

The patient continued this program for 1 month on a home program, and was checked periodically by the physical therapist. He did quite well, and after 1 month returned to full activity with the warning not to overdo his weight lifting. The approach to this case was partly based on correct classification of the pathology. Often in young, active individuals, an underlying glenohumeral joint instability is present that necessitates a slightly different approach, and is reviewed in this chapter.

Rotator Cuff Pathology in the Athlete

Rotator cuff disease or impingement that results from glenohumeral joint instability is known generally as secondary impingement. Differentiating primary impingement from secondary impingement is crucial in the proper management of the two general conditions. Secondary impingement treated as primary impingement will fail to resolve the underlying pathology (instability). The following sections review the classification of secondary impingement, which occurs primarily in the overhead and throwing athlete; the related clinical signs and symptoms; and approaches to treatment.

CLASSIFICATION

Rotator cuff pathology in the athlete represents a continuum of problems that may coexist, making the primary diagnosis difficult. General classification of rotator cuff pathology in athletes includes tensile overload, compressive impingement (Neer's classification), instability, and acute traumatic tears. Meister and Andrews[37] classify rotator cuff disease as (1) primary compressive cuff disease, (2) instability with secondary compressive disease, (3) primary tensile overload, (4) secondary tensile overload, and (5) macrotraumatic failure. Primary tensile overload is the result of deceleration forces in the absence of instability, while secondary tensile overload is precipitated by underlying instability. Neer's classification of compressive impingement is also observed in the athletic population, and has been described earlier in this chapter. Compressive rotator cuff disease can occur primarily or secondarily associated with other shoulder dysfunction. Jobe et al.[38,39] described a four-level classification of the impingement-instability complex, which focuses on instability as the central process. This classification includes (1) pure impingement without instability, (2) impingement with instability, (3) impingement with multidirectional instability, and (4) pure anterior instability without impingement. Finally, athletes sustain acute traumatic tears, and this topic will be addressed in Chapter 11.

These problems occur principally in athletes involved in overhead sports, such as swimmers, tennis players, baseball and softball players, and volleyball players. Although rotator cuff dysfunction is seen most frequently in overhead sport athletes, individuals may present with the same pathology as a result of work-related activity. The same deceleration forces observed during tennis serving can be found in various work environments. Repetitive overhead hammering or other construction activities produce similar loads to swimming or throwing. The underlying mechanics resulting in overuse must be analyzed relative to the respective signs and symptoms.

PRIMARY TENSILE OVERLOAD

Primary tensile overload can be defined as rotator cuff failure under tensile loads. These tensile loads are primarily the result of eccentric muscle contractions generally associated with activities such as throwing. In this case, the rotator cuff functions to decelerate the horizontal adduction, internal rotation, anterior translation, and distraction forces seen during deceleration.[37] During the early cocking phase of throwing, supraspinatus EMG has been shown to be 40 percent of maximum manual muscle test (MMT), with increases to 45 percent MMT during late cocking.[40] Peak infraspinatus and teres minor muscle activity have been found in the late cocking and follow-through phases of pitching.[40,41] DiGiovine et al.[42] found supraspinatus activity to peak in the early cocking phase as 60 percent MMT, and to diminish to 49 and 51 percent MMT during the late cocking and acceleration phases, respectively. Infraspinatus activity peaked at 74 percent MMT during late cocking while teres minor activity was found to be 71 percent MMT during late cocking and 84 percent MMT during deceleration. Andrews and Angelo[43] describe rotator cuff tears in throwers located from the midsupraspinatus posterior to the midinfraspinatus, consistent with the deceleration function of these muscles.

The mechanism of primary tensile overload is repetitive microtrauma during decelerative functions, resulting in fatigue and failure of the dynamic stabilizers. In addition to the rotator cuff's function in deceleration and abduction, the supraspinatus, infraspinatus, and teres minor also function to stabilize the humeral head on the glenoid. This is the dynamic component of shoulder stability, with static stabilization provided by the labrum and capsuloligamentous structures. When the rotator cuff fatigues as a result of repetitive overload, not only is the decelerative function affected, but the stabilization function is also impaired. The result may be secondary overload on the capsulolabral structures ("relative instability") and/or secondary compressive impingement. As pain persists, subtle changes in movement patterns can exacerbate the problem. Gowan et al.[40] studied the EMG patterns in amateur baseball pitchers and compared those patterns to professional pitchers. The professional pitchers used the shoulder muscles more efficiently than the amateurs, who used the rotator cuff and biceps brachii muscles during the acceleration phase.

Examination of the shoulder with primary tensile rotator cuff dysfunction reveals a stable shoulder without true compressive impingement. Resistive testing of the rotator cuff will be painful and may be weak with single or multiple repetition testing. Andrews and Gialuman[44] describe the hallmark of primary tensile cuff disease to be a partial "undersurface" rotator cuff tear. This type of tear is described as an "inside-outside" tear. Frequently no signs of compressive impingement are found at surgery.

The treatment principles are embedded in the knowledge of the underlying pathology, healing process of soft tissue, and functional demands of the shoulder. Given the premise that primary tensile overload is the result of excessive eccentric muscle contractions and resultant rotator cuff fatigue, the focus of rehabilitation should address these issues. Numerous training techniques exist that challenge the rotator cuff eccentrically. The therapist should be familiar with these techniques, as well as the muscle physiology of eccentric contractions in order to prevent exacerbation of the problem. Failure of conservative measures may result in surgery to deride the rotator cuff tear. Subacromial decompression is rarely necessary, as associated compressive cuff disease is uncommon.[37]

SECONDARY TENSILE OVERLOAD

Secondary tensile overload, like primary tensile overload, is defined as rotator cuff failure under tensile loads. In this case, excessive rotator cuff loading is due to underlying instability. The supraspinatus, infraspinatus, and teres minor function to compress the humeral head into the glenoid, providing dynamic stability.[41,45–47] This "double function" leads to early fatigue failure, tendinitis, and possible secondary mechanical impingement.[48]

The pathomechanics of secondary tensile overload are related to the rotator cuff's role in dynamic stability. In contrast to primary tensile overload, where "relative instability" may occur as a result of rotator cuff fatigue, secondary tensile overload results from the simultaneous demands of deceleration and stabilization. Although both of demands are present and generally tolerated in the normal shoulder, the unstable shoulder places an additional burden on the rotator cuff. Because the static stabilizers are compromised, the rotator cuff is overloaded, resulting in dysfunction and injury.

Evaluation of the shoulder with secondary tensile overload is similar to that of primary tensile overload, with the addition of underlying instability. Instability can be unidirectional or multidirectional and is evaluated with traditional instability testing. However, the symptoms may be those of pain rather than those of instability, and careful examination is necessary to delineate the underlying pathology. Impingement signs may be positive if secondary compressive impingement coexists. Arthroscopic findings demonstrate instability as well as an associated undersurface rotator cuff tear.

As with primary tensile overload, the treatment principles should address the underlying pathology. In this case, emphasis on dynamic stabilization will be the focus. Again, supraspinatus, infraspinatus, and teres minor strengthening will be of key importance owing to their role in both eccentric deceleration and stabilization. Additionally, the subscapularis should be trained owing to its role in opposing superior humeral head translation and contributions to the rotator cuff moment.[46,49] Failure of conservative treatment may result in surgical intervention. Stabilization procedures and debridement of a partial rotator cuff tear are the appropriate surgical measures to address the underlying pathology.

Instability–Impingement Complex

The scheme of instability and associated impingement of Jobe et al.[38,39,50] uses a four-group classification system, with instability as the central theme. In the young athlete, participation in overhead sports such as throwing, swimming, tennis, and volleyball requires large ranges, forces, and repetitions. This results in microtrauma to the static and dynamic structures, laxity in the anterior capsule, anterior humeral head subluxation, and posterior capsule tightness. This has been described as the instability–impingement complex (IIC) and can be represented by the following scheme[38]:

Instability → Subluxation → Impingement

→ Rotator cuff tear

Group 1 is considered to be the individual with pure impingement whose examination findings include positive impingement signs and negative apprehension signs. This group is generally comprised of the older recreational athlete, and is rarely seen in the younger athlete. Arthroscopic examination reveals a stable shoulder with an undersurface rotator cuff tear and associated subacromial bursitis. The labrum and glenohumeral ligaments will be normal. Treatment principles are based upon clinical examination findings, and follow the general guidelines presented in Neer's model of compressive cuff disease.

Group 2 consists of individuals with impingement-associated with labral and/or capsular injury, instability, and secondary impingement. Findings include positive impingement and apprehension and relocation signs, as well as arthroscopic findings of instability, labral damage, and an undersurface rotator cuff tear. However, the instability findings are often so subtle, even under anesthesia, that the underlying pathology may be overlooked. As with group 1 impingement, most individuals will respond to a conservative program that addresses the specific mobility, strength, and endurance deficits. Recognition of the underlying instability is the key to successful rehabilitation. In the event of failed conservative treatment, surgical intervention to stabilize the shoulder and debride any rotator cuff damage provides the best results.

Isolated acromioplasty can exacerbate underlying instability.

Those individuals classified into group 3 have hyperelastic soft tissues resulting in anterior or multidirectional instability and associated impingement. Hyperelasticity as evidenced by joint hyperextension is the distinguishing characteristic between groups 2 and 3. In this case, impingement, apprehension, and relocation signs will be positive. Arthroscopic examination reveals an unstable shoulder, an attenuated but intact labrum, and an undersurface rotator cuff tear. Jobe and Glousman[50] emphasize the difficulty in clarifying the diagnosis in groups 2 and 3. Once the diagnosis is made and the underlying pathology identified, appropriate rehabilitation measures are generally effective in returning the athlete to his or her sport.

Group 4 consists of those individuals with pure anterior instability without associated impingement. Injury is the result of a traumatic event, resulting in an acute partial or complete dislocation. Clinical and arthroscopic examination are consistent with an unstable shoulder, without impingement.

REHABILITATIVE ISSUES

Overview

Jobe and Pink[38] report that approximately 95 percent of patients with IIC will respond to conservative treatment. The remaining 5 percent will require a surgical procedure that addresses the primary pathology. Anywhere from 2 to 3 to 6 to 12 months of *appropriate* conservative rehabilitation have been recommended before considering surgical intervention, depending upon the specific impingement problem.[37,44,51,52] The rehabilitation program should be based upon the underlying pathology, the clinical examination results, and the patient goals. The concept that everyone with impingement should be treated with a stretching and strengthening program neglects the spectrum of impingement problems. Jobe et al.[39] emphasize this fact in suggesting that stretching should be performed judiciously, and only when specific musculotendinous tight-

ness can be demonstrated. Excessive stretching of already lax anterior shoulder structures may exacerbate the problem.

Rehabilitative exercises have been recommended for treating the unstable shoulder.[53,54] Burkhead and Rockwood[53] treated 140 unstable shoulders in 115 patients with an exercise program. Subjects had traumatic or atraumatic recurrent anterior, posterior, or multidirectional shoulder subluxation. In those individuals with atraumatic subluxation, 83 percent had a good or excellent result, compared with 15 percent of those with traumatic instability. The authors emphasize the importance of continuing a maintenance strengthening program, as several patients had recurrent symptoms when they stopped the exercises.

Mallon and Speer[54] recommend strengthening of the rotator cuff, specifically the supraspinatus owing to its role in preventing inferior subluxation. Short-arc strengthening is advocated, and stretching generally avoided. Kronberg et al.[55] evaluated the muscle activity and coordination in normal shoulders, and concluded that muscle activity plays a significant role in stabilization via coordinated activation of prime movers and antagonists. A subsequent study analyzed shoulder muscle activity in patients with generalized joint laxity and shoulder instability compared to the controls in the previous study.[56] Patient results demonstrated increased anterior and middle deltoid activity during flexion and abduction and decreased subscapularis activity during internal rotation as compared to controls. A nonsignificant increase in supraspinatus activity was recorded during all movements except flexion, suggesting compensatory muscle function. These findings support the supraspinatus role in stabilization, and underscore the importance of training this muscle in rehabilitation.

Evaluation

The varying muscle function throughout any upper extremity activity underscores the importance of the evaluation process. The first and most fundamental rehabilitation issue is clarification of the problem through a thorough evaluation. Subjective information should include the painful position or motion, with estimation of the force, direction, and magnitude of muscle activity. In addition to the primary movers, muscles functioning as stabilizers and antagonists must be identified. The therapist should be aware that underlying instability may be subtle and unrecognized by the athlete. Moreover, instability testing may reproduce pain but not a feeling of apprehension. The rehabilitation program will vary depending upon the absence or presence of underlying hyperelasticity, frank instability, and/or secondary compressive impingement. In all cases, the primary underlying pathology will be focus of rehabilitation, while secondary problems are simultaneously addressed. This situation is clearly more difficult than the individual presenting with a singular problem. Many athletes have returned to the clinic with a recurrence of impingement with a previously unrecognized underlying dysfunction. Realize that this underlying dysfunction may not evident in the shoulder girdle, but may be weakness in another link in the kinetic chain, resulting in excessive load on the shoulder. A lower extremity or back injury may alter movement patterns, which are amplified at the shoulder.

Itoi et al.[47] emphasize the importance of shoulder position in kinetic and kinematic analysis, as muscle function changes depending upon position. Moreover, an understanding of the differences in muscle activity between sports and among phases of the same sport is the key to designing a rehabilitation program. Electromyographic activity has been documented in swimming, throwing, golf, and tennis, and in painful and in normal shoulders.[57-63] When evaluating electromyographic data, the type of muscle contraction should be considered. The MMT on which EMG data is based is generally performed isometrically, while acquired EMG data may be from isometric, concentric, or eccentric muscle contractions, depending upon the muscle's role at any point in time. Because of the efficiency of eccentric muscle activity, the same force can be generated with fewer motor units, resulting in a lower percentage of MMT. Incorrect interpretation of this data could affect rehabilitation pro-

gram design. The type of muscle contraction required at the painful position and the number of repetitions guide rehabilitation program design.

An important aspect of the evaluation process is the determination of the specific return to activity goals. If strength or endurance are the primary issues, these should be the primary focus of rehabilitation. Dynamic stabilization and coordination drills should be at the program's core in athletes with underlying instability. Not all athletes require a plyometric program to return to their sport, and as such, the program should differ from one individual to the next most dramatically in the late stages. As the rehabilitation program proceeds, the exercise program should begin to resemble the athlete's sport. This includes body posture, exercise range, type of muscle contraction, speed, load, and repetitions. Transition to the functional progression is facilitated by appropriate program design.

Role of the Scapula

The importance of the scapula as the base of support for the glenohumeral joint is well documented.[27,48,57-60,64-66] The scapular stabilizing muscles place the scapula in an position for optimal glenohumeral function, and provide a stable base for the glenohumeral primary movers. These muscles include the rhomboids, trapezii, levator scapulae, serratus anterior, and pectoralis minor. It has been suggested that alterations in scapular positioning may contribute to the problems seen with instability and impingement.[65] As such, evaluation of scapular motion during activity as well as specific muscle testing of the stabilizers is an important component of the rehabilitation program.

Several of the scapular muscles have been studied in normal and in painful shoulders during functional activities to determine changes in firing patterns with pain. When comparing freestyle swimming EMG data between normal and painful shoulders, significant differences were found.[60,62] The painful shoulders demonstrated the following differences when compared to normals: (1) less anterior and middle deltoid activity at hand entry and exit, (2) more infraspinatus activity at the end of pull-through, (3) less subscapularis activity at midrecovery, (4) less rhomboid and upper trapezius activity at hand entry, and (5) more rhomboid and less serratus anterior activity during pulling. Decreased serratus activity during the pulling phase sets the stage for impingement symptoms, as it positions the shoulder in protraction and upward rotation to prevent impingement. Increased rhomboid activity may partially substitute for the serratus by attempting to create more subacromial space, while preparing the shoulder for early hand exit. Similar findings were noted when comparing butterfly swimmers with normal or painful shoulders.[58,59] Again, the serratus anterior, along with teres minor, demonstrated decreased activity, suggesting an unstable base of support and an inability to assist with propulsion. In normal shoulders, the subscapularis, serratus anterior, teres minor, and upper trapezius maintained high levels of activity throughout the stroke, predisposing these muscles to fatigue. As such, training programs should focus on increasing the endurance of these muscles.

Glousman et al.[67] in an EMG study of pitchers with normal shoulders and those with anterior instability, noted decreased pectoralis major, latissimus dorsi, subscapularis, and serratus anterior activity during throwing, and especially during late cocking. During this phase, the serratus anterior functions to oppose the retractors while stabilizing and protracting the scapula. Additionally, the serratus may assist in tipping the scapula to allow for maximum glenohumeral congruency during excessive external rotation.[42] Decreased serratus activity in late cocking would place additional load on the anterior static stabilizers, and may contribute to anterior instability. As such, strength and endurance of these muscles is the keystone for shoulder rehabilitation in this population.

Moseley et al.[27] analyzed the EMG activity in eight scapular muscles during 16 rehabilitation exercises. Optimal exercises for each muscle were identified by the criteria of greater than 50 percent MMT over three consecutive arcs of motion. A group of four core exercises trained each of the eight muscles at the preset criteria, and included scaption (elevation in the scapular plane), rowing, push-up with a plus (additional scapular protraction), and press-up. Closer evaluation of the data will allow the therapist to make appropriate choices regarding scapular strengthening activities. For example, the criteria for the core exercise group required that each muscle be used at the predetermined minimum level. The only qualifying exercise for the pectoralis minor was the press-up, and so it was included in the core group. The press-up did not meet minimal criteria for any other muscle group. Additionally, the highest EMG activity in the middle serratus anterior was produced during flexion and abduction, from 120° to 150°. Moreover, the standard deviations of some exercises are greater than 50 percent of the original value. As such, the therapist should choose exercises judiciously based upon the examination and activity kinetics, and should monitor the exercise quality carefully to assure proper performance (Figs. 9.8 to 9.11).

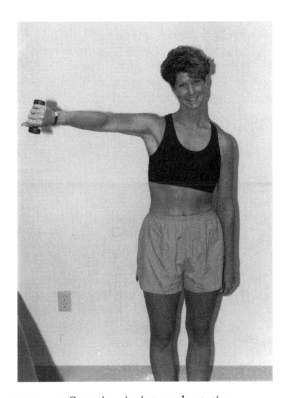

FIGURE 9.8 *Scaption in internal rotation.*

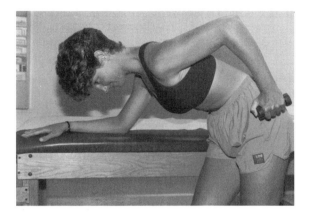

FIGURE 9.9 *Rowing.*

Open and Closed Chain Exercise

Closed chain exercises have been advocated for lower extremity rehabilitation, and have recently been suggested for the treatment of upper extremity problems.[68–71] Traditional physical therapy application of the closed kinetic chain concept assumes the distal segment to be fixed to an object that provides considerable external resistance, while in an open chain, the distal segment is free to move in space. The definition of "considerable external resistance" could potentially be met in a traditional open chain activity.[70] Dillman et al.[70] suggest a new classification of this model owing to inadequate standardized definitions, lack of quantitative-based definitions, classification of some exercises into opposing categories, and comparison of exercises with different mechanics. The authors suggest a three-level classification of (1) moveable boundary, no external load (MNL); (2) moveable boundary, external load (MEL); and (3) fixed boundary, external load (FEL). The MNL classification is like a traditional open chain exercise, the FEL like traditional closed chain exercise, and MEL the "gray" area. Activities representative of the MEL classification are a resisted bench press, hack squat, or leg press. Matched MEL and FEL exercises in a single subject demonstrated that exercises with similar biomechanics result in comparable muscular activity.

Principles of closed chain exercise in the lower extremity have been applied to the upper extremity. Further study is necessary to determine whether this application is appropriate. The supposition that closed chain shoulder exercise enhances static stability during dynamic activity via mechanoreceptor education needs further testing.[69] Specificity of exercise guidelines would suggest little carryover from closed chain exercise to open chain activity. The value of closed chain exercise in the athlete participating

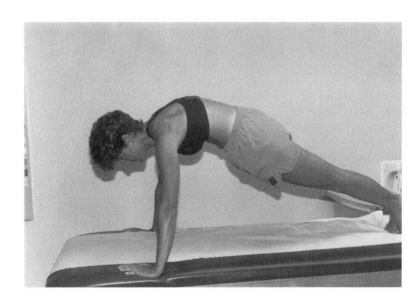

FIGURE 9.10 *Push-ups with a plus (additional scapular protraction).*

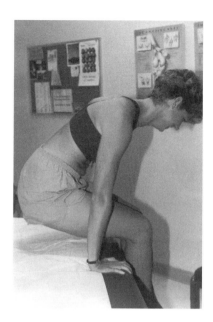

FIGURE 9.11 *Press-up.*

Closed chain exercise for the upper extremity include activities such as wall push-ups, modified and full push-ups with a plus, weight shifts in weight-bearing positions, and press-ups (Figs. 9.10 to 9.14). The progression should be from partial weight-bearing against a wall, to increasing weight-bearing on a table, to the quadriped position, to the modified and full push-up positions. Exercises may be progressed from two-arm to single-arm support, and eventually to plyometrics. Use of gymnastic balls, stair-steppers, slideboards, treadmills, rocker boards, and other traditionally lower extremity equipment challenge the shoulder dynamically. It is critical that the quality of the exercise be maintained throughout. As the scapular stabilizers fatigue, the scapulae may begin to wing, resulting in improper motor programming and possible injury. The therapist and athlete alike must be aware of and able to recognize this situation.

in a closed chain sport is evident. Closed chain exercise training in an open chain sport may be of value for reasons yet to be clarified. Muscular co-contraction in closed chain activity can provide dynamic stabilization for the individual with an unstable shoulder. Carryover of this co-contraction into an open chain is essential for the open chain sport athlete, and will be discussed in further detail in the next section.

The EMG activity during shoulder rehabilitation exercises has been well-documented.[72,73] Townsend et al.[72] studied nine muscles during 17 shoulder exercises. Exercises were considered a challenge if they produced over 50 percent MMT over three consecutive arcs, and 4 exercises were found to load each of the nine muscles at least once at the given criteria. These exercises included (1) scaption in internal rotation, (2) flexion, (3) horizontal abduction in external rota-

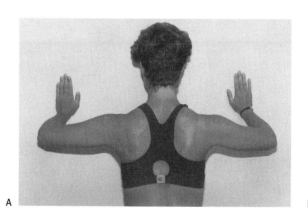
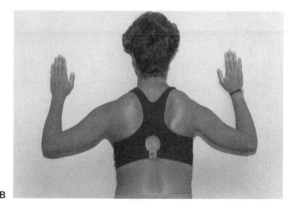

A   B

FIGURE 9.12 **(A)** *Proper performance of wall push-up.* **(B)** *Improper performance of wall push-up with excessive scapular winging. The patient should be verbally cued for proper performance.*

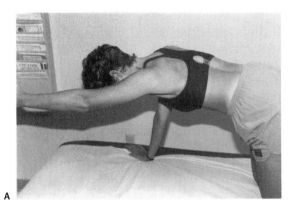
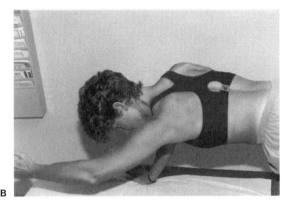

FIGURE 9.13 *Weight-bearing reaching activities.* **(A)** *Proper performance of activity with lumbar spine neutral and proper scapular stabilization.* **(B)** *Improper performance with trunk rotation and poor scapular stabilization on the right.*

tion, and (4) press-up (Figs. 9.8, 9.11, 9.15, and 9.16). As with the data from Moseley and Goldie,[30] closer scrutiny can provide the therapist with a wealth of information to guide rehabilitation. Again, the press-up was included owing to the preset criteria, when EMG activity was noted only in the pectoralis major and latissimus dorsi. For the therapist wanting to selectively train the rotator cuff, other exercises tested would be more appropriate. Although the assumption is made that the exercise with the greatest EMG activity should be chosen to strengthen a specific muscle, a different perspective is fitting. Occasionally such an activity is too strenuous for the individual recovering from an injury or surgery. In this case, the data from Townsend et al.[72] provide the therapist with a number of different choices that may be more appropriate. For example, if scaption in internal rotation is too weak or painful, scaption in external rotation requires less, but still a significant, amount of supraspinatus activity.

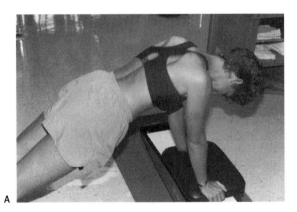
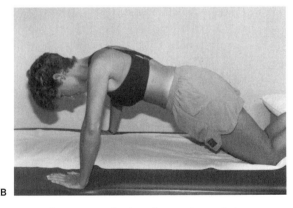

FIGURE 9.14 *Modified push-up position.* **(A)** *Improper performance during dynamic activity with excessive scapular winging during activity.* **(B)** *Return to lower level static activity to reinforce proper performance of exercise.*

Neuromuscular Retraining

Neuromuscular retraining has been advocated by many in the treatment of shoulder dysfunctions, especially the instability complex.[64,74–79] Lephart et al.[75] found decreased passive repositioning sense and threshold to detection of passive motion in individuals with anterior shoulder instability. Following reconstruction, values for these same variables were the same as the normal control group. The relationship between static and dynamic structures has been explored by Cain et al.,[80] who found contraction of the infraspinatus/teres minor reduced strain on the anterior inferior glenohumeral ligament at 90° of abduction. Guanche et al.[81] noted a reflex arc from mechanoreceptors within the glenohumeral capsule to muscles crossing the joint. These findings reinforce the synergistic activity of the static and dynamic structures about the shoulder. However, Borsa et al.[74] suggest that damage to the mechanoreceptors disables the reflexive dynamic stability, increasing the instability problem.

Exercises purporting to facilitate development of proprioception should consider the multilevel aspect of nervous system training. Reflexive patterning at the spinal cord level occurs on a subconscious level, and is only one aspect of

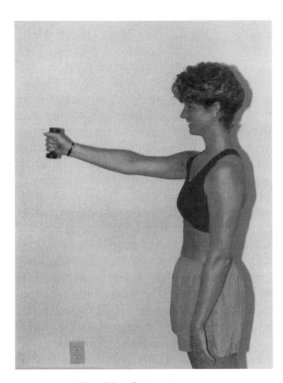

FIGURE 9.15 *Shoulder flexion.*

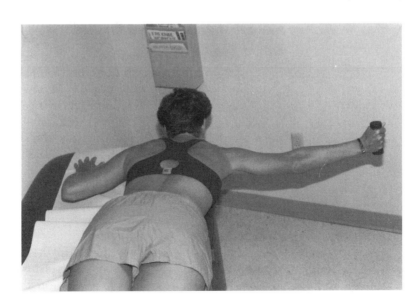

FIGURE 9.16 *Horizontal abduction in external rotation.*

neuromuscular retraining. Higher levels are involved with the planning and execution of motor tasks. The basal ganglia is involved in the more complex aspects of motor planning, and ultimately influences spinal motor neuron pool by forming a control loop with motor areas of the cortex involved with the planning and execution of voluntary motor tasks. The cerebellum regulates some of the specific parameters of motor control including synergistic coordination and background muscle tone. The question of the cognitive role in proprioceptive training deserves attention. It has been suggested that one purpose of a proprioceptive rehabilitation program is to enhance cognitive appreciation of the joint relative to position and motion, and most rehabilitation programs require cognitive attention to the task.[74] However, when throwing a ball, serving a volleyball, or swimming, the athlete is unlikely to be thinking about his or her shoulder. As such, removal of the cognitive aspect of activity must be incorporated at some time in the rehabilitation process. Mentally attending to something besides the task at hand will challenge the nervous system in a more realistic situation. Counting back by serial sevens, or engaging in unrelated conversation while performing challenging activities, will facilitate this skill. Conversion of a conscious task to unconscious motor programming, stored as central commands, is the goal.

Proprioceptive neuromuscular facilitation (PNF) exercises have been advocated for the development of kinesthetic awareness.[64,69,74] Additionally, Wilk and Arrigo[64] recommend several movement awareness drills to enhance neuromuscular control of the shoulder. These drills are performed in the advanced phase, and place the athlete in a position that challenges the stabilizing mechanisms. When performing any kinesthetic or movement awareness exercises, the therapist must closely attend to additional information derived from other sensory systems that may assist in proprioception. These factors might include tactile cueing from the supporting surface, tactile cueing from the therapist, visual cueing, and predictability of movement pattern and speed based upon previous experience. Additionally, the position during exercise becomes critical when considering the role of the cerebellum and basal ganglia in postural set and motor programming. An activity performed in supine on a table does not require the same neuromuscular coordination as when performed in standing.

The Impulse Inertial Exercise System (IES, Newnan, GA) was originally developed with neuromuscular training as the chief consideration. High-speed ballistic activities in any number of movement patterns can be repetitively performed on the IES. Rapid ballistic movements result in different patterns of agonist–antagonist muscle contractions than do slower-speed activities. Synchronous activation of agonists and antagonists occurs with ballistic movements as a result of triphasic muscle activation.[82-86] The initial burst of agonist muscle contraction initiates the activity, and this activity ceases prior to the limb reaching its final position. Subsequently the antagonist fires as a braking mechanism, and the final phase finds the agonist firing again to "clamp" the movement toward the target.[85] The same movement pattern at a slow speed demonstrates only agonist muscle contraction, with braking provided by the passive viscoelastic properties of the tissue. The timing and amplitude of antagonist activity are affected by the distance and speed of the movement. Small-amplitude movements at higher speeds resulted in substantial overlap of burst activity in agonists and antagonists during acceleration, while coactivation occurred in bursts during deceleration.[83] Finally, knowledge of the necessity for antagonist firing affects muscle activity. When a mechanical stop was placed in the testing apparatus, the antagonist burst disappeared within two to three trials, suggesting some cognitive control over the braking mechanism. This work supports the use of high-speed ballistic activities to train open chain co-contraction in an unstable shoulder. Such activities can be achieved by use of the IES or resistive tubing (Figs. 9.17 and 9.18). Any number of movement patterns can be trained, including shoulder rotation in abduction and PNF patterns.

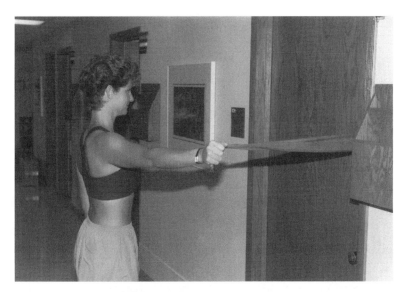

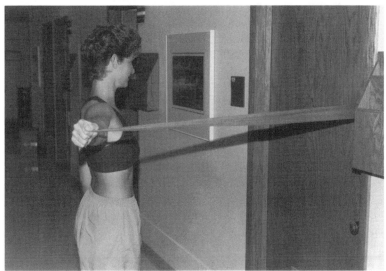

FIGURE 9.17 (A & B)
Starting and ending positions for dynamic ballistic horizontal abduction exercise using resistive tubing.

CASE STUDY 2: INSTABILITY-RELATED IMPINGEMENT

HISTORY

A 16-year-old right hand dominant high school volleyball, and softball player presented with an 8-month history of right shoulder pain. She initially felt a sharp pain while bench pressing, but had no pain after discontinuing the activity.

Shortly thereafter, she was moved from pitcher to center field, requiring longer throws. She was able to manage the remaining 2 weeks of softball. Two weeks later volleyball season started, and her shoulder pain increased. The athletic trainer at her high school placed her on a rotator cuff strengthening program, which did not relieve her symptoms. She completed the volleyball season by modifying her activity level, and had minimal trouble during basketball. However, when softball started, her symptoms again increased.

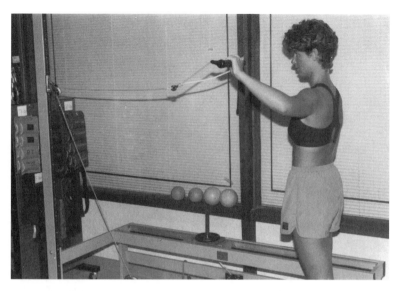

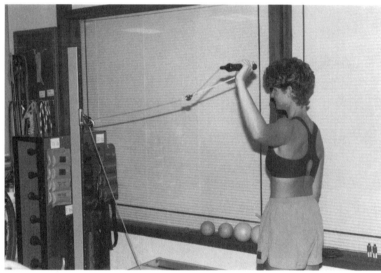

FIGURE 9.18 (A & B) *Starting and ending position for dynamic ballistic shoulder external rotation at 90° of abduction using Impulse Inertial Exercise System.*

The cocking and acceleration phases of throwing were the most painful. She was again placed on a rotator cuff strengthening program of 6 weeks duration by the athletic trainer at her high school. However, when her symptoms failed to resolve, she was referred for formal physical therapy treatment.

PHYSICAL THERAPY EVALUATION

Visual inspection: Young female, no deformities or ecchymosis; scapular posture and muscle bulk symmetrical.

AROM: Painful arc between 90° and 120° of elevation in the frontal plane; full range of motion.
PROM: Full and pain-free in all ranges.
Accessory motion of glenohumeral joint: Increased in all directions bilaterally.
Resisted testing: ⁴⁄₅ strength in resisted abduction, without pain; all other testing strong and pain-free.
Special tests: Neer's and Hawkins' impingement signs positive; horizontal crossover testing negative; biceps tension testing positive; apprehension and relocation testing positive.

Palpation: Tender over biceps tendon and rotator cuff tendon.

ASSESSMENT

Given the history and physical examination of the young athlete's shoulder, it was determined that she had impingement syndrome due to underlying instability (impingement–instability complex). The stage of clinical reactivity was subacute. She had established good rotator cuff strength due to her cuff strengthening program. However, the underlying instability had not been addressed, and was the focus of the rehabilitation program.

TREATMENT PLAN

The initial goal was to build upon her strength base without irritating her secondary impingement syndrome. She was initiated on a high-speed, short range of motion program with yellow resistive bands for shoulder external rotation and shoulder abduction, and red bands for shoulder flexion and extension. All exercises were performed in neutral abduction. After a warm-up, she performed one set for 30 seconds, attempting to perform 30 to 50 repetitions in 30 seconds. She was instructed to add an additional set of 15 seconds or more as tolerated over the next week.

On her return visit, she reported soreness for a day, with no fatigue in flexion and extension exercises after 2 days. Resisted external rotation was slightly sore but strong. Her flexion and extension exercises were progressed to 45° of abduction. One week later, she was improving steadily. She was up to 3 sets for 30 seconds of all exercises. Resisted external rotation was maintained in neutral, but progressed to red resistive bands. Flexion, extension, and abduction were discontinued, and horizontal abduction and adduction exercises at 90° of abduction with green bands were initiated. She was encouraged to try to perform up to 90 repetitions in 30 seconds.

By her fourth visit, she was feeling significantly improved. Internal and external rotation at 90° of abduction was initiated, and the resistance of the bands progressed. On visit 5, she

was progressed to PNF D2 flexion exercises and reproduction of the throwing motion. She performed over 90 repetitions of each exercise in 30 seconds, 3 sets each. On her sixth and last visit, the patient was placed on a functional progression for volleyball, as well as a maintenance strength and coordination program.

SUMMARY OF CASE

A 16-year-old high school athlete was seen for a total of six visits to treat her impingement-instability complex. The key to successful rehabilitation was the recognition of the underlying instability, with exercise protocols addressing this problem. Rotator cuff strengthening alone was ineffective in this athlete, and the incorporation of dynamic stabilization exercises provided the needed dynamic control of her unstable shoulder.

Summary

Impingement syndrome of the shoulder can result in a cascade of pathologies that primarily affect the rotator cuff and result in subacromial pain and shoulder dysfunction. The causes of impingement presented in this chapter are multifactorial but can be divided into two general categories depending on the presence of instability and/or impingement; primary impingement and secondary impingement. These categories are further subdivided based on the pathomechanics of injury, age of patient, dysfunctions, and associated pathologies. In the younger, athletic population the basic problem is instability, which leads to subluxation, impingement, and rotator cuff disease. Treatment is based on accurate classification of the pathology and is logically focused on the signs and symptoms and nature of dysfunction. For example, treatment of impingement in younger athletes is designed to restore shoulder stability and control, and correcting underlying mechanical problems associated with their sport. A systematic evaluation of the nature and extent of the injury is imperative for the clinician to properly classify the problem and design an effective rehabilitation program.

Acknowledgments

We are grateful to Anne Schwartz for providing the drawings on which our figures are based.

References

1. Neer CS: Anterior acromioplasty for the chronic impingement syndrome of the shoulder. J Bone Joint Surg 54A:41, 1972
2. Neer CS: Impingement lesions. Clin Orthop 173: 70, 1983
3. Peat M, Culham E: Functional anatomy of the shoulder complex. p. 1. In Andrews JR, Wilk KE (eds): The Athlete's Shoulder. Churchill Livingstone, New York, 1990
4. Peterson CJ, Redlund-Johnell I: The subacromial space in normal shoulder radiographs. Acta Orthop Scand 55:57, 1984
5. Weiner DS, MacNab I: Superior migration of the humeral head: a radiological aid in the diagnosis of tears of the rotator cuff. J Bone Joint Surg 52B: 524, 1970
6. Patte D: The subcorocoid impingement. Clin Orthop 254:55, 1990
7. Gerber C, Terrier F, Ganz R: The role of the corocoid process in the chronic impingement syndrome. J Bone Joint Surg 67B:703, 1985
8. Morrison DS, Bigliani LU: The clinical significance of variations in acromial morphology. Orthop Trans 11:234, 1987
9. Rathbun JB, Macnab I: The microvascular pattern of the rotator cuff. J Bone Joint Surg 52B:540, 1970
10. Rothman RH, Parke WW: The vascular anatomy of the rotator cuff. Clin Orthop 41:176, 1965
11. Neviaser RJ, Neviaser TJ: Observations on impingement. Clin Orthop 254:60, 1990
12. Codman EA: The Shoulder. 2nd Ed. Thomas Todd, Boston, 1934
13. Uhthoff HK, Hammond I, Sarkar K et al: Enthesopathy of the rotator cuff. Proceedings of 5th Open Meeting of American Shoulder and Elbow Surgeons, Las Vegas, February 1989
14. Ozaki J, Fujimoto S, Yoahiyuki N et al: Tears of the rotator cuff of the shoulder associated with pathological changes in the acromion. J Bone Joint Surg 70A:1224, 1998
15. Griegel-Morris P, Larson K, Mueller-Klaus K et al: Incidence of common postural abnormalities in the cervical, shoulder, and thoracic regions and their associations with pain in two age groups of healthy subjects. Phys Ther 72:6, 1992
16. Greenfield B, Catlin P, Coats P et al: Posture in patients with shoulder overuse injuries and healthy individuals. J Orthop Sports Phys Ther 21:287, 1995
17. Janda V: Muscles, central nervous motor regulation and back problems. p. 29. In Korr I (ed): The Neurobiologic Mechanisms in Spinal Manipulative Therapy. Plenum Press, New York, 1978
18. Kendall HD, Kendall FP, Boynton DA: Posture and Function. Williams & Wilkins, Baltimore, 1958
19. Kendall FP, McCreary EK: Muscles, Testing and Function. 3rd Ed. Williams & Wilkins, Baltimore, 1983
20. Kibler WB: Role of the scapula in the overhead throwing motion. Contep Orthop 22:5, 525, 1991
21. Diveta J, Walker ML, Skibinski B: Relationship between performance of selected scapular muscles and scapular abduction in standing subjects. Phys Ther 70:470, 1990
22. Hawkins RJ, Kennedy JC: Impingement syndrome in athletes. Am J Sports Med 8:151, 1990
23. Herring SA, Nilson KL: Introduction to overuse injuries. Clin Sports Med 6:225, 1987
24. Poppen NK, Walker PS: Normal and abnormal motion of the shoulder. J Bone Joint Surg 58A: 195, 1978
25. Inman VT, Saunders J, Abbott L: Observations on the function of the shoulder joint. J Bone Joint Surg 26:1, 1934
26. Frankel VH, Nordin M: Basic Biomechanics of the Skeletal System. Lea & Febiger, Philadelphia, 1980
27. Moseley BJ, Jobe FW, Pink M et al: EMG analysis of the scapular muscles during a baseball rehabilitation program. Am J Sports Med 20:128, 1992
28. Saha AK: Dynamic stability of the glenohumeral joint. Acta Orthop Scand 42:491, 1971
29. Culham E, Peat M: Functional anatomy of the shoulder complex. J Orthop Sports Phys Ther 18: 342, 1993
30. Moseley HF, Goldie I: The arterial pattern of the rotator cuff of the shoulder. J Bone Joint Surg 45B:780, 1963

31. Lohr JF, Uhthoff HK: The microvascular pattern of the supraspinatus tendon. Clin Orthop 254:35, 1990

32. Miklovitz SL: Thermal Agents in Rehabilitation. 2nd Ed. FA Davis, Philadelphia, 1991

33. Cyriax J: Textbook of Orthopaedic Medicine. Vol. 1: Diagnosis of Soft Tissues Lesions. 8th Ed. Bailliere Tindall, Philadelphia, 1982

34. Cofield RH, Simonet WT: Symposium in sports medicine: part 2, the shoulder in sports. Mayo Clinic Proc 59:157, 1984

35. Timmerman LA, Andrews JR, Wilk KE: Mini open repair of the rotator cuff. p. 153. In Andrews JR, Wilk KE (eds): The Athlete's Shoulder. Churchill Livingstone, New York, 1994

36. Patte D: Classification of rotator cuff lesions. Clin Orthop 254:81, 1990

37. Meister K, Andrews JR: Classification and treatment of rotator cuff injuries in the overhand athlete. J Orthop Sports Phys Ther 18:413, 1993

38. Jobe FW, Pink M: Classification and treatment of shoulder dysfunction in the overhead athlete. J Orthop Sports Phys Ther 18:427, 1993

39. Jobe FW, Tibone JE, Jobe CM, Kvitne RS: The shoulder in sports. p. 961. In Rockwood CA, Matsen FA (eds): The Shoulder. WB Saunders, Philadelphia, 1990

40. Gowan ID, Jobe FW, Tibone JE et al: A comparative electromyographic analysis of the shoulder during pitching. Am J Sports Med 15:586, 1987

41. Bradley JP, Tibone JE: Electromyographic analysis of muscle action about the shoulder. Clin Sports Med 10:789, 1991

42. DeGiovine NM, Jobe FW, Pink M, Perry J: An electromyographic analysis of the upper extremity in pitching. J Shoulder Elbow Surg 1:15, 1992

43. Andrews JR, Angelo RL: Shoulder arthroscopy for the throwing athlete. p. 79. In Paulos LE, Tibone JE (eds): Operative Techniques in Shoulder Surgery. Aspen Publishers, Gaithersburg, MD, 1991

44. Andrews JR, Giduman RH: Shoulder arthroscopy in the throwing athlete: Perspectives and prognosis. Clin Sports Med 6:565, 1987

45. Jobe FW, Moynes DR: Delineation of diagnostic criteria and a rehabilitation program for rotator cuff injuries. Am J Sports Med 10:336, 1982

46. Sharkey NA, Marder RA: The rotator cuff opposes superior translation of the humeral head. Am J Sports Med 23:270, 1995

47. Itoi E, Newman SR, Kuechle DK, Morrey BF: Dynamic anterior stabilisers of the shoulder with the arm in abduction. J Bone Joint Surg 76B:834, 1994

48. Silliman JF, Hawkins RJ: Current concepts and recent advances in the athlete's shoulder. Clin Sports Med 10:693, 1991

49. Keating JF, Waterworth P, Shaw-Dunn J, Crossan J: The relative strength of rotator cuff muscles: A cadaver study. J Bone Joint Surg 75B:137, 1993

50. Jobe FW, Glousman RE: Rotator cuff dysfunction and associated glenohumeral instability in the throwing athlete. p. 85. In Paulos LE, Tibone JE (eds): Operative Techniques in Shoulder Surgery. Aspen Publishers, Gaithersburg, MD, 1991

51. Nielsen KD, Wester JU, Lorentsen A: The shoulder impingement syndrome: The results of surgical decompression. J Shoulder Elbow Surg 3:12, 1994

52. Tibone JE, Elrod B, Jobe FW et al: Surgical treatment of tears of the rotator cuff in athletes. J Bone Joint Surg 68A:887, 1986

53. Burkhead WZ, Rockwood CA: Treatment of instability of the shoulder with an exercise program. J Bone Joint Surg 74A:890, 1992

54. Mallon WJ, Speer KP: Multidirectional instability: current concepts. J Shoulder Elbow Surg 4:54, 1995

55. Kronberg M, Nemeth G, Brostrom LA: Muscle activity and coordination in the normal shoulder: an electromyographic study. Clin Orthop 257:76, 1990

56. Kronberg M, Brostrom LA, Nemeth G: Differences in shoulder muscle activity between patients with generalized joint laxity and normal controls. Clin Orthop 269:181, 1991

57. Pink M, Jobe FW, Perry J et al: The normal shoulder during the backstroke: an EMG and cinematographic analysis of twelve muscles. Clin J Sports Med 2:6, 1992

58. Pink M, Jobe FW, Perry J et al: The painful shoulder during the butterfly stroke: an EMG and cinematographic analysis of twelve muscles. Clin Orthop 288:60, 1993

59. Pink M, Jobe FW, Perry J et al: The normal shoulder during the butterfly stroke: an EMG and cinematographic analysis of twelve muscles. Clin Orthop 288:48, 1993

60. Pink M, Perry J, Browne A et al: The normal shoulder during freestyle swimming: an EMG and cinematographic analysis of twelve muscles. Am J Sports Med 19:569, 1991

61. Jobe FW, Moynes, Antonelli DJ: Rotator cuff function during a golf swing. Am J Sports Med 14:388, 1986

62. Scovazzo ML, Browne A, Pink M et al: The painful shoulder during freestyle swimming: an EMG and cinematographic analysis of twelve muscles. Am J Sports Med 19:577, 1991

63. Ryu R, McCormick J, Jobe FW et al: An electromyographic analysis of shoulder function in tennis players. Am J Sports Med 16:481, 1988

64. Wilk KE, Arrigo C: Current concepts in the rehabilitation of the athletic shoulder. J Orthop Sports Phys Ther 118:365, 1993

65. Paine RM, Voight M: The role of the scapula. J Orthop Sports Phys Ther 18:386, 1993

66. Kelley MJ: Anatomic and biomechanical rationale for rehabilitation of the athlete's shoulder. J Sport Rehab 4:122, 1995

67. Glousman R, Jobe F, Tibone J et al: Dynamic electromyographic analysis of the throwing shoulder with glenohumeral instability. J Bone Joint Surg 70A:220, 1988

68. Lutz GE, Palmitier RA, An KN, Chao EY: Comparison of tibiofemoral joint forces during open-kinetic-chain and closed-kinetic-chain exercises. J Bone Joint Surg 75A:732, 1993

69. Davies GH, Dickoff-Hoffman S: Neuromuscular testing and rehabilitation of the shoulder complex. J Orthop Sports Phys Ther 18:449, 1993

70. Dillman CJ, Murray TA, Hintermeister RA: Biomechanical differences of open and closed chain exercises with respect to the shoulder. J Sport Rehab 3:228, 1994

71. Palmitier R, An KN, Scott S, Chao TY: Kinetic chain exercise in knee rehabilitation. Sports Med 11:402, 1991

72. Townsend H, Jobe FW, Pink M et al: Electromyographic analysis of the glenohumeral muscles during a baseball rehabilitation program. Am J Sports Med 19:264, 1991

73. Blackburn TA, McLeod WD, White B, Wofford L: EMG analysis of posterior rotator cuff exercises. Athl Training 25:40, 1990

74. Borsa PA, Lephart SM, Kocher MS, Lephart SP: Functional assessment and rehabilitation of shoulder proprioception for glenohumeral instability. J Sport Rehab 3:84, 1994

75. Lephart SM, Warner JJ, Borsa PA, Fu F: Proprioception of the unstable shoulder joint in healthy, unstable and surgically repaired shoulders. J Shoulder Elbow Surg 3:371, 1994

76. Irrgang JJ, Whitney SL, Harner CD: Nonoperative treatment of rotator cuff injuries in throwing athletes. J Sport Rehab 1:197, 1992

77. Smith FL, Brunolli J: Shoulder kinesthesia after anterior glenohumeral joint dislocation. Phys Ther 69:106, 1989

78. Blasier RB, Carpenter JE, Huston LJ: Shoulder proprioception: Effect of joint laxity, joint position, and direction of motion. Orthop Rev Jan:45, 1994

79. Allegrucci M, Whitney SL, Lephart SM et al: Shoulder kinesthesia in healthy unilateral athletes participating in upper extremity sports. J Orthop Sports Phys Ther 21:220, 1995

80. Cain RP, Mutschler TA, Fu FH, Lee SK: Anterior stability of the glenohumeral joint. Am J Sports Med 15:144, 1987

81. Guanche C, Knatt T, Solomonow M et al: The synergistic action of the capsule and the shoulder muscles. Am J Sports Med 23:301, 1995

82. Freund HJ, Budingen HJ: The relationship between speed and amplitude of the fastest voluntary contractions of human arm muscles. Exp Brain Res 31:1, 1978

83. Lestienne F: Effects of inertial load and velocity on the braking process of voluntary limb movements. Exp Brain Res 35:4407, 1979

84. Marsden CD, Obeso JA, Rothwell JC: The function of the antagonist muscle during fast limb movements in man. J Physiol 335:1, 1983

85. Wierzbicka MM, Wiegner AW, Shahani BT: Role of agonist and antagonist muscles in fast arm movements in man. Exp Brain Res 63:331, 1986

86. Desmedt JE, Godaux E: Voluntary motor commands in human ballistic movements. Ann Neurol 5:415, 1978

10

Frozen Shoulder

HELEN OWENS

Patients with a diagnosis of frozen shoulder are commonly seen in the physical therapy department. Unfortunately, frozen shoulder is often a "catch-all diagnosis"[1,2] that can imply many shoulder problems. In the literature, confusion abounds on the subject of frozen shoulder. First, there is no consensus on the name of this clinical entity. Some of the more common terms that are synonyms for frozen shoulder are adhesive capsulitis, periarthritis, stiff and painful shoulder, periarticular adhesions, Duplay's disease, scapulohumeral periarthritis, tendinitis of the short rotators, adherent subacromial bursitis,[3] painful stiff shoulder, bicipital tenosynovitis, subdeltoid bursitis, humeroscapular fibrositis, shoulder portion of shoulder-hand syndrome, bursitis calcarea, supraspinatus tendinitis, periarthrosis humeroscapularis, and a host of foreign language terms.[4]

Confusion in terminology probably reflects the confusion in the definition, pathology, etiology, and treatment of this clinical entity that is so evident in the literature. One of the difficulties in reviewing the literature of evaluation and treatment of frozen shoulder, the main thrust of this chapter, was that few studies defined frozen shoulder in the same way. As a result, inconsistencies in patient selection based on their varied definitions made it difficult to assess the value of the treatment being examined. In addition, most studies did not discuss the evaluative procedures used to reach the diagnosis of frozen shoulder. The goals of this chapter are (1) to present a literature review of the pathology, etiology, and clinical features of frozen shoulder; (2) to establish a

working definition of frozen shoulder; and (3) to present evaluative and treatment procedures for frozen shoulder. I hope that the reader can readily apply this information to clinical practice, thereby improving patient care.

Literature Review

Frozen shoulder is loosely defined as a painful stiff shoulder.[1] This definition appears to be more of a description of symptoms than a diagnosis.[5] McLaughlin states that frozen shoulder is a popular medical colloquialism and not a diagnosis.[5] In this literature review, a working definition of frozen shoulder will be established.

PATHOLOGY AND DEFINITION

Historically, Duplay[6] in 1872 was first credited with describing the painful stiff shoulder, referring to the condition as *humeroscapular periarthritis* (periarthritescapulohumerale) secondary to subacromial bursitis. In 1934, Codman[7] coined the term *frozen shoulder*, attributing the painful stiff shoulder to a short rotator tendinitis. Codman devoted only nine pages of his textbook on the shoulder to frozen shoulder, summarizing this condition as difficult to define, explain, and treat. In 1945, Neviaser[3] surgically explored 10 cases of frozen shoulder, finding absence of the glenohumeral synovial fluid and the redundant axillary fold of the capsule, as well as thickening and contraction of the capsule, which had become adherent to the humeral head, thus, he used the term *adhesive capsulitis*. As Neviaser rotated these shoulders, it appeared at first as if the humeral head and capsule were glued together but could be separated with one or two rotational movements, thus freeing joint movement. Microscopic examinations in all 10 cases revealed reparative inflammatory changes in the capsule. Based on this work, Neviaser suggested that adhesive capsulitis described the pathology of frozen shoulder.

In 1938, McLaughlin[5] reported that in surgical exploration of a number of frozen shoulders, he found no histologic evidence of inflammation. He too observed a loss of the inferior redundant fold, but the adhesions between the folds were easily separated and separation did not increase shoulder motion. McLaughlin consistently found that the rotator cuff tendon was contracted and shrunken, holding the humeral head tight in the glenoid and allowing little motion at this articulation. Although unsupported by examination, McLaughlin postulated that the tissue changes in the cuff were related to collagen stiffening. This appeared reasonable, because McLaughlin observed that prolonged disuse of the extremity preceded a frozen shoulder. He recognized that the reason for shoulder disuse may be in or removed from the shoulder. Although many studies cite disuse of the extremity as a contributing factor,[1,8–11] McLaughlin's study is one of a few that address collagen changes as a result of immobility in the frozen shoulder. Research documents that changes in periarticular connective tissue collagen result from immobilization. The effects of immobilization and its relationship to frozen shoulder will be addressed later.

In 1949, Simmonds,[12] like Codman, proposed that patients with frozen shoulder exhibited inflammation in the rotator cuff, particularly in the supraspinatus tendon. Inflammation of the supraspinatus tendon is secondary to degenerative changes in the tendon caused by impaired blood supply, as the tendon is repeatedly traumatized by rubbing against the acromion process and coracoacromial ligament. Histologic examination of four patients with frozen

shoulder confirmed the above clinical findings, showing evidence of degeneration of the supraspinatus tendon with hyperemia, a definite inflammatory reaction.

Similarly, in 1973, Macnab[13] illustrated that degenerative changes in the supraspinatus occurred first at the zone of impaired blood supply where the tendon passes over the humeral head. This area is relatively avascular, as the humeral head pressure on the tendon "wrings out" the blood vessels. The lack of circulation in this area could cause degeneration of the supraspinatus tendon. The degeneration process produces a local irritation of the tendon. In response to tissue inflammation, the body produces antibodies affecting the adjacent rotator cuff tendons. This autoimmune reaction produces a diffuse capsulitis, or frozen shoulder.

Lippmann,[14] in 1943, confirmed both Schrager and Pasteur's theory that bicipital tenosynovitis preceded frozen shoulder. In examining 12 surgical cases of frozen shoulder, Lippmann consistently found tenosynovitis of the long head of the biceps tendon. The tendon sheath was typically thickened and edematous, and the tendon was roughened and adherent to the sheath. Lippmann proposed that the progression of the frozen shoulder could be determined by the extent of tendinous adhesion: the more advanced the condition, the more adherent the tendon. He attributed stiffness of the shoulder to the upward spread of the tenosynovitis into the shoulder joint, causing adherence of the intracapsular tendon to the capsule and the articular surface of the humeral head. Ultimately, the intracapsular tendon would disintegrate and gradual improvement of shoulder function would occur.

Turek[15] theorized that continual trauma of the rotator cuff and biceps tendon as they are forced against the acromial arch results in degeneration and edema. The tendons thicken as a result, creating a barrier to humeral head movement under the arch. If trauma persists, healing by granulation tissue results in fibrous adhesions of the biceps tendon, rotator cuff, subacromial bursa, capsule, humeral head, and acromion. The result is loss of motion at the glenohumeral joint.

DePalma[16] stated that the pathologic process of frozen shoulder primarily involves the fibrous capsule. The normally flexible capsule becomes nonelastic and shrunken. The mechanism responsible for these changes is unknown. As the condition progresses, the synovial fluid, fascial covering, rotator cuff, biceps tendon, biceps tendon sheath, and subacromial bursa can all become involved. DePalma observed involvement of these structures in various stages of frozen shoulder.[16] In the early stages, the capsule becomes contracted, with loss of the inferior capsular fold. In the later phases, increased capsular fibrosis occurs. The synovial membrane becomes thickened and hypervascular. These tissues lose their elasticity and easily tear as the humerus is rotated or abducted. The coracohumeral ligament becomes a thick, contracted cord as it spans the tuberosities to the coracoid process. The subscapularis tendon also becomes fibrotic, thereby limiting shoulder external rotation. In addition to the subscapularis, the supraspinatus and infraspinatus are also tight, resulting in restricted glenohumeral motion as the head is held high in the glenoid by these fibrotic tendons, thereby limiting downward humeral excursion. The biceps tendon was found to be adhered to the sheath and the groove. Like Lippmann,[14] DePalma[16] speculated that once the gliding mechanism of the biceps tendon is gone as the tendon becomes anchored to the humerus by adhesions, shoulder function begins to return.

Like DePalma, Ozaki et al.,[17] Neer et al.,[18] and Kieras and Matsen[19] have cited a shortened coracohumeral ligament as contributing to a frozen shoulder. Ozaki also noted contracture of the rotator interval and joint capsule in his study but found no intra-articular adhesions.

The rotator interval is a space between the anterior border of the supraspinatus and the superior border of the subscapularis. The coracohumeral ligament originates from the coracoid process and passes forward and downward in the rotator interval to insert with the joint capsule into both tuberosities, bridging the bicipital groove. Normally, the rotator interval contains elastic membranous tissue. With adhesive capsulitis, both the rotator interval and coracohumeral ligament are converted into a thick fibrous cord, which holds the humeral head tightly against the glenoid fossa, restricting humeral motion.[17]

More recently, several studies of the pathology associated with frozen shoulder have used the arthroscope for direct viewing of the joint. In 1991, Hsu and Chan[20] scoped 25 patients with frozen shoulder. The authors noted synovial hypotrophy in 10 of the cases, obliteration of the inferior recess in 3 cases, rotator cuff tears in 6, and intra-articular adhesions in 4. Many patients had concomitant pathologies.

Uitvlugt et al.[21] in 1993 performed diagnostic glenohumeral joint arthroscopy before and immediately after manipulation on 20 patients with frozen shoulder. The pathologies documented were vascular synovitis in all cases, with capsular contracture primarily in the anterior and inferior capsule. Unlike Neviasar, there were no intra-articular adhesions noted. The subacromial bursa was not inspected in this study.

Pollock et al.[22] in 1994, inspected 30 frozen shoulders arthroscopically and noted subacromial bursal adhesions in all patients. He stated that a contracted glenohumeral joint capsule is the primary structure responsible for frozen shoulder.

In 1991, Wiley[23] treated 37 patients with frozen shoulder using arthroscopy. He noted a vascular reaction around the biceps tendon and the subscapularis bursa opening. He found no intra-articular adhesions or obliteration of the inferior recess. Noteworthy in this study is the careful patient selection, including only those with "primary" frozen shoulder. Primary frozen shoulder as defined by Lippmann are those patients with no findings in the history, clinical examination, or radiographs that could explain the decreased range of motion.[14] Wiley also used local anesthetic blocks, CT scans, and arthrograms to rule out other pathologies such as rotator cuff tears or impingement that could be at fault. Patients with these later pathologies are classified as having "secondary" frozen shoulder[14] and were excluded from this study.

Rizk et al.[24] selected 21 patients with "idiopathic adhesive capsulitis" to examine under arthrography. Like Lippmann, Rizk classified these patients as having no history of trauma, no neurologic, bony, or arthritic condition to account for the limited and painful shoulder. During arthrography, Rizk noted a loss of joint volume due to a constricted capsule, serrations of the synovium, nonfilling of the bicipital tendon sheath, and obliteration of the subscapular or axillary recesses. Like Wiley, he found no intra- or extracapsular adhesions.

Various pathologies have been postulated to be the cause of frozen shoulder. Both contractile and noncontractile structures have been incriminated. Cyriax[25] has outlined an examination that differentiates a contractile from a noncontractile element in shoulder dysfunction. Cyriax states that the term *frozen* describes a symptom of stiffness and not a pathology. According to Cyriax, frozen shoulder is arthritis, which implies that the entire glenohumeral joint capsule is affected, limiting both active and passive movement.

His examination includes selective tension testing of the shoulder complex whereby different structures are stressed by active, passive, and resisted motions to determine the site of the lesion. Both contractile elements (muscle, tendon, tendoperiosteal unit, and musculoperiosteal unit) and noncontractile or inert elements (ligaments, synovial membrane, joint capsule, articular surfaces, bursa, dura, fascia, nerve root, and fat pads) are tested.

In the examination, active shoulder motion in initially tested. Although active motion may incriminate both contractile and noncontractile elements, the results, when correlated with passive and resistive testing, frequently can give additional information about the soft tissue lesion. Second, passive shoulder motion is tested to evaluate the inert tissues, because the contractile elements are totally relaxed during passive testing. Last, with resisted shoulder motion, only the contractile elements are evaluated, because the tests are performed isometrically, thus preventing joint movement. Based on this examination

procedure, Cyriax observed that patients with "arthritis" causing glenohumeral stiffness have pain and limitation of movement with active and passive testing only. Resisted testing is negative, thereby ruling out any of the contractile structures previously mentioned as the cause of frozen shoulder.

Limitation in both active and passive glenohumeral movement has been observed by others.[8,9,26–28] Cyriax[25] further clarifies that arthritis exhibits limitation of passive motion in characteristic proportions, which he calls the capsular pattern. The capsular pattern of frozen shoulder is most limited in external rotation, followed by abduction, and then by internal rotation. Both Neviaser[3] and Kozin[26] noted limitations in these same motions. Others observed loss of glenohumeral movement in all directions[12,15,24,29,30], in external rotation and abduction only,[31] and in abduction, external rotation, and flexion.[32,33]

Reeves[34] substantiated the capsular pattern in arthrograms of 17 patients with frozen shoulder. He consistently noted that more contrast dye was deposited posteriorly than in any other areas of the joint capsule, and that the joint capacity was grossly reduced and the inferior capsular fold, subscapularis bursa, and biceps sheath were obliterated. Therefore, based on the arthrokinematics of shoulder motion, it follows that if the anterior capsule were more contracted than the posterior capsule, external rotation would be more limited than internal rotation. In addition, abduction would be limited by the loss of the inferior redundant fold and limited external rotation.

Likewise, Ozaki et al.[17] found a diminished joint capacity and restricted inferior axillary fold and subscapularis bursa in 17 patients with frozen shoulder due to a shortened coracohumeral ligament. As mentioned, both Ozaki et al.[17] and Neer et al.[18] substantiated that a shortened coracohumeral ligament limits external rotation. Without external rotation, abduction is also limited; hence the capsular pattern.

Scientific research points to many different structures as the cause of frozen shoulder. One common observation is that the capsule becomes contracted around the humeral head. The clinical observation of limited and painful active and passive motion in the capsular pattern substantiates that a noncontractile structure is at fault. This, however, does not rule out that the patient may have had a contractile structure initially involved and that a frozen shoulder is the end result of such a lesion.

In closing, the author would like to postulate a working definition for frozen shoulder as glenohumeral stiffness resulting from a noncontractile element. Both active and passive motion is painful and restricted. Passive mobility is limited in a capsular pattern, with external rotation being limited most, followed by abduction, and then internal rotation. A frozen shoulder does not exhibit objective findings of a contractile lesion unless the lesion is concurrent with a noncontractile lesion.

ETIOLOGY

Although much has been reported on the pathogenesis of frozen shoulder, its exact cause remains unknown. However, certain factors—pain, disuse, and a periarthritic personality—are considered to contribute to the development of frozen shoulder.

Pain in the shoulder can result from various intrinsic and extrinsic sources.[10,35–37] Whatever the source, pain usually forces the patient to protect the arm from use. Immobilization of a synovial joint has been shown to have detrimental effects on the periarticular connective tissue.[38–46]

Lundberg[47] examined the synovial membrane and fibrous layer of the anterior-inferior capsule of 14 frozen and 13 normal shoulders. He found an increased amount of hexosamine in the frozen shoulder as compared with normal shoulders. This difference was caused by an increase in the total content of glycosaminoglycans (GAG), namely, an increase in heparan sulfate, chondroitin-6 sulfate, and dermatan sulfate, and a decrease in hyaluronic acid in the frozen shoulders. These changes in GAG content reflect a process of fibrosis occurring in the tissue. There was marked fibroblastic proliferation, indicating re-

modeling of the collagenous portion of the connective tissue. The cause for the increased collagen production is unknown.

Ozaki et al.[17] also noted fibrosis in the contracted coracohumeral ligament and rotator interval in histologic studies of 17 frozen shoulders. The end result of increased fibrosis is a "subsequent loss of biologic properties of the connective tissue" in the shoulder joint, namely, "loss of capsular flexibility and toughness."[47] Therefore, the clinically observed loss of shoulder motion resulting from disuse may be the result of underlying capsular connective tissue changes.

The third factor associated with the development of frozen shoulder is that of the periarthritic personality. Some investigators[5,8,9,16] state that psychological factors, especially depression, apathy, and emotional stress, contribute to frozen shoulder. Patients with periarthritic personalities have a low pain threshold[9]; therefore, any shoulder pain will probably lead to early voluntary immobilization of the extremity. These patients take no active role in any treatment, such as exercise for shoulder pain,[9] and are therefore more likely to develop a more severe case of frozen shoulder. Wright and Haq,[48] however, tested 186 patients with frozen shoulder and found no such personality.

CLINICAL FEATURES

In the literature, a few clinical features appear consistently in patients with frozen shoulder. These common observations include arthrographic and radiographic findings, age of onset, type of onset, and course of the condition.

Arthrographic findings appear to be one of the most prevalent characteristics of frozen shoulder. So that the abnormal arthrogram may be better understood, the normal shoulder arthrogram is discussed first.

The joint capsule consists of relatively loose connective tissue with a surface area more than twice that of the humeral head.[49] The capsule normally attaches to the humeral head just proximal to the greater tuberosity, and then extends medially at the level of the anatomic neck of the

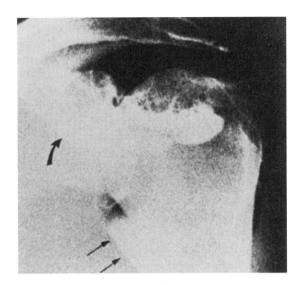

FIGURE 10.1 *Normal shoulder arthrogram. An external rotation view shows the insertion along the humeral neck, the axillary recess (straight arrows), and the subscapularis bursa (curved arrow). Note that the capsular insertion has a smooth contour. (From Goldman,[50] with permission.)*

to rule out other shoulder lesions in addition to confirming frozen shoulder.[50,53] Arthrography, however, gives no clues to what initiates the capsular changes.

Plain film findings in frozen shoulder are usually negative, except that they occasionally show some osteoporosis from disuse.[17,30,32,50–52,61,62] Seldom is frozen shoulder encountered in a patient less than 40 years of age.[4,11,16,50,51,59,61] Wright and Haq[48] and DePalma[16] speculate that this age coincides with normal degenerative changes of connective tissue, a factor that may precipitate frozen shoulder. Reeves' study[63] confirms that the strength of the anterior-inferior capsule and capsular ligament decreases with age, especially in the fifth decade. Some investigators associate frozen shoulder with the postmenopausal stage, when hormonal changes may alter connective tissue also. Most studies of frozen shoulder consider the onset to be insidious. Trauma including minor injuries was only occasionally recalled by some patients.

humerus and inserts into the bony rim of the glenoid.[50] The redundant fold of the capsule hangs in the axilla (Fig. 10.1). In addition, the shoulder joint can accept 28 to 35 ml of solution, with 16 ml of contrast fluid allowing the best viewing of the normal joint.[50]

In frozen shoulder arthrograms, the contrast dye is injected posteriorly, because the capsule is usually contracted superiorly, anteriorly, and inferiorly.[51] Abnormal findings include retraction of the joint capsule away from the greater tuberosity (Fig. 10.2),[48,52] a ragged and irregular outline of the capsule,[50,52] and absence of the axillary redundant fold (Fig. 10.2).[53–56] The joint volume is markedly decreased to less than 10 ml, and pain is usually experienced as the capacity is reached. Frequently, there is no filling of the subscapularis bursa and bicipital sheath.[23,24,52,53,55,57]

Some investigators believe that arthrography is essential in diagnosing frozen shoulder.[56,58–60] Others find it helpful but not essential

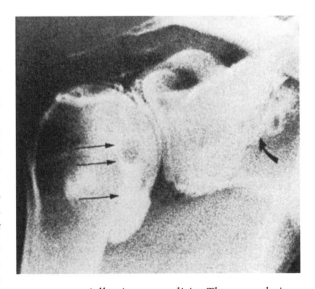

FIGURE 10.2 *Adhesive capsulitis. The capsule is retracted away from the tuberosities (straight arrows). The axillary recess is small, and extravasation has occurred prior to exercise (curved arrows). (From Goldman,[50] with permission.)*

Although many studies describe frozen shoulder as being self-limiting,[12,27,30,64,65] there are very few documented studies of the natural course of frozen shoulder.[29,64] Reeves[29] studied 41 patients with frozen shoulder for 5 to 10 years (average, 30 months), always to their greatest recovery. He defined frozen shoulder as an "idiopathic condition of the shoulder characterized by the spontaneous onset of pain with restriction of movement in every direction." He noted three consecutive stages of frozen shoulder: pain, stiffness, and recovery. The total time for greatest recovery was between 1 and 4 years after the onset of symptoms. More than half of the patients had permanent loss of shoulder motion, as compared with the uninvolved "normal" shoulder's range of motion (ROM), but had no limitation in any functional activities.

Shaffer et al.[66] followed 62 patients with idiopathic frozen shoulder for 2 to 11 years (average, 7 years). Although 60 percent of the patients had restricted ROM only 11 percent reported mild functional limitations due to pain and stiffness. These studies contradict other research indicating full recovery or slight loss of motion in 18 to 24 months from the onset of symptoms.[11,15,27,61,64]

Cyriax also classified frozen shoulder into three stages.[25] The first stage exists when the pain is confined to the deltoid area or at least does not extend distal to the elbow, when the patient can lie on the involved extremity at night, when pain is present only with movement, and when the end-feel is elastic. The second stage is present if only some of the criteria in the first stage are met. The third stage is characterized by severe pain extending from the shoulder to the forearm and wrist, inability to lie on the involved extremity at night, pain at rest and greatest at night, and an abrupt end-feel. Treatment varies according to the stage of the condition and will be addressed later.

In a small series of 21 patients with frozen shoulder, Simmonds[12] observed that after 3 years, only 6 regained normal function, 9 had weakness and pain, and 6 had either weakness or decreased mobility. Gray[64] noted that 24 of 25 patients regained normal glenohumeral motion

within 2 years from the onset of symptoms. This success was achieved with treatment of reassurance, occasional simple analgesics, and hypnosis.[64] Lippmann and colleagues[61] noted that it is uncommon to outwait the natural course of frozen shoulder without intervention. Simon[30] further emphasized that simply outwaiting the condition does not assure the patient a full painless ROM.

In addition to the previously mentioned clinical features, others are found with less consistency. Opinion varies on their relationship to the incidence of frozen shoulder. These features include sex, side involved, occupation (manual versus sedentary),[27,48] the presence of immunologic factors such as HLA-B27,[58,67,68] serum IgA levels,[69] raised C-reactive protein and immune complex levels,[68] and association with other diseases (hemiparesis,[31,48] ischemic heart disease, thyroid disease,[70,71] pulmonary tuberculosis, chronic bronchitis,[48] and diabetes[62,72–74].

Diabetes and the incidence of frozen shoulder have been under closer scrutiny, with some interesting results. Lequesne et al.[62] tested 60 consecutive patients with frozen shoulder and found that 17 of these had diabetes. In a larger sample, Bridgman[72] found that more than 10 percent of 800 diabetics had frozen shoulder compared with 2 percent of 600 nondiabetic control subjects. These authors contend that the prevalence of diabetes in frozen shoulder is significant.

In summary, the onset of frozen shoulder is usually insidious and occurs in patients more than 40 years of age. The course of the condition has been documented to be as long as 10 years. During this time, the level of pain and restriction can vary greatly. Other typical features of frozen shoulder include abnormal arthrograms with marked capsular changes and normal radiographs.

Examination

A complete description of the examination of the frozen shoulder is beyond the scope of this chapter. Emphasis will be placed on the physical therapist's objective assessment and the way in which findings relate to treatment of frozen shoulder.

SUBJECTIVE FINDINGS

In my clinical experience, most patients with frozen shoulder have had the condition for several weeks to several months before seeking treatment. When referred to physical therapy, the patient probably has taken or is currently taking a course of anti-inflammatory medication and has used self-treatment with a heating pad warm showers, aspirin, and rest of the extremity. Pain motivates the patient to seek medical attention,[9,16] as does decreased function of the extremity.[75] Subjectively, the patient complains of a vague, dull pain over the deltoid that increases with motion[2,51,61] and disturbs sleep.[29,31,32,51,61,76] Functionally, the patient will be unable to sleep on the affected side,[2,6,17,25] hook a brassiere in the back, comb the hair, or reach for a wallet in a back pocket. The patient usually cannot recall an injury and frequently is unable to determine when the pain and/or loss of function began. If the condition is more advanced, the patient may complain of pain spreading from the shoulder down the forearm,[12,25] up to the cervical spine, and into the ipsilateral scapula, and pain at rest.[25]

These complaints correspond well to Cyriax's stages of capsular lesions.[25] Although the study by Reeves[29] documents arthrographic changes in the first and last stages of frozen shoulder, from a practical standpoint Cyriax's division is more clinically applicable. In the patient population that I saw, very few patients were examined arthrographically. It appears that arthrography was reserved for those patients who did not respond to a long-term conservative program of physical therapy and medication. Even if arthrography is performed, Cyriax's stages can also be clinically helpful in treatment planning.

During the interview, it is also important to ask questions concerning the patient's general health to assess any other disease process that may be referring pain to the shoulder. The same applies to pertinent questioning concerning the shoulder complex, cervical spine, and brachial plexus structures, although these areas will be examined.

OBJECTIVE FINDINGS

Initial observation of the patient frequently reveals a stooped posture with rounded shoulders; the involved extremity is adducted and internally rotated, resting in the patient's lap.[77]

In gait, the arm swing is usually limited or absent on the affected side. A therapist observing the patient disrobe will notice that the patient's shirt is usually removed as though the arm were in a cast. The uninvolved extremity is removed first, with very little movement of the opposite side. The reverse occurs when the patient dresses. The patient usually wears shirts that button down the front and require no overhead action to remove.

The levels of the shoulders are frequently uneven, with the involved side usually elevated in a protective manner. As a result of maintaining this posture, there may be tender points along the ipsilateral upper trapezius, with perceived pain along its course to the suboccipital area. The scapula on the involved side is usually elevated, laterally rotated, and abducted as a result of excessive scapular motion to compensate for the impaired glenohumeral motion. The abnormal scapular position can cause stretch weakness of the rhomboids[77] and levator scapulae tightness, giving rise to local pain. If the condition is long-standing and there has been a long period of disuse, muscle atrophy around the involved shoulder and scapula may be evident.

Because cervical spine dysfunction can refer pain to the shoulder, this area must be assessed.[10,35,36] It is not the objective of this chapter to outline a complete cervical examination, but a few important tests are mentioned. If active cervical ROM is normal, overpressure should be applied at the end of each range.[78] This involves a gentle passive movement at the end of the available range. There should be a slight pain-free increase in the ROM. If active ROM and active ROM with overpressure are negative for provocation of symptoms, the cervical quadrant test can be performed. This involves guiding the head into extension toward one side and then adding cervical rotation to the same side.[78]

Individual cervical segmental mobility should then be tested to ascertain any joint dysfunction. Physical therapists trained in these methods have a variety of testing techniques that can be performed to check segmental mobility in all directions of motion. Cervical compression and traction tests complete the passive cervical spine examination. Additional information concerning the cervical influence on the shoulder pain may be obtained by having the patient elevate the involved shoulder while traction is being applied to the cervical spine and noting if there is any improvement in shoulder pain or ROM.[35] Finally, resistive testing of cervical ROM will provide information concerning the contractile structures of the neck.

The integrity of the brachial plexus must be evaluated in case of shoulder pain.[35] The standard Addson, hyperabduction, and costoclavicular tests may not be valid with limited shoulder motion. Elvey[35] developed a brachial plexus tension test that can be performed adequately despite restricted shoulder motion. The reader is encouraged to refer to this text for the details.

Acromioclavicular, sternoclavicular, and scapulothoracic dysfunction and first rib syndrome can also give rise to shoulder pain.[35,79] Acromioclavicular joint pain is usually very localized and can easily be pinpointed by the patient.[25] This local pain differs from the diffuse dull pain common with frozen shoulder. Scapulothoracic dysfunction usually results from excessive scapular compensatory motion, and sternoclavicular dysfunction usually results from abnormal shoulder mechanics. First rib dysfunction can result from a variety of problems. The mobility of the sternoclavicular, scapulothoracic,[35,79] acromioclavicular, and first rib[79] should be tested to rule out their involvement in shoulder pain. In summary, careful examination of the cervical spine, brachial plexus, acromioclavicular, sternoclavicular, scapulothoracic joints, and first rib is essential in a complete assessment of shoulder pain.

Much of the remaining objective assessment of the shoulder is based on Cyriax's[25] examination principles. The entire examination is presented because the negative findings are as important as the positive findings in assessing frozen shoulder. All examination procedures mentioned should be performed bilaterally, using the uninvolved extremity as "normal" for the individual who is being assessed.

Twelve movements are included in the examination, and the order of their performance is important. Active motion assesses both contractile an noncontractile elements, passive motion assesses inert structures, and resisted motion assesses contractile structures.

1. *Active elevation.* Elevation is movement away from the side in the coronal plane, with 180° possible. During active elevation, the patient's willingness to move, the muscular power, and the ROM can be assessed.

2. *Passive elevation.* The ROM, the location in the range in which pain is produced, and the end-feel should be noted. End-feel is the sensation detected by the examiner at the extreme of the passive ROM.[25,80] The normal end-feel of the shoulder is capsular, which is similar to the sensation encountered when two pieces of tough rubber are squeezed together. There is a firm arrest to movement, but some "give" is noted.[25] Both the end-feel and the point in the range where pain is provoked are important in deciding treatment. This will be further discussed in the section on stretching as treatment.

3. *Painful arc.* This can only be tested when 90° of abduction is present actively or passively. Abduction is defined as the amount of movement between the scapula and humerus, with 90° being normal. The patient actively elevates the extremity and notes if there is a painful point in the range bordered on either side by nonpainful motion. The same arc of pain can be felt as the arm is brought down from the elevated position or if elevation is performed pas-

sively. A positive finding indicates that a structure is being pinched during the movement.

4. *Passive scapulohumeral abduction.* The scapula is stabilized at its inferior angle as the therapist passively elevates the extremity, noting when the inferior angle begins to move; 90° is the normal range before the scapula moves.

5. *Passive lateral rotation.* As with passive elevation, ROM, the point in the range at which pain is provoked, and the end-feel should be noted.

6. *Passive medial rotation.* See the comment for 5, above.

Note that all resisted tests are performed isometrically. Both pain and muscle weakness are noted. The resisted tests are the following.

7. *Resisted adduction.*
8. *Resisted abduction.*
9. *Resisted lateral rotation.*
10. *Resisted medial rotation.*
11. *Resisted elbow extension.*
12. *Resisted elbow flexion.*

As previously mentioned, confusion occurs when more than one lesion exists. With this concise examination, both contractile and inert structures can be assessed.

In summary, because frozen shoulder involves a noncontractile structure, active elevation and all passive testing are limited and painful. In addition, limitation of passive movement is in a capsular proportion, with most limitation in external rotation, followed by abduction, then internal rotation.

Further information in determining which areas of the capsule are involved in frozen shoulder can be obtained by assessing motions of glenohumeral joint play. Mennel[79] coined the term *joint play* and defines it as small, involuntary movement essential for normal joint motion. He based this definition on joint mechanics, in which rotations, glides, and long axis extension (traction) are normal joint play motions. Joint play motion is often not more than 1/8 inch of movement in any plane. When joint play is lost, joint dysfunction exists. Mennel proposes that

manipulation is the preferred treatment to restore joint play.

According to Mennel, there are seven joint play motions at the glenohumeral joint. He recognizes that normal glenohumeral movement depends on normal acromioclavicular, sternoclavicular, and scapulothoracic joint movement. The reader is referred to Chapter 1 for review of this necessary harmony. All of the joint play motions are actually rolls and glides of the humeral head within the glenoid. In the shoulder, where the convex humeral head is moving on the stationary glenoid, roll and glide occur in opposite directions.[80] Any discrepancies in joint play assessment will direct the therapist with a knowledge of normal joint mechanics to the involved area of the capsule. Furthermore, treatment can be directed to these specific areas.

The normal joint play motions of the glenohumeral joint are anterior glide, posterior glide, lateral glide, inferior and posterior glide, lateral and posterior glide, external rotation of the humeral head within the glenoid fossa, and posterior glide of the humeral head within the glenoid fossa with the shoulder flexed to 90°.[65] Although the joint play motions mentioned are assessment techniques, they are also treatment techniques that can be used to restore normal shoulder mechanics by stretching the involved portions of the capsule. This will be discussed in the treatment section.

All joint play motions can be quantified using a scale from 0 to 6.[81] Although the assessment of the joint play is subjective, grading the movement allows easy documentation of the motion. Again, the univolved extremity should be tested to assess "normal" for the patient. Grade O indicates no joint movement as in an ankylosed joint; grade 1 indicates marked loss of motion; grade 2, a slight limitation in motion; grade 3, normal mobility; grade 4, a slight increase in mobility; grade 5, a marked increase in motion; and grade 6, joint instability. In frozen shoulder with capsular restrictions, grades 1 and 2 will be encountered most frequently.

A final examination tool is palpation. Cyriax[25] cautions that palpation gives very little information and is often irritating to the involved structures. For these reasons, palpation is reserved until the very end of the examination. In frozen shoulder, palpatory findings are generally negative. There may be tenderness over the acromioclavicular joint as a result of improper shoulder mechanics. In addition, any secondary muscular involvement resulting from posture or abnormal scapular motion may exhibit tender painful points. In a contractile lesion coexisting with frozen shoulder, there will probably be tenderness over the lesioned structure.

Although this evaluation is lengthy, it is imperative that an accurate assessment of the shoulder lesion be made. Proper treatment is based on an accurate assessment.[34,79,82]

Treatment

Prevention is the best treatment of frozen shoulder.[27,51] Although there is little agreement on its treatment when it occurs, there is agreement on the treatment goals; pain relief and restoration of normal shoulder movement.[65,83] Unfortunately, few controlled studies in the literature examine treatment of frozen shoulder. One of the problems in studies of frozen shoulder is the variable patient selection due to the variable definitions of what constitutes frozen shoulder. Another problem, so frequently encountered in any human subject study, is the ethics of the necessity of an untreated control group.

Hazleman[65] studied 130 cases of frozen shoulder retrospectively and found no difference in treatment of local corticosteroid injections, physical therapy consisting of pendulum and pulley exercises with short-wave diathermy, or manipulation under anesthesia. Binder and colleagues[84] followed 42 patients with forzen shoulder for 8 months and found no long-term difference in treatment by intra-articular steroids, Maitland-type passive mobilization, ice, or no treatment. Hamer and Kirk[85] documented no significant advantage in ice or ultrasound treatments, but both were beneficial in decreasing the painful stage and hastening recovery. Lee et al.[86] found no difference in patients who received local hydrocortisone and exercises or infrared irradiation and exercises. However, both groups receiving exercises did significantly better than patients receiving analgesics alone. Dacre et al., following 66 cases for 6 months, concluded that local steroid injection, physical therapy with mobilization, or a combination of both were all effective in decreasing pain and increasing shoulder function. They also concluded that the steroid injection was cost-effective.[87]

Biswas et al.[75] found that patients receiving intra-articular hydrocortisone, short-wave diathermy, and aspirin as well as active and passive mobilization exercises all benefited. Furthermore, these investigators concluded that exercise is the most important treatment in frozen shoulder. Liang and Lien[88] found no difference in active exercises when combined with intra-articular injection and heat (short-wave diathermy, ultrasound, or moist heat), with heat alone, or with injection alone. Similarly, they concluded that exercises were probably the only useful treatment for frozen shoulder. Rizk et al.[89] found that transcutaneous electrical nerve stimulation with prolonged pulley traction was superior to a variety of heat modalities and exercises.

TRANSCUTANEOUS ELECTRICAL NERVE STIMULATION

Various treatments can be used to achieve the goals of pain relief and restoration of mobility, but documentation of their effectiveness in frozen shoulder is lacking. Transcutaneous electrical nerve stimulation (TENS) can be used to decrease the symptoms of pain in both the early and later stages of frozen shoulder. Figure 10.3 illustrates an effective TENS application for frozen shoulder.[90] The analgesia provided by TENS allows other therapeutic procedures, such as exercises, to be performed more comfortably. For maximal effectiveness, TENS should be applied before and/or during the exercises.[90] Decreasing the pain during stretching of the frozen shoulder will gain the confidence of the patient as well as facilitate joint relaxation, which is essential for passive joint manipulation.

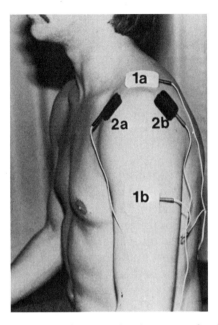

FIGURE 10.3 *TENS electrode placement for frozen shoulder. (**1a**) In depression bordered by the acromion laterally, spine of scapula posteriorly, and clavicle anteriorly; acupuncture point LI 16. (**1b**) Insertion of deltoid at lateral aspect of arm; acupuncture point LI 14 (channel 1). (**2a**) In depression below acromion anteriorly; actupuncture point LI 15. (**2b**) In depression below acromion posteriorly; acupuncture point TW 14 (channel 2). Adapted from Mannheimer and Lampe,[90] with permission.)*

TENS is significantly more effective in reducing the acute pain.[90] Therefore, TENS is an excellent treatment choice when the patient is in too acute a stage for active treatment. Such is the case in stage 3 of frozen shoulder as defined by Cyriax.[25] If TENS can reduce the discomfort, the patient will use the extremity more and probably avoid the stiffening results of disuse.

Other useful acupuncture points that can be used as electrode sides for TENS include a combination of ST 38 and UB 57 or a combination of LI 15, SI 10, GB 34, and LI 11.[91] Yun et al. found acupuncture or novocaine blocking at GB 34 to be 93 to 96 percent effective in eliminating pain and restoring full mobility in 60 patients

followed for 2 years.[92] Pothmann et al. found that one acupuncture treatment of ST 38 cured acute frozen shoulder.[93] (See reference 91 for exact point location.)

HEAT

Heat application is a very common treatment used to decrease pain and increase soft tissue extensibility. A variety of modalities, including short-wave and microwave diathermy, ultrasound, moist packs, paraffin baths, whirlpools, and infrared irradiation, create hyperthermia in the tissue.[90] The result of hyperthermia is increased circulation and vasodilation to the tissues.[90] Other investigators recommend heating the joint capsule prior to stretching, because the increased circulation acts as an analgesic.[25] The analgesic effect, however, tends to be temporary.[90]

Leclaire et al.[94] compared patients receiving hot packs, passive joint stretching, and pulley exercises to patients receiving these same treatments plus magnetotherapy. After 12 weeks there was no difference between either group in the pain scores, ROM, or functional status. Leclaire concluded that electromagnetic therapy was not beneficial in treating frozen shoulder

ULTRASOUND

Ultrasound research in frozen shoulder began in the 1950s when ultrasound was a new form of therapy. Mueller and colleagues[95] found that ultrasound at 2 W/cm^2 was of no value in treating subacute frozen shoulder. Quin[96] found no difference in groups receiving ultrasound at 0.5 W/cm^2 and exercises and those receiving diathermy and exercises.

Clinically, ultrasound is used for its thermal and mechanical effects on tissue.[96] In frozen shoulder, it is often used prior to stretching of the capsule. Because the sound waves are so focal, the therapist must be very specific as to the target tissue.[97] With the inferior capsule so frequently involved in frozen shoulder, the extremity may need to be positioned in abduction and external rotation to reach the inferior portion effectively. Similarly, any portion of the capsule can be treated specifically with proper positioning of the joint. The therapist may also put the target capsule on stretch as ultrasound is applied.

A home program of heat before exercises can be helpful, especially when the patients can exercise with less discomfort. Warm showers and warm moist compresses are easily applied. Heating pads, especially those with a moist head feature, are useful as long as the patient does not apply a pad for long periods.[82] Patients frequently abuse heating pads by falling asleep with them. Even with the pad on the lowest setting, the patient should be strictly instructed to apply it only for short intervals. Most of us have seen the mottled skin of a patient who has abused the heating pad.

CRYOTHERAPY

Cryotherapy, like heat application, produces increased circulation and vasodilation to the area. There is, however, an initial vasoconstriction with cold application.[90] Ice packs, ice massage, ice whirlpools, and vapocoolant sprays are all effective cold treatments.

Ice packs can be easily constructed at home with a plastic bag. A proportional amount of rubbing alcohol added to ice keeps it from refreezing solidly. Convincing a patient to use ice at home—especially a patient who thrives on warm showers and a heating pad—is often difficult. Ice, like heat, before exercises will help the patient perform with less pain. Pain after exercises for more than 1 to 2 hours[25] is abnormal. Ice can prove beneficial in reducing any postexercise soreness.

In the acute phase, when the extremity is generally rested, ice for its analgesic effect is very useful. In addition, if there is a concurrent lesion, such as a rotator cuff tendinitis or bicipital tenosynovitis, ice can combat the inflammation and edema, thereby decreasing pain. With lessened pain, the patient will be more willing to use the extremity and prevent subsequent stiffness.

EXERCISE

Exercise is the most useful treatment in frozen shoulder.[56,75,88] In the acute stage or stage 3 as defined by Cyriax,[25] all active treatment is contraindicated. Treatment in this stage should be directed at pain relief. As mentioned, rest, ice, and TENS are helpful at this time. In the subacute stage or stage 2, both active and passive exercises may be cautiously initiated, but the patient's reaction must be constantly monitored. Increased pain or pain lasting more than 2 hours after exercise is abnormal.[25] In stage 1, active and passive exercises can be performed, usually safely and vigorously. A good physical therapist must be able to judge when to initiate exercise, the amount and vigor of exercises, and when the patient is aggravated by exercise. Experience helps in this decision making, but each patient is different and must be individually evaluated.

Other guidelines to determine when and to what degree exercise should be used can be based on the end-feel and the pain and resistance sequence.[25] An end-feel other than the capsular resistance is abnormal at the shoulder. With the limited range of frozen shoulder, the end-feel is still capsular only in that it will occur at the end of the reduced ROM.

During passive motion testing, both the location of pain in the range and the end-feel are noted.[25] Combining these two factors will indicate the severity of the condition, thereby guiding treatment. If during passive movement the patient perceives pain before the therapist reaches the end of range, the joint is probably acute and active exercises are contraindicated. During this situation, the therapist will obviously not have a chance to evaluate the end-feel, but this can be done in subsequent visits as the pain subsides. If pain is experienced as the end of range is reached, the patient is less acute and exercises may be cautiously attempted. If exercises exacerbate the pain, they should be delayed. Last, if the end of the limited range is reached and no pain is provoked, exercises will probably be tolerated without problems.[25]

In summary, certain factors can help the therapist determine when and what exercises are indicated for the patient with frozen shoulder. The three stages as outline by Cyriax, the end-feel, and the pain/resistance sequence are three such guides.[25] A good therapist paces the patient through a graded active and passive exercise program and constantly reassesses the effect of the program on pain and stiffness.

MANIPULATION

Manipulation, or mobilization as it is frequently called, is a form of passive exercise designed to restore joint play motions of roll, glide, and joint separation.[79] Very few controlled studies involve joint manipulation in the treatment of frozen shoulder. Nicholson[98] compared treatment with mobilization and active exercises to active exercises alone in 20 patients with frozen shoulder After 4 weeks of treatment, passive abduction improved significantly in the mobilization group. There was, however, no significant difference in pain scores between the two groups. Nicholson noted that inferior glide of the humerus was the most severely restricted motion.

Bulgen et al.[99] found no superiority of Maitland-type manipulative techniques in patients with frozen shoulder for more than 1 month over treatment with ice, intra-articular steroid injections, or no treatment. In fact, after 6 weeks of treatment, the group receiving manipulation had greater loss of motion than did the other groups. Bulgen et al. explained that the detrimental effect of physical therapy occurred when manipulation was performed during the active stage, an error that must be avoided.[99]

For normal shoulder function, all areas of the capsule must be extensible to allow joint play motion. Capsular extensibility depends on friction-free sliding of the collagen fibers within the capsule.[38] Hyaluronic acid with water is the lubricant between the collagen fibers[38,100,101] that allows this free gliding to occur.

Lundberg's study of the capsular changes in frozen shoulder revealed a marked increase in fibroblastic formation of collagen, a loss of hyaluronic acid, and an increase in sulfated GAGs.[47] The newly formed collagen in the capsule depends on motion for proper alignment and deposition. Without movement, the new collagen is laid down in a haphazard manner. Abnormal collagen deposition occurs between the newly synthesized fibril and preexisting collagen fibers,[38] resulting in a mechanical block to collagen movement. Multiple adhesions between collagen fibrils and fibers is manifested as joint stiffness. In addition, with the decrease in hyaluronic acid, the lubricant between the fibers is lost, contributing to further impairment of free collagen movement.

Based on these considerations, it seems reasonable to assume that movement of the joint will prevent or limit adhesive formation. Although this is not documented, movement to prevent adhesions is a clinical goal of exercise. In the event that capsular adhesions have formed, manipulation can be used to break the adhesions and restore joint play. Further research is obviously needed in this area.

It is beyond the scope of this chapter to outline every manipulative technique for frozen shoulder. Demonstrations can be found in the texts of Maitland,[78] Mennel,[79] and Kaltenborn.[81] Techniques for each area of the shoulder capsule, acromioclavicular, sternoclavicular, and scapulothoracic joints are illustrated here. Physical therapists benefit by becoming as familiar as possible with as many techniques as possible to afford better treatment to their patients. Any of the techniques illustrated can be adapted as oscillatory or static stretching techniques and can be performed in any part of the range. The goal of treatment, whether for pain relief or increasing ROM, will influence the choice of treatment technique. The mobilization techniques are illustrated in Chapter 16.

Cervical as well as shoulder pain may be present. This may result from overuse of the upper trapezius and levator scapula with excessive scapular elevation to compensate for the loss of glenohumeral motion.[77] The upper trapezius and levator scapula are usually shortened and will need treatment to decrease pain and restore normal physiologic length. Any of the physical modalities are useful to decrease pain. Massage is relaxing as well as beneficial in moving any excessive fluid accumulation. It also can assist

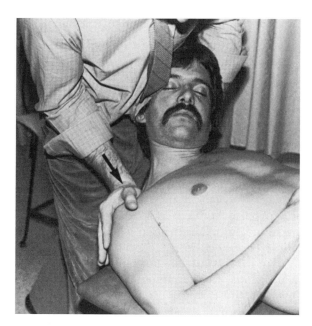

FIGURE 10.4 *Right upper trapezius stretch.* Patient position: *Supine with the head off the edge of the table.* Therapist position: *Left hand under the occiput with the head on the forearm stabilizing the head and neck in the desired amount of flexion and sidebending left and rotation right. Right palm over the clavicle and scapula medial to the acromioclavicular joint.* Technique: *Left hand maintains head and neck position. Right hand pushes the clavicle and scapula inferiorly.*

in mobilizing the soft tissue. Stretching of the upper trapezius can be done in a number of ways. Figure 10.4 illustrates a passive upper trapezius stretch.

In a good home exercise for stretching the upper trapezius, the patient simply reaches behind the back and grasps the involved distal humerus. The patient should side-bend away from and rotate toward the involved side, and flex the neck to a comfortable position. Once positioned, the stretch is imparted by pulling downward on the involved humerus.

Frequently, pain may be provoked while the shoulder is being manipulated. Although such pain is not desirable, it is often difficult to manip-

ulate a frozen shoulder without some discomfort to the patient. "Shaking" the extremity and momentary pauses will help decrease pain and maintain patient relaxation.[81] Simple gentle shaking of the extremity while in any position will stimulate the joint mechanoreceptors and decrease nociceptive input.[102]

Both Maitland[78] and Kaltenborn[81] offer guidelines to the amount of manipulation to perform in one session. Reassessment is important before and during each treatment session. Treatment can continue as long as pain is decreased and motion is improved.[81] Overtreating can cause increased pain and inflammatory reactions,[77] and may push the patient into an acute stage. The therapist should progress slowly until familiar with the patient's response to treatment. It is well documented that the course of frozen shoulder is slow[29,64]; therefore, the therapist should not expect too much improvement too quickly. A patient who is informed that improvement will be slow will be less frustrated.

Liebolt[103] has recommended four passive stretches that, performed over a period of time, will increase shoulder ROM in frozen shoulder. The four exercises are glenohumeral abduction, external rotation, flexion with external rotation, and flexion performed at the end of the available ROM. These exercises, however, do not deal with the loss of joint play. I have found that these exercises in the cardinal planes often provoke pain and do little to increase ROM.

Mechanical exercises with shoulder wheels, pulleys, and wands are often standard exercises in treating frozen shoulder. Unfortunately, like stretching in the cardinal plane, these do not address the loss of joint play. Murray[77] outlines three disadvantages of the overhead pulley system: (1) there is no stabilization of the scapula to avoid excessive abduction and upward rotation, (2) there is no force to depress the humeral head, and (3) there is a tendency for the patient to extend the spine to decrease glenohumeral motion. These same three points are applicable to the shoulder wheel, finger ladder, and wand exercises. To improve the use of these apparatuses, stabilization of the scapula can be improved by placing a strap around the scapula and the chair. The therapist or a reliable family member who has been taught the exercises can depress the humeral head while using the apparatus. Last, the patient can be instructed to keep the spine flat against the chair while performing these exercises. Despite these efforts to improve the exercises, Murray[77] contends that these apparatuses should be used only when normal gliding is present.

Active exercises allow more patient control than do mechanical exercises. Active exercises are essential in maintaining the capsular extensibility obtained through manipulation. They are best performed in a pain-free range to prevent any inflammatory reaction by forcing joint movement. The same principles of mechanical exercises apply to forced active exercises; that is, the active range will not be available if normal joint play is lacking.

Codman or pendulum[7] exercises performed with gravity are usually painfree. With the patient bent at the waist and extremity dangling, the weight of the extremity produces joint separation and eliminates a fulcrum at the glenoid or acromion with movement.[7] With traction at the joint, the patient will usually find the exercises more comfortable. For additional traction, the patient can grasp a light weight, such as an iron. The exercises include forward and backward, medial to lateral, and circular motions made with the entire extremity. The object is to have the patient increase the arc of movement within a painful ROM.

Cardinal plane or diagonal active motion can be performed as a home program if the necessary joint play movements are available. Home exercise programs should be kept simple and to a minimum, requiring no special equipment, so that the patient will comply with the program, which in frozen shoulder is usually a long course. The number of repetitions as well as the vigor will have to be determined for each patient. As mentioned, for their analgesic effects, preparatory heat or ice may be used prior to performance of exercises.

Last, muscle reeducation and strengthening may be needed to restore normal physiologic balance to the entire shoulder complex and spine.

"Muscles cannot be restored to normal if the joints which they move are not free to move."[79] Because there is often excessive scapular motion, stabilization exercises to the scapular area can be performed before full glenohumeral motion is restored. Otherwise, I do not advise strengthening exercises until near normal ROM is achieved. This will avoid strengthening a muscle in a shortened range that may impede the restoration of motion.

Isometric, isotonic (both concentric and eccentric), and isokinetic exercises, free weights, and proprioceptive neuromuscular facilitation are all useful in restoring muscle strength. Various exercise equipment such as Cybex, Universal, and Nautilus is commonplace in many health clubs, and individual programs should be developed for the patients. After pain abates and ROM is restored, most patients will not continue physical therapy for a strengthening program. Therefore, intermittent follow-up visits should be made to review and alter the exercise program as needed and to assess the patient's progress.

OTHER TREATMENTS

Cortisone injections, manipulation, joint distention, or a combination of any of these are other treatments for frozen shoulder. The literature is filled with arguments for and against manipulation under anesthesia[104–118] and cortisone injections.[59,83,111–116]

Rizk et al.[116] reported no significant improvement in ROM in patients receiving intrabursal or intra-articular steroid or lidocaine, or a combination of both. The steroid group noted a temporary relief of pain only.

Loyd and Loyd[59] advocate the use of arthrography for accurate intra-articular injections as opposed to blind clinical injections. They found that a combination of steroid injection followed by gentle manipulation was useful in treating frozen shoulder.

Mulcahy et al.[33] and Ekelund and Rydell[60] successfully treated frozen shoulder with a combination of arthrographic joint distention, intra-articular steroid injection, and gentle joint manipulation. Ekelund and Rydell noted that full

ROM was not always restored with this treatment; instead manipulation under general anesthesia would be in order.

Rizk[24] advocates capular distention through arthrography in treating frozen shoulder. He noted no intra- or extracapsular adhesion in adhesive capsulitis. In all cases, distention caused the capsule to rupture at particularly constricted sites, namely the subacromial or subscapular bursa.

Sharma et al.[117] compared joint distention and steroid injections to manipulation under general anesthesia in treatment of frozen shoulder. Distention gave better results with decreased pain and improved ROM. They suggest distention be performed early in frozen shoulder to expedite recovery.

Arthroscopy is being employed more recently in the treatment of frozen shoulder. There is disagreement in the literature about its usefulness, but some feel that it allows visualization and treatment of associated pathologies.

Hsu and Chan[20] compared arthroscopic distention, manipulation under general anesthesia and physical therapy, and physical therapy alone. The first two had better results in pain reduction and improvement in motion. The authors favor distention because it is more controllable than manipulation and any intra-articular pathology can be seen.

Pollock[22] advocates arthroscopic examination following manipulation. This allows for joint debridement and treatment of associated pathologies, which may range from acromioplasty to sectioning of the coracohumeral ligament.

Open surgical release is recommended for patients who have failed to improve with conservative treatment, including manipulation, or who have contraindications to manipulation, such as significant osteopenia, history of fracture or dislocation, or recurrence after manipulation.[118] Several authors cite a contracted coracohumeral ligament as the source of frozen shoulder and recommend releasing this ligament.[17-19] In addition to sectioning the coracohumeral ligament, Kieras and Matsen[19] also excise subdeltoid adhesions, lengthen the subscapularis, and release the anteroinferior capsule.

Several nonoperative and operative treatments of frozen shoulder have been presented. Various manipulative procedures were used in many of the treatment studies mentioned. A short lever arm with gentle force during manipulation avoids complications, such as a fractured humerus. Some investigators have reported rotator cuff tears following manipulation.[55]

Clinically, if a patient has been treated with manipulation, it is helpful to know the ROM obtained and the complications, if any, that were encountered during the procedure. It is very common for a patient to have less motion following manipulation even if therapy is initiated immediately. This may be owing to an acute inflammatory reaction and muscle splinting due to pain. Pain is frequently increased for several days following manipulation. TENS and ice are very helpful at this stage. Exercises are essential following manipulation under anesthesia. The therapist frequently sees the patient four times a day in the hospital, beginning on the day of the procedure. Reassurance and encouragement are needed to motivate the patient to exercise in the presence of pain.

In the cases of steroid injection treatment, the physical therapist should be aware of the location, number, and frequency of cortisone injections administered to the patient. Because of reports of spontaneous tendon ruptures following multiple injection, care should be exercised with these patients. Knowledge of any procedure performed on the patient enhances treatment decisions.

Summary

This chapter has presented the varied theories on pathogenesis, definition, etiology, clinical features, and treatment of the frozen shoulder. Physical therapy management for frozen shoulder may include prepatory modalities to decrease pain, passive manipulation, muscle reeducation and strengthening, and a home exercise program. The course is long and often tedious to both the patient and therapist, because progress is very slow. The goal of treatment is the restoration of normal pain-free shoulder function. Further research in all of the above areas is needed to prevent and better treat the common musculoskeletal complaint of frozen shoulder.

CASE STUDY

A 65-year-old white male presented with a 2-year history of left shoulder stiffness. Over the past 6 months, he had noted limitation in function due to the progressive stiffness with pain at the extreme of the available range. His first indication of loss of function was the inability to raise the arm to wash the axilla. Three years prior he had stiffness in the right shoulder, which resolved after a steroid injection. He denied injury to either shoulder.

Objectively, the patient exhibited a forward head posture with the left shoulder internally rotated. Active shoulder ROM was 25° of external rotation, 85° of abduction, 45° of internal rotation, 90° of flexion, and adduction to neutral. Passive elevation to 85° was painful at the end of the range with a capsular end-feel. There was compensatory scapular motion with active and passive abduction past 75° and pain at the end of the range. Passive lateral and medial rotation met with resistance and then pain at the end of the ROM with a capsular end-feel. All resisted upper extremity testing was within normal limits. Joint play motion testing revealed grade 2 for inferior, anterior, and lateral glides, and external rotation of the humeral head within the fossa. The remainder of the upper quarter evaluation was unremarkable.

Treatment included ultrasound to the glenohumeral joint for 8 minutes at 1.5 W/cm², soft tissue mobilization, and joint play manipulation. Initially, the manipulations used included inferior, anterior, and lateral glide techniques. They were applied as grade 2 oscillatory movements because the patient had pain only as the end of the range was approached. As the treatments progressed, he tolerated grades 3 and 4 of these maneuvers. He was instructed in Codman and pain-free active ROM exercises for home to be done 5 times per day. Postural awareness was also emphasized.

After 3 weeks of therapy at a frequency of 3 times per week, the patient's active ROM improved to 55° of external rotation, 120° of abduction, 65° of internal rotation, 140° of flexion, and 10° adduction. He began a home strengthening program with tubing to be performed three times daily within the pain-free ROM.

By the fifth week, the patient's ROM improved to 70° of external rotation, 145° of abduction, 75° of internal rotation, 160° of flexion, and 15° of adduction. He noted no functional limitation and resumed bowling. He voluntarily discontinued treatment, and a follow-up phone call 1 month later revealed less than full ROM but no pain or loss of function.

In my experience, this patient is typical in discontinuing treatment as soon as there is no pain or loss of function, even though lacking full ROM. The rapid return of motion is atypical for a frozen shoulder with a 2-year history.

Acknowledgments

I wish to thank Rita K. Owens-Skau, B.S., P.T., for assistance in the preparation of the manuscript, and William Boissonnault, M.S., P.T., and Steve Janos, M.S., P.T., for their assistance with the photographs.

References

1. Bateman J: The Shoulder and Neck. WB Saunders, Philadelphia. 1978
2. Neviaser JS: Adhesive capsulitis and the stiff and painful shoulder. Orthop Clin North Am 11:327, 1980
3. Neviaser JS: Adhesive capsulitis of the shoulder: study of pathological findings in periarthritis of the shoulder. J Bone Joint Surg 27:211, 1945
4. Meulengracht E, Schwartz M: The course and

prognosis of periarthrosis humeroscapularis with special regard to cases with general symptoms. Acta Med Scand 143:350, 1952

5. McLaughlin HL: The "frozen shoulder." Clin Orthop 20:126, 1961

6. Rizk TE, Pinals RS: Frozen shoulder. Semin Arthritis Rheum 11:440, 1982

7. Codman EA: The Shoulder. Kreiger, Malabar, FL, 1934

8. Coventry MB: The problem of the painful shoulder. JAMA 151:177, 1953

9. Cailliet R: Shoulder Pain. 2nd Ed. FA Davis, Philadelphia, 1981

10. Neviaser RJ: Painful conditions affecting the shoulder. Clin Orthop 173:63, 1983

11. Thompson M: The frozen shoulder and shoulder-hand syndromes. Practitioner 189:380, 1962

12. Simmonds FA: Shoulder pain with particular reference to the "frozen" shoulder. J Bone Joint Surg 31B:426, 1949

13. Macnab I: Rotator cuff tendinitis. Ann R Coll Surg Engl 53:271, 1973

14. Lippmann RK: Frozen shoulder; periarthritis; bicipital tenosynovitis. Arch Surg 47:283, 1943

15. Turek S: Orthopaedics. Principles and Their Application: JB Lippincott, Philadelphia, 1977

16. DePalma AF: Surgery of the Shoulder. JB Lippincott, Philadelphia, 1983

17. Ozaki J, Nakagawa Y, Sakurai G et al: Recalcitrant chronic adhesive capsulitis of the shoulder. J Bone Joint Surg 71A:1511, 1989

18. Neer CS, Satterlee CC, Dalsey RM et al: On the value of coracohumeral ligament release. Orthop Trans 13:235, 1989

19. Kieras DM, Matsen FA: Open release in the management of refractory frozen shoulder. Orthop Trans 15:801, 1991

20. Hsu SYC, Chan KM: Arthroscopic distention in the management of frozen shoulder. Int Orthop 15:79, 1991

21. Uitvlugt G, Detrisac DA, Johnson LL et al: Arthroscopic observations before and after manipulation of frozen shoulder. Arthroscopy 9:181, 1993

22. Pollock RG, Duralde XA, Flatow EL et al: The use of arthroscopy in the treatment of resistant frozen shoulder. Clin Orthop 304:30, 1994

23. Wiley AM: Arthroscopic appearance of frozen shoulder. Arthroscopy 7:138, 1991

24. Rizk, TE, Gavant MS, Pinals RS: Treatment of adhesive capsulitis (frozen shoulder) with arthrographic capsular distention and rupture. Arch Phys Med Rehabil: 75,803, 1994

25. Cyriax J: Textbook of Orthopaedic Medicine. 7th Ed. Vol. 1. Bailliere Tindall, London, 1978

26. Kozin F: Two unique shoulder disorders. Adhesive capsulitis and reflex sympathetic dystrophy syndrome. Postgrad Med 73:207, 1983

27. Jayson MV: Frozen shoulder: adhesive capsulitis. Br Med J 283:1003, 1981

28. Morgensen E. Painful shoulder. Aetiological and pathogenetic problems. Acta Med Scand 155:195, 1956

29. Reeves B: The natural history of the frozen shoulder syndrome. Scand J Rheumatol 4:193, 1975

30. Simon WH: Soft tissue disorders of the shoulder. Frozen shoulder, calcific tendinitis, and bicipital tendinitis. Orthop Clin North Am 6:521, 1975

31. Bruckner FE, Nye CJS: A prospective study of adhesive capsulitis of the shoulder "frozen shoulder" in a high risk population. QJ Med 198:191, 1981

32. Flicker PL: The painful shoulder. Prim Care 7:271, 1980

33. Mulcahy KA, Baxter AD, Oni OOA et al: The value of shoulder distention arthrography with intraarticular injection of steroid and local anaesthetic: a follow-up study. BR J Radiol 67:263, 1994

34. Reeves B: Arthrographic changes in frozen shoulder and post-traumatic stiff shoulders. Proc Soc Med 59:827, 1966

35. Elvey RL: The investigation of arm pain. p. 530. In Grieve GP (ed): Modern Manual Therapy of the Vertebral Column. Churchill Livingstone, Edinburgh, 1986

36. Leach RE, Schepsis AA: Shoulder pain. Clin Sports Med 2:123, 1983

37. Neviaser JS: Musculoskeletal disorders of the shoulder region causing cervicobrachial pain. Differential diagnosis and treatment. Surg Clin North Am 43:1703, 1963

38. Akeson WH, Amiel D, LaViolette D: The connective tissue response to immobility: a study of the chondroitin 4- and 6-sulphate and dermatan sulphate changes in periarticular connective tissue of control and immobilized knees of dogs. Clin Orthop 51:183, 1967

39. Akeson WH, Amiel D, LaViolette D et al: The connective tissue response to immobility: an accelerated aging response. Exp Gerontol 3:289, 1968

40. Akeson WH, Amiel D, Mechanic GL et al: Colla-

gen crosslinking alterations in joint contractures: changes in reducible crosslinks in periarticular connective tissue collagen after nine weeks of immobilization. Connect Tissue Res 5: 5, 1977

41. Akeson WH, Amiel D, Woo S: Immobility effects of synovial joints: the parthomechanics of joint contracture. Biorheology 17:95, 1980
42. Enneking W, Horowitz M: The intra-articular effects of immobilization on the human knee. J Bone Joint Surg 54A:973, 1972
43. Evans E, Eggers G, Butler J et al: Immobilization and remobilization of rats' knee joints. J Bone Joint Surg 42A:737, 1960
44. LaVigne A, Watkins R: Preliminary results on immobilization: induced stiffness of monkey knee joints and posterior capsule. In: Perspectives in Biomedical Engineering. Proceedings of a symposium of Biological Engineering Society, University of Strathclyde, Glasgow, June 1972. University Park Press, Baltimore, 1973
45. Woo S, Matthews JV, Akeson WH et al: Connective tissue response to immobility: correlative study of biomechanical and biochemical measurements of normal and immobilized rabbit knees. Arthritis Rheum 18:257, 1975
46. Schollmeier G, Uhthoff HK, Sarkar K et al: Effects of immobilization on the capsule of the canine glenohumeral joint. Clin Orthop 304:37, 1994
47. Lundberg BJ: Glycosaminoglycans of the normal and frozen shoulder-joint capsule. Clin Orthop 69:279, 1970
48. Wright V, Haq AMMM: Periarthritis of the shoulder. Aetiological considerations with particular reference to personality factors. Ann Rheum Dis 35:213, 1976
49. Anton HA: Frozen shoulder. Can Fam Phys 39: 1773, 1993
50. Goldman A: Shoulder Arthrography. Technique, Diagnosis, and Clinical Correlation. Little, Brown, Boston, 1982
51. Neviaser JS: Adhesive capsulitis of the shoulder (frozen shoulder). Med Times 90:783, 1962
52. Kaye JJ, Schneider R: Positive contrast shoulder arthrography p. 137. In Freiberger RH, Kay JJ, Spiller J (eds): Arthrography. Appleton-Century-Crofts, New York, 1979
53. Neviaser JS: Arthrography of the Shoulder. The Diagnosis and Management of the Lesions Visualized. Charles C Thomas, Springfield, IL, 1975
54. Lundberg BJ: Arthrography and manipulation in

rigidity of the shoulder joint. Acta Orthop Scand 36:35, 1965
55. Samilson RL, Raphael L, Post L et al: Arthrography of the shoulder joint. Clin Orthop 20:21, 1961
56. Neviaser RJ: The frozen shoulder diagnosis and management. Clin Orthop 223:59, 1987
57. Neviaser RJ: Arthrography of the shoulder joint. Study of the findings in adhesive capsulitis of the shoulder. J Bone Joint Surg 44A: 1321, 1962
58. Rizk TE, Christopher RP, Pinals RS et al: Arthrographic studies in painful hemiplegic shoulder. Arch Phys Med Rehabil 65:254, 1984
59. Loyd JA, Loyd HM: Adhesive capsulitis of the shoulder: arthrographic diagnosis and treatment. South Med J 76:879, 1983
60. Ekelund AL, Rydell N: Combiniation treatment for adhesive capsulitis of the shoulder. Clin Orthop 282:105, 1992
61. Lippmann K, Bayley I, Young A: The upper limb. The frozen shoulder. Br J Hosp Med 25:334, 1981
62. Lequesne M, Dang N, Bensasson M et al: Increased association of diabetes mellitus with capsulitis of the shoulder and shoulder-hand syndrome. Scand J Rheumatol 6:53, 1977
63. Reeves B: Experiments on the tensile strength of the anterior capsular structures of the shoulder in man. J Bone Joint Surg 50B:858, 1968
64. Gray RG: The natural history of "idiopathic" frozen shoulder. J Bone Joint Surg 60B:564, 1978
65. Hazleman BL: The painful stiff shoulder. Rheumatol Phys Med 11:413, 1972
66. Shaffer B, Tibone JE, Kerlan RK: Frozen shoulder. A long term follow-up. J Bone Joint Surg 74A:738, 1992
67. Bulgen DY, Hazleman BL, Voak D: HLA-B27 and frozen shoulder. Lancet 1:1042, 1976
68. Bulgen DY, Binder A, Hazleman BL et al: Immological studies in frozen shoulder. J Rheumatol 9:893, 1982
69. Bulgen DY, Hazleman B, Ward M et al: Immunological studies in frozen shoulder. Ann Rheum Dis 37:135, 1978
70. Bowman CA, Jeffcoate WJ, Pattrick M et al: Bilateral adhesive capsulitis, oligoarthritis and proximal myopathy as presentation of hypothyroidism. Br J Rheumatol 27:62, 1988
71. Wohlgethan JR: Frozen shoulder in hyperthyroidism. Arthritis Rheum 30:936, 1987
72. Bridgman JF: Periarthritis of the shoulder and diabetes mellitus. Ann Rheum Dis 31:69, 1972
73. Erhard R: Diabetic capsulitis of the shoulder. p.

101. In: Proceedings of the 4th International Federation of Orthopaedic Manipulative Therapists. International Federation of Orthopedic Manipulative Therapists, Christchurch, New Zealand, 1980

74. Fisher L, Kurtz A, Shipley M: Association between cheiroarthropathy and frozen shoulder in patients with insulin-dependent diabetes mellitus. Br J Rheumatol 25:141, 1986

75. Biswas AK, Sur BN, Gupta CR: Treatment of periarthritis shoulder. J Indian Med Assoc 72:276, 1979

76. Olsson O: Degenerative changes of the shoulder joint and their connection with shoulder pain. Acta Chir Scand suppl. 181:104, 1935

77. Murray W: The chronic frozen shoulder. Phys Ther Rev 40:866, 1960

78. Maitland GD: Peripheral Manipulation. 2nd Ed. Butterworth, Publishers, Boston, 1977

79. Mennel J: Joint Pain. Diagnosis, Treatment Using Manipulative Techniques. Little, Brown, Boston, 1964

80. Warwick R. Williams PL: Gray's Anatomy. 35th British Ed. WB Saunders, Philadelphia 1973

81. Kaltenborn FM: Mobilization of the Extremity Joints. Examination and Basic Treatment Techniques. Ilaf Bokhandel, Oslo, 1980

82. Nelson PA: Physical treatment of the painful arm and shoulder. JAMA 169:814, 1959

83. Valtonen E: Subacromial betamethasone therapy. The effect of subacromial injection of betamethasone in cases of painful shoulder resistant to physical therapy. Ann Chir Synaecol Fenn, suppl. 63:5, 1974

84. Binder Al, Bulgen DY, Hazleman BL et al: Frozen shoulder: a long-term prospective study. Ann Rheum Dis 43:361, 1984

85. Hamer J, Kirk JA: Physiotherapy and the frozen shoulder: a comparative trial of ice and ultrasonic therapy. NZ Med J 83:191, 1976

86. Lee M, Haq AMMM, Wright V et al: Periarthritis of the shoulder: a controlled trial of physiotherapy. Physiotherapy 59:312, 1972

87. Dacre JE, Beeney N, Scott DL: Injections and physiotherapy for the painful stiff shoulder. Ann Rheum Dis 48:322, 1989

88. Liang H, Lien I: Comparative study in the management of frozen shoulder. J Formosan Med Assoc 72:243, 1973

89. Rizk TE, Christopher RP, Pinals RS et al: Adhesive capsulitis (frozen shoulder): a new approach

to its management. Arch Phys Med Rehabil 64: 29, 1983

90. Mannheimer J, Lampe G: Clinical Transcutaneous Electrical Nerve Stimulation. FA Davis, Philadelphia, 1984

91. The Academy of Traditional Chinese Medicine: An Outline of Chinese Acupuncture. Foreign Languages Press, Peking, 1975

92. Yun W, Wei W, Shugin W: Treatment of periarthritis humeroscapularis with acupuncture and acupoint blocking. J Trad Chinese Med 13: 262, 1993

93. Pothmann R, Weigel A, Stux G: Frozen shoulder: differential acupuncture therapy with point ST-38. A J Acupuncture 8:65, 1980

94. Leclaire R, Bourgouin J: Electromagnetic treatment of shoulder periarthritis: a randomized controlled trial of the efficiency and tolerance of magnetotherapy. Arch Phys Med Rehabil 7:284, 1991

95. Mueller EE, Mead S, Schulz B et al: A placebo-controlled study of ultrasound treatment for periarthritis. Am J Phys Med 33:31, 1954

96. Quin CE: Humeroscapular periarthritis. Observations on the effects of x-ray therapy and ultrasonic therapy in cases of "frozen shoulder." Ann Phys Med 10:64, 1967

97. Hayes KW: Manual for Physical Agents. 3rd Ed. Northwestern University Press, Chicago, 1984

98. Nicholson GG: The effects of passive joint mobilization on pain and hypomobility associated with adhesive capsulitis of the shoulder. JOSPT 6:238, 1985

99. Bulgen DY, Binder AI, Hazleman BL et al: Frozen shoulder: prospective clinical study with an evaluation of three treatment regimens. Ann Rheum Dis 43:353, 1984

100. Ham A, Cormack D: Histology. 8th Ed. JB Lippincott, Philadelphia, 1979

101. Swann D, Radin E, Nazimiec M: Role of hyaluronic acid in joint lubrication. Ann Rheum Dis 33: 318, 1974

102. Wyke BW: Articular neurology—a review. Physiotherapy 58:94,1972

103. Liebolt FL: Frozen shoulder. Passive exercises for treatment. NY State J Med 70:2085, 1970

104. Haggart GE, Dignam RJ, Sullivan TS: Management of the "frozen" shoulder. JAMA 161:1219, 1956

105. Srivastava KP, Bhan FB, Bhatia IL: Scapulohumeral periarthritis. A clinical study and evalu-

ation of end results of its treatment. J Indian Med Assoc 59:275, 1972

106. Quigley TB: Indications for manipulation and corticosteroids in the treatment of stiff shoulders. Surg Clin North Am 43:1715, 1963

107. Heibig B, Wagner P, Dohler R: Mobilization of frozen shoulder under general anaesthesia. Acta Orthop Belg 49:267, 1983

108. Coombes WN: Frozen shoulder. JR Soc Med 76: 711, 1983

109. Quigley TB: Treatment of checkrein shoulder by use of manipulation and cortisone. JAMA 161: 850, 1956

110. Weiser HI: Painful primary frozen shoulder mobilization under local anesthesia. Arch Phys Med Rehabil 58:406, 1977

111. Steinbocker O, Argyros TG: Frozen shoulder: treatment by local injections of depot corticosteroids. Arch Phys Med Rehabil 55:209, 1974

112. Murnaghem GF, McIntosh D: Hydrocortisone in painful shoulder. Lancet 1:798, 1955

113. Roy S, Oldham R: Management of painful shoulder. Lancet 1:1322, 1976

114. Cyriax J, Trosier O: Hydrocortisone and soft tissue lesions. Br Med J 2:966, 1953

115. Crisp EJ, Kendall PH: Treatment of periarthritis of the shoulder with hydrocortisone. Br Med J 1:1500, 1955

116. Rizk TE, Pinals RS, Talaiver AS: Corticosteroid injections in adhesive capsulitis: investigation of their value and site. Arch Phys Med Rehabil 72: 20, 1991

117. Sharma RK, Bajekal RA, Bhan S: Frozen shoulder syndrome. A comparison of hydraulic distention and manipulation. Int Orthop 17:275, 1993

118. Hulstyn MJ, Weiss APC: Adhesive capsulitis of the shoulder. Orthop Rev 22:425, 1993

11

Etiology and Evaluation of Rotator Cuff Pathology and Rehabilitation

TODD S. ELLENBECKER

The integral functions of the rotator cuff musculature, combined with the large multiplanar movement patterns inherent in both activities of daily living and sport activity in the glenohumeral joint, make the rotator cuff vulnerable to injury, commonly requiring treatment in both orthopaedic and sports physical therapy. The rotator cuff musculature functions to stabilize the glenohumeral joint in four primary ways: (1) by its passive bulk, (2) by developing muscle tensions that compress the joint surfaces together, (3) by moving the humerus with respect to the glenoid and thereby tightening the static stabilizers (capsular-ligamentous restraints), and (4) by limiting the arc of motion of the glenohumeral joint by muscle tensions.[1] As one of the primary dynamic stabilizing structures of the glenohumeral joint, high-intensity concentric and eccentric rotator cuff muscular activity has been reported during simple elevation in the scapular plane,[2] as well as during the tennis serve[3-5] and throwing motion.[6,7] To better understand the rehabilitation process required to restore normal shoulder joint arthrokinematics and pain-free glenohumeral joint function, the etiology and

classification of rotator cuff pathology must first be developed.

Etiology and Classification of Rotator Cuff Pathology

The etiology of rotator cuff pathology can be described along a continuum, ranging at one end from overuse microtraumatic tendonosis, to macrotraumatic full-thickness rotator cuff tears. A second continuum of rotator cuff etiology consists of glenohumeral joint instability and primary impingement or compressive disease.[8] The clinical challenge of treating the patient with a rotator cuff injury begins with a specific evaluation and clear understanding of the underlying stability and integrity of not only the components of the glenohumeral joint, but the entire upper extremity kinetic chain.

There are several ways of classifying rotator cuff pathology. One classification method is based upon the suspected or proposed pathophysiology.[9] For the purpose of this chapter, four classifications of rotator cuff pathology will be

---

Etiologic factors associated With rotator cuff pathology

Microtrauma
Tendonosis
Instability
Macrotrauma
Rotator cuff tear
Compressive disease

---

discussed: primary compressive disease, secondary compressive disease, tensile disease/injury, and macrotraumatic failure.

PRIMARY COMPRESSIVE DISEASE

Primary compressive disease or impingement is a direct result of compression of the rotator cuff tendons between the humeral head and the overlying anterior third of the acromion, coracoacromial ligament, coracoid, or acromial-clavicular joint.[10,11] The physiologic space between the inferior acromion and superior surface of the rotator cuff tendons is termed the subacromial space. It has been measured using anteroposterior radiographs and found to be 7 to 13 mm in size in patients with shoulder pain[12] and 6 to 14 mm in normal shoulders.[13]

Biomechanical analysis of the shoulder has produced theoretical estimates of the compressive forces against the acromion with elevation of the shoulder.[14–16] Poppen and Walker[14] calculated this force at 0.42 times body weight, with Lucas[15] estimating this force at 10.2 times the weight of the arm. Peak forces against the acromion were measured between 85° and 136° of elevation,[16] a position inherent in sport-specific movement patterns[7,17] as well as commonly incurred in ergonomic and daily activities. The position of the shoulder in forward flexion, horizontal adduction, and internal rotation during the acceleration and follow-through phases of the throwing motion are likely to produce subacromial impingement due to abrasion of the supraspinatus, infraspinatus, or biceps tendon.[7]

These data provide scientific rationale for the concept of impingement or compressive disease as an etiology of rotator cuff pathology.

Neer[10,11] has outlined three stages of primary impingement as it relates to rotator cuff pathology. Stage I, edema and hemorrhage, results from the mechanical irritation of the tendon from the impingement incurred with overhead activity. This is characteristically observed in younger patients who are more athletic, and is described as a reversible condition with conservative physical therapy. The primary symptoms and physical signs of this stage of impingement or compressive disease are similar to the other two stages and consist of a positive impingement sign, painful arc of movement, and varying degrees of muscular weakness.[11]

The second stage of compressive disease outlined by Neer is termed fibrosis and tendinitis. This occurs from repeated episodes of mechanical inflammation, and can include thickening or fibrosis of the subacromial bursae. The typical age range for this stage of injury is 25 to 40 years. Neer's stage III impingement lesion, is termed *bone spurs and tendon rupture*, and is the result of continued mechanical compression of the rotator cuff tendons. Full-thickness tears of the rotator cuff, partial-thickness tears of the rotator cuff, biceps tendon lesions, and bony alteration of the acromion and acromioclavicular joint may be associated with this stage.[10,11] In addition to bony alterations that are acquired with repetitive stress to the shoulder, the native shape of the acromion is of relevance.

The specific shape of the overlying acromion process, termed *acromial architecture*, has been studied in relation to full-thickness tears of the rotator cuff.[18,19] Bigliani et al.[18] described three types of acromions: type I (flat), type II (curved), and type III (hooked). A type III or hooked acromion was found in 70 percent of cadaveric shoulders with a full-thickness rotator cuff tear, and type I acromions were only associated with 3 percent.[18] In a series of 200 clinically evaluated patients, 80 percent with a positive arthrogram had a type III acromion.[19]

Surgical treatment for primary compressive disease generally consists of decompression of 8 mm of the anterior acromion with preservation of the insertion of the deltoid, and beveling of approximately 2 cm posteriorly to provide additional space for the inflamed tendons.[9] Open repairs of associated full-thickness tears of the rotator cuff are routinely performed.

SECONDARY COMPRESSIVE DISEASE

Impingement or compressive symptoms may be secondary to underlying instability of the glenohumeral joint.[8,9] Attenuation of the static stabilizers of the glenohumeral joint, such as the capsular ligaments and labrum from the excessive demands incurred in throwing or overhead activities, can lead to anterior instability of the glenohumeral joint. Due to the increased humeral head translation, the biceps tendon and rotator cuff can become impinged secondary to the ensuing instability.[8,9] A progressive loss of glenohumeral joint stability is created when the dynamic stabilizing functions of the rotator cuff are diminished from fatigue and tendon injury.[9] The effects of secondary impingement can lead to rotator cuff tears as the instability and impingement continue.[8,9]

TENSILE OVERLOAD

Another etiologic factor in rotator cuff pathology is repetitive intrinsic tension overload. The heavy, repetitive eccentric forces incurred by the posterior rotator cuff musculature during the deceleration and follow-through phases of overhead sport activities can lead to overload failure of the tendon.[9,20] The pathologic changes referred to as "angiofibroblastic hyperplasia" by Nirschl[20] occur in the early stages of tendon injury and can progress to rotator cuff tears from the continued tensile overload.[9]

The tensile stresses incurred by the rotator cuff during the arm deceleration phase of the throwing motion to resist joint distraction, horizontal adduction, and internal rotation are reported to be as high as 1090 N with biomechanical study of highly skilled pitchers.[7] The presence of either acquired or congenital capsular laxity, as well as labral insufficiency, can greatly increase the tensile stresses to the rotator cuff muscle tendon units.[8,9]

MACROTRAUMATIC TENDON FAILURE

Unlike the previously mentioned rotator cuff classifications, cases involving macrotraumatic tendon failure usually entail a previous or single traumatic event in the clinical history.[9] Forces encountered during the traumatic event are greater than the normal tendon can tolerate. Full-thickness tears of the rotator cuff with bony avulsions of the greater tuberosity can occur from single traumatic episodes. According to Cofield,[21] normal tendons do not tear, as 30 percent or more of the tendon must be damaged to produce a substantial reduction in strength. Although a single traumatic event that resulted in tendon failure is often reported by the patient in the subjective exam, repeated microtraumatic insults and degeneration over time may have created a substantially weakened tendon that ultimately failed under the heavy load. Full-thickness rotator cuff tears require surgical treatment and aggressive rehabilitation to achieve a positive functional outcome.[9,11] Further specifics of rotator cuff surgical treatment will be discussed later in this chapter.

Additional Etiologic Factors in Rotator Cuff Pathology

In addition to the etiologic factors of rotator cuff pathology already mentioned, other factors inherent in the rotator cuff have relevance with respect to injury. The vascularity of the rotator cuff, specifically the supraspinatus, has been extensively studied beginning in 1934 by Codman. In his classic monograph on ruptures of the supraspinatus tendon, Codman described a critical zone of hypovascularity located one-half inch proximal to the insertion on the greater tuberosity.[22] This region appeared anemic with the appearance of an infarction. The biceps long head tendon was found to have a similar region of hypovascularity in its deep surface 2 cm from its insertion.[23] Rathburn and MacNab[24] reported the effects of position on the microvascularity of the rotator cuff. With the glenohumeral joint in a position of adduction, a constant area of hypovascularity was found near the insertion of the supraspinatus tendon. This consistent pattern was not observed with the arm in a position of abduction. These authors termed this the "wringing out phenomenon" and also noticed a similar response in the long head tendon of the biceps. This positional relationship has clinical ramifications for both exercise positioning and immobilization. Brooks et al.[25] found no significant difference between the tendinous insertions of the supraspinatus and infraspinatus tendons with both being hypovascular with quantitative histologic analysis.

Contradictory research published by Swiontowski et al.[26] does not support this region of hypovascularity or critical zone. Blood flow was greatest in the critical zone in living patients with rotator cuff tendonitis from subacromial impingement measured with Doppler flowmetry.

Anatomic Description of Rotator Cuff Tears

There are several primary types of rotator cuff tears commonly described in the literature. Full-thickness tears in the rotator cuff consist of tears that comprise the entire thickness (from top to bottom) of the rotator cuff tendon or tendons. Full-thickness tears are often initiated in the critical zone of the supraspinatus tendon and can extend to include the infraspinatus, teres minor, and subscapularis tendons.[27] Often associated with a tear in the subscapularis tendon is subluxation of the biceps long head tendon from the intertubercular groove, or either partial or complete tears of the biceps tendon. Histologically, full-thickness rotator cuff tears show a variety of findings ranging from almost entirely acellular and avascular margins to neovascularization with cellular infiltrate.[27]

The effects of a full-thickness rotator cuff tear on glenohumeral joint stability were studied by Loehr et al.[28] Changes in stability of the glenohumeral joint were assessed with selective division of the supraspinatus and/or infraspinatus tendons. Their findings indicated that a one-tendon lesion of either the supraspinatus or infraspinatus did not influence the movement patterns of the glenohumeral joint, whereas a two-tendon lesion induced significant changes compatible with instability of the glenohumeral joint.[28] Therefore, patients with full-thickness rotator cuff tears may have additional stress and dependence placed on the dynamic stabilizing function of the rotator cuff, due to increased humeral head translation and ensuing instability.

Additional research on full-thickness rotator cuff tears has significant clinical ramifications. One hundred consecutive patients with full-thickness tears of the rotator cuff were prospectively evaluated to determine the incidence of associated intra-articular pathology by Miller and Savoie.[29] Seventy four of 100 patients had one or more coexisting intra-articular abnormalities, with anterior labral tears occurring in 62, and biceps tendon tears in 16. The results of this study clearly indicate the importance of a thorough clinical examination of the patient with rotator cuff pathology.

A second type of rotator cuff tear is an incomplete or partial-thickness tear. Partial-thickness tears can occur on the superior surface (bursal side) or undersurface (articular side) of the rotator cuff. Although both bursal and articular side tears are partial-thickness tears of the rotator cuff, significant differences in etiology are proposed for each.[9]

Neer[10,11] and Fukoda et al.[30] have both emphasized that superior surface (bursal side) tears in the rotator cuff are the result of subacromial impingement. In the classification scheme listed earlier in this chapter, tears on the superior or bursal side of the rotator cuff are generally associated with both primary and secondary compressive disease as well as macrotraumatic tendon failure. The progression of the mechanical irritation on the superior surface can produce a partial-thickness tear that can ultimately progress to a full-thickness tear.[9-11]

Partial-thickness tears on the undersurface

or articular side of the rotator cuff are generally associated with tensile loads and glenohumeral joint instability.[9,31] Tears on the undersurface of the rotator cuff are commonly found in over-head-throwing athletes, where anterior instability, capsular and labral insufficiency, and dynamic muscular imbalances are often reported. To further understand the differing etiologies of rotator cuff tears, Nakajima et al.[31] performed a histologic and biomechanical study of the rotator cuff tendons. Biomechanically, their results showed greater deformation and tensile strength of the bursal side of the supraspinatus tendon. The bursal side of the supraspinatus tendon was comprised of a group of longitudinal tendon bundles that could disperse a tensile load and generate greater resistance to elongation than the articular or undersurface of the tendon. These authors found the articular surface to be comprised of a tendon, ligament, and joint capsule complex that elongated poorly and tore more easily.[31] The results of this study further reinforce the proposed etiology of tensile stresses producing undersurface rotator cuff tears.

One additional etiology for the undersurface tear of the rotator cuff in the young athletic shoulder is termed "inside or under surface impingement."[32,33] Placement of the shoulder in a position of 90° of abduction and 90° of external rotation causes the supraspinatus and infraspinatus tendons to rotate posteriorly, to rub on the glenoid lip, and become pinched between the humeral head and the posterosuperior glenoid rim (Fig. 11.1).[32] The presence of anterior translation of the humeral head with maximal external rotation and 90° of abduction, which has been confirmed arthroscopically during the subluxation-relocation test, can produce mechanical rubbing and fraying on the undersurface of the rotator cuff tendons. Additional harm can be caused by the posterior deltoid if the rotator cuff is not functioning properly. The posterior deltoid's angle of pull pushes the humeral head against the glenoid, accentuating the skeletal, tendinous, and labral lesions.[32] Walch et al.[33] arthroscopically evaluated 17 throwing athletes with shoulder pain during

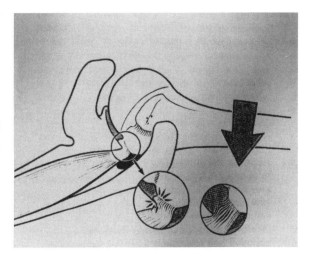

FIGURE 11.1 *Schematic representation of posterosuperior glenoid impingement between the posterior edge of the glenoid and the deep surface of the supraspinatus and infraspinatus tendons. (From Walch et al.,[33] with permission.)*

throwing and found undersurface impingement that resulted in 8 partial-thickness rotator cuff tears and 12 lesions in the posterosuperior labrum. Impingement of the undersurface of the rotator cuff on the posterosuperior glenoid labrum may be a cause of painful structural disease in the overhead athlete.

One final type or classification of rotator cuff tear is the intratendinous or interstitial rotator cuff tear. This tear develops between the bursal and articular side layers of the degenerated tendon.[34] Shear within the tendon appears to be responsible in the pathogenesis of this rotator cuff tear.

Rotator cuff pathology has several underlying etiologic factors, as evidenced by the classification schemes and scientific research in the literature. Although it is imperative to understand the common causes and classifications of rotator cuff pathology and types of rotator cuff tears, it is of paramount importance that a structured, scientifically based evaluation procedure is used not only to identify rotator cuff pathology but to ultimately identify the cause.

Clinical Evaluation of the Shoulder for Rotator Cuff Pathology

It is beyond the scope of this chapter to completely cover a comprehensive evaluation of the shoulder; this is provided in Chapter 3. A brief discussion of specific aspects of the evaluation process that are of critical importance in identification and delineation of rotator cuff pathology, however, is warranted. The multiple etiologies and specific types of rotator cuff pathology are reflected in the types of clinical tests routinely employed.

During the subjective exam, specific questioning, particularly for the overhead athlete, can greatly assist in understanding the probable cause and type of rotator cuff injury. Merely establishing that the patient has pain with overhead throwing or during the tennis serve does not provide the optimal level of information that more specific questioning aimed at identifying what stage or phase of the overhead activity would. Specific muscular activity patterns and joint kinetics inherent in each stage of these sport activities can assist in the identification of compressive disease or tensile type injuries. The presence of instability, however subtle, during the cocking phase of overhead activities can produce impingement or compressive symptoms,[9,32,33] whereas a feeling of instability or loss of control during the follow-through phase during predominantly eccentric loading can indicate a tensile rotator cuff injury.[9] Additional questions regarding a change in sport equipment, ergonomic environment, and training history provide information that is imperative in understanding the stresses leading to injury.

Objective evaluation of the patient with rotator cuff pathology must include postural testing and observation.[35] Tests to identify scapular winging in multiple positions (waist level, and 90° of flexion or greater) with an axial load via the arms are indicated. Testing for scapular dyskinesia can be performed using the Kibler scapular slide test in both neutral and 90° elevated positions.[36] A tape measure is used to measure the distance from a thoracic spinous process to the inferior angle of the scapula. A difference of more than 1 cm is considered abnormal, and may indicate scapular muscular weakness and poor overall stabilization of the scapulothoracic joint.[36]

A detailed, isolated assessment of glenohumeral joint range of motion is a key ingredient to a thorough evaluation. Identification of selective internal rotation range of motion loss on the dominant extremity was consistently reported in elite tennis players[37,38] and professional baseball pitchers. (Ellenbecker TS: unpublished data, 1991). A goniometric method using an anterior containment force by the examiner (Fig. 11.2) to minimize the scapulothoracic contribution and or substitution is recommended by this author. The loss of internal rotation range of motion is significant for two reasons. The relationship between internal rotation range of motion loss (tightness in the posterior capsule of the shoulder) and increased anterior humeral head translation has been scientifically identified. The increase in anterior humeral shear force reported by Harryman et al.[39] was manifested by a horizontal adduction cross-body maneuver, similar to that incurred during the follow-through of the throwing motion or tennis serve. Tightness of the posterior capsule has also been linked to increased superior migration of the humeral head during shoulder elevation.[40] Anterior translation of the humeral head and superior migration are two key factors indicated in rotator cuff pathology.[8,9] Internal rotation range of motion loss has also been consistently identified in a population of patients with glenohumeral joint impingement.[41]

Measurement of active and passive internal and external rotation at 90° of abduction along with scapular plane elevation, forward flexion, and abduction are performed during the evaluation of the patient with rotator cuff injury. Documentation of combined functional movement patterns (Apley's scratch test),[42] such as internal rotation with extension, and abduction and external rotation, is important, but specific, isolated testing of glenohumeral joint motion is a

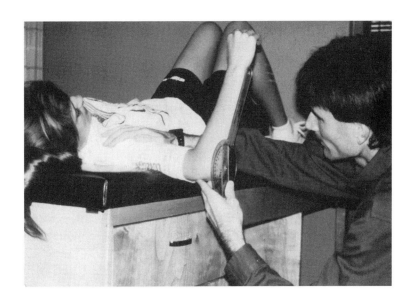

FIGURE 11.2 *Goniometric measurement of internal rotation range of motion.*

necessary requirement to identify important glenohumeral joint motion restrictions.[37]

Determination of isolated and gross muscular strength during the evaluation of the patient with rotator cuff pathology not only has a major impact on the determination of the underlying cause, but assists in the formulation of a specific, objectively based rehabilitation program. Isolated testing in the "empty can" position for the supraspinatus is performed in the scapular plane, 30° anterior to the coronal plane (Fig. 11.3).[43,44] Testing for the infraspinatus and teres minor is done with resisting external rotation in both the neutral adducted and 90° abducted position. Resisted internal rotation in the neutral adducted position is generally recommended for the subscapularis.[44] Care must be taken when interpreting normal grade static manual muscle tests of the internal and external rotators. Normal grade ⅗ muscular strength has shown large variability when compared to isokinetic testing in patients with rotator cuff pathology, and in normal controls.[45] Regardless of this reported variability, the consistent application of manual muscle testing for the rotator cuff, deltoid, scapular stabilizers, and distal upper extremity muscle groups is highly recommended. For the patient with subtle symptoms and apparently

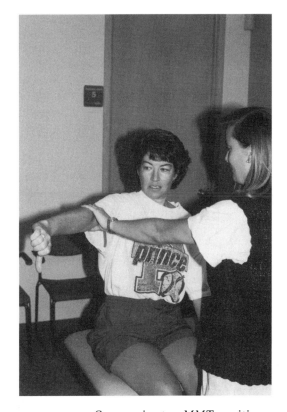

FIGURE 11.3 *Supraspinatus MMT position.*

normal muscular strength, more specific, dynamic, isokinetic testing is indicated to better identify muscular weakness or unilateral strength imbalances.[46]

Special Tests

The classic tests for evaluation of a patient with rotator cuff pathology are the impingement tests. The impingement test reported by Neer[10,11] places the shoulder in full forward flexion with overpressure. This places the supraspinatus under the coracoacromial arch, and can compress the tendon and reproduce the patient's symptoms. A second impingement test, reported by Hawkins and Kennedy,[47] involves 90° of forward flexion with full internal rotation. This test passes the rotator cuff under the coracoacromial arch, with pain and a facial grimace being indicative of a positive test. A final impingement test is the crossed arm adduction test, which involves horizontally adducting the humerus starting in 90° of elevation. These impingement tests primarily indicate the presence of rotator cuff injury from compressive or impingement etiology.[10,48] Tests to determine the integrity of the static stabilizers of the glenohumeral joint are a vital part of the comprehensive evaluation.[8,9] Rotator cuff injury caused by instability of the glenohumeral joint is a common occurrence in younger individuals and in overhead athletes.[8,9]

Clinical tests for instability must be routinely performed on the patient with rotator cuff pathology, to determine the underlying mobility status and/or degree of instability in the glenohumeral joint. Clinical tests for instability of the glenohumeral joint include the apprehension and MDI sulcus signs, as well as the fulcrum, load and shift, and subluxation relocation tests. (Further discription of these clinical tests can be found in Chapter 3). The subluxation relocation test popularized by Jobe[8,32] is performed with the patient supine, with 90° of glenohumeral joint abduction and 90° of external rotation. The examiner pushes the humeral head forward, using one hand on the posterior aspect of the patient's shoulder. This places tension on the anterior capsule and can produce a subtle anterior subluxation of the humeral head, often reproducing the patient's shoulder pain.[8] The relocation portion of the test consists of a posteriorly directed force produced by the examiner, by placing the heel of the hand over the humeral head anteriorly. This posterior force centralizes the humeral head in the glenoid fossa. A positive subluxation/relocation sign consists of provocation of the patient's symptoms, with the anterior translation in the position of 90° of abduction and external rotation, with cessation of the symptoms with the relocation (posterior centralization force).

Capsular mobility testing with the patient supine at 30°, 60°, and 90° of abduction is also performed with both anterior and posterior stresses imparted. The anterior stress applied at 30°, 60°, and 90° tests the integrity of the superior, middle, and inferior glenohumeral ligaments, respectively.[48] The degree of translation of the humeral head relative to the glenoid, as well as endfeel, are bilaterally compared and recorded.[9,49] Capsular mobility testing with the shoulder in 90° of abduction is particularly important, due to the important hammock-like stabilizing function of the inferior glenohumeral ligament complex. The anterior band of the inferior glenohumeral ligament provides critical reinforcement against anterior translation of the humeral head (subluxation) with the arm in a position of 90° of abduction and 90° of external rotation.[48]

An additional test to determine the degree of anterior capsular laxity is the Lachman test of the shoulder.[9] With the patient supine and the shoulder abducted 90° with 45° of external rotation, an anterior force is applied to the humeral head to assess anterior translation of the glenohumeral joint and note the end point of the anterior capsule.[9]

The consistent use of these instability tests will provide the clinician with greater insight regarding the relationship, if any, between the patient's rotator cuff pathology and glenohumeral joint instability. The identification of either anterior or multidirectional glenohumeral joint laxity should lead to the formulation of a treatment plan addressing the instability.[9] The special tests listed above are by no means comprehensive, with many other areas of significant emphasis, such as tests to determine the integrity of the biceps and glenoid labrum, being of paramount importance. Interpretation of the results of a comprehensive evaluation will allow the clinician to develop an objectively based rehabilitation program for rotator cuff pathology.

Biomechanical Concepts for Rehabilitation of Rotator Cuff Pathology

Several biomechanical concepts have significant applications in the formulation and application of rehabilitative exercise for the patient with rotator cuff pathology. One important concept is the force couple. A force couple consists of a pair of forces acting on an object that tends to produce rotation, even though the forces may act in opposing directions.[50] An example of a force couple in the shoulder is the deltoid-rotator cuff force couple outlined by Inman et al.[51] The force vector of the deltoid, if contracting unopposed, is superior, which would create superior migration of the humeral head.[52] The supraspinatus muscle has a compressive function when contracting, creating an approximation of the humerus into the glenoid (Fig. 11.4). The infraspinatus, teres minor, and subscapularis produce a caudal force that resists the superior migration of the humeral head. One factor of key importance when clinically interpreting the force couple concept is the muscle's force potential in relation to its physiologic cross-sectional area.[50] Research shows the subcapularis to have the greatest force potential, followed closely by the infraspinatus-teres minor group.[50] The smallest physiologic cross-sectional area is exhibited by the supraspinatus. These small rotator cuff cross-sectional areas pale in comparison to the larger force-generating capacities of the deltoid muscle. The presence of a force couple imbal-

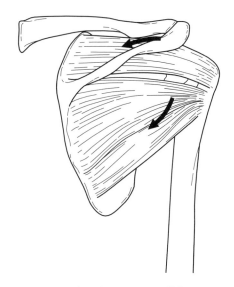

FIGURE 11.4 *Deltoid-rotator cuff force couple.*

ance is often identified on initial evaluation of the patient with rotator cuff pathology.[35,41] Weakness of the rotator cuff, coupled with hypertrophy or training enhancement of the deltoid through uneducated exercise prescription by the patient using traditional "large shoulder muscle group dominant" resistive training exercises, further perpetuates this force couple imbalance.

The coordinated interplay between the rotator cuff and deltoid musculature is further demonstrated in EMG analysis by Kronberg et al.[2] This study illustrates that all of the rotator cuff muscles are involved, to some extent, with basic shoulder movements, acting to assist in the movement and counterbalance the micromotions of the humeral head to keep it stable within the glenoid.

Additional force couples described in the literature[8,50] are the serratus anterior-trapezius and internal-external rotator couples. The serratus anterior-trapezius force couple is also important in rotator cuff pathology, as it produces upward rotation of the scapula,[8] moving the overlying acromion superiorly out of the path of the elevating proximal humerus. The internal-external rotator force couple is another commonly imbalanced pair in the overhead athlete, due to selective development of internal rotation strength, which overpowers the controlling and decelerative influence of the external rotators.[50,53,54]

Further evidence of the rotator cuff's vital function in glenohumeral joint arthrokinematics has been demonstrated by Cain et al.[55] and Blaiser[1] in cadaveric studies. These studies have shown the rotator cuff's ability to reduce the strain on the anterior capsule (inferior glenohumeral ligament) with the shoulder in 90° of abduction and external rotation. This important stabilizing function to resist anterior translation demonstrates the rotator cuff's critical contribution to joint stability. Additional biomechanical research by Clark et al.[56] identifies the intimate, adherent association of the rotator cuff to the capsuloligamentous structures, and the ability of rotator cuff muscular contraction to create tension and effect orientation of the capsuloligamentous complex. Muscular force vectors have been studied with the shoulder in the functional position of 90° of abduction and external rotation.[57] In this abducted position, the subscapularis functions as a flexor and internal rotator, the supraspinatus as an extensor, and the infraspinatus as an adductor. This study demonstrates the importance of working the dynamic stabilizers of the shoulder in both neutral and functional positions to most closely simulate the actual muscular length, tension, and contraction specificity incurred in ADL and overhead sport movement patterns.

Rehabilitation of Rotator Cuff Pathology

Both nonoperative and postoperative rehabilitation of the rotator cuff involve the following principles.

REDUCTION OF OVERLOAD AND TOTAL ARM REHABILITATION

The initial goal of any treatment program includes the reduction of pain and inflammation by protection of the extremity from stress, but not complete function.[20] Application of modalities and modification of, or complete cessation of, sport and ergonomic movement patterns is often required. Care should be taken to identify the presence of any compensatory actions in the upper extremity kinetic chain, such as excessive scapular movement and/or elbow kinematics.[58] Early use of distal strengthening of the elbow, forearm, and wrist is indicated, particularly in postoperative cases where the degree and length of immobilization is greater. Mobilization of the scapulothoracic joint and submaximal strengthening of the scapular stabilizers is indicated, taking great care not to impart inappropriate stresses or loads to the injured tissues.

RESTORATION OF NORMAL JOINT ARTHROKINEMATICS

Thorough evaluation to determine the degree of hyper or hypomobility of the glenohumeral joint, coupled with isolated joint range of motion measurements, predicates the progression of and inclusion of stretching and joint mobilization in treatment. The presence of increased anterior capsular laxity and underlying instability of the glenohumeral joint, a finding consistently found in overhead athletes, contraindicates the application of joint accessory mobilization and stretching techniques that attenuate the anterior capsule. Posterior capsular mobilization and stretching techniques to improve internal rotation range of motion are often indicated and applied. The consequences of posterior capsular tightness have been outlined earlier in the chapter.

In postoperative rehabilitation of rotator cuff repairs, the use of joint mobilization techniques to both retard and address the effects of immobilization is recommended. In addition to the posterior capsular mobilization described, specific emphasis on the caudal glide in varying positions of abduction is applied assertively, to stress the inferior capsule and prevent both adhesions and functional elevation range of motion loss.

PROMOTION OF MUSCULAR STRENGTH BALANCE AND LOCAL MUSCULAR ENDURANCE

The addition of resistive exercise is begun as inflammation and pain levels allow. Early submaximal resistive exercise in the rotator cuff and scapular muscles is initiated in the form of multiple-angle isometrics, progressing rapidly to submaximal isotonic exercises, because of their inherent dynamic characteristics.[46] The presence or lack of pain over the joint or affected tendon(s) determines the speed of progression and intensity of exercise. Resistive exercises that emphasize concentric and eccentric muscular contributions from the key dynamic stabilizers of the shoulder are used. Movement patterns requiring high activation levels from the rotator cuff based on EMG confirmation via biomechanical study are applied.[59-61] The proper use of these patterns using a low-resistance (never greater than 5 pounds and typically initiated with either no weight or as little as 1 pound) high-repetition format is recommended to enhance local muscular endurance[62] of the rotator cuff musculature. The movement patterns pictured in Figure 11.5 have been biomechanically studied, and produce high levels of rotator cuff activation. These positions also do not place the shoulder in a potential position of impingement, nor do they place excessive stress to the often attenuated anterior capsuloligamentous complex. The movement patterns recommended for strengthening the rotator cuff do not place the shoulder in elevation beyond 90° or posterior to the coronal plane.

Similar positional limitations are applied in this stage of rehabilitation for strengthening the scapular stabilizers. Patterns resisting scapular protraction and retraction, elevation and depression produce considerable muscular activity in the serratus anterior, trapezius, and rhomboids.[63] Use of closed-chain exercise, which approximates the glenohumeral joint and produces co-contraction of the proximal stabilizing musculature of the scapulothoracic joint, is also recommended in both non- and postoperative rehabilitation of the rotator cuff. Progression to advanced-level plyometric exercises for the

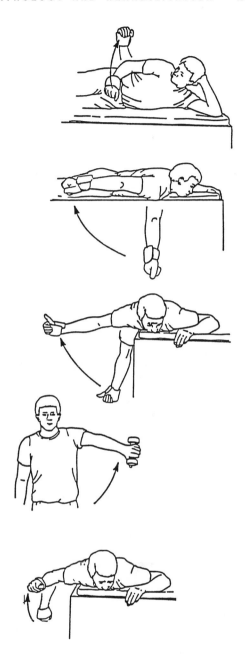

FIGURE 11.5 *Rotator cuff exercises predicated on electromyographic research.*

upper extremity is also indicated. Commonly applied are medicine balls and therapeutic Swiss balls in exercise patterns that utilize the stretch-shortening cycle of the scapulothoracic musculature, such as chest passes, and various throw and catch maneuvers that alter the position of the glenohumeral joint.[64]

Resistive exercises with emphasis on the biceps muscle are recommended in rotator cuff rehabilitation, due to the glenohumeral joint stabilizing and humeral head depression actions.[65–67] Strengthening of the biceps in neutral and 90° of shoulder flexion is recommended, with concentric and eccentric contractions implemented.

The use of isokinetic exercise is warranted in later stages of both non- and postoperative rehabilitation. As patients tolerate medium-resistance surgical tubing exercise and can perform isolated rotator cuff exercise with a 3-pound weight, they are considered for this progression.

The Davies modified base position is initially used for all patients for internal and external rotation.[35,46] Submaximal intensities at speeds ranging from 210° to 300°/sec are used, with specific emphasis on the external rotators because of their important role in functional activities[3,5,7] and in the maintenance of dynamic glenohumeral joint stability.[1,56]

Progression from the modified position in patients who will return to aggressive overhead activity is followed, using tissue tolerance as the guide. Isokinetic internal and external rotation in the scapular plane, with 80° to 90° of abduction using fast contractile velocities, has been successfully used as an end-stage rotator cuff exercise, to prepare the rotator cuff musculature for the demands of overhead activity (Fig. 11.6).

Interpretation of isokinetic test data typically focuses on bilateral comparisons and unilateral strength ratios.[46] Unilaterally dominant

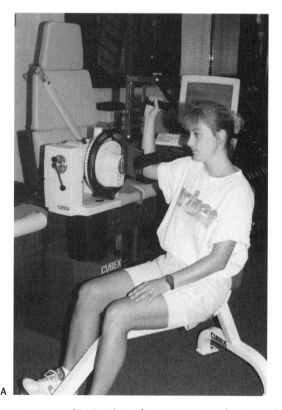
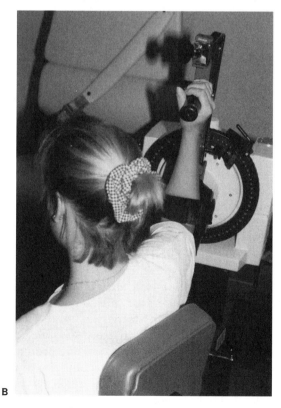

A   B

FIGURE 11.6 (A & B) *Isokinetic internal/external rotation with 90° of abduction in the scapular plane.*

upper extremity sport athletes often demonstrate 15 to 30 percent greater internal rotation strength on the dominant arm, with bilaterally symmetrical external rotation strength.[35,46,53,54] Although bilateral comparison does provide important baseline comparison for the individual, the unilateral strength ratio may be of even greater importance.[35,41,46] The unilateral external/internal rotation ratio in healthy shoulders has been reported at 66% throughout the velocity spectrum.[46] Patients with rotator cuff impingement and glenohumeral joint instability have significant alterations of this normal 66 percent ratio.[41] The unilateral strength ratio is also altered (< 66 percent) in the dominant arm in overhead throwing and racquet sport athletes due to the selective internal rotation strength development.[35,46,53,54] Isokinetic exercise and isolated joint testing is an objectively quantifiable method to address the force couple imbalances often inherent in the shoulder with rotator cuff pathology.

Specific Factors Influencing the Rehabilitation of Rotator Cuff Tears

SURGICAL APPROACH

The type of surgical approach used during open repairs of rotator cuff tears has a considerable influence on several aspects of the rehabilitative process. Two surgical approaches commonly seen in rehabilitation will be briefly discussed. The "deltopectoral approach" consists of an anterolateral incision beginning just below the middle one third of the clavicle, crosses the coracoid tip, and continues distally in an oblique lateral fashion to the anterior aspect of the humerus.[68] Nearly all anterior surgical procedures can be accomplished using this surgical exposure, including open rotator cuff tears.

In some cases, anterior surgical exposure of the shoulder requires detachment of the deltoid origin from the anterior aspect of the acromion.[69] This is particularly common if an open subacromial decompression is performed. The

subacromial decompression is used to remove a portion of the overlying offending structure, and provide both protection for the rotator cuff and prevention of further disease progression following its repair.[69]

Another commonly used surgical exposure for rotator cuff repair is the lateral "deltoid-splitting" approach. This surgical approach begins with a transverse incision through the skin, 4 to 6 cm in length, beginning at the anterolateral corner of the acromion and continuing posteriorly to the posterolateral corner.[70] A straight longitudinal incision based off the lateral aspect of the acromion, along the line of the deltoid fibers, is also frequently used. Regardless of the orientation of the skin incision, the deltoid is then split in line with its fibers near the anterolateral corner of the acromion. The deltoid's origin is protected and not detached. The deltoid is not split further distally than 5 cm to avoid damage to the axillary nerve.[70]

The type of surgical approach used in an open rotator cuff repair dictates the progression of both range of motion and resistance exercise following surgery. With the anterior deltopectoral approach (where the deltoid can be detached from its origin), restrictions regarding the application of active or resistive exercise are normally given, to allow the deltoid's origin to heal and become viable before the larger stresses incurred with active or resistive movements are applied. Active-assistive movement following surgery with the mini-arthrotomy technique, using the lateral deltoid splitting approach, can normally commence on the first postoperative day.[70] Preservation of the deltoid's origin allows more aggressive range of motion and earlier application of strengthening exercises during the rehabilitation process. This author's protocol for rehabilitation following open rotator cuff repair with a deltoid splitting surgical approach is given in Case Study 1 later in the chapter.

Progression of both range of motion and resistive exercise is much faster following arthroscopic rotator cuff debridement (Case Study 2). Active, active-assistive, and passive range of motion all commence on the first postoperative day following arthroscopy unless associated surgical procedures were performed such as anterior capsulorrhaphy, repair of a Bankart lesion with suture tacks, laser capsulorrhaphy, or extensive subacromial decompression. Submaximal intensity resistive exercise is also initiated rapidly, following debridement of partial rotator cuff tears. Because arthroscopic approaches to the shoulder do not disturb the deltoid origin or the trapezo-deltoid fascia, resistive exercise using a low-resistance, high-repetition format is recommended early, to retard atrophy and begin to normalize muscular strength imbalances.[70]

LENGTH OF IMMOBILIZATION

The degree and length of immobilization of the shoulder following rotator cuff repair can greatly affect early rehabilitation emphasis. Traditional immobilization in a sling or sling and swathe for up to 6 weeks following open rotator cuff repairs results in a capsular pattern of range of motion limitation that requires extensive joint mobilization and passive stretching. Extensive limitation in active and passive elevation, as well as external rotation of the shoulder, are commonly present following this degree and length of immobilization. Patients seen following arthroscopic debridement of partial rotator cuff tears often receive no immobilization other than a sling for one to two postoperative days, and hence often require minimal accessory mobilization to restore normal joint arthrokinematics. The common finding of associated instability and capsular laxity in the overhead athlete with partial undersurface rotator cuff tears, coupled with minimal immobilization time following arthroscopic debridement, often deemphasize the importance of accessory joint mobilization, especially to the anterior capsule. As stated earlier, the loss of internal rotation range of motion does indicate the application of posterior capsular mobilization and passive stretching techniques in this population.[39,40]

SURGICAL PROCEDURE

Debate in the literature regarding the surgical management of rotator cuff tears exists. Open repair of the torn rotator cuff tendon versus arthroscopic debridement and subacromial decompression are two options frequently discussed.[71–73] Rockwood and Burkhead[71] followed 93 patients who underwent open debridement and subacromial decompression for irreparable rotator cuff tears. Minimal deterioration in function and no degenerative changes were reported with an 8-year average follow-up evaluation. Burkhart[73] studied 25 patients who underwent arthroscopic debridement and subacromial decompression of massive rotator cuff tears with an average 30 month follow-up. Eighty-eight percent of the patients in this series were found to have good or excellent results, with no deterioration of results over time. Finally, Montgomery et al.[72] compared the results of open surgical repair to arthroscopic debridement in 87 consecutive patients with full-thickness rotator cuff tears. A 2- to 5-year follow-up revealed that the open surgical repair group had superior results as compared to the arthroscopic group. The literature contains an extensive array of research demonstrating the efficacy of various surgical procedures for rotator cuff pathology which is far beyond the scope of discussion of this chapter. One consistent finding is the important role of physical therapy in both the conservative treatment[74,75] as well as postoperative management of rotator cuff disease.

Factors Influencing the Results of Nonoperative Rehabilitation of Rotator Cuff Tears

Several factors are consistently reported in the literature as having a significant relationship to the outcome of nonoperative treatment of rotator cuff disease. Clinical findings and prognostic factors associated with unfavorable clinical outcomes in a sample of 136 patients with impingement syndrome and rotator cuff disease were (1) rotator cuff tear greater in size than 1.0 cm^2, (2) a history of pretreatment symptoms greater than 1 year, and (3) significant functional impairment at initial evaluation.[75] Itoi and Tabata[74] reported on the clinical outcome of conservative treatment of 124 shoulders with a full-thickness rotator cuff tear with a follow-up of 3 years. The primary factors relating to an unsatisfactory result were identified in their sample as limited abduction range of motion and significant abduction muscular weakness on initial evaluation of the patient. Factors not associated with clinical outcome included patient age, gender, occupation, associated instability, dominance, and chronicity of onset.

Summary

Rehabilitation of rotator cuff pathology requires an extensive, objectively based evaluation and thorough understanding of the complex biomechanical principles and etiologic factors associated with rotator cuff injury. A rehabilitation program aimed at restoring normal joint arthrokinematics and normal muscular strength, endurance, and balance is supported by the scientific principles currently present in the literature. Isolated treatment and evaluative focus on the rotator cuff and glenohumeral joint must be combined with a more global upper extremity kinetic chain approach to comprehensively address rotator cuff pathology.

CASE STUDY 1
REHABILITATION FOLLOWING ARTHROSCOPIC ROTATOR CUFF DEBRIDEMENT OF AN UNDERSURFACE TEAR OF THE SUPRASPINATUS

SUBJECTIVE INFORMATION

The patient is a 27-year-old professional baseball pitcher who started having left anterior shoulder pain in early April following a normal, uneventful spring training. Although the patient denies any particular incident of injury, he reported initially decreased recovery following pitching and pain in the anterior aspect of his shoulder during the acceleration phase and continued pain during

ing follow-through of his pitching motion. In addition to localized anterior left shoulder pain, the patient complained of weakness, loss of velocity in his throwing performance, and eventually an inability to tolerate repeated repetitions of overhead activity. His pertinent history includes previous bouts of what he calls impingement dating back to his high school and collegiate baseball years. He denies any dislocations of his left shoulder. After 2 months of nonoperative treatment, including nonsteroidal anti-inflammatory medication and physical therapy for rotator cuff and general upper extremity strengthening, he was scheduled for further diagnostic testing.

Diagnostic testing revealed an undersurface (articular side) tear in the supraspinatus tendon. He underwent an arthroscopic procedure to debride the margins of the partial-thickness tear. He is referred to physical therapy one day following arthroscopic surgery.

INITIAL FINDINGS

Examination of the patient postop reveals no obvious atrophy with the exception of a hollowing in the infraspinous fossa on the left. Passive motion on the second day postop is 120° in forward flexion, 100° of abduction, 75° of external rotation, and 20° of internal rotation. Good distal strength is present, and intact neurologic status is confirmed. Passive accessory mobility of the patient's left shoulder reveals a 2+ anterior translation at 60° and 90° of abduction, as compared to a 1+ on the right uninjured shoulder. Posterior and caudal mobility are equal bilaterally. Additional special tests such as labral and impingement test are deferred due to the patients acute postoperative nature.

TREATMENT
WEEK 1

Modalities are applied (electric stimulation and ice) to decrease pain and swelling, with a primary goal initially of restoring normal joint motion. Passive, active assistive and active ROM are used to terminal ranges as tolerated. Accessory mobilization is applied in the posterior and caudal directions to facilitate the return of flexion, abduction, and internal rotation ROM. Anterior glides are not indicated due to the hypermobility assessed on initial evaluation. Application of isometric and manually resisted rotator cuff strengthening is initiated along with scapular stabilization techniques (rhythmic stabilization, manual protraction/retraction). At the end of the first postoperative week, the patient has 175° of forward flexion and abduction, 90° of external rotation, and 35° of internal rotation measured with 90° of abduction.

WEEKS 2–4

Continued use of ROM techniques at terminal ranges of motion are indicated, with posterior glides and emphasis on stretching of the posterior musculature to increase internal rotation. Progression of the patient's rotator cuff strengthening program includes concentric and eccentric isotonic exercise using the patterns with high levels of scientifically documented rotator cuff activation. Initially a 1-pound weight is tolerated with progression to 3 pounds by 3 weeks postop. Advancement of the patient's scapular strengthening program includes the use of closed-chain Swiss ball exercise, seated rows, shrugs, and serratus anterior dominant activities including a protraction punch movement pattern with tubing and manual resistance. Distal strengthening is of key importance, and bicep/tricep and forearm/wrist isotonics are performed both in the clinic and in the home program. Continued progress of this patient is documented with AROM of the left shoulder at 175° of forward flexion and abduction, 95° of external rotation, and 40° of internal rotation.

WEEKS 4–8

Addition of isokinetic exercise in the modified base position is warranted with this patient. Tolerance of a minimum of 3-pound isolated rotator cuff exercises, negative impingement tests, and functional range of motion make him a candidate between 4 to 6 weeks postop. A submaximal introduction to the isokinetic form of resistance is recommended, with an isokinetic test to document internal and external rotation strength ap-

plied during this time frame. Results of the patients initial isokinetic test show 10 to 15 percent greater internal rotation strength when compared to the uninjured extremity and 5 to 10 percent weaker external strength at 5 weeks postop. External/internal rotation ratios range between 45 and 50 percent, revealing a relative weakness or imbalance of external rotation strength on the dominant extremity. A plyometric program with medicine balls to simulate functional muscular contractions and facilitate scapulothoracic strength is initiated during this stage.

WEEKS 8–12

Continued mobilization and PROM to normalize glenohumeral joint motion are performed, with continued emphasis on the posterior capsule and posterior musculature. Isotonic rotator cuff exercise is progressed to not more than 5 pounds, and advancement of the scapular programs in isotonic, closed-chain, and plyometric venues continues. Isokinetic testing at 8 to 9 weeks postop shows 25 percent greater internal rotation strength, and equal external rotation strength measured in the modified position. At this time the patient is progressed to an interval throwing program, carried out at the clinic on alternate days beginning with tossing at a 30-foot distance, progressing over the next 3 to 4 weeks to 60, 90, and 120-foot stages. Once the patient tolerates 120 feet with as many as 75 to 100 repetitions, he is progressed to throwing off the mound at 50 percent intensities. The isokinetic strengthening is progressed to a more functional 90° abducted position in the scapular plane. The continuation of a total arm strength program both in-clinic and at home is followed.

CASE STUDY 2
OPEN ROTATOR CUFF REPAIR (DELTOID SPLITTING APPROACH)

SUBJECTIVE HISTORY

The patient is a 51-year-old male competitive tennis player with a 1 year history of shoulder tendonitis/impingement symptoms reported as intermittent based on his level of activity. One month ago the patient was hitting a serve early in a match with minimal warm-up and felt a deep, sharp pain in the anterolateral aspect of his shoulder as his arm was accelerating forward just prior to impacting the ball. He was unable to continue playing, and following the match was unable abduct or flex his arm more than 90°. Continuous pain was reported, even with rest and sleeping, and he was evaluated by an orthopedic surgeon 2 days later. An MRI was scheduled, which revealed a full-thickness tear of the supraspinatus tendon. He subsequently underwent an open surgical repair using a deltoid splitting approach, and is referred for postoperative rehabilitation 2 days following surgery.

INITIAL FINDINGS

The patient presents with his right arm immobilized in a sling. Initial orders are for passive range of motion for the initial 2 weeks within the limitations of 100° of flexion and abduction, 30° to 40° external rotation. The patient has no distal radiation of symptoms and full light touch sensation and strong distal grip. The initial exam consists primarily of a neurologic screening and passive range of motion measurement. The patient's contralateral extremity has a 1° load and shift and anterior translation. The patient expressly denies any instability in either shoulder prior to this injury. Instability or impingement tests are not performed on the postop shoulder at this time.

INITIAL PHASE *(Weeks 0–6)*

Modalities consisting of electric stimulation and ice are applied as needed to control pain and increase local blood flow. Passive range of motion is performed using the above guidelines as maximal ranges. Evaluation of the patient's accessory movement reveals a decreased caudal glide and posterior glide relative to the contralateral extremity. Accessory mobilizations are applied using the caudal and posterior directions along with passive stretching. Mobilization of the scapulothoracic joint is also used. Passive stretching

of the elbow, particularly into extension because of the continued use a sling for immobilization, is indicated, as well as the use of grip putty to prevent disuse atrophy of the forearm and wrist musculature during the immobilization period. The patients initial range of motion at 1 week status post open rotator cuff repair is 90° of flexion and abduction, 50° of internal rotation, and 30° of external rotation. During the third postoperative week, passive range of motion is progressed to active-assistive range of motion. The use of overhead pulleys and the upper body ergometer are added within the range of motion restrictions listed. Submaximal multiple angle isometrics are performed for shoulder IR/ER, as well as manual resistance exercise for the biceps and triceps, scapular protractors/retractors, and elevators, and distal forearm and wrist musculature.

PHASE II: TOTAL ARM STRENGTH *(WEEKS 6–12)*

The patient's range of motion is advanced from active assistive to active, and terminal ranges of flexion, abduction, and internal and external rotation are included. Current range of motion of the patient is 120° of flexion, 105° of abduction, 60° of external rotation, and 60° of internal rotation. Continued mobilization of the glenohumeral joint is combined with end-range passive stretching techniques to restore normal joint arthrokinematics. Initiation of resistive exercise in the form of isotonic internal and external rotation, prone extension, horizontal abduction, and eventually scaption are performed with no resistance, progressing the resistance level as tolerated. Advancement of the scapular strengthening program to include plyometrics with a Swiss ball and eventually a medicine ball are included during this time frame. Concentric and eccentric muscular work are performed using surgical tubing and controlled execution of the resistive exercise patterns with isotonic resistance. At 10 days postop this patient has 155° of forward flexion, 145° of abduction, and 85° of external rotation with 90° of abduction. Sixty degrees of internal rotation is present with 90° of abduction. Tolerance of 3-pound isolated rotator cuff exercises (mentioned earlier) is demonstrated. The patient is progressed to isokinetic internal and external rotation in the modified base position for a trial of submaximal isokinetic exercise. Continued use of home exercise for the rotator cuff using tubing as well as the use of tubing and a counterbalanced weight for a forearm and wrist program, to begin to prepare the distal upper extremity for the return to tennis play in the later stages of rehab.

RETURN TO ACTIVITY PHASE *(WEEKS 12–16)*

Continued accessory mobilization to achieve full ranges of elevation is applied to this patient, as well as passive stretching in physiologic range of motion patterns. An isokinetic test is performed in the modified base position, revealing equal internal rotation strength bilaterally, with a 35 percent external rotation deficit identified. The patient's ER/IR ratio is 54 percent, well below the desired 66 percent balance. Range of motion for this patient has continued to improve to 175° of flexion and 160° of abduction, 95° of external rotation, and 60° of internal rotation. Advancement of the patient's strengthening program includes the 90° abducted position for both isokinetic IR/ER and surgical tubing strengthening. Plyometric exercise with medicine balls intensifies, as does the entire scapular program, including the use of closed chain push-ups and step-ups with emphasis on protraction for serratus strengthening. The patient continues with rehabilitative exercise and close adherence to a home program to reinforce the concepts of total arm strength in preparation for the interval return to tennis play. Achievement of greater external rotation muscular strength and endurance is recommended before this patient begins the interval tennis program. The guided return to tennis will include groundstroke activity initially, with progression to volleys and serving based on tolerance to the forehand and backhand groundstrokes. Typically the interval program following an open repair of a full-thickness rotator cuff tear takes up to 6 to 8 weeks before protected match play can resume. Emphasis on continued use a rotator cuff and scapular strength maintenance program is followed upon discharge of the patient from formal physical therapy.

References

1. Blaiser RB, Guldberg RE, Rothman ED: Anterior stability: Contributions of rotator cuff forces and the capsular ligaments in a cadaver model. J Shoulder Elbow Surg 1:140, 1992
2. Kronberg M, Nemeth F, Brostrom LA: Muscle activity and coordination in the normal shoulder: An electromyographic study. Clin Orthop 257:76, 1990
3. Rhu KN, McCormick J, Jobe FW et al: An electromyographic analysis of shoulder function in tennis players. Am J Sports Med 16:481, 1988
4. Vangheluwe B, Hebbelinck M: Muscle actions and ground reaction forces in tennis. Int J Sports Biomechan 2:88, 1986
5. Miyashita M, Tsunoda T, Sakurai S et al: Muscular activities in the tennis serve and overhead throwing. Scand J Sports Sci 2:52, 1980
6. Jobe FW, Moynes DR, Tibone JE et al: An EMG analysis of the shoulder in pitching. Am J Sports Med 12:218, 1984
7. Fleisig GS, Andrews JR, Dillman CJ, Escamilla RF: Kinetics of baseball pitching with implications about injury mechanisms. Am J Sports Med 23:233, 1995
8. Jobe FW, Kivitne RS: Shoulder pain in the overhand or throwing athlete: The relationship of anterior instability and rotator cuff impingement. Orthop Rev 28:963, 1989
9. Andrews JR, Alexander EJ: Rotator cuff injury in throwing and racquet sports. Sports Med Arthroscop Rev 3:30, 1995
10. Neer CS: Anterior acromioplasty for the chronic impingement syndrome in the shoulder. A prelimonary report. J Bone Joint Surg 54A:41, 1972
11. Neer CS: Impingement lesions. Clin Orthop 173:70, 1983
12. Golding FC: The shoulder: The forgotten joint. Br J Radiol 35:149, 1962
13. Cotton RE, Rideout DF: Tears of the humeral rotator cuff: a radiological and pathological necropsy survey. J Bone Joint Surg 46B:314, 1964
14. Poppen NK, Walker PS: Forces at the glenohumeral joint in abduction. Clin Orthop 135:165, 1978
15. Lucas DB: Biomechanics of the shoulder joint. Arch Surg 107:425, 1973

16. Wuelker N, Plitz W, Roetman B: Biomechanical data concerning the shoulder impingement syndrome. Clin Orthop 303:242, 1994

17. Elliot B, Marsh T, Blanksby B: A three dimensional cinematographic analysis of the tennis serve. Int J Sports Biomechan 2:260, 1986

18. Bigliani LU, Ticker JB, Flatow EL et al: The relationship of acromial architecture to rotator cuff disease. Clin Sports Med 10:823, 1991

19. Zuckerman JD, Kummer FJ, Cuomo et al: The influence of coracoacromial arch anatomy on rotator cuff tears. J Shoulder Elbow Surg 1:4, 1992

20. Nirschl RP: Shoulder tendonitis. In Pettrone FP (ed): Upper Extremity Injuries in Athletes. American Academy of Orthopaedic Surgeons Symposium. Mosby, Washington, DC, 1988

21. Cofield R: Current concepts review of rotator cuff disease of the shoulder. J Bone Joint Surg 67A: 974, 1985

22. Codman EA: The Shoulder. 2nd Ed. Thomas Todd, Boston, 1934

23. Chansky HA, Iannotti JP: The vascularity of the rotator cuff. Clin Sports Med 10:807, 1991

24. Rathburn JB, MacNab I: The microvascular pattern of the rotator cuff. J Bone Joint Surg 52B: 540, 1970

25. Brooks CH, Revell WJ, Heatley FW: A quantitative histological study of the vascularity of the rotator cuff tendon. J Bone Joint Surg 74B:151, 1992

26. Swiontowski MF, Iannotti JP, Boulas HJ et al: Intraoperative assessment of rotator cuff vascularity using laser doppler flowmetry. p. 208. In Post M, Morrey BF, Hawkins RJ (eds): Surgery of the Shoulder. St. Louis, Mosby Year Book, 1990

27. Iannotti JP: Lesions of the rotator cuff: Pathology and Pathogenesis. In Matsen FA, Fu FH, Hawkins RJ (eds): The Shoulder: A Balance of Mobility and Stability. American Academy of Orthopaedic Surgeons, Rosemont, IL, 1993

28. Loehr JF, Helmig P, Sojbjerg JO, Jung A: Shoulder instability caused by rotator cuff lesions: An in vitro study. Clin Orthop 303:84, 1994

29. Miller C, Savoie FH: Glenohumeral abnormalities associated with full-thickness tears of the rotator cuff. Orthop Rev 23:February 1994, 159

30. Fukada H, Hamada K, Yamanaka K: Pathology and pathogenesis of bursal side rotator cuff tears viewed from en bloc histologic sections. Clin Orthop 254:75, 1990

31. Nakajima T, Rokumma N, Kazutoshi H et al: Histologic and biomechanical characteristics of the supraspinatus tendon: Reference to rotator cuff tearing. J Shoulder Elbow Surg 3:79, 1994

32. Jobe FW, Pink M: The athlete's shoulder. J Hand Ther April-June 1994, 107

33. Walch G, Boileau P, Noel E, Donell ST: Impingement of the deep surface of the supraspinatus tendon on the posterosuperior glenoid rim: An arthroscopic study. J Shoulder Elbow Surg 1:238, 1992

34. Fukuda H, Hamada K, Nakajima T, Tomonaga A: Pathology and pathogenesis of the intratendinous tearing of the rotator cuff viewed from en bloc histologic sections. Clin Orthop 304:60, 1994

35. Ellenbecker TS: Rehabilitation of shoulder and elbow injuries in tennis players. Clin Sports Med 14:87, 1995

36. Kibler WB: Role of the scapula in the overhead throwing motion. Contemp Orthop 22:525, 1991

37. Ellenbecker TS, Roetert EP, Piorkowski P: Shoulder internal and external rotation range of motion of elite junior tennis players: a comparison of two protocols, abstracted. J Orthop Sports Phys Ther, 17:65, 1993

38. Chandler TJ, Kibler WB, Uhl TL et al: Flexibility comparisons of elite junior tennis players to other athletes. Am J Sports Med 18:134, 1990

39. Harryman DT, Sidles JA, Clark JM, et al: Translation of the humeral head on the glenoid with passive glenohumeral joint motion. J Bone Joint Surg 72A:1334, 1990

40. Matsen FA III, Artnz CT: Subacromial impingement. p. 623. In Rockwood CA Jr, Matsen FA III (eds): The Shoulder. WB Saunders, Philadelphia, 1990

41. Warner JJP, Micheli LJ, Arslanian LE, et al: Patterns of flexibility, laxity, and strength in normal shoulders and shoulders with instability and impingement. Am J Sports Med 18:366, 1990

42. Hoppenfeld S: Physical examination of the spine and extremities. Prentice-Hall, Norwalk, CT, 1976

43. Saha AK: Mechanism of shoulder movements and a plea for the recognition of "zero position" of glenohumeral joint (reprinted). Clin Orthop 173:3, 1983

44. Daniels L, Worthingham C: Muscle Testing: Techniques of Manual Examination. 5th Ed. WB Saunders, Philadelphia, 1986

45. Ellenbecker TS: Muscular strength relationship between normal grade manual muscle testing and isokinetic measurement of the shoulder internal and external rotators, abstracted. J Orthop Sports Phys Ther 19:72, 1994

46. Davies GJ: A compendium of isokinetics in clinical usage. 4th Ed. S & S Publishers, LaCrosse, WI, 1992

47. Hawkins RJ, Kennedy JC: Impingement syndrome in athletes. Am J Sports Med 8:151, 1980

48. Obrien SJ, Neves MC, Arnoczky SJ et al: The anatomy and histology of the inferior glenohumeral ligament complex of the shoulder. Am J Sports Med 18:449, 1990

49. Altchek DW, Skyhar MJ, Warren RF: Shoulder arthroscopy for shoulder instability. p. 187. In: Instructional Course Lectures. The Shoulder. American Academy of Orthopaedic Surgeons, Rosemont, Illinois

50. Dillman CJ: Biomechanics of the rotator cuff. Sports Med Arthroscop Rev 3:2, 1995

51. Inman VT, Saunders JB, de CM Abbot LC: Observations on the function of the shoulder joint. J Bone Joint Surg 26A:1, 1994

52. Weiner DS, MacNab I: Superior migration of the humeral head. J Bone Joint Surg 52B:524, 1970

53. Ellenbecker TS: Shoulder internal and external rotation strength and range of motion of highly skilled junior tennis players. Isokinet Exercise Sci 2:1, 1992

54. Ellenbecker TS, Mattalino AJ: Concentric isokinetic shoulder internal and external rotation strength in professional baseball pitchers. J Orthop Sports Phys Ther (submitted)

55. Cain PR, Mutschler TA, Fu F et al: Anterior stability of the glenohumeral joint. A dynamic model. Am J Sports Med 15:144, 1987

56. Clarke J, Sidles JA, Matsen FA: The relationship of the glenohumeral joint capsule to the rotator cuff. Clin Orthop 254:29, 1990

57. Bassett RW, Browne AO, Morrey BF, An KN: Glenohumeral muscle force and moment mechanics in a position of shoulder instability. J Biomechanics 23:405, 1990

58. Cooper JE, Shwedyk E, Quanbury AO et al: Elbow joint restriction: effect on functional upper limb motion during performance of three feeding activities. Arch Phys Med Rehabil 74:805, 1993

59. Ballantyne BT, O'Hare SJ, Paschall JL et al: Electromyographic activity of selected shoulder muscles in commonly used therapeutic exercises. Phys Ther 73:668, 1993

60. Blackburn TA, McLeod WD, White B et al: EMG analysis of posterior rotator cuff exercises. Athletic Training 25:40, 1990

61. Townsend H, Jobe FW, Pink M et al: Electromyographic analysis of the glenohumeral muscles during a baseball rehabilitation program. Am J Sports Med 19:264, 1991

62. Fleck S, Kraemer W: Designing Resistance Training Programs. Human Kinetics, Champaign, IL, 1987

63. Moesley JB, Jobe FW, Pink M: EMG analysis of the scapular muscles during a shoulder rehabilitation program. Am J Sports Med 20:128, 1992

64. Wilk KE, Voight ML, Keirns MA et al: Stretch-shortening drills for the upper extremities: theory and clinical application. J Orthop Sports Phys Ther 17:225, 1993

65. Glousman R, Jobe FW, Tibone JE et al: Dynamic electromyographic analysis of the throwing shoulder with glenohumeral joint instability. J Bone Joint Surg 70A:220, 1988

66. Itoi E, Kuechle DK, Newman SR et al: Stabilising function of the biceps in stable and unstable shoulders. J Bone Joint Surg 75B:546, 1993

67. Rodosky MW, Harner CD, Fu FH: The role of the long head of the biceps muscle and superior glenoid labrum in anterior stability of the shoulder. Am J Sport Med 22:121, 1994

68. Harryman DT: Common approaches to the shoulder. p. 3. In: Instructional Course Lectures. Upper Extremity. American Academy of Orthopaedic Surgeons, Rosemont, Illinois

69. Kunkel SS, Hawkins RJ: Open Repair of the rotator cuff. In Andrews JR, Wilk KE (eds): The Athlete's Shoulder. Churchill Livingstone, New York, 1994

70. Timmerman LA, Andrews JR, Wilk KE: Mini-open repair of the rotator cuff. In Andrews JR, Wilk KE (eds): The Athlete's Shoulder. Churchill Livingstone, New York, 1994

71. Rockwood CA Jr, Burkhead WZ: Management of patients with massive rotator cuff defects by acromioplasty and rotator cuff debridement. Orthop Trans 12:190, 1988

72. Montgomery TJ, Yerger B, Savoie FH: Management of rotator cuff tears: a comparison of arthroscopic debridement and surgical repair. J Shoulder Elbow Surg 3:70, 1994

73. Burkhart SS: Arthroscopic debridement and decompression for selected rotator cuff tears. Clinical results, pathomechanics, and patient selection based on biomechanical parameters. Orthop Clin North Am 24:111, 1993

74. Itoi E, Tabata S: Conservative treatment of rotator cuff tears. Clin Orthop 275:165, 1992

75. Bartolozzi A, Andreychik D, Ahmad S: Determinants of outcome in the treatment of rotator cuff disease. Clin Orthop 308:90, 1994

12

Visceral Pathology Referring Pain to the Shoulder

JOHN C. GRAY

An important component of the initial orthopedic evaluation is to differentiate the etiology of a patient's pain complaints as neuromusculoskeletal in origin versus visceral pathology or disease. Screening for visceral disease is important for several reasons: (1) many diseases mimic orthopedic pain and symptoms, and a subsequent delay in diagnosis and treatment may lead to severe morbidity or death; (2) there is a significant increase in the number of patients over the age of 60 seeking orthopedic medical care; and (3) there is an increase in the managed care environment that encourages fewer referrals to specialists, fewer referrals for diagnostic testing, and less time given to primary care physicians to make an accurate diagnosis of every patient complaining of musculoskeletal pain. Consequently, the physical therapist in an outpatient orthopedic setting is evaluating and treating patients who have greater morbidity and are more acutely ill than the patients who presented for therapy 10 or 15 years ago. Recent research has found that approximately 50 percent of all the patients referred for outpatient orthopedic physical therapy have at least one of the following diagnoses: high blood pressure, depression, asthma, chemical dependency, anemia, thyroid problems, cancer, diabetes, rheumatoid arthritis, kidney problems, hepatitis, or heart attack.[1]

Two important aspects of the orthopedic evaluation that will help detect visceral pathology or disease are a careful history and palpation. A sampling of important questions related to the history-taking portion of the evaluation is listed below[2]:

1. Describe the first and last time you experienced these same complaints.

2. Are your symptoms the result of a trauma, or are they of a gradual or insidious onset?

3. Was it a macrotrauma (motor vehicle accident, fall, sports injury) or repeated microtrauma (overuse injury, cumulative trauma disorder)?

4. What was the mechanism of injury?

5. Do you have any other complaints of pain throughout the rest of your body—head, neck, chest, back, abdomen, arms, or legs?

6. Do you have any other symptoms throughout the rest of your body—headaches, nausea, vomiting, dizziness, shortness of breath, weakness, fatigue, fever, bowel or bladder changes, numbness, tingling, pins or needles?

7. Is your pain worse at night?

8. Are there positions or activities that change your pain, either aggravating or relieving your symptoms?

9. Does eating or digesting a meal affect your pain?

10. Does bowel or bladder activity affect your pain?

11. Does coughing, laughing, or deep breathing affect your pain?

12. Does your shoulder pain get worse with exertional activities (climbing stairs) that don't directly involve your shoulder?

The following are some warning signs, gathered during the history and interview, that may indicate possible visceral pathology or disease.[3,4]

1. Pain is constant.

2. The onset of pain is not related to trauma or overuse.

3. Pain is described as throbbing, pulsating, deep aching, knifelike, or colicky.

4. There is no relief of pain or symptoms with rest.

5. Symptoms are bilateral.

6. Constitutional symptoms are present: fever, night sweats, nausea, vomiting, pale skin, dizziness, fatigue, or unexplained weight loss.

7. Pain is worse at night.

8. Pain does not change with body position or activity.

9. Extraordinary relief of pain is obtained with aspirin (bone cancer).

10. Pain changes in relation to organ function (eating, bowel or bladder activity, coughing or deep breathing, menstrual cycle).

11. Indigestion, diarrhea, constipation, or rectal bleeding are present.

12. Shoulder pain increases with exertion that does not stress the shoulder (walking or climbing stairs).

A self-administered patient questionnaire (Fig. 12.1) is useful as a screen for possible visceral pathology or disease. For example, if a patient has a few checks under the "yes" column for pulmonary, then refer to the section below titled "lung." In this way you can analyze the patient's signs and symptoms to see if they correlate with a Pancoast tumor or a pulmonary infarct. The idea is not to diagnose visceral pathology, which should be left to the physician, but to assess whether or not the patient's symptoms are orthopedic in origin.

The second important aspect of the evaluation is palpation. Palpation should include the lymph nodes (for infection or neoplasm), which are normally up to 1 to 2 cm, in the cervical (medial border of sternocleidomastoid, anterior to upper trapezius muscle), supraclavicular, axilla, and femoral triangle regions.[3,5] Abnormal findings are swollen, tender, or immovable lymph nodes.[5] Palpate the abdomen for muscle rigidity and significant local tenderness (possible visceral disease), or a large pulsatile mass (indicative of an aortic aneurysm).[3,5] Palpation in the right upper abdominal quadrant will reveal the liver, gallbladder, and portions of the small and large intestines (Plate 12.1). The left upper abdominal quadrant will reveal the stomach, spleen, tail of the pancreas, and portions of the small and large intestines (Plate 12.1).[6] The kidneys lie deep posteriorly in the left and right upper abdominal quadrants.[6] The appendix and large intestine are found in the right lower quadrant, and other portions of the large intestine may be found in the left lower quadrant.[6] A tender mass in the femoral triangle or groin area may indicate a hernia.[6] A pulsating mass in the midline may indicate an aortic aneurysm.[6] When evaluating abdominal tenderness it is important to differentiate the source as originating from the superficial myofascial wall or from the deep viscera. If palpable tenderness is again elicited with the abdominal wall contracted and the head and neck flexed off the table, then the symptoms are originating from the myofascial abdominal wall.[6] If, however, the palpable tenderness disappears in the above situation, then you should suspect deep visceral pathology.[6]

The ability to palpate and interpret peripheral pulses is another important diagnostic tool for the orthopedic manual therapist. When palpating a pulse, the therapist needs to compare the amplitude and force of pulsations in one artery with those in the corresponding vessel on the opposite side.[7] Palpation of the artery should be performed with a light pressure and a sensitive touch. If the pressure is firm, then there is a risk of not being able to perceive a weak pulse or misinterpreting your own pulse as that of the patient's.[7] Pulsations may be recorded as normal (4), slightly (3), moderately (2), or markedly reduced (1), or absent (0).[7] Palpate the arterial pulses for cardiovascular and peripheral vascular disease. The arterial pulses may be palpated in the upper extremity (axillary artery in the axilla, brachial artery in the cubital fossa, ulnar and radial arteries at the wrist) and lower extremity (femoral artery at femoral triangle, popliteal artery at popliteal fossa, posterior tibialis artery posterior to medial malleolus, and dorsal pedis artery at the base of the first and second metatarsal bones).[3,5,7,8]

Be aware of the easy and common diagnoses of osteoarthritis, degenerative joint or disc disease, and spondylosis in the elderly population. Many asymptomatic elderly persons have positive radiographs for these diseases. Also, the elderly in our society are at a greater risk for visceral pathology and disease. In addition, old asymptomatic orthopedic injuries may become symptomatic due to facilitation from a segmentally related visceral organ in a diseased state.[9,10]

Pain may be defined as an unpleasant sensory and emotional experience associated with actual or potential tissue damage.[11] True visceral pain can be experienced within the involved viscus.[3,12] It is described as deep, dull, achy, colicky, and poorly localized.[3,12,13] There is also a strong autonomic reflex phenomenon, including sudomotor (increased sweating) changes, vasomotor (blood vessel) responses, changes in arterial pressure and heart rate, and an intense psychic alarm reaction.[11,12,14] Viscera are innervated by nociceptors (Plate 12.2)[3,15] These free nerve endings are found in the loose connective tissue walls of the viscus, including the epithelial and serous linings, as well as the walls of the local blood vessels in the viscus.[3] After activation of

these nociceptors by sufficient chemical or mechanical stimulation, neural information is transmitted along small unmyelinated type C nerve fibers within sympathetic and parasympathetic nerves.[3,15–17]

This information is subsequently relayed to the mixed spinal nerve, dorsal root, and into the dorsal horn of the spinal cord (Plate 12.2). Second-order neurons in the dorsal horn project in the anterolateral system.[15] Within the anterolateral system, nociceptive impulses ascend in the spinothalamic, spinoreticular, and spinomesencephalic tracts.[15] The targets in the brain for these tracts are the thalamus, recticular formation, and midbrain, respectively.[15]

Chemical stimulation of nociceptors may result from a buildup of metabolic end products, such as bradykinins or proteolytic enzymes, secondary to ischemia of the viscus.[3] Prolonged spasm or distension of the smooth muscle wall of viscera can cause ischemia secondary to a collapse of the microvascular network within the viscus.[3] Chemicals, such as acidic gastric fluid, can leak through a gastric or duodenal ulcer into the peritoneal cavity, resulting in local abdominal pain.[3,18]

Mechanical stimulation of visceral nociceptors can occur secondary to torsion and traction of the mesentery, distention of a hollow viscus, or impaction.[3,11–14] Distention may result from a local obstruction such as a kidney stone or from local edema due to infection or inflammation.[3] Spasm of visceral smooth muscle may also be a sufficient mechanical stimulus to activate the nociceptors of the involved viscus.[3,13,18]

Visceral pain is not uncommon in patients suffering from neoplastic disease. Pain complaints from cancer patients have several origins. Somatic pain occurs as a result of activation of nociceptors in cutaneous and deep tissues (tumor metastasis to bone) and is usually constant and localized.[11] Visceral pain results from stretching and distending or from the production of an inflammatory response and the release of algesic chemicals in the vicinity of nociceptors.[3,11,12] Metastatic tumor infiltration of bone and gastrointestinal and genitourinary tumors that invade abdominal and pelvic viscera are very common causes of pain in the cancer pa-

PATIENT QUESTIONNAIRE

	YES	NO
NAME _____ DATE _____		
AGE	_____	
HEIGHT	_____	
WEIGHT	_____	
FEVER AND/OR CHILLS	_____	_____
UNEXPLAINED WEIGHT CHANGE	_____	_____
NIGHT PAIN/DISTURBED SLEEP	_____	_____
EPISODE OF FAINTING	_____	_____
DRY MOUTH (DIFFICULTY SWALLOWING)	_____	_____
DRY EYES (RED, ITCHY, SANDY)	_____	_____
HISTORY OF ILLNESS PRIOR TO ONSET OF PAIN	_____	_____
HISTORY OF CANCER	_____	_____
FAMILY HISTORY OF CANCER	_____	_____
RECENT SURGERY (DENTAL ALSO)	_____	_____
DO YOU SELF INJECT MEDICINES/DRUGS	_____	_____
DIABETIC	_____	_____
PAIN OF GRADUAL ONSET (NO TRAUMA)	_____	_____
CONSTANT PAIN	_____	_____
PAIN WORSE AT NIGHT	_____	_____
PAIN RELIEVED BY REST	_____	_____

PULMONARY

	YES	NO
HISTORY OF SMOKING	_____	_____
SHORTNESS OF BREATH	_____	_____
FATIGUE	_____	_____
WHEEZING OR PROLONGED COUGH	_____	_____
HISTORY OF ASTHMA, EMPHYSEMA OR COPD	_____	_____
HISTORY OF PNEUMONIA OR TUBERCULOSIS	_____	_____

CARDIOVASCULAR

	YES	NO
HEART MURMUR/HEART VALVE PROBLEM	_____	_____
HISTORY OF HEART PROBLEMS	_____	_____
SWEATING WITH PAIN	_____	_____
RAPID THROBBING OR FLUTTERING OF HEART	_____	_____
HIGH BLOOD PRESSURE	_____	_____
DIZZINESS (SIT TO STAND)	_____	_____
SWELLING IN EXTREMITIES	_____	_____
HISTORY OF RHEUMATIC FEVER	_____	_____
ELEVATED CHOLESTEROL LEVEL	_____	_____
FAMILY HISTORY OF HEART DISEASE	_____	_____
PAIN/SYMPTOMS INCREASE WITH WALKING OR STAIR CLIMBING AND RELIEVED WITH REST	_____	_____

PREGNANT WOMEN ONLY

	YES	NO
CONSTANT BACKACHE	_____	_____
INCREASED UTERINE CONTRACTIONS	_____	_____
MENSTRUAL CRAMPS	_____	_____
CONSTANT PELVIC PRESSURE	_____	_____
INCREASED AMOUNT OF VAGINAL DISCHARGE	_____	_____
INCREASED CONSISTENCY OF VAGINAL DISCHARGE	_____	_____
COLOR CHANGE OF VAGINAL DISCHARGE	_____	_____
A INCREASED FREQUENCY OF URINATION	_____	_____

FIGURE 12.1 (A & B) *A self-administered patient questionnaire. (Figure continues.)*

PATIENT QUESTIONNAIRE

FEMALE UROGENITAL SYSTEM (WOMEN ONLY)

	YES	NO
DATE OF LAST MENSES		
ARE YOU PREGNANT		
PAINFUL URINATION		
BLOOD IN URINE		
DIFFICULTY CONTROLLING URINATION		
CHANGE IN THE FREQUENCY OF URINATION		
INCREASE IN URGENCY OF URINATION		
HISTORY OF URINARY INFECTION		
POST-MENOPAUSAL VAGINAL BLEEDING		
VAGINAL DISCHARGE		
PAINFUL MENSES		
PAINFUL INTERCOURSE		
HISTORY OF INFERTILITY		
HISTORY OF VENEREAL DISEASE		
HISTORY OF ENDOMETRIOSIS		
PAIN CHANGES IN RELATION TO MENSTRUAL CYCLE		

GASTROINTESTINAL

DIFFICULTY IN SWALLOWING		
NAUSEA		
HEARTBURN		
VOMITING		
FOOD INTOLERANCES		
CONSTIPATION		
DIARRHEA		
CHANGE IN COLOR OF STOOLS		
RECTAL BLEEDING		
HISTORY OF LIVER OR GALLBLADDER PROBLEMS		
HISTORY OF STOMACH OR GI PROBLEMS		
INDIGESTION		
LOSS OF APETITE		
PAIN WORSE WHEN LYING ON YOUR BACK		
PAIN CHANGE DUE TO BOWEL/BLADDER ACTIVITY		
PAIN CHANGE DURING OR AFTER MEALS		

MALE UROGENITAL SYSTEM (MEN ONLY)

PAINFUL URINATION		
BLOOD IN URINE		
DIFFICULTY CONTROLLING URINATION		
CHANGE IN FREQUENCY OF URINATION		
INCREASE IN URINARY URGENCY		
DECREASED FORCE OF URINARY FLOW		
URETHRAL DISCHARGE		
HISTORY OF URINARY INFECTION		
HISTORY OF VENEREAL DISEASE		
IMPOTENCE		
PAIN WITH EJACULATION		
HISTORY OF SWOLLEN TESTES		

B

FIGURE 12.1 *(Continued).* **(B)**.

tient.[11] Deafferentation pain results from injury to the peripheral and/or central nervous system as a result of tumor compression or infiltration of peripheral nerve or the spinal cord, or injury to peripheral nerve as a result of surgery, chemotherapy, or radiation therapy for cancer.[11] Examples are metastatic or radiation-induced brachial or lumbosacral plexopathies, epidural spinal cord and/or cauda equina compression, and postherpetic neuralgia.[11]

Somatic, visceral, and deafferentation pain may be complicated by sympathetically maintained pain, in which efferent sympathetic activity promotes persistent pain, hyperpathia, and vasomotor and sudomotor changes.[11] Also, nociceptors may be facilitated following injury, leading to lower threshold of activation, greater intensity of response to injury, and the emergence of spontaneous activity within the interneuron pool of the dorsal horn.[11,19]

The observation has been made that visceral disease produces not only orthopedic pain, but true orthopedic dysfunction.[20,21] For example, pain referred to the T4 spinal segment from cardiac tissue (angina) may cause reflex muscle guarding of the muscles supplied by T4, which will interfere with the normal mobility of that segment of the spine. This may then produce movement around a nonphysiologic axis at that segment and subsequently lead to joint injury, locking, or hypomobility.

Theories on Visceral Referred Pain

1. Referred pain is pain experienced in tissues that are not the site of tissue damage, and whose afferent or efferent neurones are not physically involved in any way.[22]

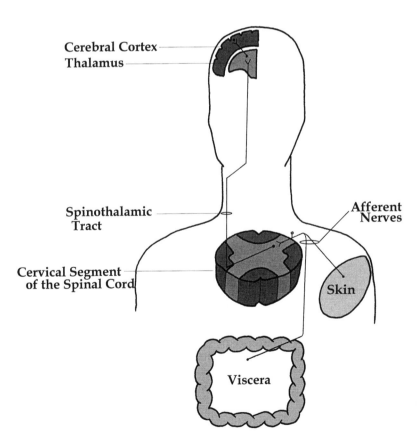

FIGURE 12.2 *Schematic drawing of a single afferent nerve fiber receiving input from both skin and viscera.*

2. Pain happens within the central nervous system, not in the damaged tissue itself. Pains do not really happen in hands or feet or heads; they happen in the images of heads and feet and hands.[22]

3. Referred pain from deep somatic structures is often indistinguishable from visceral referred pain.[23]

4. Visceral pain fibers constitute less than 10 percent of the total afferent input to the lower thoracic segments of the spinal cord and are rarely activated.[15] In this way, a visceral stimulus may be mistaken for the more familiar somatic pain.[15]

5. Visceral referred pain may be due to misinterpretation by the sensory cortex.[24] Over the years, specific cortical cells are repeatedly stimulated by nociceptive activity from a specific area of the skin. When nociceptors of a viscus are eventually stimulated, chemically or mechanically, these same sensory cortex cells may become stimulated with the cortex interpreting the origin of this sensory input based on past experience. The pain, therefore, is perceived to arise from the area of skin that has repeatedly stimulated these cortical cells in the past. The referred pain may lie within the dermatome of those spinal segments that receive sensory information from the visceral organ.[24]

6. Sensory fibers dichotomize as they "leave" the spinal cord, one branch passing to a visceral organ as the other branch travels to a site of reference in muscle or skin (Fig. 12.2).[25,26]

7. Visceral nociceptor activity converges with input from somatic nociceptors into com-

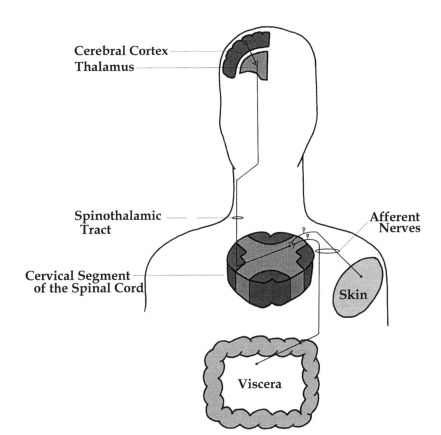

Cerebral Cortex
Thalamus

Spinothalamic Tract

Cervical Segment of the Spinal Cord

Afferent Nerves

Skin

Viscera

FIGURE 12.3 *Schematic drawing of a visceral afferent nerve and a somatic afferent nerve converging onto the same spinothalamic tract cell in the dorsal horn of the spinal cord.*

mon pools of spinothalamic tract cells in the dorsal horn of the spinal cord. Visceral pain is then referred to remote cutaneous sites because the brain "misinterprets" the input as coming from a peripheral cutaneous source, which normally bombards the central nervous system with sensory stimuli (Fig. 12.3).[6,11–15,23,27–29]

Viscera Capable of Referring Pain to the Shoulder

DIAPHRAGM

The central portion of the diaphragm, which is segmentally innervated by cervical nerves C3 to C5 via the phrenic nerve,[3,30] can refer pain to the shoulder.[25,29–34] Although the diaphragm is a musculotendinous structure and not a viscus, it is interesting in terms of the distance it refers its pain to the shoulder. Also, many viscera (liver, esophagus, stomach and pancreas) can refer pain to the shoulder through contact with the diaphragm (Plates 12.1, 12.3, and Fig. 12.4).[3] In the rat, cervical (C3, C4) dorsal root ganglion cells were seen that had collateral nerve fibers that emanated from both the diagphragm and the skin of the shoulder (Fig. 12.2).[25]

Symptoms

Pain in the shoulder is most often felt at the superior angle of the scapula, in the suprascapular region, and in the upper trapezius muscle.[30,31] Normally there are no complaints of pain in the region of the diaphragm, unless the patient suffered trauma or a musculoskeletal strain to the surrounding tissues.

Diagnosis

Local tenderness or shoulder pain during palpation of the diaphragm. Full active and passive shoulder girdle elevation may cause pain,

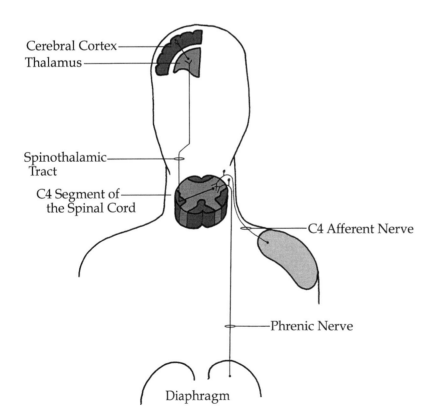

FIGURE 12.4 *Schematic drawing of an afferent nerve from the diaphragm converging onto the same spinothalamic tract cell as is a somatic afferent nerve from the skin of the shoulder.*

because this motion changes the shape of the thoracic cage and subsequently puts tension on the diaphragm.[32] Shoulder pain is reproduced or exacerbated by deep breathing, coughing, or sneezing.[32,35]

CASE STUDY 1

HISTORY

A 24-year-old right-handed male presented to physical therapy (February 1992) with a diagnosis of "left shoulder pain." His only complaint was periodic, and severe, localized left shoulder pain at the acromioclavicular joint (Fig. 12.5). He denied neck pain, headaches, weakness, arm pain, or paresthesias. The patient denied any other complaints or symptoms throughout the rest of his body. He reported he was a competitive racquetball and volleyball player. He played either sport three to four times a week. The patient reported pain for the 6 days prior to presentation, but denied any trauma. Nine days prior to evaluation he participated in a 2-day walleyball (volleyball on a racquetball court) tournament. Six days prior to presentation the patient was involved in two competitive racquetball league matches.

He reported a constant low-intensity ache that never went away, regardless of what he did. He was able, however, to produce a sudden and sharp pain with certain movements. He was able to sleep on his left side without much difficulty. Eating and bowel or bladder activity had no affect on his symptoms. Coughing, laughing, and deep inhalation did, however, produce a sudden sharp pain in the shoulder.

PAST MEDICAL HISTORY

1991: Muscle strain on left side of rib cage
1990: Muscle strain on left side of rib cage
1987: Low back injury—sprain/strain

PHYSICIAN-ORDERED TESTS

No radiographs were ordered.

GENERAL HEALTH

The patient questionnaire (Fig. 12.6) did not produce any significant "red flags" to indicate visceral involvement. The patient was young and appeared fit and healthy.

CERVICAL SCREEN

Active and passive ROM was WNL and painless. Cervical axial compression (see Fig. 4.14) and Spurling's quadrant compression tests (see Fig. 4.16) were negative.

SHOULDER AROM AND PROM

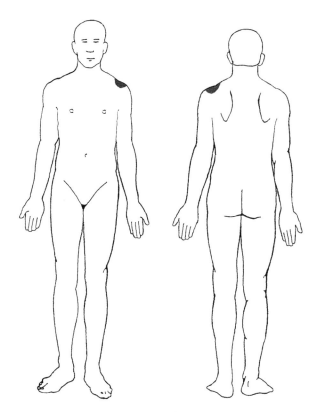

FIGURE 12.5 *Pain diagram from a 24 year-old right-handed male with a presenting diagnosis of "left shoulder pain."*

Left shoulder active and passive ROM was WNL with minimal discomfort and no reproduction of symptoms.

PATIENT QUESTIONNAIRE

	YES	NO
NAME __Case Study #1__ DATE __02/15/92__		
AGE	24	
HEIGHT	5'11"	
WEIGHT (lbs)	165	
FEVER AND/OR CHILLS		X
UNEXPLAINED WEIGHT CHANGE		X
NIGHT PAIN/DISTURBED SLEEP		X
EPISODE OF FAINTING		X
DRY MOUTH (DIFFICULTY SWALLOWING)		X
DRY EYES (RED, ITCHY, SANDY)		X
HISTORY OF ILLNESS PRIOR TO ONSET OF PAIN		X
HISTORY OF CANCER		X
FAMILY HISTORY OF CANCER		X
RECENT SURGERY (DENTAL ALSO)		X
DO YOU SELF INJECT MEDICINES/DRUGS		X
DIABETIC		X
PAIN OF GRADUAL ONSET (NO TRAUMA)	X	
CONSTANT PAIN	x	
PAIN WORSE AT NIGHT		x
PAIN RELIEVED BY REST		x

PULMONARY

	YES	NO
HISTORY OF SMOKING		X
SHORTNESS OF BREATH		X
FATIGUE		X
WHEEZING OR PROLONGED COUGH		X
HISTORY OF ASTHMA, EMPHYSEMA OR COPD		X
HISTORY OF PNEUMONIA OR TUBERCULOSIS		X

CARDIOVASCULAR

	YES	NO
HEART MURMUR/HEART VALVE PROBLEM		X
HISTORY OF HEART PROBLEMS		X
SWEATING WITH PAIN		X
RAPID THROBBING OR FLUTTERING OF HEART		X
HIGH BLOOD PRESSURE		X
DIZZINESS (SIT TO STAND)		X
SWELLING IN EXTREMITIES		X
HISTORY OF RHEUMATIC FEVER		X
ELEVATED CHOLESTEROL LEVEL		X
FAMILY HISTORY OF HEART DISEASE	X	
PAIN/SYMPTOMS INCREASE WITH WALKING OR STAIR CLIMBING AND RELIEVED WITH REST		X

PREGNANT WOMEN ONLY

	YES	NO
CONSTANT BACKACHE		
INCREASED UTERINE CONTRACTIONS		
MENSTRUAL CRAMPS		
CONSTANT PELVIC PRESSURE		
INCREASED AMOUNT OF VAGINAL DISCHARGE		
INCREASED CONSISTENCY OF VAGINAL DISCHARGE		
COLOR CHANGE OF VAGINAL DISCHARGE		
INCREASED FREQUENCY OF URINATION		

FIGURE 12.6 *Patient questionnaire for Case Study 1.*

RESISTED TESTING

There was no reproduction of symptoms.

THORACIC SPINE AROM AND PROM

Thoracic motion was minimally limited in flexion and extension. Sharp left shoulder pain, however, was noted with movement into the end range of flexion or extension.

RESISTED TESTING

There was no reproduction of symptoms.

PALPATION

There was no tenderness or reproduction of symptoms with palpation of musculoskeletal structures throughout the cervical spine, chest, and shoulder. Palpation of the lymph nodes and arterial pulses in the cervical spine and upper extremities was negative. Palpation of the abdomen revealed local pain and tenderness along the left anterolateral border of the diaphragm and costal margin, just under the rib cage. Palpation of this peripheral portion of the diaphragm did not reproduce shoulder pain.

RIB AROM AND PROM

Active deep inhalation and passive lower rib cage compression reproduced left shoulder pain.

RESISTED TESTING

There was no reproduction of symptoms.

NEUROLOGIC EXAMINATION

Sensation, deep tendon reflexes and strength testing of the upper extremities was WNL.

SPECIAL TESTS

Passive flexion with humeral internal rotation (IR) or external rotation (ER) was negative; glenohumeral, sternoclavicular, and acromioclavicular joint compression and distraction were negative; upper limb nerve tension tests were negative. Immediate and sharp left shoulder pain, however, was reproduced with deep inhalation, coughing, or laughing.

JOINT MOBILITY

Glenohumeral, scapulothoracic, sternoclavicular, and acromioclavicular joint mobility were all WNL, grade 3, with no symptom reproduction.

ASSESSMENT

The patient's signs and symptoms were consistent with an extrinsic source of shoulder pain. This extrinsic source appeared to be from an irritation of the central left hemidiaphragm with subsequent referred pain to the left shoulder.

PNEUMOPERITONEUM

Pneumoperitoneum, or air in the peritoneal cavity, can refer pain to the shoulder due to pressure on the central portion of the diaphragm (Plate 12.3 and Fig. 12.4).[30–32,36–41] Air may become trapped within the peritoneal cavity in a number of different ways.

Perforation of an abdominal viscus can release air into the peritoneum.[30,38,42] Examples of this are a peptic ulcer, acute pancreatitis, perforated appendix, and a splenic infarct or rupture.[32,38,42]

Symptoms

The patient may complain of acute or spasmodic shoulder and/or abdominal pain. In the case of a splenic infarct or rupture, the pain will be in the left shoulder.[42] There will be a variety of symptoms depending on which viscus is perforated. See the associated symptoms under "Diaphragm" earlier in the chapter.

Diagnosis

Pain and/or rigidity will be noted with abdominal palpation. An upright plain anterior-posterior radiograph will demonstrate free intraperitoneal air under one or both hemidiaphragms.[36] See the associated diagnostic clues under "Diaphragm" earlier in the chapter.

Abdominal or vaginal surgery that allows operative free air to enter and become trapped within the peritoneal cavity, is another source of referred pain to the shoulder.

Symptoms

Pain in the shoulder. See the associated symptoms under "Diaphragm."

Diagnosis

There will be a history of recent abdominal or vaginal surgery. The abdomen is not tender to palpation and rigidity is absent. An upright plain anterior-posterior radiograph will demonstrate free intraperitoneal air under the diaphragm.[36] See the associated diagnostic clues under "Diaphragm."

For females, certain activities during pregnancy, within 6 weeks postpartum, or following abdominal or vaginal surgery, can lead to pneumoperitoneum. These include menstruation, effervescent vaginal douching, vigorous sexual intercourse, orogenital insufflation, and knee to chest stretching exercises.[36,37,39,40] The last three

activities can be fatal due to an air embolism.[36,37,39–41] To create pneumoperitoneum, air must first enter the vagina before it passes through a patent os cervix to enter the body cavity of the cervix and subsequently travel through the uterine tube prior to escaping into the peritoneal cavity (Fig. 12.7).

Symptoms

Pain in the shoulder. See the associated symptoms under "Diaphragm."

Diagnosis

There will be a history of current or recent pregnancy or recent abdominal or vaginal surgery. The abdomen is not tender to palpation and rigidity is absent. An upright plain anterior-posterior radiograph will demonstrate free intraperitoneal air under the diaphragm.[36] See the associated diagnostic clues under "Diaphragm."

LUNG

The lung, which is innervated by thoracic nerves T5 to T6,[3] is capable of referring pain from two distinct diseases to the shoulder.[30,32,33,35,43–46]

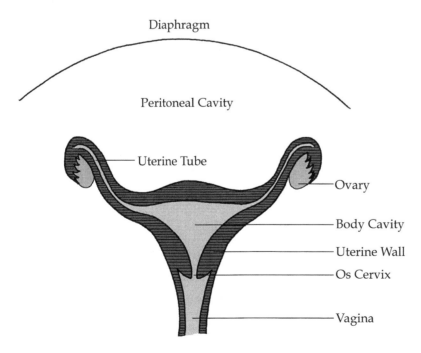

FIGURE 12.7 *Schematic drawing of the pathway that air must travel in order to create a pneumoperitoneum.*

The first is pulmonary infarction that is often secondary to a pulmonary embolism.[32,46] The second is a Pancoast tumor. The most common cause of pulmonary embolism is a deep venous thrombosis (DVT) originating in the proximal deep venous system of the lower legs.[46] Risk factors for DVT include blood stasis due to bed rest, endothelial (blood vessel) injury from surgery or trauma, and a state of hypercoagulation.[46] Other risk factors include congestive heart failure, trauma, surgery (especially of the hip, knee, and prostate), more than 50 years of age, infection, diabetes, obesity, pregnancy, and oral contraceptive use.[46] Pain is referred to the shoulder due to contact with the central portion of the diaphragm (Plate 12.3 and Fig. 12.4).[30–32]

Symptoms

Pain in the shoulder is most often felt at the superior angle of the scapula, in the supraclavicular region, and in the upper trapezius muscle.[30,31] Patients will usually report the relief of pain when lying on the involved shoulder.[2] Symptoms related directly to the pulmonary embolism may include swollen and painful legs with walking, acute dyspnea or tachypnea, chest pain, tachycardia, low-grade fever, rales, diffuse wheezing, decreased breath sounds, persistent cough, restlessness, and acute anxiety.[46–48] See the associated symptoms under "Diaphragm" earlier in the chapter.

Diagnosis

There is a history of recent surgery. Chest radiographs, arterial blood gas studies, pulmonary angiography, and ventilation-perfusion (V/Q) scintigraphy are diagnostic tools available for the physician.[49] Plain radiographs may not demonstrate the infarct, however, which may be hidden by the dome of the diaphragm.[32] This is a potentially fatal condition that needs rapid referral for emergency medical attention. See the associated diagnostic clues under "Diaphragm."

The second disease state is a Pancoast tumor that occurs in the apical portion of the lung (Plate 12.4).[30,32,35,43,45,46,50,51] Lung cancer is the most common fatal cancer in both men and women.[50] It commonly refers pain to the supraclavicular fossa, usually on the right side.[32] Pain from a Pancoast tumor may be referred to the shoulder due to the involvement of the upper ribs.[51] Shoulder and arm pain may also occur secondary to contact between the cancerous lobes of the lung with the eighth cervical (C8) and first thoracic (T1) nerves, resulting in shoulder and upper extremity symptoms similar to thoracic outlet syndrome or a C8 radiculopathy.[35,43,45,46,50,51] The chest wall and subpleural lymphatics are often invaded by the tumor.[51] Other structures that may be involved include the subclavian artery and vein, internal jugular vein, phrenic nerve, vagus nerve, common carotid artery, recurrent laryngeal nerve, sympathetic chain, and stellate ganglion.[43,45,51] Cancer can metastasize to the lungs from carcinomas in the kidney, breast, pancreas, colon, or uterus.[46]

The lung itself is a common source of metastatic cancer to bone, the liver, adrenal glands, and the brain.[46,50] Symptoms associated with cancer of the spine include a deep, dull ache that may be unrelieved by rest.[50] Pain often precedes a pathologic fracture.[50] If a fracture is present, then the pain may be sharp, localized, and associated with swelling.[50] Pain will be reproduced with mechanical stress, thereby simulating a pure musculoskeletal dysfunction. Neurologic signs and symptoms will be present in some patients due to compression of the spinal cord. Pain is exacerbated by percussion of the spinous process, with a reflex hammer, of the involved vertebrae.[50]

Symptoms

Shoulder pain is the presenting symptom in over 90 percent of patients with a Pancoast tumor.[43,46] Arm pain is common, often involving the medial aspect of the forearm and hand, including the fourth and fifth digits.[43,45,51] Paresthesias may be felt in the arm and hand due to compression of the subclavian artery and vein.[51] Patients will often report relief of pain when lying on the involved shoulder.[2] Associated symptoms include Horner syndrome (contraction of the pupil, partial ptosis of the eyelid, and sometimes a loss of sweating over the affected side of the face; Plate 12.4), supraclavicular fullness, hand intrinsic atrophy, and discoloration or edema of the arm.[32,43,45,46,51] Also, some patients will complain of a sore throat, fever, hoarseness, bloody sputum, unexplained weight loss, chronic cough, dyspnea, and/or wheezing.[35,45–47]

Diagnosis

Smoking is a risk factor.[35,46] Peak incidence occurs in smokers around 60 years of age.[35] Refer the patient for a chest radiograph (Plate 12.4). However, bone lesion of the spine may be detected before lung lesion on plain radiograph, because lung cancer metastasizes to bone early.[46,50]

CASE STUDY 2

HISTORY

A 66-year-old right-handed female presented to physical therapy (May 1994) with complaints of severe ($^7/_{10}$) right shoulder pain that radiated down her arm and along the ulnar border of her forearm and hand to include the third through fifth digits (Fig. 12.8). The patient presented with a diagnosis of "frozen shoulder." She denied neck pain, headaches, or chest pain. About 6 weeks prior to her evaluation she reported an episode in which it felt like her whole right arm went numb. This symptom did not return. She did, however, report periodic mild numbness along the ulnar border of her right hand. On further discussion she admitted that she forgot to tell her physician about the numbness. The patient stated that her shoulder pain started gradually sometime in January 1994. Her pain was aggravated by reaching into the back seat of her car from the driver's seat. Relief of pain occurred when she lay down on her right side.

The patient denied that there was any change in her symptoms following stair climbing, a greasy meal, or a bowel movement. Except for what she described on the patient questionnaire,

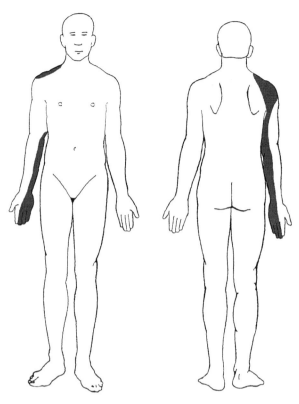

FIGURE 12.8 *Pain diagram from a 66-year-old right-handed female with a presenting diagnosis of "frozen shoulder."*

the patient denied any other complaints or symptoms throughout her body.

PAST MEDICAL HISTORY

1994: Surgery to R. TMJ (2 months ago) for a malignant melanoma.
1991: Fell on right shoulder, no fracture, resolved in 4 months.
1975: Lumbar disc surgery.

PHYSICIAN-ORDERED TESTS

Cervical spine and right shoulder radiographs were negative per physician.

GENERAL HEALTH

The patient questionnaire (Fig. 12.9) revealed a family history of cancer. Her grandmother had throat cancer, her father had prostate cancer,

PATIENT QUESTIONNAIRE

	YES	NO
NAME __Case Study #2__ DATE __5/31/95__		
AGE	66	
HEIGHT	5'4"	
WEIGHT (lbs)	85	
FEVER AND/OR CHILLS		X
UNEXPLAINED WEIGHT CHANGE	X	
NIGHT PAIN/DISTURBED SLEEP		X
EPISODE OF FAINTING		X
DRY MOUTH (DIFFICULTY SWALLOWING)		X
DRY EYES (RED, ITCHY, SANDY)		X
HISTORY OF ILLNESS PRIOR TO ONSET OF PAIN		X
HISTORY OF CANCER	X	
FAMILY HISTORY OF CANCER	X (3)	
RECENT SURGERY (DENTAL ALSO)	X	
DO YOU SELF INJECT MEDICINES/DRUGS		X
DIABETIC		X
PAIN OF GRADUAL ONSET (NO TRAUMA)	X	
CONSTANT PAIN	X	
PAIN WORSE AT NIGHT	X	
PAIN RELIEVED BY REST		X

PULMONARY

	YES	NO
HISTORY OF SMOKING	X	
SHORTNESS OF BREATH	X	
FATIGUE		X
WHEEZING OR PROLONGED COUGH	X	
HISTORY OF ASTHMA, EMPHYSEMA OR COPD		X
HISTORY OF PNEUMONIA OR TUBERCULOSIS		X

CARDIOVASCULAR

	YES	NO
HEART MURMUR/HEART VALVE PROBLEM		X
HISTORY OF HEART PROBLEMS		X
SWEATING WITH PAIN	X	
RAPID THROBBING OR FLUTTERING OF HEART	X	
HIGH BLOOD PRESSURE		X
DIZZINESS (SIT TO STAND)		X
SWELLING IN EXTREMITIES		X
HISTORY OF RHEUMATIC FEVER		X
ELEVATED CHOLESTEROL LEVEL		X
FAMILY HISTORY OF HEART DISEASE	X (1)	
PAIN/SYMPTOMS INCREASE WITH WALKING OR STAIR CLIMBING AND RELIEVED WITH REST		X

PREGNANT WOMEN ONLY

	YES	NO
CONSTANT BACKACHE		
INCREASED UTERINE CONTRACTIONS		
MENSTRUAL CRAMPS		
CONSTANT PELVIC PRESSURE		
INCREASED AMOUNT OF VAGINAL DISCHARGE		
INCREASED CONSISTENCY OF VAGINAL DISCHARGE		
COLOR CHANGE OF VAGINAL DISCHARGE		
INCREASED FREQUENCY OF URINATION		

FIGURE 12.9 *Patient questionnaire for Case Study 2.*

and her sister had pancreatic cancer. It also revealed that she is a 100 pack-year smoker (packs per day × number of years she smoked). The pulmonary part of the questionnaire was significant.

CERVICAL SCREEN

Active and passive extension and, separately, right rotation reproduced shoulder pain. Cervical axial compression testing was positive only in extension (see Fig. 4.14). Valsalva was negative. Spurling's quadrant compression test was positive on the right for reproduction of right arm pain (see Fig. 4.16).

SHOULDER AROM AND PROM

Active and passive ROM were equally limited. Abduction and ER were moderately limited with minimal limitations in IR and flexion. Minimal shoulder pain and no arm pain was reproduced.

RESISTED TESTING

The shoulder girdle muscles tested strong and painless in the three muscle lengths tested.

PALPATION

Swelling and tenderness were noted in the supraclavicular fossa. There was no edema or skin discoloration noted in the extremities. Palpation of the lymph nodes, arterial pulses, and the abdomen was negative.

NEUROLOGIC EXAMINATION

Sensation to light touch and pinprick was decreased in the right C8 and T1 dermatome. Deep tendon reflexes were (2+) and equal at the biceps, brachioradialis, and triceps tendons. The right abductor digiti minimi tendon reflex was (1+). Strength was decreased as follows: right triceps ($^4/_5$), wrist flexion and extension ($^4/_5$), and the intrinsics of the hand were ($^3/_5$).

SPECIAL TESTS

Glenohumeral joint compression and distraction were negative. Passive shoulder flexion with IR or ER was minimally painful at the shoulder in both cases. Passive right shoulder girdle depression with cervical left sidebending produced shoulder and arm pain; brachial plexus tension stretch also reproduced the symptoms. Thoracic outlet tests were negative.

JOINT MOBILITY

The acromioclavicular, sternoclavicular, and scapulothoracic joint mobility was WNL, grade 3. The glenohumeral joint was minimally restricted, grade 2, in distraction only. This was mostly due to muscle guarding.

ASSESSMENT

The patient's signs and symptoms appeared to be consisted with a right C8 radiculopathy. A brachial plexus lesion could not be ruled out.

Suspicions were raised with respect to the insidious onset of symptoms, age of the patient, constant pain, night pain, family history of cancer, patient history of cancer, pulmonary symptoms, and a 100 pack-year smoking history. The patient was referred back to her physician during the initial course of physical therapy, during which minimal progress was made. Following a chest radiograph the patient was diagnosed with a Pancoast tumor in her right lung.

ESOPHAGUS

The esophagus, which is segmentally innervated by thoracic nerves T4 to T6, is able to refer pain to the shoulder through contact with the central portion of the diaphragm (Fig. 12.4).[3,6,52] Esophageal pain is transmitted via afferents in the splanchnic and thoracic sympathetic nerves.[15] The primary afferent fibers, both A-delta and C fiber neurons, pass through the paravertebral sympathetic chain and the rami communicans to join the spinal nerve and enter the dorsal root ganglia before entering the dorsal horn of the spinal cord (Plate 12.2).[15] Referred pain is thought to occur through convergence of visceral (cardiac and esophageal) and somatic afferents onto the same dorsal horn neurons (Fig. 12.3).[15,53]

Symptoms

Pain in the shoulder that may be exacerbated during or following meals.[3] There may be substernal chest, neck, or back pain.[47] Other symptoms include difficulty swallowing, weight loss, and (in the late stages) drooling.[47] Symptoms associated with cancer are bloody cough, hoarseness, sore throat, nausea, vomiting, fever, hiccups, and bad breath.[47] Symptoms associated with reflux esophagitis are regurgitation, frequent vomiting, and a dry nocturnal cough.[47] The patient will complain of heartburn that is aggravated by strenuous exercise, or by bending over or lying down, and is relieved by sitting up or taking antacids.[47] See the associated symptoms under "Diaphragm" earlier in the chapter.

Diagnosis

Positive 24-hour intraesophageal pH and pressure recordings, acid perfusion, edrophonium stimulation, balloon distension, and ergonovine stimulation.[3,54,55] See the associated diagnostic clues under "Diaphragm."

HEART

The heart, which is innervated by thoracic nerves T1 to T5,[3] is capable of referring pain to the shoulder.[30–33,52,56] Cardiac afferent fibers have shown evidence of convergence with esophageal afferents and somatic afferents in the upper thoracic spinal cord.[23] In fact, esophageal chest pain is known to mimic angina pectoris.[54] In addition, convergence has been demonstrated between cardiac afferents, abdominal viscera (gallbladder, for example) afferents, and somatic afferents in the lower thoracic spinal cord.[23,53] Convergence has also been noted with proximal somatic afferents (shoulder), phrenic (diaphragm), and cardiopulmonary spinal afferents onto the cervical spinothalamic tract neurons (Fig. 12.10).[29] This explains how diaphragmatic disease and cardiac disease are both able to refer

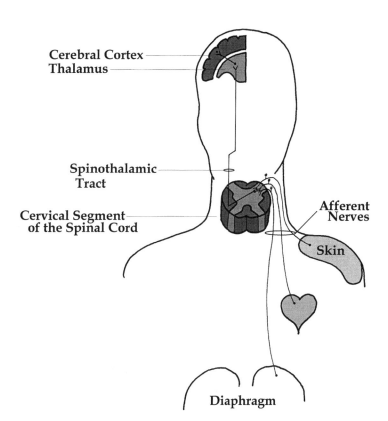

FIGURE 12.10 *Schematic drawing of a somatic afferent nerve (shoulder), a phrenic nerve (diaphragm), and a cardiopulmonary afferent nerve all converging onto the same spinothalamic tract neuron.*

pain to the shoulder and other cervically related dermatomes.

Symptoms

The patient may complain of pain in the left shoulder that is often associated with reports of numbness and tingling in the left hand.[8,31,47,57] Pain may also be felt in the chest, neck, arm (usually the left and a C8 and T1 distribution), jaw, posterior thorax, or epigastrium.[8,35,47,57] The patient may describe tightness, pressure sensations, throbbing, cramping, or aching in the above areas.[8,35] Other symptoms include exertion and nocturnal dyspnea, ankle edema, palpitations, easy fatigability, syncope, weakness, anxiety, profuse sweating, nausea, vomiting, tachycardia, or bradycardia.[8,35,47]

Diagnosis

A history of shoulder or chest pain (angina) on effort or exercise, such as a brisk walk, not associated with movements of the shoulder.[8] Relief of symptoms with rest.[8] There may be a resting pulse greater than 100 or less than 50 beats per minute.[35] Blood pressure consistently higher than 160/90 is a positive sign.[35] Nitroglycerin will provide immediate relief of symptoms. Refer for ECG, blood test (increased CPK), treadmill with echocardiogram, and/or angiography. Heart disease is most common in men over 40 and is associated with smoking, obesity, high blood pressure, diabetes, and physical inactivity.[35,57] Timely recognition of a cardiac problem cannot be overstated; coronary artery disease presents as angina, myocardial infarction, heart failure, and sudden death.[35]

CASE STUDY 3

HISTORY

A 48-year-old obese left-handed male presented to physical therapy (December 1994) with a diagnosis of "shoulder pain-bursitis," and complaining of moderate (%10) pain in his left shoulder

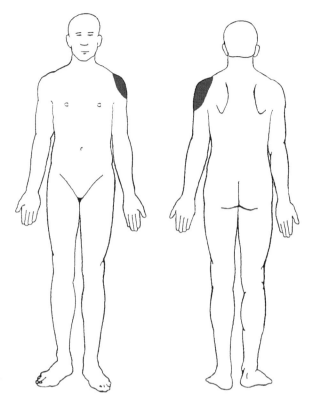

FIGURE 12.11 *Pain diagram from a 48-year-old left-handed male with a presenting diagnosis of "shoulder pain-bursitis."*

(Fig. 12.11). He reported the pain was not constant and did not radiate down his arm. He denied neck pain or upper extremity numbness. He did admit that his left hand "tingled" every once in a while. His shoulder pain started 2 months ago. The patient reported that his symptoms started 2 days after an afternoon of throwing and catching a football with his son. His shoulder pain was aggravated by activities of waxing his car, carrying groceries, or climbing stairs. He reported relief of symptoms with rest.

The patient denied a change in symptoms after eating a greasy meal, bowel movement, coughing, laughing, or deep inhalation. Other than what he reported on the patient questionnaire, he denied any other complaints or symptoms throughout his body.

PAST MEDICAL HISTORY

1993: Arthroscopic surgery to the right knee.
1993: Fell onto left shoulder, sprained, resolved in 3 months.
1985: Lumbar disc surgery.

PHYSICIAN-ORDERED TESTS

No radiographs or special lab tests ordered.

GENERAL HEALTH

The patient questionnaire (Fig. 12.12) was significant for the pulmonary and cardiovascular sections. At the time of evaluation he was a 35 pack-year smoker, had a history of heart problems (palpitations and tachycardia), and both his father and grandfather died prematurely of heart attacks.

CERVICAL SCREEN

Active and passive ROM was WNL and painless. Cervical axial compression and Spurling's quadrant compression tests (see Fig. 4.16) were negative.

SHOULDER AROM AND PROM

Active and passive ROM were WNL and painless.

RESISTED TESTING

Shoulder girdle muscles were strong ⅘ and painless.

PALPATION

No significant musculoskeletal tenderness was found throughout the shoulder girdle. Palpation of the lymph nodes and the abdomen was negative. Palpation of the arterial pulses in the left upper extremity revealed that they were of normal (grade 4) strength.

NEUROLOGIC EXAMINATION

Sensation, deep tendon reflexes, and strength testing of the upper extremities was WNL.

SPECIAL TESTS

Passive flexion with humeral IR or ER was negative; glenohumeral compression and distraction were negative; upper limb nerve tension tests were negative.

JOINT MOBILITY

No restrictions or hypermobilities were found in any of the joints in the shoulder girdle.

ASSESSMENT

The patient's symptoms were not reproduced during a thorough neuromusculoskeletal examination, and therefore his complaints were not consistent with an orthopedic dysfunction or injury. A return to the interview process revealed that the patient periodically felt a tightness or pressure on his chest at the same time he felt the shoulder pain. Both symptoms rapidly went away when he sat down and relaxed. The symptoms were reproduced when he climbed a hill behind his house.

Subsequently the patient was referred back to the physician for follow-up to rule out cardiopulmonary disease. He was subsequently diagnosed with myocardial ischemia with associated angina pectoralis. His symptoms disappeared with nitroglycerin.

PERICARDITIS

The heart, which is innervated by thoracic nerves T1 to T5, is capable of referring pain to the shoulder in cases of pericarditis.[3,35,57] Pericarditis is an inflammation of the sac surrounding the heart.[35,57]

Symptoms

There is usually a sharp burning pain in the chest or left shoulder.[35,47,57] Pain may be aggravated by deep breathing, coughing, or lying flat; and relieved by sitting up and leaning forward.[8,35,47,57] Other symptoms include fever, tachycardia, and dyspnea.[47] Symptoms of chronic pericarditis include pitting edema of the arms and legs, serous fluid in the peritoneal cavity, enlarged liver, distended veins in the neck, and a decrease in muscle mass.[47]

Diagnosis

There will often be a pericardial friction rub, which has different characteristics than a heart murmur, noted during auscultations of the

PATIENT QUESTIONNAIRE

	YES	NO
NAME **Case Study #3** DATE 12/11/94		
AGE	48	
HEIGHT	5'10"	
WEIGHT (lbs)	245	
FEVER AND/OR CHILLS		X
UNEXPLAINED WEIGHT CHANGE		X
NIGHT PAIN/DISTURBED SLEEP		X
EPISODE OF FAINTING		X
DRY MOUTH (DIFFICULTY SWALLOWING)		X
DRY EYES (RED, ITCHY, SANDY)		X
HISTORY OF ILLNESS PRIOR TO ONSET OF PAIN		X
HISTORY OF CANCER		X
FAMILY HISTORY OF CANCER		X
RECENT SURGERY (DENTAL ALSO)		X
DO YOU SELF INJECT MEDICINES/DRUGS		X
DIABETIC		X
PAIN OF GRADUAL ONSET (NO TRAUMA)	X	
CONSTANT PAIN		X
PAIN WORSE AT NIGHT		X
PAIN RELIEVED BY REST	X	

PULMONARY

	YES	NO
HISTORY OF SMOKING	X	
SHORTNESS OF BREATH	X	
FATIGUE	X	
WHEEZING OR PROLONGED COUGH		X
HISTORY OF ASTHMA, EMPHYSEMA OR COPD		X
HISTORY OF PNEUMONIA OR TUBERCULOSIS		X

CARDIOVASCULAR

	YES	NO
HEART MURMUR/HEART VALVE PROBLEM		X
HISTORY OF HEART PROBLEMS	X	
SWEATING WITH PAIN	X	
RAPID THROBBING OR FLUTTERING OF HEART ...		X
HIGH BLOOD PRESSURE	X	
DIZZINESS (SIT TO STAND)		X
SWELLING IN EXTREMITIES		X
HISTORY OF RHEUMATIC FEVER		X
ELEVATED CHOLESTEROL LEVEL	X	
FAMILY HISTORY OF HEART DISEASE	X	
PAIN/SYMPTOMS INCREASE WITH WALKING OR STAIR CLIMBING AND RELIEVED WITH REST	X	

PREGNANT WOMEN ONLY

	YES	NO
CONSTANT BACKACHE		
INCREASED UTERINE CONTRACTIONS		
MENSTRUAL CRAMPS		
CONSTANT PELVIC PRESSURE		
INCREASED AMOUNT OF VAGINAL DISCHARGE		
INCREASED CONSISTENCY OF VAGINAL DISCHARGE		
COLOR CHANGE OF VAGINAL DISCHARGE		
INCREASED FREQUENCY OF URINATION		

FIGURE 12.12 *Patient questionnaire for Case Study 3.*

thorax.[8,47] Patients with chronic pericarditis will demonstrate pulsus paradoxus, which is an exaggerated decline in blood pressure during inspiration.[47] There are a variety of etiologies including viral and bacterial infection, trauma, cancer, collagen vascular disease, uremia, postcardiac surgery, myocardial infarction, radiation therapy, and aortic dissection.[8,35,57]

BACTERIAL ENDOCARDITIS

Bacterial endocarditis is another source of pain in the region of the shoulder girdle.[57–59] It is an inflammation of the cardiac endothelium overlying a heart valve due to a bacterial infection.[8,57] If left undiagnosed and untreated, bacterial endocarditis can be fatal.[58,59] Risk groups for this illness include patients with abnormal cardiac valves, congenital heart disease, or degenerative heart disease (calcific aortic stenosis); parenteral drug abusers; and those with a history of bacteremia.[57–59] Treatment is with antibiotics.[57–59]

History will often reveal no trauma or previous occurrence of these symptoms. Plain radiograph may show destructive changes indicative of an infection.[58,59] Symptoms are not due to referred pain; therefore the patient will have a positive musculoskeletal examination of the involved joint. Monarticular involvement is thought to be secondary to deposition of large particulate masses (emboli) that contain immune complexes.[57–59]

Symptoms

Pain is most common in the glenohumeral, sternoclavicular, or acromioclavicular joints, and is usually monarticular.[57–59] Low back pain, which may mimic a herniated disc, and sacroiliac joint pain are often reported.[57] In approximately 25 to 27 percent of patients, musculoskeletal complaints are the first symptoms of this disease.[57–59] There may be an abrupt onset of intermittent shaking chills with fever.[47,57] The patient may also complain of dyspnea and chest pain with cold and painful extremities.[57] Other symptoms include pale skin, weakness, fatigue, night sweats, tachycardia, and weight loss.[8,47,57]

Diagnosis

Palpation of the involved joint will reveal warmth, redness and tenderness.[57–59] An acute synovitis in a single joint, especially the metacarpalphalangeal, sternoclavicular, or acromioclavicular joints—which are not commonly involved in other diseases—should raise suspicions of bacterial endocarditis.[58,59] There is a heart murmur, positive blood test for anemia, elevated erythrocyte sedimentation rate (ESR), decrease in serum albumin levels, increase in serum globulin concentration, and microhematuria.[58,59] There is relief of symptoms with antibiotics. Fever will be present at some time during the illness.[57–59] Associated signs are dyspnea, peripheral edema, fingernail clubbing, enlarged spleen, anorexia, Roth's spots (small white spots in the retina, usually surrounded by areas of hemorrhage), petechiae (small purplish hemorrhagic spots on the skin), and Janeway lesions (small red-blue macular lesions) on the palm of the hands or the soles of the feet.[47] Diagnosis may be difficult in elderly patients who have a higher frequency of nonpathologic heart murmurs and are less likely to develop a fever in response to infection.[57–59]

CASE STUDY 4

HISTORY

A 64-year-old right-handed female presented to physical therapy (September 1993) with a diagnosis of "right shoulder pain." She reported the sudden onset, without trauma, of right shoulder and upper trapezius pain approximately 1 month prior to presentation (Fig. 12.13). She denied neck pain, headaches, arm pain, or numbness and tingling. The patient also stated that her low back had been stiff during the week prior to presentation.

The patient denied a change in her symptoms after eating a greasy meal, bowel movement, coughing, laughing, or deep inhalation. Other than what she reported on the patient questionnaire, she denied any other complaints or symptoms throughout her body.

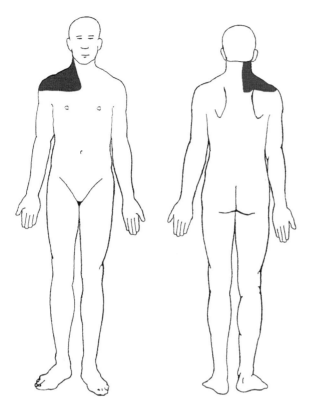

FIGURE 12.13 *Pain diagram from a 64-year-old right-handed female with a presenting diagnosis of "right shoulder pain."*

PAST MEDICAL HISTORY

1993: Root canal, 6 weeks ago.
1993: Surgery (March) to implant a prosthetic heart valve.
1975: Hysterectomy.

PHYSICIAN-ORDERED TESTS

No imaging studies were ordered.

GENERAL HEALTH

The patient questionnaire (Fig. 12.14) revealed recent surgery, fever, shortness of breath, and a prosthetic cardiac valve. On further questioning the patient admitted to an episode of chest pain 2 weeks ago, but she related this to muscle soreness from washing her windows.

CERVICAL SCREEN

Active and passive ROM into flexion or left side-bending produced a "stretching ache" in the right upper trapezius. Cervical spine axial compression was negative in the flexed, neutral, and extended postures (see Fig. 4.14). Spurling's quadrant compression test was also negative (see Fig. 4.16).

SHOULDER AROM AND PROM

Active and passive flexion, extension, abduction, horizontal adduction, and horizontal abduction reproduced pain. In addition, specific active and passive scapular motions of elevation, depression, protraction, and retraction were also reproductive of the patient's pain.

RESISTED TESTING

There was no muscle or group of muscles that reproduced pain in all three muscle lengths (shortened, mid, and lengthened).

PALPATION

The right sternoclavicular joint was slightly warm and red, with exquisite tenderness noted. A palpable band of tender tissue was noted in the right upper trapezius muscle. There was no tenderness or enlargement noted with palpation of the lymph nodes. Palpation of the abdomen did not reveal rigidity or viscus enlargement. Palpation of the arterial pulses in the right upper extremity revealed that they were of normal (grade 4) strength. There were no petechia or Janeway lesions on her skin. Ankle edema was noted bilaterally.

NEUROLOGIC EXAMINATION

Upper extremity sensation, DTR, and strength were all WNL.

SPECIAL TESTS

Glenohumeral compression and distraction were negative; passive flexion with IR or ER were equally painful; the empty can sign was also negative.

PATIENT QUESTIONNAIRE

	YES	NO
NAME **Case Study #4** DATE 9/16/93		
AGE	64	
HEIGHT	5'5"	
WEIGHT (lbs)	125	
FEVER AND/OR CHILLS	X	
UNEXPLAINED WEIGHT CHANGE		X
NIGHT PAIN/DISTURBED SLEEP		X
EPISODE OF FAINTING		X
DRY MOUTH (DIFFICULTY SWALLOWING)		X
DRY EYES (RED, ITCHY, SANDY)		X
HISTORY OF ILLNESS PRIOR TO ONSET OF PAIN	X	
HISTORY OF CANCER		X
FAMILY HISTORY OF CANCER	X	
RECENT SURGERY (DENTAL ALSO)	X	
DO YOU SELF INJECT MEDICINES/DRUGS		X
DIABETIC		X
PAIN OF GRADUAL ONSET (NO TRAUMA)..sudden onset.	X	
CONSTANT PAIN		X
PAIN WORSE AT NIGHT		X
PAIN RELIEVED BY REST	X	

PULMONARY

	YES	NO
HISTORY OF SMOKING		x
SHORTNESS OF BREATH	X	
FATIGUE		x
WHEEZING OR PROLONGED COUGH		X
HISTORY OF ASTHMA, EMPHYSEMA OR COPD		X
HISTORY OF PNEUMONIA OR TUBERCULOSIS		X

CARDIOVASCULAR

	YES	NO
HEART MURMUR/HEART VALVE PROBLEM	x	
HISTORY OF HEART PROBLEMS	X	
SWEATING WITH PAIN		x
RAPID THROBBING OR FLUTTERING OF HEART		X
HIGH BLOOD PRESSURE	X	
DIZZINESS (SIT TO STAND)		X
SWELLING IN EXTREMITIES	x	
HISTORY OF RHEUMATIC FEVER		X
ELEVATED CHOLESTEROL LEVEL	X	
FAMILY HISTORY OF HEART DISEASE	X	
PAIN/SYMPTOMS INCREASE WITH WALKING OR STAIR		
CLIMBING AND RELIEVED WITH REST		x

PREGNANT WOMEN ONLY

	YES	NO
CONSTANT BACKACHE		
INCREASED UTERINE CONTRACTIONS		
MENSTRUAL CRAMPS		
CONSTANT PELVIC PRESSURE		
INCREASED AMOUNT OF VAGINAL DISCHARGE		
INCREASED CONSISTENCY OF VAGINAL DISCHARGE ...		
COLOR CHANGE OF VAGINAL DISCHARGE		
INCREASED FREQUENCY OF URINATION		

FIGURE 12.14 *Patient questionnaire for Case Study 4.*

JOINT MOBILITY

The mobility of the glenohumeral, acromioclavicular, and scapulothoracic joints was graded WNL, grade 3. The right sternoclavicular joint was graded hypomobile, grade 2, in all directions. Pain was reproduced with both compression and distraction of the sternoclavicular joint.

ASSESSMENT

The patient's signs and symptoms were consistent with an irritable right sternoclavicular joint with capsular and articular cartilage or meniscus involvement. The patient's history of prosthetic valve surgery, recent surgery, shortness of breath, fever, chest pain, and sudden onset of pain without trauma were of concern. She was referred back to her primary care physician in order to rule out cardiac disease. The patient was subsequently diagnosed with bacterial endocarditis. After a week on antibiotics her shoulder pain disappeared.

VASCULAR

An aneurysm within a subclavian vessel, or an aortic orifice of a subclavian vessel, can result in pain at the shoulder.[30–32,47,52] This is a potentially dangerous arterial condition.[35] An aneurysm is an abnormal widening of the arterial wall caused by the destruction of the elastic fibers of the middle layer of that wall or due to a tear in the inner lining of the arterial wall that allows blood to flow directly into the wall and subsequently widen it.[35] Aortic aneurysms can enlarge and compress pain-sensitive structures in the upper mediastinum, leading to shoulder pain.[30] They generally occur in the elderly and slowly enlarge over a period of many years.[35] Rapid morbidity or mortality is expected if an aneurysm ruptures.[35]

Symptoms

Pain in the shoulder that may include throbbing and cramping. The patient may also report paresthesias, neck pain, and/or chest pain.[47] Other symptoms include night sweats, pallor,

nausea, weight loss, Raynaud's phenomenon, diplopia, dizziness, and syncope.[47] Symptoms may be aggravated by an increase in activity level (climbing stairs, fast walk, or upper extremity repetitive motions), and relieved by rest.[32]

Diagnosis

There will be a prolonged capillary refill time for the fingers, systemic hypotension, and a weak or absent distal pulse.[47] Bilateral dilation of the pupils will occur late.[47] A chest radiograph may or may not allow visualization of the aneurysm.

Arterial occlusion, usually due to atherosclerosis or compression of the subclavian artery, as in thoracic outlet syndrome, of the shoulder can present as a deep constant pain or lead to ischemic pain with exercise.[30,60]

Symptoms

Patients will complain of pain in the region of the shoulder girdle that may mimic a nerve root compression.[61] Other symptoms include paresthesias, coldness, weakness, and fatigue in the involved extremity.[47,61]

Diagnosis

Systolic blood pressure will be higher while diastolic blood pressure remains unchanged in the involved extremity.[47] Claudication will be noted with a distal pulse that is weak or absent.[47,61] The extremity will be cool, cyanotic, and demonstrate a prolonged capillary refill time.[47] Tachycardia and angina pectoris may also be present.[47] Contrast angiography will demonstrate arterial occlusion that is best seen with the extremity elevated.[61] In the case of thoracic outlet syndrome, one of the following tests will be positive: Adson's, costoclavicular, hyperabduction, pectoralis minor, or the 3-minute flap-arm test.[60–62]

Thrombophlebitis of the axillary and subclavian veins can also cause shoulder pain (Fig. 12.15).[30,52,63] Thrombophlebitis is an inflammation of a vein in the presence of a blood clot. This is a serious situation, because an emboli may

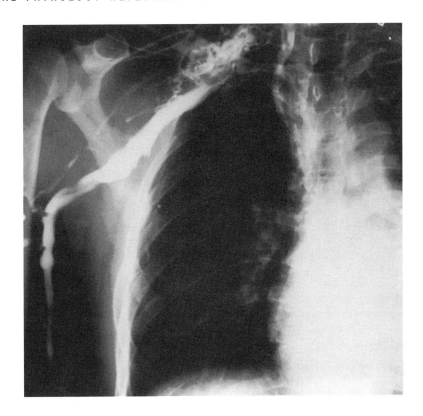

FIGURE 12.15 *Thrombosis of the subclavian vein at the level of the thoracic outlet. (From Rohrer,[63] with permission.)*

break free and travel to the lung, a potentially fatal condition. The risk of pulmonary embolization for persons with a subclavian thrombosis is approximately 12 percent.[63] Deep vein thrombosis of the upper extremity is often due to venous trauma from repetitive motions of the shoulder, which is referred to as effort thrombosis, in persons with an abnormal thoracic outlet.[63] Other causes of venous thrombosis include the presence of indwelling venous catheters (central lines or pacemaker leads), local compression, radiation, or hypercoagulability.[63]

Symptoms

There will be pain in the region of the shoulder girdle. Fever and chills may be present.[47] The patient may complain of cold and swollen fingers.[64] Patients with effort thrombosis complain of the sudden onset of swelling and cyanosis involving the entire arm.[63] These patients will often report a history of upper extremity exertion such as weightlifting.[63] Symptoms of shortness of breath, pleuritic chest pain, hemoptysis, or a new nonproductive cough are suggestive of a pulmonary embolus.[63]

Diagnosis

Edema, coldness, and cyanosis will be noted in the fingers, hand, and upper arm.[47,63,64] Distension of the superficial veins is usually seen in the hand, upper arm, shoulder, or anterior chest wall.[63,64] Effort thrombosis is usually seen in young, healthy individuals with an athletic physique.[63] It is also seen frequently in hikers who carry backpacks.[63] Exertion of the involved extremity will lead to a significant exacerbation of the pain and swelling.[63] Physician-ordered tests include duplex ultrasound scanning and venography.

The shoulder–hand syndrome, also known as reflex sympathetic dystrophy or minor causalgia, is another source of shoulder pain and dysfunction from a vascular disorder.[60] This syndrome is precipitated by trauma to the upper extremity (sprain, laceration, fracture, or rotator cuff tear), cervical disc disease, cervical spondylosis, hemiplegia, herpes zoster, and cardiovascular disease.[60] These disorders are responsible for a reflex stimulation of the sympathetic nerve supply to the extremity with a resultant increase in vasomotor tone.[60]

Symptoms

Patients will complain of shoulder pain and tenderness in conjunction with aching, paresthesias, swelling, coldness, and stiffness in the hand and fingers.[60] The symptoms are constant, even at rest.[60]

Diagnosis

Limited mobility (active and passive) of the shoulder, wrist, hand, and fingers will be noted in association with cyanosis, coldness, nonpitting edema, and hyperhidrosis in the hand and fingers.[60] Eventually the fingers will demonstrate stiffness, weakness, muscular atrophy, flexion deformity, and trophic changes of the nails.[60] After 6 months, plain radiographs will show spotty osteoporosis of the head of the humerus, carpus, and sometimes the phalanges.[60] After 9 months, the skin of the hand becomes smooth and glossy, and there is atrophy of the subcutaneous tissue and intrinsic muscles, flexion contractures of the fingers, and osteoporosis of the entire extremity.[60]

Additional diagnostic tests that may be indicated for a variety of vascular disorders include Allen's test, Doppler ultrasonic flow detector, systolic blood pressure, pulse volume recording, angiography, and auscultation of the major arteries.[7,62]

LIVER

The liver, which is segmentally innervated by thoracic nerves T7 to T9, is able to refer pain to the right shoulder through its contact with the central portion of the diaphragm (Plate 12.1 and Fig. 12.4).[3,6,32,52,65] Cancer of the liver is more common in men and women over the age of 50.[3] The liver is one of the most common sites of metastasis from primary cancers elsewhere in the body (colorectal, stomach, pancreas, esophagus, lung, and breast cancers).[65] Hepatitis, or inflammation of the liver, can range from the subclinical to the rapidly progressive and fatal stage.[6,65]

Symptoms

Right shoulder pain may be acute or spasmodic in nature.[3] The patient may also complain of headache, myalgias, and arthralgias.[6] Other symptoms include indigestion, nausea, vomiting, unexplained weight loss, and fatigue.[3,6,47,65] Pain from cancer of the liver may be described as deep, gnawing, and poorly localized to the upper abdomen or back.[3] See the associated symptoms under "Diaphragm" earlier in the chapter.

Diagnosis

There may be an upper abdominal mass, an enlarged liver, or tenderness in the right upper quadrant of the abdomen.[3,6,47,65] Associated signs are jaundice, pale skin, purpura, ecchymosis, spider angiomas, palmar erythema, anorexia, and the accumulation of serous fluid in the peritoneal cavity.[6,47,65] Refer the patient for radiograph, diagnostic ultrasound, CT scan, or MRI of the abdomen.[65] See the associated diagnostic clues under "Diaphragm."

PANCREAS

The pancreas, which is segmentally innervated by thoracic nerves T6 to T10, can refer pain to the left shoulder through contact with the central portion of the diaphragm (Plate 12.1 and Fig. 12.4).[3,6,30,52] Shoulder pain is usually at the left scapula or supraspinous area.[6] Cancer of the pancreas is more common in men and women over 50 years of age.[3] Pancreatic cancer has been linked to diabetes, alcohol use, a history of pancreatitis, and a high-fat diet.[42] Pancreatitis, or inflammation of the pancreas, may be caused by heavy alcohol use, gallstones, viral infection, or blunt trauma.[6,42] Acute pancreatitis can be fatal.[42]

Symptoms

Pain in the left shoulder, mid epigastrium, and/or back.[6,42] Patients with a pancreatic abscess, cancer, or pancreatitis may complain of fever, weight loss, jaundice, tachycardia, nausea, and/or vomiting.[42,47] In addition, patients with a pancreatic abscess may also report an abrupt rise in temperature, diarrhea, and hypotension.[47] Patients with pancreatic cancer may also complain of fatigue, weakness, and gastrointestinal bleeding.[47] A patient with pancreatitis will often bend forward or bring the knees to the chest in order to relieve the pain.[42,47] These patients will report an exacerbation of pain with walking or lying supine.[42] In addition, these latter patients will complain of a waxing and waning pain in the epigastric and left upper quadrant of the abdomen.[6] Pain will be exacerbated by eating, alcohol intake, or vomiting.[6] See the associated symptoms under "Diaphragm" earlier in the chapter.

Diagnosis

There may be an abdominal mass, enlarged liver or spleen, or tenderness in the epigastric area.[3,6,47] Diagnostic ultrasound, CT scan, or MRI may be necessary for an accurate diagnosis. See the associated diagnostic clues under "Diaphragm."

GALLBLADDER

The gallbladder (Plate 12.1), which is innervated by thoracic nerves T7 to T9, is capable of referring pain to the right shoulder.[3,6,30–32,47,52,65] Afferent fibers (T6 to T11) from the gallbladder pass into hepatic and coeliac plexuses and then enter the major splanchnic nerves, through which they pass to the sympathetic chain into the spinal cord.[27] Common diseases of the gallbladder include cholecystitis (inflammation) and cholelithiasis (stones).[3] Risk factors for the latter include age (increases with age), sex (more

common in women), pregnancy, oral contraceptive use, obesity, diabetes, a high-cholesterol diet, and liver disease.[65] Gallbladder cancer is more common in men and women over the age of 50.[3]

Symptoms

Cramping pain or a deep, gnawing, poorly localized pain in the back or right shoulder may be the first symptoms.[3,6,47,65] Pain is usually referred to the right scapula.[3,6,65] Other symptoms include chronic epigastric or right upper abdominal pain after meals, nausea, vomiting, and fever.[6,47,65] Patients suffering with cholelithiasis, the passage of a stone through the bile or cystic duct, will complain of sudden and severe paroxysmal pain in addition to chills and restlessness.[47]

Diagnosis

Gallbladder cancer is characterized by weight loss, anorexia, and/or jaundice.[47,65] Patients with cholecystitis will have a fever, jaundice, tenderness over the gallbladder, and abdominal rigidity.[47,65] Cholelithiasis will produce a low-grade fever in the patient.[6,47] Fatty or greasy foods will exacerbate the symptoms of gallbladder disease.[3,65] There will be tenderness, and occasionally a palpable mass, in the right upper abdominal quadrant.[6] Refer for radiograph, diagnostic ultrasound, and/or CT scan.[65] These disorders are more common in obese women over 40 years of age.[3,6]

CASE STUDY 5
HISTORY

A 51-year-old right-handed obese female presented to physical therapy (May 1995) with a diagnosis of "right shoulder strain." She complained of a periodic severe, deep, and generalized ache across the back of her right

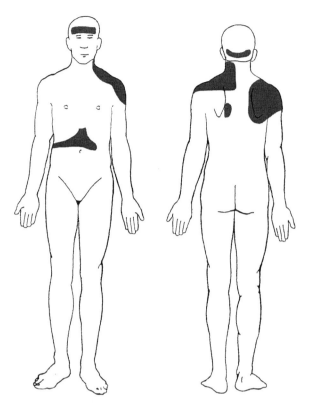

FIGURE 12.16 *Pain diagram from a 51-year-old right-handed female with a presenting diagnosis of "right shoulder strain."*

shoulder (Fig. 12.16). The patient reported the sudden onset of a severe ache in her right shoulder after a day of housecleaning 2 weeks ago. She admitted to a chronic history (5 years) of headaches, neck pain, and left shoulder pain with tingling in her left hand. The symptoms in her neck and left shoulder did not change after cleaning her house, and they remained mild in intensity. She stated that she had never had significant pain in the right shoulder prior to the 2 weeks before her evaluation. She did admit that there was an occasional ache in her right shoulder blade over the past 2 months before presentation to physical therapy. The pain in her left shoulder was not the same as the pain in the right. The left shoulder pain was sharp, shooting, and localized.

She reported her pain was worse at night.

The patient denied having more shoulder pain during prolonged walks or climbing stairs. According to the patient, coughing, laughing, or deep breathing did not increase her symptoms. Other than the information she provided on the questionnaire, the patient denied any other complaints or symptoms throughout her body.

PAST MEDICAL HISTORY

1994: Arthroscopic decompression of right shoulder (August).
1993: Diagnosis of hepatitis.
1990: MVA with diagnosis of cervical sprain/strain, whiplash.
1983: Diagnosis of diabetes.

PHYSICIAN-ORDERED TESTS

Cervical spine radiographs demonstrated mild to moderate spondylosis throughout the cervical spine; right shoulder radiographs were negative.

GENERAL HEALTH

The patient questionnaire (Fig. 12.17) was significant for gastrointestinal symptoms. Further questioning revealed that she had a low-level fever for the 3 weeks prior to the evaluation. She also admitted having upper abdominal pain after greasy meals. The patient also stated that her right shoulder pain was worse following a large meal.

CERVICAL SCREEN

Active and passive cervical extension, left side-bending, or left rotation reproduced neck and left shoulder pain. Cervical spine axial compression was negative in flexion and neutral; there was reproduction of left shoulder pain in extension. Spurling's quadrant compression was negative on the right; left sided testing was positive for left shoulder pain and tingling in the left hand (see Fig. 4.16). None of the cervical provocational tests reproduced right shoulder pain.

SHOULDER AROM AND PROM

Active and passive ROM testing of the right shoulder did not reproduce pain, although mild restrictions were noted with flexion, abduction, and external rotation.

PATIENT QUESTIONNAIRE

	YES	NO
NAME **Case Study #5** DATE 5/21/95		
AGE	51	
HEIGHT	5'3"	
WEIGHT (lbs)	175	
FEVER AND/OR CHILLS	X	
UNEXPLAINED WEIGHT CHANGE	X	
NIGHT PAIN/DISTURBED SLEEP	X	
EPISODE OF FAINTING		X
DRY MOUTH (DIFFICULTY SWALLOWING)		X
DRY EYES (RED, ITCHY, SANDY)		X
HISTORY OF ILLNESS PRIOR TO ONSET OF PAIN		X
HISTORY OF CANCER		X
FAMILY HISTORY OF CANCER	x (1)	
RECENT SURGERY (DENTAL ALSO)	X	
DO YOU SELF INJECT MEDICINES/DRUGS	X	
DIABETIC	X	
PAIN OF GRADUAL ONSET (NO TRAUMA)		X
CONSTANT PAIN		X
PAIN WORSE AT NIGHT	X	
PAIN RELIEVED BY REST		X

GASTROINTESTINAL

	YES	NO
DIFFICULTY IN SWALLOWING		X
NAUSEA	X	
HEARTBURN		X
VOMITING		X
FOOD INTOLERANCES	X	
CONSTIPATION		X
DIARRHEA	X	
CHANGE IN COLOR OF STOOLS		X
RECTAL BLEEDING		X
HISTORY OF LIVER OR GALLBLADDER PROBLEMS	X	
HISTORY OF STOMACH OR GI PROBLEMS	X	
INDIGESTION	X	
LOSS OF APETITE		X
PAIN WORSE WHEN LYING ON YOUR BACK		X
PAIN CHANGE DUE TO BOWEL/BLADDER ACTIVITY		X
PAIN CHANGE DURING OR AFTER MEALS	X	

FIGURE 12.17 *Patient questionnaire for Case Study 5, modified to show significant portions of both pages.*

RESISTED TESTING

Resistive testing of the muscles throughout the right shoulder girdle did not reproduce pain.

PALPATION

Mild tenderness, without reproduction of significant shoulder pain, was noted in the left upper trapezius, left middle trapezius and rhomboids, and the right infraspinatus muscle belly. Lymph nodes and arterial pulses in the neck and upper extremity were WNL. Palpation of the abdomen revealed rigidity and exquisite tenderness in the right upper abdominal quadrant.

NEUROLOGIC EXAMINATION

Increased sensitivity to light touch and pin-prick was noted in the left C6 dermatome. Hyperreflexia (3 +) was noted for the left brachioradialis

DTR. Isometric manual muscle testing of the upper extremities was WNL.

SPECIAL TESTS

Right glenohumeral compression and distraction tests were negative; passive flexion with IR or ER was negative; the empty can sign was also negative.

JOINT MOBILITY

The right acromioclavicular and scapulothoracic joints were graded 3, WNL, in mobility. The right sternoclavicular joint was hypomobile, grade 2, in distraction and inferior gliding. The right glenohumeral joint was hypomobile, grade 2, in all directions, probably due to muscle guarding.

ASSESSMENT

The patient's signs and symptoms were inconsistent with an active orthopedic injury of the right shoulder. Chronic joint dysfunction was noted in the right shoulder girdle. The left shoulder and hand symptoms were thought to be secondary to a mild and chronic left cervical radiculopathy. The cervical spine did not appear to be a source of right shoulder symptoms. Of concern was the patient's history of diabetes, hepatitis, fever, shoulder pain associated with greasy meals, and the exquisite tenderness in the right upper abdominal quadrant. The patient was referred back to her primary care physician to rule out any gastrointestinal problems. The patient was subsequently diagnosed with cholecystitis.

KIDNEY

The kidney (Plate 12-1), which is innervated by thoracic nerves T10 to L1,[3] may refer pain to the shoulder girdle region.[32,66] There are several pathologies to consider with respect to the kidney, including cancer, perinephric abscess, and other disease processes such as kidney stones. Associated disorders are pyelonephritis, nephritis, nephropathy, nephrotic syndrome, renal artery occlusion, renal failure, renal infarction, and renal tuberculosis.[47]

Symptoms

Some of the following complaints may be noted: acute or spasmodic ipsilateral shoulder, lower abdominal, groin, low back, or flank pain; weakness, fatigue, or generalized myalgia; unexplained weight loss; nausea, vomiting, or chills; or painful, frequent, or urgent urination or hematuria.[3,47,66,67]

Diagnosis

Tenderness will be noted at the costovertebral angle and, in the case of inflammation, there will be a fever.[47,66] Musculoskeletal pain is rarely the primary complaint. Cancer of the kidney is most common between the ages of 55 and 60.[50] It can metastasize to the lung, brain, or liver.[50] Metastasis to bone occurs late in the disease process.[50]

In patients with a perinephric abscess, there is no tenderness over the renal areas of the back, and only mild distension is noted during abdominal palpation.[67] There will be an elevated ESR, white cell count, and fever.[67] A plain anteroposterior KUB (view of the kidney, ureters, and bladder) radiograph will demonstrate the following: (1) difficulty identifying the psoas stripe, (2) absence of the renal outline, and (3) curvature of the spine towards the side of the disease.[67] Refer for an intravenous pyelogram and/or CT scan.

Kidney stones may produce a severe cramping pain.[3] Chronic kidney disease may be associated with poor calcium deposits in bone, which will lead to a weak bone structure.[3] For all of the diseases of the kidney that have been discussed, patients may benefit by referrals for diagnostic ultrasound, CT scan, or MRI.

STOMACH

The stomach, which is segmentally innervated by thoracic nerves T6 to T10, can refer pain to the shoulder through contact with the central portion of the diaphragm (Plate 12.1.2 and Fig. 12.4).[3,30] Cancer of the stomach is more common in men and women over 50 years of age.[3] Risk factors for an ulcer or gastritis include heavy alcohol use, smoking, and the use of nonsteroidal anti-inflammatory drugs (NSAIDs).[6,42]

Symptoms

Pain is most often described in the right shoulder.[42] The patient may also complain of epigastric or right upper abdominal quadrant pain.[6,42] Patients with cancer, an ulcer, or gastritis may complain of weight loss, night pain, or chronic dyspepsia—painful digestion, a sense of fullness after eating, heartburn, nausea, vomiting, and a loss of appetite.[6,42,47] Patients with stomach cancer may complain of a deep, gnawing and poorly localized pain in the upper abdomen or back.[3] Persons with an ulcer may also complain of gastrointestinal bleeding and epigastric pain 1 to 2 hours after a meal, which occurs with vomiting, fullness, or abdominal distention.[42,47] Patients with gastritis may also report belching, fever, malaise, anorexia, or bloody vomit.[47] See the associated symptoms under "Diaphragm" earlier in the chapter.

Diagnosis

There may be an abdominal mass or tenderness.[3,47] Abdominal CT scan or MRI may be necessary for an accurate diagnosis. See the associated diagnostic clues under "Diaphragm."

COLON AND LARGE INTESTINE

The colon and large intestine, which is innervated by thoracic and lumbar nerves T11 to L1,[3] is capable of referring pain to the right shoulder (Plate 12.1).[68] The gastrointestinal tract (GI) has dual innervation (Plate 12.2). There are afferent fibers that join sympathetic nerves and afferent fibers that join parasympathetic nerves.[69] Pain from the GI is predominately mediated by afferent activity in sympathetic nerves such as the splanchnic and hypogastric nerves.[69] These afferent nerve fibers have their cell bodies in thoracolumbar spinal ganglia and their central projections enter the spinal cord at levels between T2 and L3.[69] Disorders relevant to this region include ulcerative colitis, irritable bowel syn-

drome, spastic colon, obstructive bowel disease, diverticulitis, and cancer. Colon cancer is the most frequently diagnosed cancer in the United States.[6] Cancer in this region is most common in men and women over the age of 50.[3,50] Metastasis to the spine, liver, and lung are common.[6,50] Smoking, alcohol, NSAIDs, and caffeine may increase the risk of disease.[3] The NSAIDs may also mask the symptoms.[3] Other risk factors include a prior history of inflammatory bowel disease, prior cancer of another organ, and benign polyps of the colon.[6]

Symptoms

Pain is referred to the right shoulder from the hepatic flexure of the colon (Plate 12.1).[68] A cramping pain is often described in the lower midabdominal region.[6,42,47] There may also be a fluctuation of pain with eating habits, painful bowel movements, diarrhea, indigestion, nausea, vomiting, change in bowel habits, bloody stools, jaundice, and weight loss.[3,47] Irritable bowel syndrome is the most common gastrointestinal disorder in Western society.[42] Symptoms are aggravated or precipitated by emotional stress, fatigue, or alcohol, or by eating a large meal with fruit, roughage, or a high fat content.[42] In addition to the above symptoms there may be constipation, foul breath, and flatulence.[42] The predominant symptom with ulcerative colitis is rectal bleeding and diarrhea.[42] With obstructive bowel disease the patient will complain of constipation, rapid heart rate, and short episodes of intense cramping pain.[47] Diverticulitis, an inflammation in the wall of the colon, will produce constant left lower abdominal pain with radiation commonly to the low back, pelvis, or left leg.[6] In cases of cancer, there may be a change in the frequency of bowel movement, a sense of incomplete evacuation, bloody stools, unexplained weight loss, weakness, fatigue, exertional dyspnea, and vertigo.[6,47,50]

Diagnosis

Patients may exhibit abdominal distension, abdominal tenderness, rectal bleeding, anorexia, and abnormal bowel sounds.[47] Diagnosis is confirmed by a positive colonoscopy.

POSTVIRAL FATIGUE SYNDROME

Postviral fatigue syndrome (PFS) is yet another source of pain in the region of the shoulder girdle.[30,70–77] Recent research has suggested a relationship between PFS and fibromyalgia.[72,78] The criteria for a diagnosis of fibromyalgia syndrome includes neck and shoulder pain as well as a specific tender point in the supraspinatus muscle.[78–81]

There appears to be an association between PFS and the abnormal early onset of intracellular acidosis during exercise.[71,75,76] This is thought to represent excessive lactic acid production secondary to a problem with metabolic regulation.[71,75–78] It also appears to be a problem with muscle metabolism.[70,71,75,77] There is speculation that this disease is related to destruction of the mitochondria within the cell.[71,78] This subsequently leads to an inability to perform aerobic glycolysis, so that the patient is stuck in perpetual anaerobic glycolysis, which results in a build-up of lactic acid leading to early fatigue and complaints of muscle soreness.[71,76,78] Mitochondrial damage and fibromyalgia have been associated with the irritable bowel or "leaky gut" syndrome.[78,81,82] A healthy intestinal wall is coated with hundreds of different species of microorganisms. This protective coating of microorganisms acts in concert with the physical barrier provided by the cells lining the intestinal tract to provide the body with important filter-like protection. Damaging substances like unhealthy bacteria, toxins, chemicals, and wastes are filtered out and eliminated. Persons with "leaky gut" syndrome, however, are not able to filter out all of the damaging substances. Subsequently, unhealthy bacteria, toxins, chemicals, and wastes leak through the intestinal wall and into the bloodstream. One very well known risk factor for the development of intestinal mucosal damage is the use of nonsteroidal anti-inflammatory drugs (NSAIDs).[83–89]

Persons with PFS are more susceptible to viruses and have a harder time fighting viruses due to their inability to metabolize essential fatty acids.[74] The essential fatty acids are proposed to have a strong antiviral effect.[74] In addition, omega-3 fatty acids have successfully been used to treat ulcerative colitis.[90] Postviral fatigue syndrome is also known as myalgic encephalomyelitis; Epstein-Barr virus syndrome; chronic fatigue syndrome; and Iceland, Akureyri, or royal free disease.

Symptoms

Insidious onset of severe muscle fatigue and myalgia, exacerbated by exercise.[47,70] Most common in cervical, thoracic, and shoulder regions.[70] There may be associated headaches, dizziness, cognitive dysfunction, sore throat, and/or disturbed sleep.[47,70]

Diagnosis

Postviral fatigue syndrome is most common in young and middle-aged adults, especially women. It always follows a viral infection (coxsackie, Epstein-Barr, rubella, or varicella) and primarily affects skeletal muscle. There is usually mild lymphadenopathy and fever.[47] Plain radiographs and laboratory studies, such as ESR, are not helpful. Range of motion in the spine or extremities is usually within normal limits. Muscle biopsies are not diagnostic, but abnormalities in fatty acid metabolism have been noted.[70,74] Single-fiber EMG studies have demonstrated prolonged jitter values.[70] There may be associated psychological problems, such as depression, in patients with chronic complaints.[71–73]

Note: The case studies used in this chapter have been modified for instructional purposes.

Summary

The best way to determine if a patient has visceral pathology is to first eliminate all possible neuromusculoskeletal tissues as a source of the symptoms. This requires skill, confidence, and experience in performing your own orthopedic evaluation. If you cannot reproduce a patient's symptoms or have difficulty identifying a tissue in lesion, or if a patient does not respond to treatment, then ruling out visceral pathology becomes imperative. An orthopedic patient who demonstrates signs and symptoms of visceral pathology can be saved from severe morbidity or death by early referral to the appropriate physician.

Acknowledgements

I wish to thank Ola Grimsby and Jim Rivard for their contributions and hard work on the illustrations for this chapter.

References

1. Boissonnault WG, Koopmeiners MB: Medical history profile: orthopaedic physical therapy outpatients. J Orthop Sports Phys Ther 20:2, 1994
2. Goodman CC, Snyder TEK: Systemic origins of musculoskeletal pain: associated signs and symptoms. p. 522. In: Differential Diagnosis in Physical Therapy. 2nd Ed. WB Saunders, Philadelphia, 1995
3. Boissonnault WG, Bass C: Pathological origins of trunk and neck pain, 1. Pelvic and abdominal visceral disorders. J Orthop Sports Phys Ther 12:192, 1990
4. Goodman CC, Snyder TEK: Introduction to differential screening in physical therapy. p. 1. In: Differential Diagnosis in Physical Therapy. 2nd Ed. WB Saunders, Philadelphia, 1995
5. Boissonnault WG, Janos SC: Screening for medical disease: physical therapy assessment and treatment principles. p. 1. In Boissonnault WG (ed): Examination in Physical Therapy Practice: Screening for Medical Disease. 2nd Ed. Churchill Livingstone, New York, 1995
6. Koopmeiners MB: Screening for gastrointestinal system disease. p. 101. In Boissonnault WG (ed): Examination in Physical Therapy Practice: Screening for Medical Disease. 2nd Ed. Churchill Livingstone, New York, 1995
7. Abramson DI, Miller DS: Clinical and laboratory tests of arterial circulation. p. 51. In: Vascular Problems in Musculoskeletal Disorders of the Limbs. Springer-Verlag, New York, 1981
8. Michel TH, Downing J: Screening for cardiovascular system disease. p. 31. In Boissonnault WG (ed): Examination in Physical Therapy Practice: Screening for Medical Disease. 2nd Ed. Churchill Livingstone, New York, 1995
9. Natkin E, Harrington G, Mandel M: Anginal pain referred to the teeth: report of a case. Oral Surg 40:678, 1975
10. Henry J, Montuschi E: Cardiac pain referred to site of previously experienced somatic pain. Br Med J 9:1605, 1978
11. Payne R: Cancer pain: anatomy, physiology, and pharmacology. Cancer 63:2266, 1989
12. Procacci P, Maresca M: Clinical aspects of visceral pain. Funct Neurol 4:19, 1989
13. Cervero F: Mechanisms of acute visceral pain. Br Med Bull 47:549, 1991
14. Gebhart G, Ness T: Central mechanisms of visceral pain. Can J Physiol Pharmacol 69:627, 1991
15. Lynn R: Mechanisms of esophageal pain. Am J Med 92:11S, 1992
16. Cousins M: Introduction to acute and chronic pain: implications for neural blockade. In Cousins M, Bridenbaugh P (eds): Neural Blockade in Clinical Anesthesia and Management of Pain. JB Lippincott, Philadelphia, 1988
17. Raj P: Prognostic and therapeutic local anesthetic block. In Cousins M, Bridenbaugh P (eds): Neural Blockade in Clinical Anesthesia and Management of Pain. JB Lippincott, Philadelphia, 1988
18. Ruch T: Visceral sensation and referred pain. In Fulton J (ed): Textbook of Physiology. WB Saunders, Philadelphia, 1949
19. Korr IM: Sustained sympatheticotonia as a factor in disease. p. 229. In Korr IM (ed): The Neurobiologic Mechanisms in Manipulative Therapy. Plenum, New York, 1978
20. Lewit K: The contribution of clinical observation to neurobiological mechanisms in manipulative therapy. p. 3. In Korr IM (ed): The Neurobiologic Mechanisms in Manipulative Therapy. Plenum, New York, 1978
21. Patterson M: A model mechanism for spinal segmental facilitation. J Am Osteop Assoc 76:62, 1976
22. Grieve G: Clinical features. p. 159. In: Common Vertebral Joint Problems. Churchill Livingstone, New York, 1981
23. Lewis T, Kellgren J: Observations relating to referred pain, visceromotor reflexes and other associated phenomena. Clin Sci 4:47, 1939
24. Cyriax J: Referred pain. p. 22. In: Textbook of Orthopaedic Medicine. Vol. 1. Diagnosis of Soft Tissue Lesions. 8th Ed. Bailliere Tindall, London, 1982

25. Laurberg S, Sorensen K: Cervical dorsal root ganglion cells with collaterals to both shoulder skin and the diaphragm. A fluorescent double labelling study in the rat. A model for referred pain? Brain Res 331:160, 1985

26. Bahr R, Blumberg H, Janig W: Do dichotomizing afferent fibers exist which supply visceral organs as well as somatic structures? A contribution to the problem of referred pain. Neurosci Lett 24:25, 1981

27. Doran F: The sites to which pain is referred from the common bile-duct in man and its implication for the theory of referred pain. Br J Surg 54:599, 1967

28. Hobbs S, Chandler M, Bolser D et al: Segmental organization of visceral and somatic input onto C3-T6 spinothalamic tract cells of the monkey. J Neurophysiol 68:1575, 1992

29. Bolser D, Hobbs S, Chandler M et al: Convergence of phrenic and cardiopulmonary spinal afferent information on cervical and thoracic spinothalamic tract neurons in the monkey: implications for referred pain from the diaphragm and the heart. J Neurophysiol 65:1042, 1991

30. Campbell S: Referred shoulder pain: an elusive diagnosis. Postgrad Med 73:193, 1983

31. Calliet R: Visceral referred pain. p. 262. In: Shoulder Pain. 3rd Ed. FA Davis, Philadelphia, 1981

32. Leland J: Visceral aspects of shoulder pain. Bull Hosp Jt Dis 14:71, 1953

33. Capps J: An Experimental and Clinical Study of Pain in the Pleura, Pericardium, and Peritoneum. Macmillan, New York, 1932

34. Bateman J: Applied physiology of the shoulder and neck. p. 67. In: The Shoulder and Neck. WB Saunders, Philadelphia, 1978

35. Boissonnault W, Bass C: Pathological origins of trunk and neck pain, 2. Disorders of the cardiovascular and pulmonary system. J Orthop Sports Phys Ther 12:208, 1990

36. Angel J, Sims C, O'Brien W et al: Postcoital pneumoperitoneum. Obstet Gynecol 71:1039, 1988

37. Christiansen W, Danzl D, McGee H: Pneumoperitoneum following vaginal insufflation and coitus. Ann Emerg Med 9:480, 1980

38. Rucker C, Miller R, Nov H: Pneumoperitoneum secondary to perforated appendicitis: a report of two cases and a review of the literature. Am J Surg 33:188, 1967

39. Lozman H, Newman A: Spontaneous pneumoperitoneum occurring during postpartum exercises in the knee chest position. Am J Obstet Gynecol 72:903, 1956

40. Aronson M, Nelson P: Fatal air embolism in pregnancy resulting from an unusual sex act. Obstet Gynecol 30:127, 1967

41. Quigley J, Gaspar I: Fatal air embolism on the eighth day of puerperium. Am J Obstet Gynecol 32:1054, 1936

42. Goodman CC, Snyder TEK: Overview of gastrointestinal signs and symptoms. p. 215. In: Differential Diagnosis in Physical Therapy. 2nd Ed. WB Saunders, Philadelphia, 1995

43. Vargo M, Flood K: Pancoast tumor presenting as cervical radiculopathy. Arch Phys Med Rehabil 71:606, 1990

44. Welch WC, Erhard R, Clyde B et al: Systemic malignancy presenting as neck and shoulder pain. Arch Phys Med Rehabil 75:918, 1994

45. Kovach SG, Huslig EL: Shoulder pain and Pancoast tumor: a diagnostic dilemma. J Manipulative Physiol Ther 7:25, 1984

46. Goodman CC, Snyder TEK: Overview of pulmonary signs and symptoms. p. 147. In: Differential Diagnosis in Physical Therapy. 2nd Ed. WB Saunders, Philadelphia, 1995

47. Loeb S: Professional Guide to Signs and Symptoms. Springhouse Corp, Springhouse, Pennsylvania, 1993

48. Arnall D, Ryan M: Screening for pulmonary system disease. p. 69. In Boissonnault WG (ed): Examination in Physical Therapy Practice: Screening for Medical Disease. 2nd Ed. Churchill Livingstone, New York, 1995

49. Niethammer JG, Hubner KF, Buonocore E: Pulmonary embolism: how V/Q scanning helps in diagnosis. Postgrad Med 87:263, 1990

50. Boissonnault W, Bass C: Pathological origins of trunk and neck pain, 3. Diseases of the musculoskeletal system. J Orthop Sports Phys Ther 12:216, 1990

51. Netter FH: Diseases and pathology. p. 105. In: The Ciba Collection of Medical Illustrations: Respiratory System. 2nd Ed. Vol. 7. Ciba-Geigy Corporation, West Caldwell, NJ, 1980

52. Coventry MB: Problem of painful shoulder. JAMA 151:177, 1953

53. Ammons W: Cardiopulmonary sympathetic afferent input to lower thoracic spinal neurons. Brain Res 529:149, 1990

54. Nevens F, Janssens J, Piessens J et al: Prospective study on prevalence of esophageal chest pain in patients referred on an elective basis to a cardiac

unit for suspected myocardial ischemia. Dig Dis Sci 36:229, 1991

55. Lagerqvist B, Sylven C, Beermann B: Intracoronary adenosine causes angina pectoris like pain—an inquiry into the nature of visceral pain. Cardiovasc Res 24:609, 1990

56. Askey JM: The syndrome of painful disability of the shoulder and hand complicating coronary occlusion. Am Heart J 22:1, 1941

57. Goodman CC, Synder TEK: Overview of cardiovascular signs and symptoms. p. 77. In: Differential Diagnosis in Physical Therapy. 2nd Ed. WB Saunders, Philadelphia, 1995

58. Churchill M, Geraci J, Hunder G: Musculoskeletal manifestations of bacterial endocarditis. Ann Intern Med 87:754, 1977

59. Hunder G: When musculoskeletal symptoms point to endocarditis. J Musculoskel Med 9:33, 1992

60. Abramson DI, Miller DS: Clinical entities with both vascular and orthopedic components. p. 181. In: Vascular Problems in Musculoskeletal Disorders of the Limbs. Springer-Verlag, New York, 1981

61. Wilgis EFS: Compression syndromes of the shoulder girdle and arm. p. 69. In: Vascular Injuries and Diseases of the Upper Limb. Little, Brown, Boston, 1983

62. Wilgis EFS: Diagnosis. p. 15. In: Vascular Injuries and Diseases of the Upper Limb. Little, Brown, Boston, 1983

63. Rohrer MJ: Vascular problems. p. 77. In Pappas AM (ed): Upper Extremity Injuries in the Athlete. Churchill Livingstone, New York, 1995

64. Abramson DI, Miller DS: Vascular complications of musculoskeletal disorders produced by trauma. p. 263. In: Vascular Problems in Musculoskeletal Disorders of the Limbs. Springer-Verlag, New York, 1981

65. Goodman CC, Snyder TEK: Overview of hepatic and biliary signs and symptoms. p. 284. In: Differential Diagnosis in Physical Therapy. 2nd Ed. WB Saunders, Philadelphia, 1995

66. Goodman CC, Snyder TEK: Overview of renal and urologic signs and symptoms. p. 254. In: Differential Diagnosis in Physical Therapy. 2nd Ed. WB Saunders, Philadelphia, 1995

67. Davidson R, Lewis E, Daehler D et al: Perinephrenic abscess and chronic low back pain. J Fam Pract 15:1059, 1982

68. Swarbrick E, Hegarty J, Bat L et al: Site of pain from the irritable bowel. Lancet 1980:443, 1980

69. Cervero F: Neurophysiology of gastrointestinal pain. Baillieres Clin Gastroenterol 2:183, 1988

70. Behan P, Behan W: Postviral fatigue syndrome. Crit Rev Neurobiol 4:157, 1988

71. Behan P, Behan W, Bell E: The postviral fatigue syndrome—an analysis of the findings in 50 cases. J Infect 10:211, 1985

72. Whelton C, Salit I, Moldofsky H: Sleep, Epstein-Barr virus infection, musculoskeletal pain, and depressive symptoms in chronic fatigue syndrome. J Rheumatol 19:939, 1992

73. Holmes G, Kaplan J, Gantz N et al: Chronic fatigue syndrome: a working case definition. Ann Intern Med 108:387, 1988

74. Horrobin D: Post-viral fatigue syndrome, viral infections in atopic eczema, and essential fatty acids. Med Hypotheses 32:211, 1990

75. Dowsett E, Ramsay A, McCartney R et al: Myalgic encephalomyelitis—a persistent enteroviral infection? Postgrad Med J 66:526, 1990

76. Arnold D, Bore P, Radda G et al: Excessive intracellular acidosis of skeletal muscle on exercise in a patient with a post-viral exhaustion/fatigue syndrome. Lancet 1984:1367, 1984

77. Jamal G, Hansen S: Electrophysiological studies in the postviral fatigue syndrome. J Neurol Neurosurg Psychiatry 48:691, 1985

78. Bland JS, Thompson T: Fibromyalgia and myofascial pain syndromes. p. 1. In: Applying New Essentials in Nutritional Medicine. HealthComm, Gig Harbor, Washington, 1995

79. Fan PT, Blanton ME: Clinical features and diagnosis of fibromyalgia. J Musculoskel Med 9:24, 1992

80. St. Claire SM: Diagnosis and treatment of fibromyalgia syndrome. J Neuromusculoskel Syst 2:101, 1994

81. Wolfe F: Fibromyalgia. Semin Spine Surg 7:200, 1995

82. Veale D, Kavanagh G, Fielding JF et al: Primary fibromyalgia and the irritable bowel syndrome: different expressions of a common pathogenetic process. Br J Rheumatol 30:220, 1991

83. Rainsford KD: Leukotrienes in the pathogenesis of NSAID-induced gastric and intestinal mucosal damage. Agents Actions 39:C24, 1993

84. Gabriel SE, Jaakkimainen L, Bombardier C: Risk for serious gastrointestinal complications related to use of nonsteroidal anti-inflammatory drugs: a meta-analysis. Ann Intern Med 115:787, 1991

85. Rainsford KD, James C, Johnson DM et al: Effects of chronic NSAIDs on gastric mucosal injury re-

lated to mucosal prostanoids, and plasma drug concentrations in human volunteers. Agents Actions 39:C21, 1993

86. Hirschowitz BI, Lanas A: NSAID association with gastrointestinal bleeding and peptic ulcer. Agents Actions 35(suppl):93, 1991

87. Melarange R, Gentry C, O'Connell C et al: Anti-inflammatory efficacy and gastrointestinal irritancy: comparative 1 month repeat oral dose studies in the rat with nabumetone, ibuprofen and diclofenac. AAS 32:33, 1991

88. Bateman DN, Kennedy JG: Non-steroidal anti-inflammatory drugs and elderly patients: the medicine may be worse than the disease. Br Med J 310: 817, 1995

89. Nicholson AA, Bennett JR: Case report: radiological appearance of colonic stricture associated with the use of nonsteroidal anti-inflammatory drugs. Clin Radiol 50:268, 1995

90. Simopoulos AP: Omega-3 fatty acids in health and disease and in growth and development. Am J Clin Nutr 54:438, 1991

13

Manual Therapy Techniques

ROBERT A. DONATELLI

TIMOTHY J. McMAHON

The primary goal of the clinician is to optimize function, decrease pain, restore proper mechanics, facilitate healing, and assist regeneration of tissues. Manual therapy has been demonstrated clinically to be an important part of rehabilitation and assessment of restricted joint movement. Clinical application of manual techniques is based on an understanding of joint mechanics, tissue histology, and muscle function. Significant advancement has been made in describing the benefits of passive movement by such researchers as Akeson, Woo, Mathews, Amiel, and Peacock.[1-3] With this knowledge in hand the clinician can apply manual therapy techniques during critical stages of wound healing to influence extensibility of scar tissue, reduce the development of restrictive adhesions, and provide foundations of neuromuscular mechanisms to restore homeostasis.[1] Through an understanding of the effects of immobilization and soft tissue healing constraints we can establish criteria for phases of manual therapy techniques.

This chapter will focus on manual therapy for the shoulder complex from a basic science and problem-solving approach. Manual therapy will be discussed in relation to soft tissue and joint mobilization and muscle reeducation. Management of the shoulder patient will be discussed from a perspective of protective versus nonprotective injuries.

Normal joint function includes a dynamic combination of arthrokinematics (intimate mechanics of joint surfaces), osteokinematics (the movement of bones), muscle function, fascial extensibility, and neurobiomechanics (addressed in Chap. 6). Dysfunction and pain of the shoulder can result from altered function of any or all of these systems. A detailed sequential evaluation that hypothesizes particular impairments dictates which particular manual therapy strategies are appropriate. Please refer to Chapter 3 for shoulder evaluation procedures. Clearing the cervical and thoracic spine and brachial plexus is reviewed in Chapter 4 and 5. Manual techniques discussed will focus on the shoulder complex.

DEFINITIONS

Several terms must be defined when mobilization is discussed. Articulation, oscillation, distractions, manipulation and mobilization all describe a specialized type of passive movement.

Articulatory techniques are derived from the osteopathic literature. They are defined as passive movement applied in a smooth rhythmic fashion to stretch contracted muscles, ligaments, and capsules gradually.[4] They include gentle techniques designed to stretch the joint in each of the planes of movement inherent to the joint.[4] The force used during articular techniques is usually a prolonged stretch into the restriction or tissue limitation.

Oscillatory techniques are best defined by Maitland, who describes oscillations as passive movements to the joint, which can be a small or large amplitude and applied anywhere in a range of movement, and which can be performed while the joint surfaces are held distracted or compressed[5]. There are four grades of oscillations. Grade 1 is a small-amplitude movement performed at the beginning of range. Grade 2 is a large-amplitude movement performed within the range, but not reaching the limit of the range. Grade 3 is a large-amplitude movement up to the limit of range. Grade 4 is a small-amplitude movement performed at the limit of range[5]. Grades 1 and 2 are used primarily for neurophysiologic effects and do not engage detectable resistance. Grades 3 and 4 are designed to initiate mechanical changes in the tissue and do engage tissue resistance.

Distraction is defined as "separation of surfaces of a joint by extension without injury or dislocation of the parts."[6] Distraction techniques are designed to separate the joint surface attempting to stress the capsule.

Manipulation is defined by *Dorland's Illustrated Medical Dictionary* as "skillful or dexterous treatment by the hand. In physical therapy, the forceful passive movement of a joint beyond its active limit of motion."[7] Maitland describes two manipulative procedures. Manipulation is a sudden movement or thrust, of small amplitude, performed at a speed that renders the patient powerless to prevent it.[5] Manipulation under anesthesia is a medical procedure used to restore normal joint movement by breaking adhesions.

Mobilization is defined as "the making of a fixed or ankylosed part movable. Restoration of motion to a joint."[6] To the clinician, mobilization is passive movement that is designed to improve soft tissue and joint mobility. It can include oscillations, articulations, distractions, and thrust techniques.

Mobilization, in this chapter, is defined as a specialized passive movement, attempting to restore the arthrokinematics and osteokinematics of joint movement. Mobilization includes articulations, oscillations, distractions, and thrust techniques. The techniques are built on active and passive joint mechanics and are directed at the periarticular structures that have become restricted secondary to trauma and immobilization. These same techniques can be effective tools in assessment of specific joint impairments.

Soft tissue mobilization (STM) for purposes of this chapter will be as defined by Johnson: "STM is the treatment of soft tissue with consideration of layers and depth by initially evaluating and treating superficially proceeding to bony prominence, muscle, tendon, and ligament."[8]

Effects of Passive Movement on Scar Tissue: Indications and Contraindications for Mobilization

Research indicates that mobilization is most effective in reversing the changes that occur in connective tissue following immobilization.[1] Additionally, mobilization after trauma must be carefully analyzed. When is it safe to apply stress to scar tissue? How much stress should be applied to the scar in order to promote remodeling? What direction should stress be applied? These important questions must be answered before we can determine the indications for mobilization of scar tissue. Indications for mobilization will be discussed in regards to protective and nonprotective categories of shoulder injuries. A case study format will be used for each category to illustrate changes in treatment and discuss the rationale of each phase.

CASE STUDY 1
PROTECTIVE INJURY

Protective injuries are from surgery and/or trauma with significant soft tissue damage or repair. Examples of protective injuries include anterior capsular shift, Bankart repair, rotator cuff repair, and shoulder dislocation. Rehabilitation for patients with protective injuries is divided into six phases: maximum protection, protected mobilization, moderate protection, late moderate protection, minimum protection, and return to function. This case study will illustrate the concepts of phased rehabilitation in a patient with a protective shoulder injury.

HISTORY

A 16-year-old female basketball player was referred for postoperative rehabilitation of a right anterior capsulolabral reconstruction. The procedure performed was a mini-open procedure that include a rotator cuff interval reduction and anterior capsular shift with labral cartilage repair. Prior to surgery the patient had recurrent anterior dislocations for the past 3 years. Functional limitations included weakness and instability, especially with basketball activities, and difficulty sleeping on the effected side. Additional past medical history includes previous arthroscopic surgery to repair torn cartilage to the same shoulder 2 years prior with little change in symptoms. The patient presented 2 weeks postoperatively with stiffness, weakness, and some mild pain.

SUMMARY OF INITIAL FINDINGS

See Table 13.1 for ROM measurements.

- Slightly elevated and protracted scapula R
- Decreased fascial mobility of suture, and along fascia of inferior clavicle.

- Palpable tenderness and trigger points on subscapularis, serratus anterior, levator scapula, pectoralis minor, and lower portions of longus colli muscles.

- Scapular gliding revealed pectoralis major and minor tightness, and excessive mobility of the scapula in an anterior direction.

- Hypermobility of wrist, knee bilaterally, and left shoulder joints.

ASSESSMENT

Adolescent female athlete with a protective shoulder injury and reconstructive surgery. Patient is currently in the protective mobilization phase. Patient appears to have anterior pectoral tightness and middle trapezious stretch weakness. Inherent ligament laxity throughout other joints.

PHASE 1: MAXIMUM PROTECTION PHASE (*1 to 10 Days Postwound*)

TREATMENT

Patient was immobilized in a sling postoperatively for the first 5 to 7 days. AAROM and PROM in the following protected ranges: Up to 90° of flexion, 45° of internal rotation, 90° of abduction, and neutral external rotation to be started 1 to

TABLE 13.1 *Protective injury case study 1: Summarization of ROM measurements*

	WEEKS POSTOPERATIVELY				
	2	4	6	8	16
PROM (degrees)					
Flexion	80	130	140	165	176
Abduction	58	90	102	160	170
External rotation, neutral position	−5	14	25	45	64
External rotation, 45° abd. position	−10	18	30	53	75
External rotation, 90° abd. position	NT	NT	38	56	80
Internal rotation, 45° abd. position	43	63	63	65	70
Extension	NT	NT	60	69	78
AROM (degrees)					
Flexion	NT	NT	125	160	170
Scaption	NT	NT	130	165	175

Abbreviation: NT, not tested.

2 weeks postoperatively. Ice and rest with arm supported for pain reduction.

RATIONALE

Immobilization during the first 3 to 5 days is critical to allow the inflammatory and proliferation stages to proceed. The inflammatory stage begins 1 hour postwound and continues for 72 hours, during which vasodilation, edema, and phagocytosis of debris in and around the wound are occurring.[9] The matrix and cellular proliferative stage begins 24 hours postwound and is characterized by endothelial capillary buds, with fibroblasts synthesizing extracellular matrix.[9,10] The scar is still quite cellular with presence of macrophages, mast cells, and fibroblasts. Little to no motion should occur during the first 3 to 5 days in order to protect the newly forming network of capillaries.[2] Excessive motion too early can result in a prolonged inflammatory stage and excessive scarring. Heat should also be avoided secondary to vascular stress on capillary budding. Ice can be used to control swelling and pain.

By the 7th to 10th day postwound gentle stress to the tissues is initiated. The fibroblastic stage of healing has already begun with presence of fibroblasts in the wound.[9,10] Gentle early motion, such as with grades 1 and 2 joint mobilization and PROM in protected positions, helps to facilitate aligning of newly forming collagen fibers, aid muscle relaxation, and prevent adhesion formation. In protected injuries with surgical involvement, it is helpful to have an operative report to inform the therapist of the specific tissues involved in the procedure. For this case study, the anterior capsule, a small portion of the subscapularis, and the labrum were primarily involved.

PHASE 2: PROTECTED MOBILIZATION *(10 Days to 3 Weeks) See Table 13.1 for current ROM measures.*

TREATMENT

Continued grades 1 and 2 joint mobilization progressing toward grades 3 and 4 by 3 weeks. Scapular gliding passive and active assistive. Strain counterstrain an indirect positional release technique[11] to spinal and rib dysfunctions. PROM and AAROM in protected positions described in the previous phase.

RATIONALE

The goal of this phase is to promote a functional scar and attempt to decrease other compensatory or contributing dysfunctions. Early mobilization is critical in effecting scar tissue length, glide, and tensile strength. As the inflammatory phase ends, the fibroplasia stage of healing has already begun. The production of scar tissue begins on the fourth day of wound healing and increases rapidly during the first 3 weeks.[2,12] Peacock has substantiated this peak production of scar by the increased quantities of hydrxyproline.[2] Hydryxyproline is a byproduct of collagen synthesis.[2,13] Collagen production begins and continues to increase for up to 6 weeks.[2,9,10]

The newly synthesized collagen fibrils are weak against tensile force. Intramolecular and intermolecular cross-linking of collagen develop[5], designed to resist tensile forces.[2,13] The first peak in tensile strength occurs around the 21st day postwound.[2]

Gentle mobilization techniques can be effective during early fibroplasia due to the immaturity of the collagen tissue. Arem and Madden demonstrated that after 14 weeks of scar maturation, elongation of scar was no longer possible.[14] In contrast, the 3-week-old scar was significantly lengthened when subject to the same tension.[14] Peacock hypothesizes that the mechanism by which the length of the scar is increased becomes critical for the restoration of the gliding mechanism.[2] Stretching, or an increase in length of the scar, is a result of straightening or reorientation of the collagen fibers, without a change in their dimensions.[2] For this to occur, the collagen fibers must glide on each other. The gliding mechanism is hampered in unstressed scar tissue by the development of abnormally placed cross-links and a random orientation of the newly synthesized collagen fibrils.[12] Early gentle passive motion starting around the 10th day and progressing to the 21st day facilitates the development of tissue tensile strength by helping align newly synthesized collagen. Additionally, improved tensile strength allows for early AROM in the next phase.

PHASE 3: MODERATE PROTECTION PHASE (*3 to 6 Weeks*)

REEVALUATION

See Table 13.2 for PROM measures. Continued muscle guarding of subscapularis. Serratus anterior, first rib, longus colli, and scalenes with little to no tenderness. Subjective reports of decreasing soreness and pain of GH joint at rest. Sutures have been removed and superficial closure complete. Patient continues with anterior chest muscle tightness and decreased scapular excursion.

TREATMENT

PROM stretching and physiologic oscillations to 30° of external rotation in neutral and 45° abducted positions, joint mobilization GH joint with grades 3 and 4 in a posteroanterior (PA) direction and gentle posterior capsule stretching. STM to superficial scar (suture), inferior clavicle, fascial restricitons between pectoralis major and minor and between rib cage and pectoralis minor. Muscle reeducation initiated with proprioceptive neuromuscular facilitation PNF scapular techniques with active, eccentric, and concentric patterns (primarily posterior elevation and depression). Gentle AAROM and AROM initiated but continuing to avoid combination of external rotation and abduction. At 5 weeks isometrics begun in the Plane of the Scapula (30° to 45° arterior to frontal plane) for internal and external rotation, extension, and abduction.

RATIONALE

The moderate protection phase allows for more AAROM progressing toward AROM by the 4th week. Collagen production continues to be high until the 6th week.[2,9,10] The goal of rehabilitation at this stage is to further facilitate extensibility of newly synthesized collagen, realign randomly oriented collagen, and enhance fiber glide between collagen fibers. Tensile strength has reached its first peak, allowing gentle AROM as early as 3 weeks[2] in protected positions (rotation before elevation especially in contractile component injuries). STM to sutures and surrounding fascial planes facilitates suture scar extensibility and proper muscle function, and decreases pain.

An additional goal of rehabilitation for this phase is to prevent muscle atrophy, inhibition, and effects of immobilization. PNF scapular patterns with a progression towards resisted patterns during this phase foster activation and restoration of scapular muscle activity, providing dynamic proximal stability. Progressive isometric exercises in protected positions can be used around 5 weeks by the patient at home or work to stimulate inhibited muscle and provide dynamic tension to healing soft tissue.

PHASE 4: LATE MODERATE PROTECTION (*6 to 12 Weeks*)

REASSESSMENT

Decreased tenderness and improved fascial glide of suture scar and surrounding superficial fascia. Scapular mobility within normal limits. Refer to Table 13.1 for ROM measures.

TREATMENT

Six to eight weeks PROM stretching with emphasis on external ROM in the plane of the scapular and 45° abducted position. Continuing PNF scapular patterns working on any areas of weakness. AROM PNF patterns for upper extremity initiated with some resistance in weak aspects of the pattern. Active scapular stabilization and movement patterns incorporating closed kinetic chain exercises.

At 8 to 12 weeks, AROM exercises begun in unrestricted ROM (no loading of joint in external and abduction). (Progressive resistive exercises) (PREs) in protected ROM with emphasis on rotator cuff strengthening progressing to overhead exercises. Submax isokinetic internal/external rotation in the plane of the scapula (limited external rotation to 45°).

TABLE 13.2 *Summarization of phases of rehabilitation for protective shoulder injuries*

PHASES	MAXIMUM PROTECTION	PROTECTED MOBILIZATION	MODERATE PROTECTION	LATE MODERATE PROTECTION	MINIMUM PROTECTION	RETURN TO FUNCTION
Time	1–10 days	10 days to 3 weeks	3–6 weeks	6–12 weeks	12–16 weeks	+16 weeks
Stage of healing	Inflammatory, proliferative early fibroplasia	Early fibroplasia	Fibroplasia, maturation	Maturation	Maturation	Maturation
Goals	Protect newly formed scar	Facilitate functional scar, aligning new collagen fibers; clear spinal and rib dysfunction	Enhance tensile strength of scar	Stress scar; restore force couples; proximal, distal	Same as previous phase; increase strength rotator cuff, parascapular muscles	Return to function progressively
Manual therapy techniques	7–10 days postwound, grades 1 and 2 joint mobs	Joint mobs— grades 1 and 2 progress to 3, 4; STM surrounding tissue; PNF scapular patterns; protected PROM	As previous, STM to suture, scapular release tech.; PNF scapular patterns	Scapular release tech.; PNF UE patterns; low-load prolonged stretch	PNF UE patterns with significant resistance; low-load prolonged stretch if needed	As needed for any deficits
Other therapeutic interventions	Position education; anti-inflammatory modalities; ice	Home program of PROM in protected ranges	Codman exercises, T-bar, Swiss ball, foam roller; AAROM and AROM exercises	Isokinetics in protected ROM— submax; active scapular stabilization exercises; PREs	Same as previous, increasing effort and ROM; plyoball throwing	Progressive return to sport drills, light recreational activities

RATIONALE

At 6 weeks collagen production tapers off. The maturation or remodeling phase of healing begins around 3 weeks and continues for up to 12 to 18 months.[9] Maximizing scar extensibility is essential, because by 14 weeks scar deformability may be greatly decreased.[13] Strengthening is emphasized more during this phase.

Some strengthening has already begun using PNF scapular patterning to reestablish balance of function of the parascapular muscles in the previous phase. During the first 2 to 3 weeks of this phase, active and reactive scapular stabilization activities are initiated. These exercises help to restore force couples around the scapula and usually involve some co-contraction or synergy patterns of the rotator cuff. During the last 3 to 4 weeks of this phase, emphasis shifts toward strengthening the rotator cuff throughout the full range of movement. Through the progressions described, proximal stability and force couples are established before distal force couples. Low-level weights or theraband resistance for this case study for internal and external rotation effected healing subscapularis tendon and enhanced dynamic GH joint stability.

PHASE 5: MINIMAL PROTECTION *(12 to 16 Weeks)*

REEVALUATION

See Table 13.1 for ROM measurements. Patient demonstrating some elevation of scapula with late elevation phase; excessive scapula elevation increased with resistance. Activities of daily living within normal limits. No pain with most activities and exercises.

TREATMENT

Continued progression of weights and reps of previous phase of exercises. Chest pass throwing against plyotrampoline with 2.5-1b, ball. STM performed to apparent remaining fascial restrictions along the inferior clavicle followed by manual and PRE strengthening of lower trapezious and serratus anterior. PNF resistive patterns performed close to end-range abduction and external rotation.

RATIONALE

Multiple repetitions in unrestricted ROM continue to provide stress to the maturing scar. Manual techniques during this phase are used to further fine-tune function and clear any remaining restrictions. Neuromuscular control at end-range abduction and external rotation is essential to help protect capsular reconstruction and return to sport.

PHASE 6: RETURN TO FUNCTION *(16 Weeks +)*

REEVALUATION

Isokinetic testing reveals external/internal rotators ratio at 81 percent and 20 percent stronger than uninvolved side.

TREATMENT

Patient began progressive basketball shooting and drill activities at 18 weeks. Patient was instructed not to begin team play until 22 weeks postoperatively. Patient was discharged at 18 weeks with an extensive program of rotator cuff strengthening and scapular stabilization exercises.

RATIONALE

The return to function phase begins usually around 16 weeks if elements of movement are free of abnormal patterns and pain. This phase happens sooner based on patient response, specific trauma, and level of function required. Exercises are more functionally based and maximal efforts are used. Isokinetic testing of rotator cuff muscles inform the therapist of any deficits in particular internal External ratio's, that may indicate increased hazard for return to function. Currently reimbursement issues and managed care policies may not allow physical therapists to follow a patient completely through all phases of rehabilitation.

In summary, protected shoulder injuries can be safely progressed through a phased program of rehabilitation based on stages of soft tissue healing. Table 13.2 summarizes the various stages. Manual therapy techniques used at specific stages of healing can enhance the strength and extensibility of scar, reestablish force couples, and restore functional movement patterns.

CASE STUDY 2
NONPROTECTIVE INJURY

Nonprotective shoulder injuries are primarily shoulder dysfunctions that have no significant soft tissue healing constraints. Examples of nonprotective injuries include postacromioplasty, prolonged immobilization, adhesive capsulitis, and impingement syndromes. Often these patients present with pain, stiffness, and limited function. This case study will illustrate the concepts of rehabilitation for a patient with a non-protective injury.

HISTORY

A 46-year-old female homemaker presents with left shoulder pain and stiffness. Patient was referred 5 days postarthroscopic surgery and closed manipulation. Patient began having pain and stiffness several months prior possibly due to overworking in her yard. Left L shoulder became increasingly stiff and painful the 5 to 6 weeks prior to surgery. Diagnosis given was adhesive capsulitis. Past medical history: "stiff neck" 2 to 3 years ago.

SUMMARY OF INITIAL FINDINGS

See Table 13.3 for initial ROM measurements.

- Functionally, patient is unable to reach overhead, fasten bra. Moderate difficulty with dressing, placing hand behind back, and washing opposite axilla
- Upper quarter screening: Extension and sidebending L of cervical spine were limited by 50 percent and painful actively and passively with over pressure.
- L scapula protracted, downwardly rotated, and winging
- Tenderness and muscle spasm: Posterior cervical spine C1–2, anterior cervical spine along longus colli muscles at C5–6 L, Posterior aspects of ribs 2–4 L, L subscapularis, supraspinatus, infraspinatus, teres minor, and levator scapula
- Capsular testing revealed restricted motion in all directions

ASSESSMENT

Patient with nonprotective shoulder injury. Adhesive capsulitis with strong muscle guarding and possible adaptive shortening of subscapularis. Unable to fully assess capsular restrictions secondary to muscle guarding of rotator cuff and subscapularis muscles.

INITIAL PHASE

TREATMENT

Indirect techniques such as strain and counterstrain used on cervical, rib, and shoulder musculature. PROM stretching to tolerance in external and internal rotation, flexion and abduction with scapula stabilized. Joint mobilization of grades 1 and 2. Patient instructed in positioning comfort for L shoulder and cervical spine.

RATIONALE

The initial phase of rehabilitation for nonprotected injuries primarily focuses on anti-inflammatory modalities, grades 1 and 2 joint mobiliza-

TABLE 13.3 *Nonprotective injury case study 2: Summarization of ROM measurements*

TIME	INITIAL	2 WEEKS	4 WEEKS	6 WEEKS	10 WEEKS
PROM (degrees)					
Flexion	102	112	140	150	174
Abduction	70	80	120	150	170
External rotation, neutral position	−20	5	30	36	62
External rotation, 45° abd. position	10	20	45	56	70
External rotation, 90° abd. position	NT	NT	40	46	75
Internal rotation, 45° abd. position	52	54	52	53	71
Hyperextension	48	50	53	53	71
AROM (degrees)					
Scaption	70	90	112	132	155

Abbreviation: NT, not tested.

tion, and education. Patients often will perform habitual patterns of movement, maintaining current state of dysfunction. Correction, modification, or cessation of predisposing activities is essential. Goals of rehabilitation during this phase are to reduce inflammation and pain, restore proximal stability spine, scapula muscle activity, and avoid painful positions. Clearing spinal and rib dysfunctions that contribute or are source problems for shoulder signs and symptoms is essential during this phase for an optimal functional outcome.

INTERMEDIATE PHASE

R E E V A L U A T I O N

By the third treatment, patient reports decreased soreness of the L shoulder at rest. Still experiencing pain with reaching and overhead activities. See Table 13.3 for ROM measurements. Decreased pain and stiffness of cervical spine but ROM still restricted. Continued abnormal position of L scapula.

T R E A T M E N T

Continued **PROM** stretching, joint mobilization as previous. Patient started on low-load prolonged stretch with heat in the plane of the sca-pula using theraband and a 1-lb weight initially for 10 minutes progressing to 20 minutes over a series of 4 to 5 treatment sessions. High-speed (200°/s) isokinetics were initiated for internal and external rotation in the plane of the scapula in the available ROM. Scapular release techniques used to mobilize fascial restrictions within subscapularis, serratus anterior, and levator scapula. Joint mobilization, myofascial release techniques used to address facet joint irritation C5–6 and suboccipitally. PNF scapular patterns progressing from passive to resistive movements with emphasis on posterior depression, as illustrated in Figure 13.1.

R A T I O N A L E

The intermediate phase of rehabilitation begins when patient reactivity allows for more aggressive progression of techniques. Goals of this phase are to maximize ROM of all components of shoulder movement and normalize force couples of scapula and GH joint. Emphasis is placed on restoring rotation at the GH joint and then on elevation.

Traditional manual therapy techniques used to treat limited shoulder ROM have followed the arthokinematic movements of joint surfaces oc-

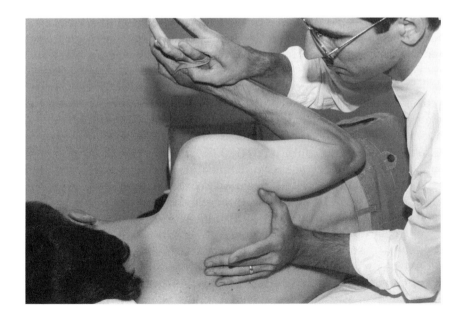

FIGURE 13.1

curring at the glenohumeral. Kaltenborn determined the appropriate method of applying a gliding mobilization technique by the convex concave rule.[15] For example, sliding of the convex humeral head an a concave glenoid surface occurs in the opposite direction of the humerus. Therefore, during elevation of the shoulder, the humeral is sliding inferiorly as the bone moves superiorly. However, data are now available that challenge the concave-convex rule of arthrokinematic motion.

Poppen and Walker[16] report a movement of the humeral head in a superior and inferior direction during elevation of the shoulder. Howell et al. demonstrated translatory motion of head of the humerus to be opposite of that predicted by the concave-convex rule. Only patients with instability demonstrated translation in the direction predicted by the concave-convex rule.[17] Soft tissue tension capsular, ligament rather than joint surface geometry may be a greater determinant of the arthrokinematics of the GH joint.

The type and frequency of force used to mobilize depends on the implicated tissue. In this case study, the implicated tissue of restriction is the anterior and inferior capsule, GH ligaments, and subscapularis. The authors advocate the use of low-load prolonged stretch in addition to oscillation techniques for more significant soft tissue restrictions. Connective tissue structures such as ligaments, tendons and capsules respond to mechanical stress in a time-dependent or viseoelastic manner.[18-21] Viscoelasticity is a mechanical property of materials that describes the tendency of a substance to deform at a constant rate. The rate of deformation is not dependent on speed of the external force applied. If the amount of deformation does not exceed the elastic range, the structure can return to the original resting length after the load is removed. If loading is continued into the plastic range, passing the yield point, failure of the tissue will occur. Failure is thought to be a function of breaking intermolecular cross-links rather than rupture of the collagen tissue.[22]

If permanent increase in ROM is a goal of treatment, then manual therapy should be aimed at producing plastic deformation. Taylor et al.[23] showed that there is a increased risk of tissue trauma and injury with rapid stretch rates. Rapidly applied forces will cause material to react in a stiff, brittle fashion, causing tissue tearing. Gradually applied loads result in tissue responding in a more yielding manner with plastic deformation. If the tissue is held under a constant external load and at a constant length, force relaxation occurs.[24]

In addition to increasing extensibility of GH capsular and ligamentous structures, muscle extensibility must also be addressed. Clinically the authors have found subscapularis to be commonly restricted in shoulder dysfunction. Subscapularis is the most stablizing factor during external rotation of the glenohumeral joint in 0° of abduction.[25] Additionally, most patients tend to guard or immobilize a painful shoulder by adducting and internally rotating the GH joint, thus shortening subscapularis.

In prolonged immobilization and dysfunctions such as adhesive capsulitis, subscapularis may accommodate to a shorten position. Muscles respond to immobilization by degeneration of myofilaments, change in sacromere alignment and configuration, decrease in mitochondria, and decreased ability to generate tension.[26] Muscles accommodate to immobilization in a shortened position by losing sarcomeres. Tabary et al. found that muscles immobilized in a shortened position for 4 weeks had a 40 percent decrease in total sacromeres and displayed an increased resistance to passive movement.[27] Muscles immobilized in a lengthened position had 20 percent more sacromeres and demonstrated no change in resistance to passive motion.

Functionally, limited subscapularis extensibility may effect functional elevation. Otis et al.[28] have recently documented the importance of restoring rotation to the glenohumeral joint in order to facilitate elevation. It was demonstrated that the contribution of infraspinatus moment arm to abduction is enhanced with internal rotation while that of subscapularis is enhanced with external rotation.[28] Low-load prolonged stretch and rotational exercises in the plane of the scapula in our case study are an attempt to reverse the effects of immobility, increasing the extensibility and strength of the subscapularis muscle. Restrictions of subscapularis tend to also affect parascapular muscles secondary to the altered scapulohumeral rhythm.

Scapular release techniques and STM (described later in the chapter) can be used to release fascial restrictions that have developed as a result of abnormal movement patterns. In this particular case, the patient had excessive protraction and downward rotation of the scapula with trigger points in the levator scapula, serratus anterior, and pectoralis minor. Warwick and Williams[29] report a possible fusion of the serratus anterior and levator by their fascial connection. Excessive tone of pectoralis minor effectly depresses the scapula and restricts the scapular rotation necessary for proper elevation. Furthermore, the serratus anterior and levator scapula work as a force couple to rotate the scapula. Increasing the extensibility of the fascia of these three muscles would allow proper functioning of parascapular force couples during elevation.

RETURN TO FUNCTION PHASE

REEVALUATION

See Table 13.3 for 10-week ROM measurements. All ADLs without pain and patient has started working in the yard without limitations. Patient

without cervical pain but ROM cervical spine 3/4 normal SB L and R.

TREATMENT

Patient instructed in exercise progressions for next 2 months with emphasis on rotator cuff and parascapular muscle exercises. Patient allowed to progress back to swimming and gardening activities to tolerance.

RATIONALE

Once ROM and strength are optimized, a home program is finalized to further facilitate physiologic changes such as increased sacromeres and remodeling of periarticular tissues. In the competitive and industrial athlete, form, technique, and training error correction is essential to prevent recurrence of dysfunction.

In summary, rehabilitation of nonprotective injuries depends on the implicated tissues or systems in dysfunction or restriction. Table 13.4 summarizes the phases of rehabilitation. GH joint arthrokinematics may be strongly influenced by periarticular tissue extensibility and muscle function rather than pure joint geometry. Manual techniques must comply with the type of tissue or system response desired. Continual

TABLE 13.4 *Summary of phased rehabilitation for nonprotective shoulder injuries*

PHASES	INITIAL	INTERMEDIATE	RETURN TO FUNCTION
Signs and symptoms (reactivity)	Pain at rest; difficulty sleeping; pain before resistance	No pain at rest; pain with resistance; moderate reactivity; limited rot, and elevation; weakness of rotator cuff and/or parascapular muscles	ROM maximized; functional movement pain free; muscle imbalances resolving
Goals	Decrease pain	Restore rotation ROM and strength of parascapular muscles and rotator cuff	Return to function
Manual therapy techniques	Grades 1 and 2 joint mobs	Grades 3 and 4 joint mobs; STM; scapular release techniques; PNF scapular and UE patterns; low-load prolonged stretch	Fine-tuning of functional patterns with PNF
Other therapeutic interventions	Anti-inflammatory modalities; positioning and activity education	Heat with stretch; isokinetic and isotonics working rotation before elevation in POS; isometrics; AAROM with T bars, Swiss balls, foam rollers; GH joint and scapular taping techniques	Home program, correct technique and training errors

reassessment of subjective, functional, and objective measures assists the therapist in evaluating treatment effectiveness.

Role of Mobilization

The primary role of joint mobilization is to restore joint mobility and facilitate proper biomechanics of involved structures. Joint mobilization has two proposed rationales—neurophysiologic and biomechanical.

The neurophysiologic effect is based on the stimulation of peripheral mechanoreceptors and the inhibition of nociceptors (pain fibers). Nociceptors are unmyelinated nerve fibers that have a higher threshold of stimulation than mechanoreceptors.[30,31] There is evidence that stimulation of peripheral mechanoreceptors blocks the transmission of pain to the CNS,[30] Wyke postulates that this phenomenon is due to a direct release of inhibitory transmitters within the basal spinal nucleus, inhibiting the onward flow of incoming nociceptive afferent activity. Joint mobilization is one method of enhancing the frequency of discharge from the mechanoreceptors, thereby diminishing the intensity of many types of pain.

The biomechanical effect of joint mobilization is focused on the direct tension of periarticular tissues to prevent complications resulting from immobilization and trauma. The lack of stress to connective tissue results in changes in normal joint mobility.

The periarticular tissue and muscles surrounding the joint demonstrate significant changes after periods of immobilization. Akeson et al. have substantiated a decrease in water and glycosaminoglycans (GAG, the fibrous tissue lubricant), an increase in fatty fibrous infiltrates (which may form adhesions as they mature into scar), an increase in abnormally placed collagen cross-links (which may contribute to the inhibition of collagen fiber gliding), and the loss of fiber orientation within ligaments (which significantly reduces their strength).[1,3] Passive movement or stress to the tissues can help to prevent theses changes by maintaining tissue homeostasis.[2] The exact mechanisms of prevention are uncertain.

CONTRAINDICATIONS

We can understand contraindications to joint mobilization by becoming aware of the common abuses of passive movement. The abuses of passive movement can be broken down into two categories: creation of excessive trauma to the tissues and causing undesired or abnormal mobility.[1]

Improper techniques, such as extreme force, poor direction of stress, and excessive velocity, may result in serious secondary injury. In addition, mobilization to joints that are moving normally or that are hypermobile can create or increase joint instabilities.

Ultimately, selection of a specific technique will determine contraindications. For example, the very gentle grade 1 oscillations, as described by Maitland, rarely have contraindications. These techniques are mainly used to block pain. They are of small amplitude and controlled velocity. In contrast, manipulative techniques have many contraindications. Haldeman describes the following conditions as major contraindications for thrust techniques: arthrides, dislocation, hypermobility, trauma of recent occurrence, bone weakness and destructive disease, circulatory disturbances, neurologic dysfunction, and infectious disease.[32]

PRINCIPLES OF JOINT MOBILIZATION TECHNIQUES

The mobilization techniques are designed to restore intimate joint mechanics. Several general principles should be remembered during application of the techniques.

Hand Position

The mobilization hand should be placed as close as possible to the joint surface, and the forces applied should be directed at the periarticular tissues. The stabilization hand counteracts the movement of the mobilizing hand by applying an equal but opposite force or by supporting or preventing movement at surrounding joints. Excessive tension in the therapist's hands during joint mobilization can result in the patient guarding against the mobilization.

Direction of Movement

The direction of movement of mobilization should take in account the mechanics of the joint mobilized, the arthrokinematic and osteokinematic impairments of the dysfunction, and the current reactivity of the tissues involved.

The direction of forces to the joint is also determined based on the response desired. Neuromuscular relaxation and pain modulation effects will be appreciated if the direction of force is opposite pain. Biomechanical effects will be appreciated if forces are directed towards resist but to patient tolerance. The resistance represents the direction of capsular or joint limitation. Movement into the restriction is an attempt to make mechanical changes within the capsule and the surrounding tissue. The mechanical changes may include breaking up of adhesions, realignment of collagen, or increasing fiber glide. Certain movements stress specific parts of the capsule. For example, arthrogram studies demonstrated that external rotation of the glenohumeral joint stresses the anterior recess of the capsule.[33]

Body Mechanics

Proper body mechanics are essential in application of mobilization techniques. The therapist is able to impart desire direction and force of movement if working from a position of stability. The therapist should stand close to the area being mobilized and use weight shifting through legs and trunk to assist movement in the vector of mobilization. The therapists hands and arms should be positioned to act as fulcrums and levers to fine-tune mobilization.

Duration and Amplitude

Several animal model studies have been performed to determine the most effective technique for obtaining permanent elongation of collagenous tissue, using different loads and loading time. The studies used rat tendons to demonstrate the elongation of tissue under varied loads. A high-load, short-duration treatment (105 g to 165 g for 5 minutes) and a low-load, long-duration treatment (5 g for 15 minutes) were compared.[34,35] The results indicated that low-load, long-duration stretch was more effective in obtaining a permanent elongation of the tissue. In humans, Bonutti et al.[36] determined that the optimal method to obtain plastic deformation and reestablish ROM is static progressive stretch (SPS). One to two 30-minute sessions per day of SPS for 1 to 3 months produced an overall average increase in motion of elbow contractures of 69 percent, with excellent compliance by the patients. As previously noted, the authors advocate the use of low-load prolonged stretch with heat to facilitate plastic deformation of shoulder capsular restrictions. Figure 13.2 depicts one method of low-load prolonged stretch for external rotation. The patient needs to be in a subacute stage of reactivity and the stretch is to patient tolerance. Heat used in conjunction with the stretch has been found to be more effective than stretch alone.[37,38] The patient's shoulder is placed in the plane of the scapula with a wedge or stack of towels. The stretch is performed by theraband resistance to assist with positioning and the use of a hand weight and gravity to stretch anterior periarticular structures. Duration of stretch can be from 20 to 30 minutes.

Little research has been performed on joint mobilization to determine the optimum duration of oscillation. Often the duration is determined by the change desired by the therapist. For example, GH joint mobilization of grades 1 or 2 performed to facilitate neuromuscular relaxation could be performed until muscle guarding was reduced and ROM increased.

Ghenohumeral Joint Techniques

FIGURE 13.3: INFERIOR GLIDE OF THE HUMERUS

Patient Position

Supine, with the involved extremity close to the edge of the table. A strap may be used to stabilize the scapula. The extremity is abducted to the desired range.

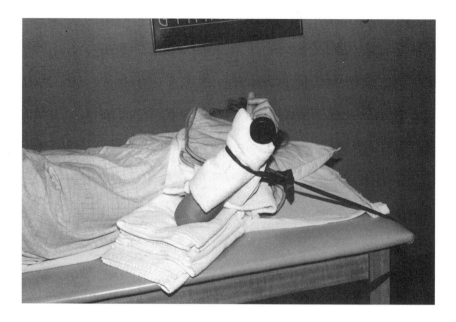

FIGURE 13.2

Therapist Position

Facing the lateral aspect of the upper arm. Cephalad hand web space is placed on superior ghenohumeral inferior to acromion. Assisting hand supports the weight of the arm by holding the distal upper arm superior to epicondyles and bracing patient's arm against therapist. Assisting hand/arm can also impart distractive force and change amount of rotation. The mobilizing hand glides the head of the humerus inferiorly, attempting to stress the axillary

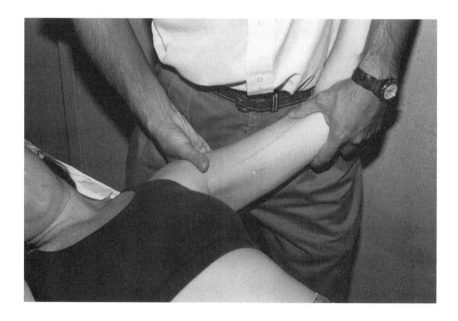

FIGURE 13.3

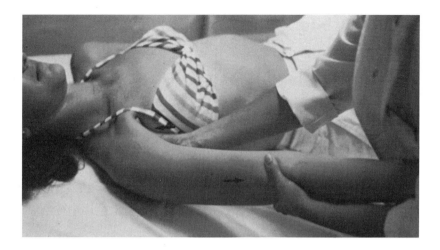

FIGURE 13.4

pouch or inferior portion of the glenohumeral capsule.

FIGURE 13.4: LONGITUDINAL DISTRACTION—INFERIOR GLIDE OF THE HUMERUS

Patient Position

Supine, with the involved extremity as close as possible to the edge of the table.

Therapist Position

Facing the joint, with inner hand up into the axilla pressing against scapulaghenoid. The outer mobilizing hand grips the epicondyles of the humerus and imparts a distractive force stressing the inferior capsule. To increase the efficiency of the pull, the therapist can weight shift and rotate the body slightly away from the patient. A prolonged stretch is often effective with this technique.

FIGURE 13.5: POSTERIOR GLIDE OF THE HUMERUS

Patient Position

Supine, with arm slightly abducted and flexed into plane of the scapula and resting on the therapist's thigh.

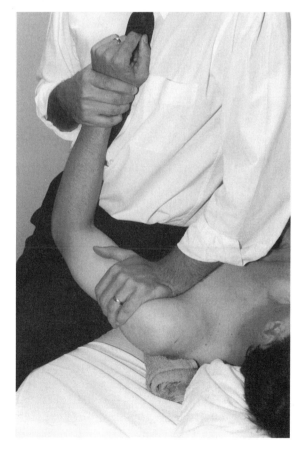

FIGURE 13.5

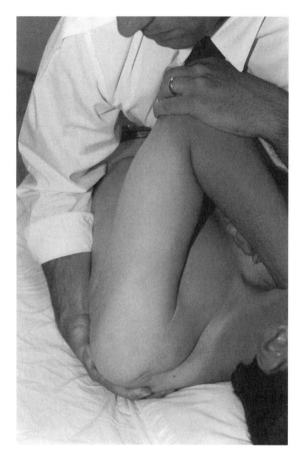

FIGURE 13.6

Therapist Position

Sitting on treatment table at 45° turn from sagittal plane. Mobilizing hand is placed on anterior humeral head, with a wedge or rolled towel under lateral scapula. Assisting hand supports distal extremity to facilitate relaxation. The mobilization is directed posterior along the plane of the glenoid. This technique is useful for reactive shoulders with posterior capsule tightness.

FIGURE 13.6: POSTERIOR GLIDE OF HUMERUS

Patient Position

Supine with involved shoulder flexed 90° and horizontal adducted to first tissue resistance.

Therapist Position

Opposite side of patient's shoulder. Mobilizing hand is same is involved shoulder. Therapist cups patient's elbow in mobilizing hand and assists mobilization with therapist sternum. Assisting hand stabilizes the scapula under patient. Mobilization movement is along 35° of glenoid tilt. The level of flexion can be changed to work the most restricted part of the capsule. This technique is useful with subacute and chronic posterior capsule tightness.

FIGURE 13.7: LATERAL DISTRACTION OF THE HUMERUS

Patient Position

Supine, close to edge of table, with the involved extremity flexed at the elbow and glenohumeral joint. The extremity rests on the therapist's shoulder. A strap and the table stabilize the scapula.

Therapist Position

Facing laterally, both hands grasp the humerus as close as possible to the joint. The therapist should assess which vector of movement is most restricted by starting laterally with mobilization and proceeding caudally. To improve delivery of oscillation or stretch, therapist should align his or her trunk along vector of mobilization.

FIGURE 13.8: ANTERIOR GLIDE OF THE HEAD OF THE HUMERUS

Patient Position

Prone, with the involved extremity as close as possible to the edge of the table. The head of the humerus must be off the table. A wedge or towel roll is placed just medial to joint line under the coracoid process. The extremity is abducted and flexed into the plane of the scapula.

Therapist Position

Distal to the abducted shoulder facing cephalad. The outer hand applies slight distraction force while the inner mobilizing hand glides

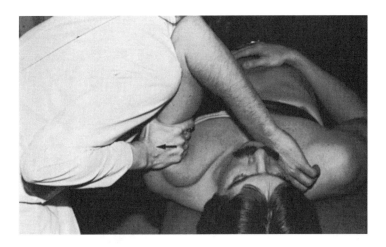

FIGURE 13.7

the head of the humerus anteriorly, stressing the anterior capsule. The tendon of the subscapularis is also stressed with this technique. The mobilization can be fine-tuned by changing the angle of the anterior force to the area most restricted.

FIGURE 13.9: ANTERIOR/POSTERIOR GLIDE OF THE HEAD OF THE HUMERUS

Patient Position

Prone, with the involved extremity over the edge of the table abducted to the desired range. A strap may be used to stabilize the scapula.

Therapist Position

Facing laterally in a sitting position, with the forearm of the involved extremity held between the therapist's knees. Both hands grasp the head of the humerus and apply anteroposterior movement oscillating the head of the humerus. Grades 1 and 2 are mainly used with this technique to stimulate mechanoreceptor activity.

FIGURE 13.10: ANTERIOR/POSTERIOR GLIDE OF THE HEAD OF THE HUMERUS

Patient Position

Supine with the involved extremity supported by the table. A towel roll, pillow, or wedge is placed under the elbow to hold the arm in the POS.

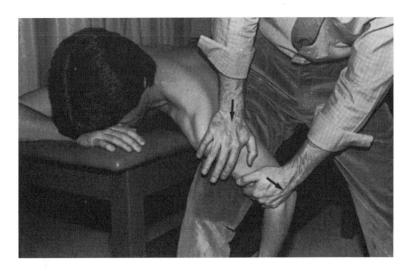

FIGURE 13.8

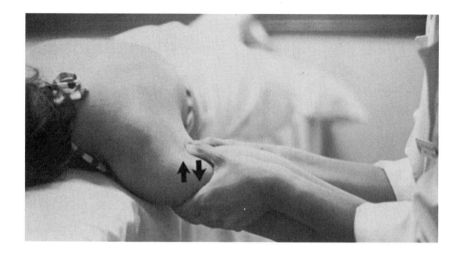

FIGURE 13.9

Therapist Position

Facing laterally in a sitting position. The fingertips hold the head of the humerus while a gentle up-and-down movement is applied. This technique is used with grades 1 and 2 oscillations.

FIGURE 13.11: EXTERNAL ROTATION OF THE HUMERUS

Patient Position

Supine with the involved extremity supported by the table. The arm is held in the plane of the scapula.

Therapist Position

Facing laterally with caudal mobilizing hand grasping the distal humerus, the heel of the cephalad mobilizing hand over the lateral aspect of the head of the humerus. Force is applied through both hands. The caudal hand rotates the humerus externally and provides long-axis distraction while the cephalad hand pushes the head of the humerus in a posterior direction.

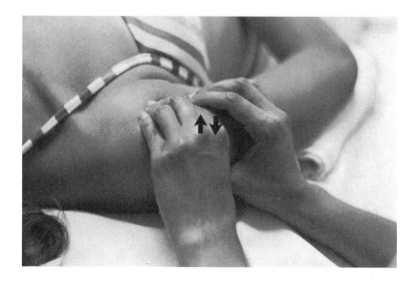

FIGURE 13.10

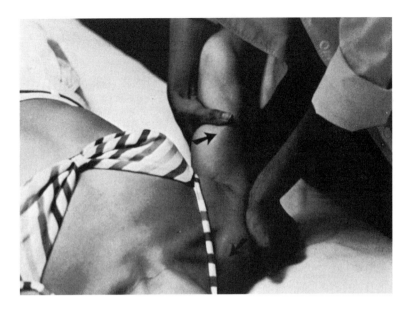

FIGURE 13.11

FIGURE 13.12: EXTERNAL ROTATION/ ABDUCTION/INFERIOR GLIDE OF THE HUMERUS

Patient Position

Supine with the involved extremity supported by the table. The arm is abducted in the plane of the scapula.

Therapist Position

Facing laterally with the caudal hand holding the distal humerus and the heel of the cephalad hand over the head of the humerus. The caudal hand abducts the arm and externally rotates the humerus while maintaining the POS. The cephalad hand simultaneously pushes the head of the humerus into external rotation and slight

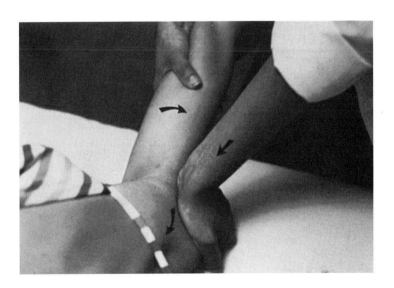

FIGURE 13.12

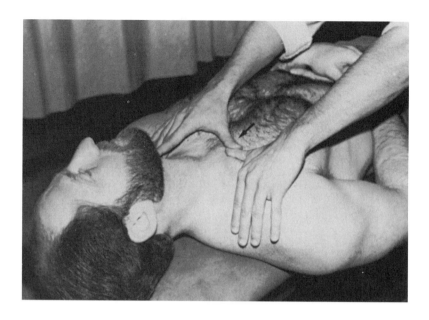

FIGURE 13.13

inferior glide. The force can be oscillated, thrusted, or a prolonged stretch.

Sternoclavicular and Acromioclavicular Techniques

FIGURE 13.13: SUPERIOR GLIDE OF THE STERNOCLAVICULAR JOINT

Patient Position

Supine with the involved extremity close to the edge of the table.

Therapist Position

Facing cranially. The volar surface left thumb pad is placed over the inferior surface of the most medial aspect of the clavicle. The right thumb reinforces the dorsal aspect of the left thumb. Both thumbs mobilize the clavicle superiorly. Graded oscillations are most successful with this technique.

FIGURE 13.14: INFERIOR/POSTERIOR GLIDE OF THE STERNOCLAVICULAR JOINT

Patient Position

Supine with the patient's head supported on a pillow. The patient's cervical spine sidebent toward and rotated away from involved side 20° to 30°.

Therapist Position

At the head of the patient, using thumb pad or pisiform contact on the most medial portion of the clavicle. Mobilization is performed in a inferior/posterior/lateral direction parallel to the joint line. Elevating the involved shoulder to a position of restriction and then performing mobilization the SC joint may assist the rotational component of clavicle motion joint.

FIGURE 13.15: ANTERIOR GLIDE OF THE ACROMIOCLAVICULAR JOINT

Patient Position

Supine at a diagonal to allow the involved acromioclavicular joint to be over the edge of the table.

Therapist Position

Mobilizing force is performed with both thumbs (dorsal surfaces together). The therapist places the distal tips of the thumbs posteriorly to the most lateral edge of the clavicle. Both thumbs push the clavicle anteriorly. Graded oscillations are mainly used with this technique.

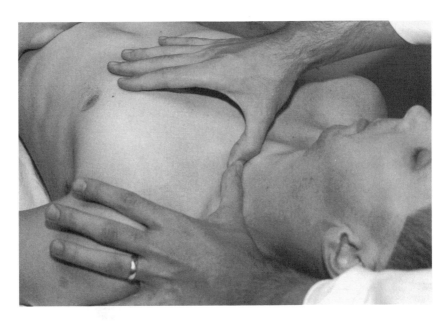

FIGURE 13.14

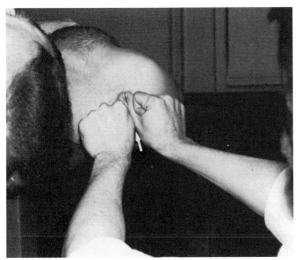

FIGURE 13.15

FIGURE 13.16: GAPPING OF THE ACROMIOCLAVICULAR JOINT

Patient Position

Sitting close to the edge of the table

Therapist Position

Facing laterally with the heel of the left hand over the spine of the scapula and the thenar eminence to the right hand over the distal clavicle.

The force is applied simultaneously. Both hands push the bones in opposite directions, obtaining a general stretch to the capsular structures of the acromioclavicular joint. Oscillations or a prolonged stretch are used with this technique.

Soft Tissue Mobilization and Scapulothoracic Release Techniques

Soft tissue mobilization for purposes of this chapter will be as defined by Johnson: "STM is the treatment of soft tissue with consideration of layers and depth by initially evaluating and treating superficially proceeding to bony prominence, muscle, tendon, ligament etc."[8] The goals of STM in the patient are similar to those of joint mobilization: development of functional scar, elongation of collagen tissue, increase in GAGs, and facilitatation of lymphatic drainage.[39]

In overuse syndromes, trauma, postsurgical conditions, and abnormal movement patterns of the shoulder, areas of tenderness and restricted extensibility of connective tissue may develop. Adhesions within the fascia may reduce the muscles' ability to broaden during contraction and

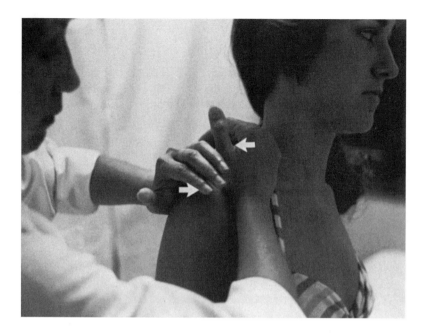

FIGURE 13.16

lengthen during passive elongation.[39] Abnormal compensations may occur, possibly leading to breakdown of compensating tissues.

Within the shoulder complex several areas are important to evaluate for fascial restrictions. Scapulothoracic releasing techniques will also be described due to the musculotendious and fascial characteristics of this articulation. The following is a description by muscle(s) or space between structures to evaluate and mobilize. Table 13.5 defines the types of techniques referred to in the figure legends.

FIGURE 13.17 SUBSCAPULARIS

Patient Position

Supine with the shoulder abducted to tolerance

Therapist Position

Facing axilla with mobilizing fingers on muscle belly of subscapularis. Parallel mobilization or perpendicular strumming or direct oscillation may be used. Assistive techniques are sustaining pressure while elevating and adducting the shoulder as in Figure 13.17B.

TABLE 13.5 *Treatment hand techniques*

Sustained pressure: Pressure applied directly to restricted tissue at the desired depth and direction of maximal restriction

Direct oscillations: Repeated oscillations on and off a restriction with uptake of slack as restriction resolves

Perpendicular mobilization: Direct oscillations and/or sustained pressure techniques performed perpendicular to muscle fiber or soft tissue play

Parallel mobilization: Pressure applied longitudinally to restrictions along the edge of the muscle belly or along bony contours

Perpendicular (transverse) strumming: Repeated rhythmical deformations of a muscle belly to improve muscle play and reduce tone

(Adapted from Johnson,[39] with permission.)

FIGURE 13.18: SUBSCAPULARIS ARC STRETCH

Patient Position

Supine

Therapist Position

Cephalad hand simultaneously elevates, externally rotates, and distracts the involved shoulder, while the caudal hand (thenar side)

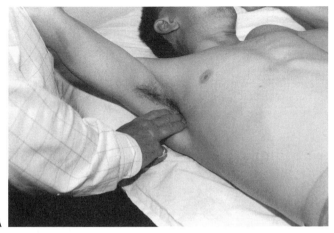

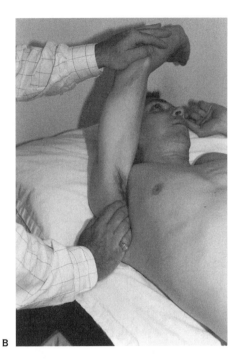

FIGURE 13.17

stabilizes the lateral border of the scapula. Both movements occur simultaneously in a slight arcing fashion.

FIGURE 13.19: PECTORALIS MINOR

Patient Position

Supine or sidelying with arm slightly abducted and flexed.

Therapist Position

Mobilizing fingers glide along in a superficial vector along ribs 3 to 5 lateral to medial underneath pectoralis major. Often pectoralis minor is bound down and tender in shoulder dysfunction. STM techniques used: direct oscillation, sustained pressure, perpendicular and parallel deformations. Assistive techniques are inhalation, contract relax with shoulder protraction.

FIGURE 13.20: SERRATUS ANTERIOR—UPPER PORTION

Patient Position

Sidelying with involved side up.

Therapist Position

Standing posterior to patient's shoulder. Caudal hand elevates the scapula in an cephalad and anterior direction off the rib cage. The therapist can use the fingers of top hand to roll over and palpate the superior fibers of the serratus anterior that attach to the 1st and 2nd ribs as well as the fascial attachments between levator scapularis and serratus anterior.[29] STM techniques: sustained pressure, direct oscillation. Assistive techniques: resistive PNF diagonal contract relax, deep breath.

FIGURE 13.21: SERRATUS ANTERIOR—LOWER PORTION

Patient Position

Sidelying.

Therapist Position

Place mobilizing fingers along an interspace of ribs 2 to 8 on interdigitations of serratus anterior. STM techniques used: parallel techniques

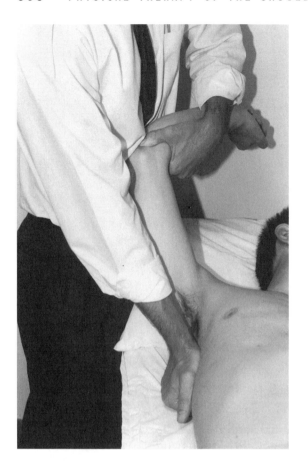

FIGURE 13.18

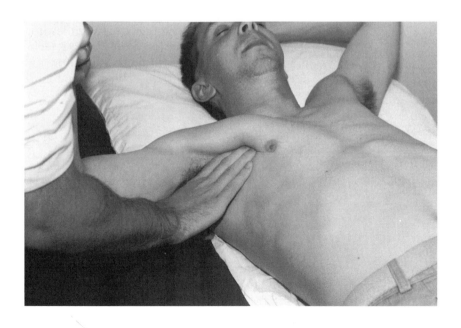

FIGURE 13.19

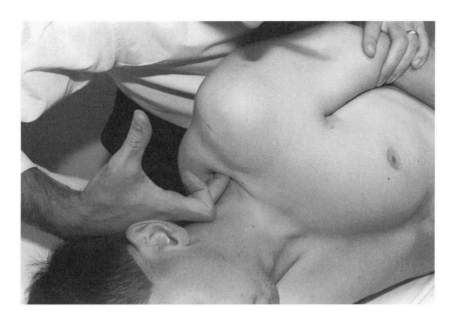

FIGURE 13.20

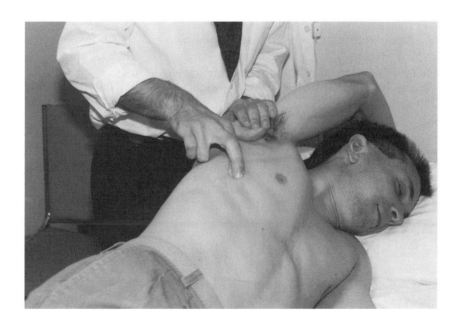

FIGURE 13.21

along rib contours medial to lateral or lateral to medial. Assistive techniques: deep breath, contract relax with scapular depression, rotation of the thoracic spine to the same side. Restrictions may be evident with previous history of rib fracture or abdominal surgery.

FIGURE 13.22: INFERIOR CLAVICLE

Patient Position

Supine with involved extremity supported by a pillow.

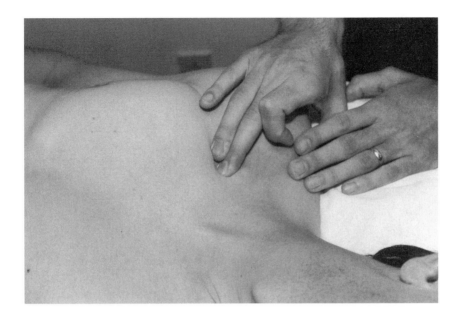

FIGURE 13.22

Therapist Position

Same side as involved shoulder. Palpating medial to lateral or vice versa along inferior clavicle, look for fascial restrictions and tenderness especially at the costoclavicular ligament, subclavius muscle, and the conoid and trapezoid ligaments. This region is important to evaluate and treat in shoulder patients who have protracted and externally rotated scapula with adaptive shortening of anterior chest musculature.

FIGURE 13.23: SCAPULAR DISTRACTION

Patient Position

Sidelying close to the edge of the table with the involved extremity accessible to the therapist. A pillow may be placed against the patient's chest to provide anterior support.

Therapist Position

Facing the patient with caudal hand underneath inferior angle of the scapula and the cephalad hand grasping the vertebral border of the scapula. Both hands tilt the scapula away from the thoracic wall along with the distraction of the scapula by the therapist leaning backward.

FIGURE 13.24: SCAPULAR DISTRACTION, POSTERIOR APPROACH

Patient Position

Sidelying as previous but closer to posterior edge of table.

Therapist Position

Posterior to patient with therapist's hips in perpendicular orientation to patient's trunk. Therapist's adjacent leg on the treatment table with knee bent and placed along midthoracic spine. Outer mobilizing hand grasps the vertebral border of the scapula. Inner hand supports the anterior GH joint. Once hand placement is achieved, the therapist leans back, distracting the scapula away from the thoracic wall. Sustained stretch most effective with this technique.

FIGURE 13.25: SCAPULAR EXTERNAL ROTATION

Patient Position

Sidelying with the involved extremity accessible to the therapist.

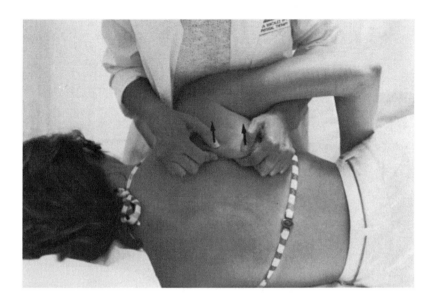

FIGURE 13.23

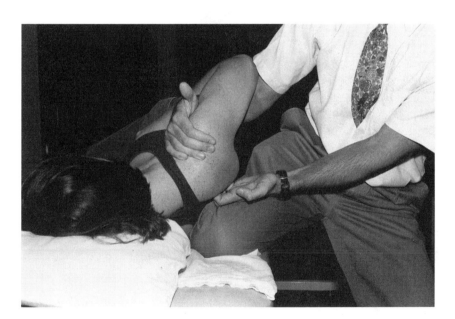

FIGURE 13.24

Therapist Position

Facing the patient with the caudal hand under the extremity through the axillary area. The cephalad hand grasps the superior aspect of the scapula while the caudal hand grasps the inferior angle. The force is applied simultaneously, producing an external rotation of the scapula. Figure 13.26 demonstrates external rotation of the scapula with soft tissue technique using the therapist's elbow to mobilize upper trapezious and levator scapula. Assistive techniques include patient actively rotating cervical spine toward and away from involved side, and spray and stretch to upper trapezious trigger points.

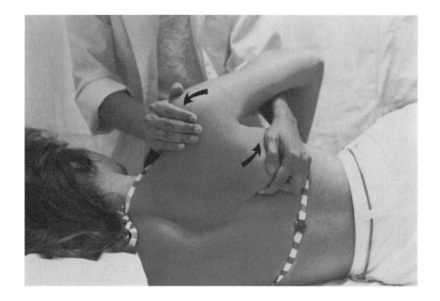

FIGURE 13.25

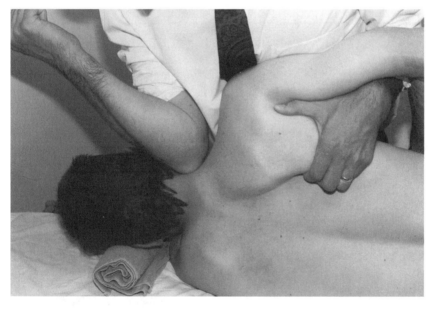

FIGURE 13.26

FIGURE 13.27: SCAPULA DISTRACTION, PRONE

Patient Position

Prone with the involved extremity supported by the table.

Therapist Position

Facing cephalad, outer hand under the head of the humerus and the adjacent mobilizing hand web space under the inferior angle of the scapula. The forces are applied simultaneously. The outer hand lifts the GH joint while the adjacent hand lifts the inferior angle of the scapula.

Summary

Rehabilitation of shoulder injuries using manual techniques is based on an understanding of

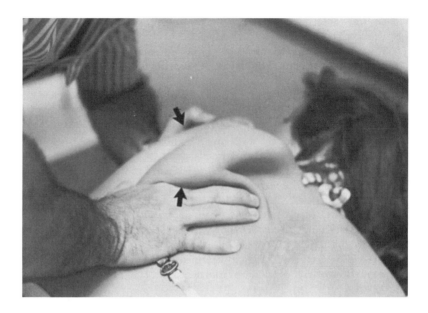

FIGURE 13.27

stages of soft tissue healing, normal and abnormal arthrokinematics and osteokinematics of the shoulder complex, effects of biomechanical stress on various tissues, and muscle function. The application of manual techniques for the shoulder is dependent on a thorough sequential evaluation and continual reassessment. Indications and contraindictions for mobilization are based on an understanding of the histology of immobilized and traumatized tissues. Clinical management of shoulder injuries has been discussed from a perspective of protective versus nonprotective injuries, and phased programs of rehabilitation have been presented. Research on the efficacy of manual therapy must be advanced and traditional concepts and techniques should comply with current and future discoveries.

Acknowledgements

We would like to thank Jill Heinzmann, R.P.T. and John Zubal, A.T.C. for their assistance with the manual technique pictures.

References

1. Frank C, Akeson WH, Woo S et al: Physiology and therapeutic value of passive joint motion. Clin Orthop 185:113, 1984

2. Peacock EE Jr: Wound Repair. 3rd Ed. WB Saunders, Philadelphia, 1984

3. Akeson WH, Amiel D, Woo SLY: Immobility effects on synovial joints. The pathomechanics of joint contracture. Biorheology 17:95, 1980

4. Stoddard A: Manual of Osteopathic Technique. Hutchinson, London, 1959

5. Maitland GD: Peripheral Manipulation. Butterworth Publishers, London, 1970

6. Clayton L (ed): Taber's Cyclopedic Medical Dictionary. FA Davis, Philadelphia, 1977

7. Friel J (ed): Dorland's Illustrated Medical Dictionary. 25th Ed. WB Saunders, Philadelphia, 1974

8. Johnson GS: Course notes, Functional Orthopedic I, Institute for Physical Art, San Francisco, March 1991

9. Andriacchi T et al: Ligament: Injury and repair. In Woo SLY, Buckwalter J (eds): Injury and Repair of the Musculoskeletal Soft Tissues. American Academy of Orthopaedic Surgeons, 1991

10. Kellet J: Acute ST injuries, a review of the literature. Med Sci Sports Exerc 18:5, 1986

11. Jones LH: Strain and Counterstrain. American Academy of Osteopathy, Colorado Springs, 1981

12. Kelly M, Madden JW: Hand surgery and wound healing. p. 49. In Wolfort FG (ed): Acute Hand Injuries: A Multispecialty Approach. Little, Brown, Boston, 1980

13. Cohen KI, McCoy BJ, Diegelmann RF: An update on wound healing. Ann Plast Surg 3:264, 1979

14. Arem AJ, Madden JW: Effects of stress on healing

wounds: intermittent noncyclical tension. J Surg Res 20:93, 1976

15. Kaltenborn FM: Mobilization of the Extremity Joints. Olaf Norris Bokhandel, Oslo, Norway, 1980

16. Poppen NK, Walter PS: Normal and abnormal motion of the shoulder. J. Bone Joint Surg 58:195, 1976

17. Howell SM, Galinat BJ et al: Normal and abnormal mechanics of the glenohumeral joint in the horizontal plane. J Bone Joint Surg 70:227, 1988

18. Vidik A: On the rheology and morphology of soft collagenous tissue. J Anat 105:184, 1969

19. Reigger LL: Mechanical properties of bone. In Davis GJ, Gould JA (eds): Orthopaedic and Sports Physical Therapy. CV Mosby, St. Louis, 1985

20. Betsch DF, Bauer E: Structure and mechanical properties of rat tail tendon. Biorheology 17:84, 1980

21. Butler DL, Grood ES, Noyes FR et al: Biomechanics of ligament and tendons. Exer Sport Sci Rev 6:126, 1979

22. Hirsh G: Tensile properties during tendon healing. Acta Orthop Scand, suppl. 153:1, 1974

23. Taylor DC, Dalton JD, Seaber AV et al: Viscoelastic properties of musculotendon units: The biomechanical effects of stretching. Am J Sports Med 18:300, 1990

24. Van Brocklin JD, Follis DG: A study of the mechanical behavior of toe extensor tendons under applied stress. Arch Phys Med 46:369, 1965

25. Turkel SJ, Panio MW, Marshall JI, Girgis FG: Stabilizing mechanisms preventing anterior dislocation of glenohumeral joint. J Bone Joint Surg 63: 1208, 1981

26. Cooper RR: Alterations during immobilization and regeneration of skeletal muscle in cats. J Bone Joint Surg 54:919, 1972

27. Tabary JC, Tabary C, Tardieu C et al: Physiological and structural changes on the cat soleus muscle due to immobilization at different lengths by plaster casts. J Physiol 224:231, 1972

28. Otis JC, Jiang CC, Wickiewicz TL et al: Changes in the movement arms of the rotator cuff and deltoid muscles with abduction and rotation. J Bone Joint Surg 76:667, 1994

29. Warwick R, Williams P (eds): Gray's Anatomy, 35th British Ed. WB Saunders, Philadelphia, 1973

30. Wyke BD: The neurology of joints. Ann R Coll Surg Engl 41:25, 1966

31. Wyke BD: Neurological aspects of pain therapy: a review of some current concepts. p. 1. In Swerdlow M (ed): The Therapy of Pain. MTP Press, Lancaster, England, 1981

32. Haldeman S: Modern Developments in the Principles and Practice of Chiropractic. Appleton-Century-Crofts, East Norwalk, CT, 1980

33. Kummel BM: Spectrum of lesion of the anterior capsule mechanism of the shoulder. Am J Sports Med 7:111, 1979

34. Warren CG, Lehman JF, Koblanski NJ: Elongation of rat tail tendon: effects of load and temperature. Arch Phys Med Rehabil 52:465, 1971

35. Warren CG, Lehman JF, Koblanski NJ: Heat and stretch tech-procedure: an evaluation using rat tail tendon. Arch Phys Med Rehabil 57:122, 1976

36. Bonutti PM, Windau BS et al: Static progressive stretch to reestablish elbow range of motion. Clin Orthop 303:128, 1994

37. Lehman JF, Masock AJ, Warren CG, Koblanski JN: Effects of therapeutic temperatures on tendon extensibility. Arch Phys Med Rehabil 51:481, 1970

38. Lentell G, Hetherington T, Eagn J, Morgan M: The use of thermal agents to influence the effectiveness of a low load prolonged stretch. Orthop Sports Phys Ther 17:200, 1992

39. Johnson GS: Soft tissue mobilization. In Donatelli R, Wooden MJ (eds): Orthopaedic Physical Therapy, Churchill Livingstone, New York, 1994

14

Strengthening Exercises

KAREN E. DAVIS

ROBERT A. DONATELLI

Strengthening is one of the most vital components of shoulder rehabilitation. Once sufficient healing occurs and adequate range of motion is obtained, strengthening often becomes the main focus of treatment. As the effects of prolonged immobilization are becoming more apparent, early mobilization and strengthening are gaining in popularity.

The present chapter defines strength, strength training principles, and exercise prescription. Muscles essential to shoulder mobility and stability are discussed along with specific strengthening exercises for the shoulder.

The case studies present treatment programs for two shoulder patients. These cases apply strengthening principles to the rehabilitation plans. Incorporating strengthening exercises and exercise prescription appropriately to each patient is as important as any other component of treatment. This chapter will provide some guidelines to follow when designing your own strengthening regime.

Strength

Strength is defined as the ability to produce force and is often used as a measure of ability.[1] Strength is important in both health and performance.[1] Strength training can positively effect the entire musculoskeletal system as bone, muscle, and associated connective tissue adapt ac-

cordingly.[2] Strength training increases the maximum strength of tendons and ligaments while stronger muscles reduce the relative daily stress placed upon joints throughout the body.[1] Strength training increases skeletal muscle mass, force-generating capability, and metabolic capacity. Strength training also increases flexibility, possibly increasing performance and reducing the potential for injury both with work-related and athletic activities.[3]

Muscular Endurance

"Absolute muscular endurance (AME) is the ability to maintain a given fixed submaximal force output during work relying primarily on anaerobic metabolism until exhaustion."[4] Factors that contribute to AME or anaerobic capacity include (1) biochemical adaptations, (2) maximal strength levels, (3) neural adaptations, and (4) muscle hypertrophy.[4] Muscle endurance has been described as performing work using moderate to heavy loads over a period of time.[1] Most clinicians are familiar with the cardiovascular factors contributing to overall endurance or aerobic capacity. Cardiovascular factors may contribute to muscle endurance; however, increases in adenosine triphosphate (ATP), creatinine phosphokinase (CP), glycogen stores, myokinase activity, and maximum strength largely comprise anaerobic capacity.[1] Concentrations of

ATP-CP and glycogen in skeletal muscle are important in maintaining high-intensity work loads and work rates.[4] Observations of increased ATP-CP and glycogen stores have been found after strength training.

Power and Agility

Power is the rate at which work is performed.[1] An increase in power allows the athlete to perform at higher work rates. Increasing maximum power would enable an athlete or patient to work at a smaller percentage of maximum and therefore endure longer work periods. The speed at which a skill is performed can be expressed in terms of Newton's second law, "force equals mass times acceleration." The velocity of a movement may be enhanced by increasing the force. Strength-speed training and speed training increase the speed of movement by general strengthening of the appropriate muscles, making movements faster.[1]

Agility, the ability to rapidly change the direction of the body, is strongly related to strength and power. Studies have shown that significant increases in the strength of the legs accompanies increases in power and velocity of movement.[1] General performance may be increased by increasing maximal strength through resistive training.

Muscle Fiber Types

The two basic fiber types found in human muscle are slow or type I muscle fibers and fast or type II muscle fibers.[5] Type I fibers are able to maintain muscle contractions for extended periods of time, deriving their energy by oxidative metabolism, aerobically. Type II fibers produce more force than type I fibers, deriving their energy from nonoxidative metabolism, anaerobically. Adenosine triphosphate is required for energy to create and maintain muscle contractions.[6] Creatinine phosphokinase and myosin kinase are required for anaerobic metabolism.

Strength Training

Strength training results in the interaction of neural, muscular, and mechanical factors.[7,8] Neural factors include motor unit activity, recruitment of motor units, and modulation of the frequency of motor unit firing. Muscular factors include the cross-sectional area of a muscle and the length–tension relationship at the time of contraction.[7] The moment arm identified and the force generated by the muscle comprise the mechanical factors. At very short and very long lengths, muscle generates low tension.[9] There is an optimal length at which a muscle is able to generate the most tension.

The most consistent finding after resistance training is an increase in the cross-sectional area of the muscle.[10] Increased cross-sectional area is a major contributor to muscle strength; however, initial gains in muscle strength are not due to this increase. During the first few weeks, neural adaptations are thought to mediate the initial strength improvements. Several of the mechanisms contributing to this initial increase in force production include (1) an increase in motor neuron excitability, (2) better co-contraction of synergists, (3) inhibition of neural protective mechanisms, and (4) an increase inhibition of antagonists.[10] Muscle fiber size does not change until approximately 8 to 12 weeks of training. The actual muscle fiber size increase is secondary to the addition of myofibril proteins to the muscle fibers.[10]

Strength training improves the strength of each motor unit, and thus fewer motor units are required at a given submaximal workload.[10] After strength training, more motor unit reserves are available for continuation of work.

Pure aerobic training will likely reduce the ability of strength-power athletes to perform.[11] Andersen and Kearney[11] demonstrate that a so-called repetition continuum exists. When strength and endurance training are performed in excess, maximal strength performance can be blunted possibly secondary to the transformation of fast twitch to slow twitch muscle fibers.[11,12]

Exercise Types

The three basic methods used in strengthening include isometrics, isotonics, and isokinetics. An isometric, or static, contraction is a muscular contraction where there is no change in the angle of the involved joint(s) and little or no change in the length of the contracting muscle.[13] Isometrics produce strength gains specific to the joint angle performed.[14] Isometric training is not effective throughout the range of motion unless many joint angles are trained. Isometric and dynamic measures of strength are not strongly related; therefore, training with isometrics for sports or activities that require dynamic strength is not recommended. Combination training, including isometrics and dynamic training, would provide the benefits of both types of strengthening.

In rehabilitation, isometric and multiangle isometrics are advantageous with protective injuries were wound healing is present. There is an approximate 20° physiologic strengthening overflow with isometrics, allowing pain-free strengthening with possible strength improvements in the affected range.[15]

An isotonic contraction is a muscular contraction where a constant load is moved through a range of motion of the involved joint(s).[13] Isotonics include concentric (shortening) and eccentric (lengthening) muscle contractions. Isotonics mimic many functional activities and, because the resistance is preset, are appropriate to use when a predetermined amount of work is to be performed. Maximal eccentric contractions produce higher tension levels than concentric contractions. Eccentric training requires longer recovery periods and alone has not been shown to be superior to concentric training.[16]

An isokinetic contraction is a muscular contraction through a range of motion at a constant velocity.[13] Isokinetics are discussed in detail in Chapter 16.

Plyometrics

Plyometrics are high-intensity training bridging the gap between speed and strength.[17] Plyometrics are exercises in which a rapid deceleration, eccentric contraction, of a mass is followed by a rapid acceleration, concentric contraction. The stretch reflex, or stretch-shortening cycle, is evoked by the rapid eccentric contraction, resulting in a greater concentric contraction.[17] The eccentric, amortization, and concentric phases comprise a plyometric exercise. Amortization occurs following the eccentric phase, prior to the active concentric or push-off phase of the activity. The shorter and quicker the amortization phase, the more power will be developed.[17]

Because plyometrics are a high-intensity type of training, adequate strength is a prerequisite. Drills should progress from basic to advanced with intensity progressing from low to high.[17] Adequate recovery time must be allowed because plyometrics incorporate maximal-effort multijoint movements. Two to four days of recovery is suggested depending on the sport and time of year. Recommendations for frequency range from one to three days per week, with 15 to 20 minutes per session depending on the sport. It is recommended that a training schedule with alternating days of heavy lifting and plyometric training be constructed to provide sufficient recovery periods.

The types of contractions used in strength training may vary; however, the principles of strength training must be considered for all programs to improve strength, power, endurance, and overall function. The principles of strength training, intensity, frequency, duration, and specificity will be discussed in the following section.

Exercise Prescription

The basic principles of training include intensity, frequency, duration, and specificity.[1] Warm-up, rest periods, periodization and maintenance must also be incorporated into a complete exercise prescription.

INTENSITY

Intensity or volume is denpendent on the number of sets and repetitions, rest between sets, duration of workout, and the amount of weight or load used.[18] Pauletto describes repetitions (reps) as "the number of times an exercise is done without resting during one set." The completion of one exercise performed consecutively without rest is known as a set. The maximal load lifted over a given number of repetitions before fatiguing is a repetition maximum, abbreviated RM.

Determining 1 RM may be feasible when the athlete is healthy. In a clinical setting, however, using a predicted RM to determine a load to be used is more appropriate and safe. Determining a 10 RM, and then calculating or using a standard chart to derive 1 RM, is a more feasible method. Once 1 RM is established, the desired percentage, usually 80 percent, may be obtained. To determine 10 RM the patient performs 10 repetitions with a weight. After a 2- to 4-minute rest period, more weight is added and additional sets of 10 repetitions are performed until a weight only allowing 10 repetitions is performed.[20]

It is known that high-intensity load training or high volume (sets and reps) will result in muscular adaptations and strength gains.[19] The specific amount of resistance required for these strength gains varies.[19] Novice trainees can increase strength with a load of 35 percent of isometric 1 RM and 45 percent of 1 RM in circuit training. Eighty percent of 1 RM is more commonly used with athletes. The 1 RM is tested weekly, and during the other training days workouts are performed at 50 to 90 percent of 1 RM, depending upon the goals of training.

Six or fewer repetitions, with weight based on a low RM (1 to 5 RM), provide the most strength and power benefits.[20] Weight based on 6 RM to 12 RM provides moderate gains, and weight based on 20 RM and above provides muscular endurance gains without strength gains. The intensity of training is categorized as high, moderate, or low with corresponding RMs of 90 percent, 70 to 90 percent and below 70 percent.[20] Moderate workloads and moderate volumes of work are suggested for athletes retraining after injury, prepubescent athletes, and hypertensive populations. The intensity of training in rehabilitation must consider tissue healing and prior physical activity of the patient and be directed towards rehabilitation goals.

FREQUENCY AND DURATION

Recommendations on training are based on experiments varying sets, repetitions, exercises, and frequency or days per week.[1] Generally, training 3 days per week is recommended. This will vary according to the muscle groups trained and the desired outcome. Lower body and larger muscle groups will require more time for recovery, whereas upper body training may be performed more often without overtraining. During the first few weeks of training, the frequency should be less. Also, eccentric loading causes more muscle damage, and the frequency of training should be less to avoid injury and overtraining. It is recommended that athletes recovering from injury should resume training at 50 to 60 percent of preinjury status and increase 10 percent per week.[20] Athletes recover faster from single-joint exercises than from multiple-joint exercises.[20] In rehabilitation, multiple-joint exercises requiring more energy should be performed prior to single-joint exercises requiring less energy. An example of this principle includes performance of multiplane PNF diagonal patterns for the shoulder prior to performance of single-plane internal-external rotation exercises of the shoulder, when both exercises are to be performed during the same workout.

SPECIFICITY

Specificity of training is the most important principle in strength training. The rehabilitation goals will determine the specificity of training and dictate the intensity, frequency, and duration of the program. The SAID (specific adaptations to imposed demands) principle indicates that the body will gradually adapt to the specific demands imposed upon it.[14] Thus, the demands must be specific to the desired goals and constantly change for continual adaptations and resultant increases in strength.

WARM-UP

General and specific warm-up methods have been demonstrated to improve performance as well as reduce the risk of injury from training.[1]

General warm-up should include stretching of all muscles crossing all joints. Specific warm-up includes light to moderate sets performed for each exercise. It is our experience that specific warm-up also allows for the observation of the proper technique for the exercise performed.

REST PERIODS

Rest periods are dependent upon the volumes and loads. They should be designed with the strengthening goals in mind. When training for absolute strength, longer rest periods (3 to 5 minutes) are used between heavy, near-maximal repetitions.[19] Brief rest periods of 30 to 60 seconds are used with higher volumes of exercise, more exercises, and moderate loads (8 RM to 12 RM).

PERIODIZATION

The periodization system is used to prevent overtraining while optimizing peak performance.[21] Periodization is a systematized and organized method of training to "peak" at the right time. With event sports, periodization is geared for peaking on a given day. With team sports, such as basketball, baseball, or football where all the games are important, periodization is geared for peaking for an entire season. Periodization involves not only in-season but also off-season and preseason.

Variation in training is important in breaking up the monotony that occurs when the body adapts to imposed demands. Overload and change in stimulus are required to optimize training. A macrocycle in periodization refers to the overall training period.[21] Two or more mesocycles can occur in a macrocycle, consisting of weeks to months in length. These mesocycles comprise the distinct periods of preseason, in-season, and off-season or transition periods. Mesocycles begin with high-volume, low-intensity training, and progress to low-volume, high-intensity training just prior to competition. The type of transition period, length, and number of mesocycles are sport or activity dependent. We believe rehabilitation goals and discharge maintenance plans can also be designed using the periodization principles.

MAINTENANCE

Maintenance programs in rehabilitation must be developed to maintain reasonable strength, power, and endurance levels to prevent reinjury. Rehabilitation maintenance programs are similar to in-season programs used in atheletics where competitive seasons are of considerable length. The volume and intensity must be sufficient enough to maintain strength, power, and or endurance levels but not producing an overload when combined with work or sport activities. Stone and O'Bryant[1] recommend using three sets of 2 to 3 reps with moderate to heavy weight for major exercises, and 3 to 5 reps with resistive exercises. We have found success in maintenance programs that comprise three sets of 8 to

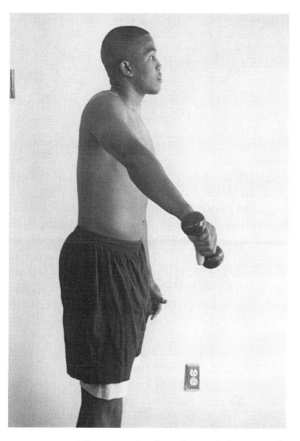

FIGURE 14.1 *Elevation in the plane of the scapula with internal rotation.*

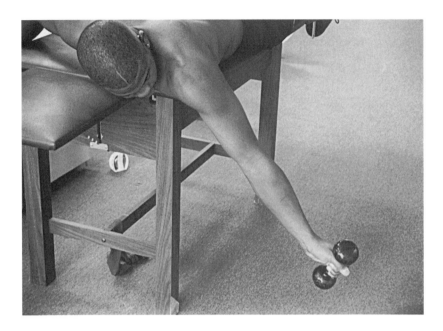

FIGURE 14.2 *Prone horizontal abduction at 100° with external rotation.*

10 repetitions performed 2 or 3 days per week with moderate weights.

Strengthening Exercises for the Shoulder

The muscles of the glenohumeral joint have been grouped into three functional categories by Saha.[22] The first group, prime movers, include the deltoid and clavicular head of the pectoralis major. The second group, steering muscles, include the supraspinatus, subscapularis, and infraspinatus. This group maintains the humeral head in the glenoid. Finally, the latissimus dorsi, teres major and minor, and sternal head of the pectoralis major are collectively the third group, the depressors.

Dynamic glenohumeral stability is provided by the rotator cuff. The rotator cuff muscles are important providers of joint stability as they approximate the humeral head in the glenoid fossa.[23] The importance of force coupling between the rotator cuff and the deltoid is best described by Inman et al.[24] The sheer forces across the joint from the deltoids' upward pull are balanced by the firing of the rotator cuff during elevation.

Townsend et al.[25] performed an electromyographic (EMG) analysis of the glenohumeral muscles. The four rotator cuff muscles and other positioners of the humerus were studied using common shoulder exercises from rehabilitation programs used by professional baseball clubs. Four exercises were found to be the most challenging for every muscle. These exercises were (1) elevation in the plane of the scapula with internal rotation (Fig. 14.1) (2) flexion, (3) prone horizontal abduction with the arm externally rotated (Fig. 14.2), and (4) press-up (Fig. 14.3). The plane of the scapula is further defined in Chapter 1.

The supraspinatus has been identified as the most frequently injured muscle of the rotator cuff group.[26] Jobe and Moynes[26] also support that the rotator cuff muscles should be evaluated and strengthened individually. They report maximal supraspinatus muscle activity at 90° of arm abduction, 30° of horizontal flexion, and full internal rotation in the upright position. Blackburn et al.[27] duplicated this test position described by Jobe and Moynes[26] and analyzed various other exercise positions, reporting the

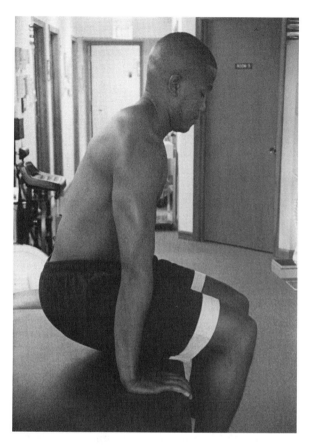

FIGURE 14.3 *Press-up.*

greatest supraspinatus EMG activity in the prone position with the humerus horizontally abducted 100° and externally rotated to thumb-up position (Fig. 14.2). The EMG activities of the infraspinatus and teres minor were maximized with (prone) external rotation with 90° of abduction at the glenohumeral joint and 90° of flexion at the elbow joint (Fig. 14.4).

Worrell et al.[28] compared the supraspinatus EMG activity during the two previously described test positions for the supraspinatus, revealing the prone position superior to standing for EMG activity. The prone position is advocated in strengthening the supraspinatus to promote more supraspinatus muscle activity. However, we suggest that the patient remain pain free while performing this or any exercise in the prone position.

The scapular rotator muscles are essential to glenohumeral mobility and stability.[29] These muscles include the upper trapezius, lower trapezius, levator scapulae, rhomboids, middle and lower serratus anterior, and pectoralis minor. The scapular rotator muscles stabilize the glenoid fossa as the humeral head articulates. Dynamic balance and coordination are provided at the scapulothoracic joint. Many force couples exist around the shoulder complex, most importantly the serratus anterior, upper trapezius, and lower trapezius at the scapulothoracic joint. These muscle act synchronously on the scapula to upwardly rotate and position the glenoid during full elevation of the humerus.[24,30] Moseley et al.[29] examined and identified four exercises that best strengthen the scapular rotators. These exercises include (1) elevation in the plane of the scapula with internal rotation (Fig. 14.1), (2) rowing (Fig. 14.5) (3) push-up with a plus (Fig. 14.6), and (4) press-up (Fig. 14.3). The roles of these muscles and exercises are further discussed in detail in Chapter 2.

Strengthening of the biceps brachii is an important component of the shoulder rehabilitation program (Fig. 14.7). The anatomic alignment of the biceps brachii allows it to function, assisting the rotator cuff, as a compressor of the humeral head.[31] As the scapula upwardly rotates, the rotator cuff and biceps brachii depress the humeral head, reducing shear forces from the deltoid.[31,32] Rodosky et al.[32] investigated the effects of tension on the long head of the biceps with the arm abducted and externally rotated. Tension in the long head of the biceps increased torsional rigidity to external rotation, increasing anterior stability of the glenohumeral joint. This increased stability is greatest during the middle ranges of elevation.

Does Strength Equal Function?

Few studies exist involving strength training specific to the shoulder and consequent improvements in function.[33-35] Wooden et al.[33] demonstrated strength gains and improvement in

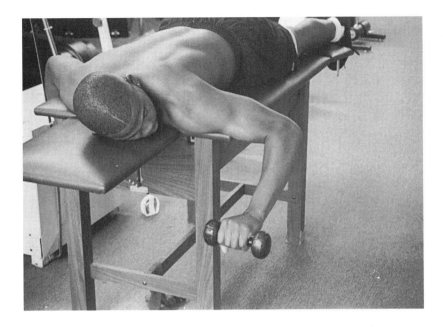

FIGURE 14.4 *Prone external rotation with 90° of abduction at the shoulder and 90° of flexion at the elbow.*

function training baseball pitchers. Isotonic concentric exercises were used on an isokinetic device. The results indicated statistically significant increases in throwing velocity and an increase in external rotator torque.

Ellenbecker et al.[34] compared the effects of concentric isokinetic versus eccentric isokinetic exercise on rotator cuff strength and power and on tennis serve velocity. Concentric strength was significantly improved in both groups after 6 weeks of training. Improvements in eccentric strength and serve velocity were only found with the concentric training group; however, not using a controlled group weakened the results of this study.

Mont et al.[37] performed a study similar to Ellenbecker's examining strength training isokinetically and functional outcomes using tennis serve velocity. Mont et al. compared isokinetic training of the shoulder internal and external rotators using concentrically trained, eccentrically trained, and control groups. Statistically significant concentric and eccentric gains were obtained with both training groups when compared to the control. The increase in serve velocity was greater than 11 percent.

All three studies illustrate sport-specific functional improvements through strength training. Several other studies have shown increases in power and velocity of movement with significant increases in the strength of the legs.[1] Extensive reviews of the physiologic effects of resistance and endurance training illustrate the effects on performance.[36–39] Muscle strength, endurance, verticle jump, and sprint speed are just a few of the variables increased with resistance and endurance training.

Summary

Strength is a measure of human performance. Strength is a result of the interaction of neural, muscular, and mechanical factors. Initial gains in muscular strength during the first few weeks are secondary to neural adaptations. Increases in cross-sectional area of muscle contribute to strength gains after the first few weeks of training. The primary cellular effects of strength training occur in the fast, type II, muscle fibers. The type II fibers are responsible for muscle strength and power and must be recruited during training to be hypertrophied. Training with

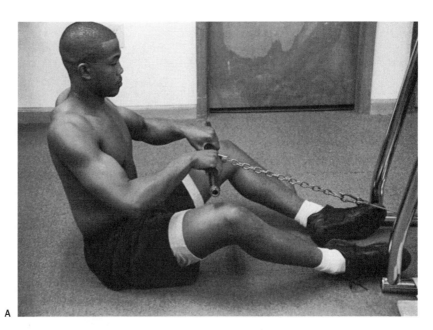

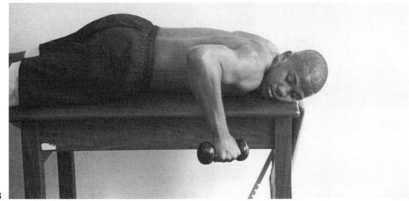

FIGURE 14.5 **(A)** *Seated rowing.* **(B)** *One-arm rowing.*

low or moderate weight will not provide this stimulus. Strength training must also be specifically designed to meet the rehabilitation goals.

Increases in maximum strength allow the athlete or worker to perform at a smaller percentage of their maximum effort and thus endure longer work rates. This ability represents an overall increase in muscular endurance. Adequate muscle strength and endurance at the shoulder complex is necessary to maintain adequate physiologic and accessory motion, and thus normal scapulohumeral rhythm.

The muscles at the shoulder complex must work together to provide adequate stability and mobility. This is achieved by synchronous activity of the rotator cuff, long head of the biceps, rotators of the scapula, and the deltoid. Fatigue or weakness of any of these muscle can lead to abnormal translation of the humeral head.[23] Weakness of the rotator cuff is also thought to trigger glenohumeral instability.[39] Scapular rotator muscle weakness allows excessive scapular movement, contributing to poor scapulohumeral rhythm. Abnormal humeral head translation of the humeral head, or altered scapulohumeral rhythm, can contribute to irritation of adjacent tissues and shoulder pathology.[23]

Proprioceptive exercises and eventually plyo-

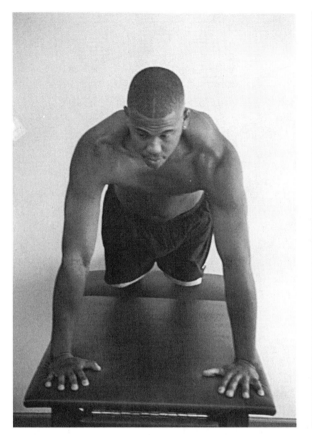

FIGURE 14.6 *Push-up with a plus.*

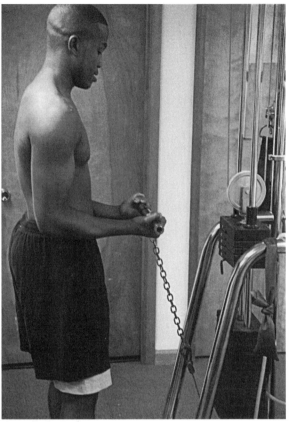

FIGURE 14.7 *Biceps curls.*

metrics must be applied to enhance neuromuscular control. All types of strengthening must coincide with the stage of rehabilitation appropriate for that patient. Progression of the strengthening program must be sequential while working to meet the patient's goals. Criteria for reduction in pain and improvement in ROM and strength must be met before the patient is progressed. Finally, to complete a rehabilitation program, some form of functional training must be incorporated prior to the return to work or sport.

The next two cases discuss two common patient types. The first case illustrates a work injury that demonstrates the importance of strength at the shoulder joint in providing stability to avoid impingement. The second case, involving an overhead athlete, demonstrates the need for strengthening to provide dynamic stability to avoid instability and overuse.

CASE STUDY 1:
IMPINGEMENT SYNDROME

The focus of this case was to restore soft tissue mobility and muscular strength and endurance to the shoulder complex and educate the patient in a maintenance program specific to his job-related tasks.

HISTORY

This case presents a 45-year-old airplane mechanic. This patient reports his job tasks require working on airplanes from supine, kneeling, and standing positions, with most activities requiring reaching in front and/or overhead. He has been performing these job duties for 15 years. He reports intermittent shoulder pain during the last 3 to 4 years that has progressively worsened over the last 3 to 4 months. He has been referred to physical therapy with a diagnosis of "impingement syndrome."

INITIAL EVALUATION

Radiographic findings did not reveal an abnormal shaped acromion; however, mild bone spurring was present on the underlying surface of the AC joint. Visual inspection revealed gross atrophy of the right shoulder complex. Gross postural changes including an increased thoracic kyphosis, forward head, and rotated humerus were apparent. Active elevation of the humerus in the plane of the scapula was approximately 80° and limited by pain. The lateral border of the scapula protracted excessively during active elevation. Passive external rotation was limited to 5° at 0° of abduction and 20° at 90° of abduction. Accessory glenohumeral motion testing revealed moderate capsular restrictions in anterior and posterior directions for the involved extremity. Overall passive scapular mobility was limited in rotation and distraction from the rib cage.

Isokinetic assessment of the rotator cuff was deferred at this point due to limited ROM for rotation; however, gross manual muscle tests revealed 4/5 internal rotator and 3/5 external rotator strength. The patient was not able to assume the prone test position for the supraspinatus. Supraspinatus testing standing revealed pain and weakness. Strength assessments revealed 3+/5 muscle grades for the scapular rotators, serratus anterior, middle and lower trapezius, rhomboids, and external glenohumeral rotators. Impingement testing was positive (see Chapter 3). Neurologic testing was normal. Palpation revealed trigger points within the subscapularis, levator scapulae, and pectoralis major muscles.

INTERPRETATION OF FINDINGS

Apparent muscle atrophy and postural and radiographic changes may be attributed to disuse and age-related changes of the glenohumeral joint. Limits in passive range of motion demonstrate limits in mobility of the subscapularis and capsular structures.[40,41] Limits in the scapulothoracic articulations were also identified. Limits in active elevation correspond to the passive findings. During this middle phase of elevation (60° to 140°), there is an increase in scapulothoracic movement.[42] Adequate glenohumeral and scapular rotator strength is critical, because maximum shearing forces of the deltoid occur at this phase. This middle range is also the range in which this patient performs the majority of his work-related tasks. The presence of trigger points in the muscle and shoulder complex correspond to overactivity of these muscles compensating for the reduced scapular motion.[43]

All of this patient's findings are contributors to a reduced suprahumeral space leading to impingement.

TREATMENT PLAN AND RATIONALE
INITIAL PHASE (WEEK 1)

This patient was placed on light duty at work and his overhead activities were limited during his rehabilitation. This patient was seen three times per week during the first 12 weeks of physical therapy. Initial treatments focused on restoring soft tissue mobility. Heat in conjunction with a low load prolonged stretch into external rotation was applied to the shoulder (Fig. 14.8). The humerus was positioned 30° anterior to the frontal plane and 1- to 3-pound weights were progressively added to patient tolerance for 10, 20, and 30 minutes in consecutive treatment sessions. Elevating tissue temperatures with superficial moist heat in conjunction with a low load prolonged stretch are thought to cause plastic deformation in connective tissues.[44] Soft tissue techniques to reduce trigger points followed by glenohumeral and scapular mobilizations were then performed.

Active stretching of the antagonistic muscles, pectoralis major, upper trapezius, and levator scapulae was performed prior to strengthening of the agonistic scapular rotators. Janda (49) describes muscle imbalances occurring from tight muscles inhibiting its antagonist. Janda[45]

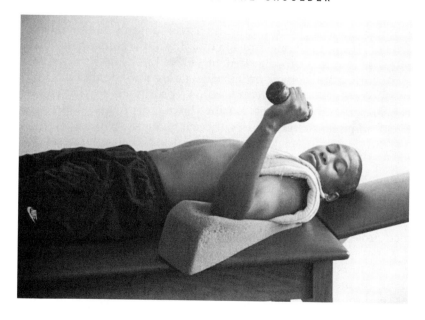

FIGURE 14.8 *Moist heat with a low load prolonged with 2 lb weight stretch into external rotation.*

stresses the importance of stretching the antagonists prior to strengthening the agonists.

After two visits, improvement in external rotation reached 45° at 0° of abduction and 60° at 90° of abduction. Scapulothoracic rhythm was improved, and excessive protrusion of the scapula with active movements was reduced. Active elevation was full; however, a painful arc was present, implicating impingement of subacromial tissues. All strengthening movements and daily tasks were limited to 90° of elevation during this phase.

A 5-minute general warm-up using an upper body ergometer was used prior to active stretching and strengthening exercises (Fig. 14.9). Stretches for both the inferior and posterior rotator cuff were incorporated with 30-second holds, repeated five times.

Isotonic strengthening exercises included the following.

1. Elevation in the plane of the scapula with the arm internally rotated (Fig. 14.1)
2. Prone horizontal abduction at 100° with arm externally rotated
3. Press-up (Fig. 14.3)
4. Seated rowing (Fig. 14.5a)
5. Biceps curls (Fig. 14.7)
6. Prone extension with internal rotation (Fig. 14.10)

Eighty percent of an estimated 1 RM was used as the load for all isotonic scapular rotator exercises. Three sets of 10 repetitions was preceded by a specific warm-up of the exercise without weight. At this time the patient's ability to perform the exercise through pain-free ROM was assessed.

Isokinetic testing of the glenohumeral rotators was performed in the plane of the scapula. Test results indicated a 45 percent deficit of the external rotators and a 22 percent deficit of the internal rotators. During the next visit, isokinetic strengthening of the rotators was begun using speeds of 90° and 120° per second for 3 sets of 10 repetitions (Fig. 14.11) Each physical therapy session concluded with ice to the shoulder for 10 minutes. Ice was applied to prevent any adverse inflammatory responses secondary to stretching, to maintain the plastic deformation gained with treatment, and to reduce delayed-onset muscle soreness.[46]

MIDDLE PHASE (WEEKS 3 TO 5)

During the following 3 weeks of physical therapy, this patient was seen three times per week. Heat with stretch and soft tissue manipulation

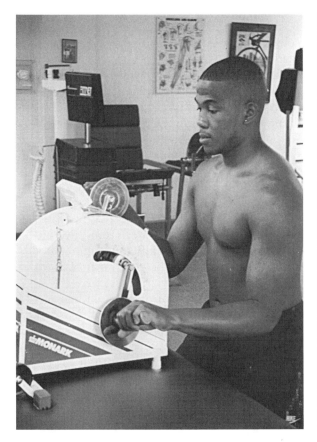

FIGURE 14.9 *Upper body ergometer.*

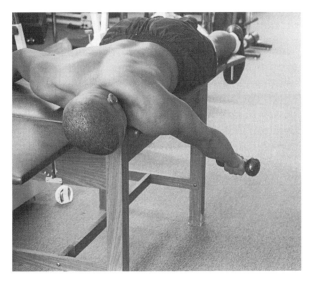

FIGURE 14.10 *Prone extension with internal rotation.*

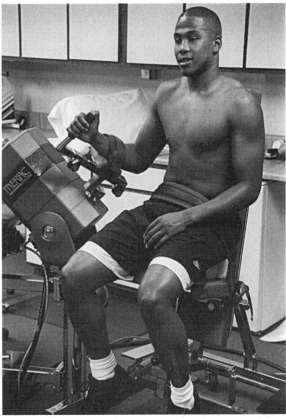

FIGURE 14.11 *Isokinetics for internal and external rotation of the shoulder in the plane of the scapula (30° anterior to frontal plane).*

continued prior to strengthening until active and passive mobility testing was within normal limits (at the end of week 3). Isotonic and isokinetic strengthening were continued. A new 1 RM was established at the beginning of each week with the load increasing accordingly. A set of 10 repetitions was added to the isokinetic strengthening weekly, progressing to six sets of 10 repetitions by the fourth week of treatment.

FINAL PHASE (WEEK 6)

Prior to discharge, manual muscle testing revealed 4/5 strength of the scapular rotators. Isokinetic reassessment demonstrated a 15 percent external rotator deficit and a 10 percent increase in internal rotator strength.

A maintenance program was reviewed prior to discharge. This program incorporated all of the isotonic strengthening exercises performed during therapy, with sidelying internal and external rotation exercises replacing the isokinetics for the glenohumeral rotators. The patient was instructed to perform three sets of 10 repetitions for each exercise 3 days a week for 6 weeks. A continued program of three sets of 10 repetitions for each exercise was recommended to be performed 2 days per week indefinitely provided this patient was performing the same job tasks.

CASE STUDY 2: ROTATOR CUFF AND BICIPITAL TENDONITIS

The focus of the case is to identify the contributing factors to rotator cuff and bicipital tendonitis, initiate the appropriate strengthening program, and return this athlete to competitive sports.

HISTORY

This case presents a 21-year-old collegiate female tennis player with a complaint of chronic right shoulder pain. Her prior history for this shoulder includes similar painful episodes, usually occurring mid to late season, during the past 3 years. Previous treatments include the use of oral anti-inflammatories and modality treatments administered in the athletic training facility on campus. Her current complaints have not subsided with these types of conservative treatment and she has been referred for physical therapy evaluation and treatment. Her current medical diagnosis is "rotator cuff and bicipital tendonitis."

INITIAL EVALUATION

Radiographic findings were normal. Visual inspection revealed moderate right scapular elevation, protraction, and atrophy of the posterior rotator cuff muscles. External rotation was limited by 30° in the adducted position, when compared to the uninvolved side. She presented with positive impingement sign. Apprehension and relocation tests were positive. Biceps brachialis testing was positive for Speed's test. Posteriorly, limited capsular mobility was detected. Manual muscle testing demonstrated pain and weakness of the supraspinatus, subscapularis, and infraspinatus/teres minor (3/5 muscle grades). The scapular rotators (serratus anterior, upper, middle, and lower trapezius, and rhomboids) demonstrated fair plus (3+/5 muscle grades) strength, but fatigued quickly with repetitive testing.

Overall this athlete reported her current shoulder pain had progressed from intermittent to constant, and was significantly aggravated by most activities using the right arm over 90° of elevation.

Isokinetic testing of the glenohumeral rotators was performed in the plane of the scapula. Test results indicated peak torque, power, and total work deficits of greater than 40 percent for the external rotators and greater than 20 percent for the internal rotators when compared to the uninvolved side. The peak torque of the external rotators was 50 percent of the internal rotators.

Palpation revealed trigger points within the subscapularis muscle belly and tenderness along the anteriosuperior aspect of the right shoulder.

INTERPRETATION OF FINDINGS

Signs and symptoms indicate a possible secondary impingement and tendonitis as a result of abnormal anterior translation of the humeral head. The abnormal or excessive translation may be secondary and/or contributing to the loss of dynamic stability from the rotator cuff and biceps tendon, evident by the tendonitis.[23] The scapular rotator weakness and posterior capsular tightness are also predisposing and/or precipitating factors.

TREATMENT PLAN AND RATIONALE
INITIAL PHASE (WEEK 1)

This athlete was restricted from tennis activities during the initial phase of treatment. She did, however, independently perform lower body and conditioning workouts. She was seen for

5 consecutive days during this initial phase. Treatment focused on decreasing the reactivity of the inflamed tissue and restoring normal soft tissue mobility within the shoulder complex.

Heat was applied to the shoulder joint in conjunction with low-voltage surged electrical stimulation to the subscapularis trigger points to begin treatment. Soft tissue and joint mobilizations were applied to the glenohumeral and scapulothoracic joints to further reduce the trigger points and improve posterior capsular mobility.

Low-voltage medium-frequency electrical simulation was applied to the supraspinatus and posterior rotator cuff while isometric were performed for external rotation in the plane of the scapula for 15 minutes. All treatments during this initial phase of treatment commenced with an iontophoresis treatment at the rotator cuff insertion site using dexamethasone sodium phosphate followed by a 10-minute application of ice.

Overall tissue reactivity and subjective report of pain were reduced by the fourth day of treatment, and the use of the upper–body ergometer (UBE) was initiated in an attempt to begin general muscular endurance training. Rhythmic stabilization exercises for the glenohumeral and scapulothoracic joints were also initiated at this point in treatment, manually performed by the therapist.

MIDDLE PHASE (WEEKS 2 TO 6)

During week 5-minute warm-up was performed on the UBE prior to active stretching and isotonic strengthening exercises as in Case 1. Isotonic exercises included the following.

1. Elevation in the plane of the scapula (Fig. 14.1)
2. Prone horizontal abduction at 100° with external rotation (Fig. 14.2)
3. Seated rowing (Fig. 14.5a)
4. Biceps curls (Fig. 14.7)
5. Serratus press (Fig. 14.12)
6. Prone extension with internal rotation (Fig. 14.10)

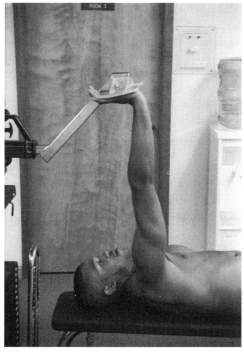
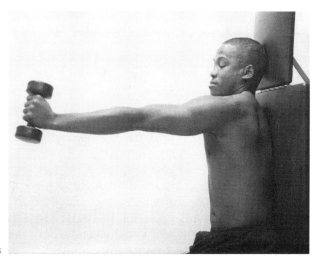

FIGURE 14.12 (A & B) _Serratus press._

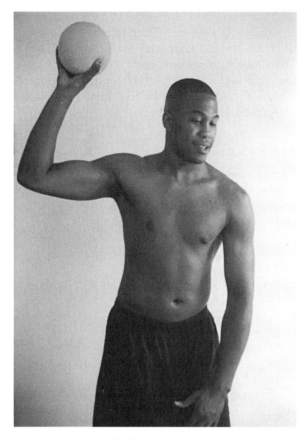

FIGURE 14.13 *Plyoball single-arm baseball throw.*

Three sets of 10 repetitions were performed using a weight equal to 80 percent of 1 RM, by the calculated 10-RM method, determined during the first session each week. An additional set for each isotonic exercise was added each week, progressing to seven sets by week 6. Thirty-second rest periods between sets and 60-second rests periods between exercises were incorporated.

Submaximal concentric training of the glenohumeral rotators was initiated during week 2 using a velocity spectrum from 120° to 300° per second (Fig. 14.11). As the atheletee tolerated, isokinetics were progressed to a maximal effort level by week 3. Isokinetic training began with 8 repetitions during weeks 2 and 3, increasing to 10 repetitions during weeks 4 and 5, and to 12 repetitions during week 6, allowing 15-second

rest periods between sets. A 10-minute application of ice terminated each session.

Proprioceptive training progressed to include the following closed kinetic chain activities.

1. Balancing on hands and knees
2. Balancing on hands and knees on the balance board
3. Balancing on hands and knees on the minitramp
4. Balancing on hands and knees on an exercise ball

FINAL PHASE (WEEKS 7 AND 8)

A reassessment of the glenohumeral rotators revealed a 5 percent deficit of external rotator strength, a 15 percent increase in internal rotator strength, and a 75 percent external to internal rotator value. Scapular rotator strength assessed by manual muscle tests were 5/5.

The upper body ergometer warm-up, three sets of 10 repetitions of isotonic exercises and the isokinetic velocity spectrum, one set of 10 repetitions at each speed, began each treatment session during the final phase. Based on the strength improvements, functional drills were safely incorporated. These drills were performed every other day, totaling 3 days per week, and included the following activities.

Drills with surgical tubing

1. PNF diagonals for D1 and D2
2. Internal and external rotation at 90° of elevation in the plane of the scapula

Modification of these exercises included adding a brief hold and varying the speed of arm movement.

Drilla with Plyoball/minitramp (beginning with 10 throws, increasing by 10 each session):

1. Overhead soccer pass with two hands
2. Chest pass
3. Single-arm baseball throw (Fig. 14.13)
4. Trunk rotations mirroring ground strokes (forehand and backhand)

5. Sit-ups with a ball toss/catch using a slanted minitramp
6. Prone trunk extension with the plyoball overhead

Two-minute rest periods were allowed between each exercise.

Prior to discharge a program was developed with the athlete and her coach. Using periodization principles, this program encompassed year-round training with in-season, off-season, and preseason guidelines.

References

1. Stone MH, O'Bryant H: Weight Training: A Scientific Approach. Burgess International, 1987
2. Kraemer WJ: General adaptations to resistance and endurance training programs. In Baechle TR (ed): Essentials of Strength Training and Conditioning/National Strength and Conditioning Association. Human Kinetics, Champaign, IL, 1994
3. Jobe FW, Moyers DR: Delineation of diagnostic criteria and rehabilitation program for rotator cuff injuries. Am J Sports Med 10:336, 1982
4. Stone MH, Wilson D, Rozenek R et al: Bridging the gap: anaerobic capacity physiological basis. NSCA J 5:40, 1984
5. Fleck SJ, Kraemer WJ: Designing Resistance Training Programs. Human Kinetics, Champaign, IL, 1987
6. Tesch PA, Colliander EB, Kaiser P: Muscle metabolism during intense, heavy-resistance exercise. Eur J Appl Physiol 55:362, 1986
7. Enoka RM: Muscle strength and its development: new perpectives. Sports Med 6:146, 1988
8. Rutherford OM, Jones DA: The role of learning and coordination in strength training. Eur J Appl Physiol 55:100, 1986
9. Lieber RL, Bodine-Fowler SC: Skeletal muscle mechanics: implications for rehabilitation. Phys Ther 73:844, 1993
10. Dudley GA, Harris RT: Neuromuscular adaptations to conditioning. In Baechle, TR (ed): Essentials of Strength Training and Conditioning/National Strength and Conditioning Association. Human Kinetics, Champaign, IL, 1994
11. Andersen T, Kearney JT: Effects of three resistance training programs on muscular strength and absolute and relative endurance. Res Q Exer Sport 53:1, 1982
12. Kraemer WJ: Exercise physiology corner; the dynamics of muscular structure and function. NSCA J 4:46, 1983
13. Lamb DR: Physiology of Exercise: Response and Adaptations. 2nd Ed. Macmillan, New York, 1984
14. Arnheim Dd, Prentice WE: Principles of Athletic Training. 8th Ed. Mosby Year Book, St. Louis, 1993
15. Atha J: Strengthening muscle. Exer Sports Sci Rev 9:1, 1981
16. Ellenbecker TS, Davies GJ, Rowinski MJ: Concentric versus eccentric isokinetic strengthening of the rotator cuff. Am J Sports Med 16:64, 1988
17. Allerheilgn WB: Speed development and plyometric training. In Baechle TR (ed): Essentials of Strength Training and Conditioning/National Strength and Conditioning Association. Human Kinetics, Champaign, IL, 1994
18. Pauletto B: Let's talk training #2: intensity. NSCA J 8:33, 1986
19. Wathen D: Training volume. In Baechle (ed): Essentials of Strength Training and Conditioning/National Strength and Conditioning Association. Human Kinetics, Champaign, IL, 1994
20. Wathen, D: Load assignment. In Baechle (ed): Essentials of Strength Training and Conditioning/National Strength and Conditioning Association. Human Kinetics, Champaign, IL, 1994
21. Wathen D: Periodization: Concepts and Applications. In Baechle (ed): Essentials of Strength Training and Conditioning/National Strength and Conditioning Association. Human Kinetics, Champaign, IL, 1994
22. Saha AK: Theory of Shoulder Mechanism. Charles C Thomas, Springfield, IL, 1961
23. Pappas A, Goss T, Kleinman P: Symptomatic shoulder instability due to lesions of the glenoid labrum. Am J Sports Med 9:11, 1981
24. Inman VT, Saunders M, Abbot LC: Observations on the function of the shoulder joint. J Bone Joint Surg 26:1, 1994
25. Townsend H, Jobe FW, Pink M, Perry J: EMG analysis of the glenohumeral muscles during a baseball rehabilitation program. Am J Sports Med 20:264, 1991
26. Jobe FW, Moynes DR: Delineation of diagnostic criteria and a rehabilitation program for rotator cuff injuries. Am J Sports Med 10:336, 1982
27. Blackburn TA, McLeod WD, White B Wofford L:

EMG analysis of posterior rotator cuff exercises. Athletic Training 25:40, 1990

28. Worrell TW, Corey BJ, York SL, Santiestaban J: An analysis of supraspinatus EMG activity and shoulder isometric force development. Med Sci Sports Exer 24:744, 1992

29. Moseley JB, Jobe FW, Pinks M: EMG analysis of the scapular muscles during a shoulder rehabilitation program. Am J Sports Med 20:128, 1992

30. Hart D, Carmichael SW: Biomechanics of the shoulder. J Orthop Sports Phys Ther 6:229, 1985

31. Peat M: Functional anatomy of the shoulder complex. Phys Ther 66:1855, 1986

32. Rodosky MW, Harner CD, Fu FH: The role of the long head of the biceps muscle and superior glenoid labrum in anterior stability of the shoulder. Am J Sports Med 22:121, 1994

33. Wooden MJ, Greenfield B, Johanson M et al: Effects of strength training on throwing velocity and shoulder muscle performance on teenage baseball players. J Orthop Sports Phys Ther 15:223, 1992

34. Ellenbecker TS, Davies GJ, Rowinski MJ: Concentric versus eccentric isokinetic strengthening of the rotator cuff. Am J Sports Med 16:64, 1988

35. Mont MA, Cohen DB, Campbell KR et al: Isokinetic concentric versus eccentric training of shoulder rotators with functional evaluation of performance enhancement in elite tennis players. Am J Sports Med 22:513, 1994

36. Kraemer WJ: Physiological and cellular effects of exercise training. p. 659. In Leadbetter WB, Buckwalter JA, Gordon SL eds: Sports-Induced Inflammation, American Academy of Orthopedic Surgeons, Park Ridge, IL, 1990

37. Kraemer WJ, Daniels WL: Physiological effects of training. p. 29. In Bernhardt DB ed: Sports Physical Therapy. Churchill Livingston, New York, 1986

38. Kraemer WJ, Deschenes MR, Fleck SJ: Physiological adaptations to resistance exercise: Implications for athletic conditioning. Sports Med 6:246, 1988

39. Stone MH, Fleck SJ, Triplett NT, Kraemer WJ: Health-and performance-related potential of resistancetraining. Sports Med 11:210, 1991

40. Turkel SJ, Panio MW, Marshall JL, Grigis FG: Stabilizing mechanisms preventing anterior dislocation of the glenohumeral joint. J Bone Joint Surg 63A:1208, 1981

41. Harryman DT, Sidles JA, Harris SL, Matsen FA: The role of the rotator cuff interval capsule in passive motion and stability of the shoulder. J Bone Joint Surg 74A:53, 1992

42. Bagg SD, Forest WJ: Electromyographic study of the scapular rotators during arm abduction in the scapular plane. Am J Phys Med 65:111, 1986

43. Travell JG, Simons DG: Myofascial Pain and Dysfunction. The Trigger Point Manual. Williams Wilkins, Baltimore, 1984.

44. Warren G, Lehman JF, Koblanski JN: Heat and stretch procedures: an evaluation using rat tail tendon. Ach Phys Med Rehab 57:122, 1976

45. Janda V: Central nervous motor regulation and back problems. In Korr IM (ed): The Neurobiologic Mechanisms in Manipulative Therapy. Plenum, New York, 1978

46. Michlovitz SL: Biophysical principles of heating and superficial heat agents. In Michlovitz SL (ed): Thermal Agents in Rehabilitation. FA Davis, Philadelphia, 1986

15

Myofascial Treatment

DEBORAH SEIDEL COBB

ROBERT CANTU

Introduction

The complexity of the shoulder joint often makes it a difficult joint for a physical therapist to evaluate and treat. The biomechanical complexity of the shoulder is a function of an interrelationship between bony structures and myofascia. Evaluation and treatment of the shoulder must therefore address both of these components.

Two highly interrelated approaches to treating the shoulder are joint manipulation and myofascial manipulation (Fig. 15.1). All of the myofascial tissues including capsule, ligament, and surrounding fascia are categorized as soft tissues. The question is, when is one performing joint mobilization and when is one performing myofascial manipulation? What is the difference between the two? Both joint mobilization and myofascial manipulation have their effects upon connective tissue.

Joint manipulation has been defined as "the skilled passive movement of a joint."[1] This movement is gained primarily by following the rules of arthrokinematics. This makes joint mobilization easier to understand and use. Myofascial mobilization, on the other hand, is not as clear-cut. Many myofascial lesions do not follow any arthrokinematic rules. The basis for myofascial mobilization is more intuitive, relying on palpation rather than arthrokinematics.

By definition, myofascial manipulation is defined as "the forceful, passive movement of musculofascial elements through its restrictive directions, beginning with its most superficial layer and progressing into depth, while taking into account its relationship to the joints concerned."[1] This definition contains several key elements:

1. Myofascial manipulation as defined for this chapter is direct technique. (Find the lesion and treat in the direction of the restriction.)
2. Awareness of the 3-dimensionality of myofascia is key to its successful implementation.
3. A strong interrelationship exists between joint mobilization and myofascial manipulation.

The primary focus of this chapter is the treatment of the myofascial tissues significant to the shoulder joint.

Histology of Connective Tissue

Connective tissue comprises 16 percent of a person's body and stores 23 percent of the body's total water content.[2] Skin, muscle, tendon, ligaments, joint capsule, periosteum, aponeuroses, and blood vessel walls all contain connective tissue. Bone, cartilage, and adipose tissue can also

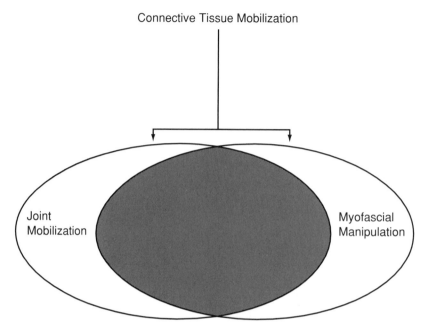

FIGURE 15.1 *Interrelationship of joint manipulation and myofascial manipulation approaches to treating the shoulder.*

histologically be considered connective tissue but are not relevant to our discussion of myofascia.[2-5] Connective tissue is comprised of cells, ground substance, and three fiber types: Collagen, elastin, and retinaculin (Table 15.1).[5,6] As therapists, we are concerned with the ordinary connective tissue that comprises the superficial and deep fascia as well as the nerve and muscle sheaths, ligaments, and tendons.

CLASSIFICATION OF CONNECTIVE TISSUE

Connective tissue can be divided into three types based on fiber density and arrangement: dense regular, dense irregular, and loose regular. Tendons and ligaments are comprised primarily of *dense regular* connective tissue, which is characterized by a high proportion of collagen fibers to ground substance, and a parallel arrangement of fibers. These characteristics allow for high tensile strength with low extensibility. Dense regular connective tissue has poor vascularity due to its compactness. Healing time is therefore significantly increased after any trauma (see Fig. 15.4).

Dense irregular connective tissue is found in joint capsule, periosteum, dermis of skin, fascial sheaths, and aponeuroses. A dense multidirectional fiber arrangement is characteristic of this type of connective tissue. Due to the structure it is able to limit forces in a three-dimensional manner. As compared to dense regular connec-

TABLE 15.1. *Components of connective tissue*

Collagen: Most tensile of connective tissue fibers
   Type I collagen: Ordinary connective tissue (loose and dense)
   Type II collagen: Hyaline cartilage
   Type III collagen: Lining of arteries and fetal dermis
   Type IV collagen: Basement membranes
Elastin: More elastic then collagen. Lining of arteries and ligamentum flavum
Reticulin: Most elastic fiber. Framework of lymph nodes and glands
Ground substance: Viscous medium in which cells and connective tissue lie
   Mechanical barrier against foreign matter
   Medium for nutrient and waste diffusion
   Maintains spacing between adjacent collagen fibers (interfiber distance) to prevent cross-links

tive tissue, it possesses a higher proportion of ground substance as well as increased vascularity.

Loose regular connective tissue is found in the superficial and deep fascia as well as nerve and muscle sheath, endomysium, and the supportive structure of the lymph system. This tissue is the most easily mobilized with myofascial techniques.[3–5,7]

Effects of Immobilization and Mobilization on Connective Tissue

With an understanding of the normal biomechanics and histology of the myofascial tissue, it is now important to see how these tissues are affected by immobilization, trauma, and remobilization. This is essential so that realistic goals can be set in the clinic. It is important to remember that most of the available information on the effects of immobilization of connective tissue has come from research done on animals, most of which were normal and nontraumatized. This is fundamentally different from patients typically seen in a orthopedic clinic.[1]

Amiel et al. performed extensive animal studies on the immobilzation of connective tissue during the 1960s and 1970s.[8–13] Their studies typically involved immobilizing a normal animal knee then analyzing the histologic effects on connective tissue. The authors found fibrofatty infiltrates, primarily in the areas of capsular folds. With longer periods of immobilization greater amounts of infiltrate developed and adhesions began to form in the connective tissue.

Under histologic examination, no significant loss of collagen was found—only loss of ground substance (glycosaminoglycans and water). With the loss of ground substance came a decreased fiber distance, leading to cross-link development between collagen fibers. Immobilization leads to a lack of stress being applied to the collagen fibers, causing them to align in a haphazard fashion.[13] This alignment leads to a decreased tissue extensibility.[8–13] When immobilization occurs for less than 12 weeks, the rate of collagen synthesis and degradation are the same. After 12 weeks of immobilization, collagen degradation exceeds collagen synthesis, resulting in a net collagen loss.[14]

In a study by Evans et al, it was found that if rat knees were experimentally immobilized, then manipulated under high velocity, partial joint mobility could be restored. If these joints were allowed to move prior to manipulation, full mobility could then be restored. This held true for immobilization of less than 30 days. Longer periods of immobilization result in less optimal return of mobility.[13]

Other Physiologic Responses To Myofascial Manipulation

Soft tissue mobilization and massage are commonly used interchangeably. Additional effects of massage on the body have been well documented in the literature. Three secondary effects are on blood flow, the basal metabolism, and the autonomic system.

Massage has been shown to increase blood flow to the extremities. Deep massage strokes increase total blood flow in both animal and human subjects. Massage causes capillaries to dilate in the region of the stroking, resulting in increased blood volume and flow. Of significance is the fact that milder massage does not produce the same effect. The type and depth of the myofascial technique may alter the effect produced on the body.[15–17]

The autonomic system has also been shown to be effected by massage. Ebner reported that connective tissue massage stimulates circulation in a region of the body, which in turn opens up increased circulatory pathways to other body regions. The mechanical friction created by massage stimulates the mast cells in connective tissue to produce histamine. Histamine causes vasodilation, resulting in increased blood flow around the body.[18,19,22]

Myofascial Evaluation of the Shoulder

When evaluating the shoulder, the physical therapist is looking for a *correlation of findings* that might be indicative of a dysfunction. History, as well as the results from visual, movement, and palpatory exams, should be considered. It is important to remember that connective tissue changes, in the absence of other objective findings, are not necessarily dysfunctional. Several consistent findings are a better indicator of a problem. For example, consider a patient who presents with a stiff and painful shoulder. External rotation and abduction are most limited. Physical evaluation reveals tightness of the internal rotators and adductors, especially pectoralis major, latissimus dorsi, and teres major. Posturally, this patient assumes a protracted position. This combination of findings is indicative of a shoulder dysfunction possibly related to postural abnormalities. The individual findings of posture or tightness were not significant until they correlated with pain and loss of motion. Treatment must then address all the significant components contributing to the dysfunction.

HISTORY

History gives valuable insight into patient conditions before a hand ever touches them. For example, myofascial pain of nonmechanical origin is usually dull and nonspecific. Myofascial pain of mechanical origin is more specific. If a patient reports specific sharp pain that is easily reproduced, a more specific pathology may be present. By knowing the behavior of the patient's pain, we can begin to isolate the nature of the problem. We then move on to try to correlate the history with objective findings.

POSTURAL EVALUATION

Body posture can give us clues as to the area of movement disturbance or where the body may have excessive stress placed upon it. The importance of posture is in how it relates to function.

For the shoulder, we must consider the trunk and neck positions in both sitting and standing as well as the relationship of the scapulae relative to the trunk. The evaluator should be looking for areas of muscle or connective tissue asymmetry as well as increased muscle activity. Because fascial planes can be restricted over large areas of the body, a head to foot evaluation may be needed. If a leg length discrepancy exists, a patient may develop muscle asymmetry due to prolonged shortening or lengthening of a muscle or group of muscles.

Vladamir Janda helped demonstrate the effects of myofascial imbalances on postural imbalances. He looked extensively at how muscles respond to dysfunction. Janda observed that changes in muscle function play an important role on the pathogenesis of many painful conditions. Janda defined a *postural muscle* as one that responds to dysfunction by tightening and a *phasic muscle* as one that responds to dysfunction by weakening. In the upper extremity we see a typical pattern of tightening of the upper trapezius, levator scapulae, and pectoralis with weakening of the deep neck flexors and lower scapular stabilizers. All of these contribute to the typical kyphotic, protracted posture often seen in the clinic, (Table 15.2).[20,21]

Tight muscles tend to act in an inhibitory way on their antagonist muscles. It does not seem reasonable to start a strengthening program for the weakened antagonist as the first step in a rehabilitation program. After stretching of the tightened muscles, the strength of the inhibited muscles may return without any further treatment. In the case of a frozen shoulder patient, it would make sense to first stretch out the

TABLE 15.2. *Postural versus phasic muscles of the shoulder girdle and upper thoracic region*

POSTURAL	PHASIC
Upper trapezius	Latissimus dorsi
Levator scapulae	Lower trapezius
Pectoralis minor	Middle traps
Pectoralis major (upper portion)	Rhomboids
Cervical erector spinae	Anterior cervical musculature

shortened internal rotators and adductors like the subscapularis before attempting to strengthen the weakened external rotators and abductors.

MOVEMENT ANALYSIS

Active movement testing may provide further information with which to correlate postural findings. It is important to consider what is happening to the entire body when looking at active shoulder motion. *Quality* as well as quantity should be considered. Do limitations in range correlate to postural findings? For example, if on postural evaluation the patient was found to have a forward head position with pectoralis major and minor shortening, we may expect to see limited forward elevation of the shoulder.

Passive range of motion should also be for both quality and quantity of movement as well as for endfeel. Is the endfeel capsular, or is there limitation by soft tissue? Proper stabilization is necessary to achieve true range of motion and proper endfeel. See Chapter 3 for a detailed evaluation sequence.

PALPATORY EXAM

Now that posture and movement have been assessed, the examiner can begin to palpate for the location of the dysfunction. As previously mentioned, palpatory findings must also correlate with postural and movement findings to be of any significance. The palpatory exam includes the myofascial structures by layer and palpation of the joint structures. Palpation of the shoulder must include the scapular, cervical, thoracic, and anterior chest wall regions.

Superficial palpation is performed on the skin and superficial connective tissues. The examiner should be assessing for temperature, moisture, and light touch to determine the extensibility of the connective tissues. Tissue rolling is one way to check the extensibility of these structures. It involves the lifting away of the superficial connective tissue and skin from the underlying structures.

Deep palpation involves palpation through the layers of tissue perpendicular to the tissues as well as moving the perpendicular tissues. The examiner should be able to palpate the tendons, muscle bellies, muscle sheath, myotendinous junctions, joint capsule, tenoperiosteal junctions, and deep periosteal layers of tissue. To assess mobility of muscle, a technique called transverse muscle play may be used. This involves bending of the muscle to assess its transverse flexibility, (see Figs. 15.3 and 15.4). Palpatory findings will change with treatment, so it is important to be constantly reassessing.

Myofascial Techniques for the Shoulder

The following therapeutic techniques are just a few of many available treatments for the shoulder. These techniques have been chosen because of their effectiveness in the clinic as witnessed by the authors. It is important to remember that any technique can be modified to suit the patient problem or needs of the clinician.

POSITIONING OF THE PATIENT AND THERAPIST

Maximum effectiveness cannot be achieved if the technique is not efficiently executed. If a therapist is not properly positioned, the patient may not be able to relax, or the therapist may be putting undue stress on the patient's body. Remember to avoid needless body contact with the patient. A pillow between the patient and therapist can provide a mechanical barrier as needed.

JOINT PROTECTION

Because the hands are the primary tool of the manual therapist, it is essential to protect them. Here are a few general suggestions on how a manual therapist can protect the hands:

1. Avoid hyperflexion or hyperextension of the joints. This will decrease the problems of hypermobility and early arthritis.

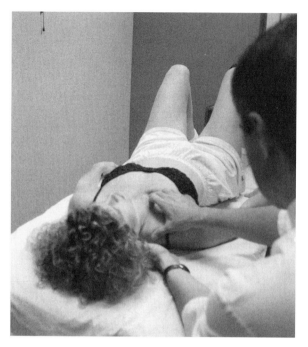

FIGURE 15.2

2. Use elbows, pisiforms, or fists on patients who are too large to safely use your fingers on. Be creative.

3. During off hours from work, try to rest your hands and protect them from excessive strain.

4. Use cold water rinses or short ice massage on your joints if inflammation occurs from vigorous treatment of a patient.

ANTEROPOSTERIOR LATERAL ELONGATION OF THE UPPER THORACIC REGION (FIG. 15.2)

Rationale

This technique is used for relaxing and lengthening the myofascia in the upper thoracic region and the shoulder girdle. This technique is of great value to patients who have protracted shoulder girdles. It should be used before trying to teach postural correction or strengthening.

Patient Position

Supine with the head in a neutral position on the treatment table.

Therapist Position

Seated near the patients' head at a 45° angle to the shoulder girdle.

Procedure

Begin stroking with the fingertips in a medial to lateral position. Once the glenohumeral joint is reached, replace the hands in the original position and repeat the stroke. The strokes may become progressively deeper.

TRANSVERSE MUSCLE PLAY OF THE PECTORALS (FIGS. 15.3, 15.4)

Rationale

Tightening of the pectorals is a common problem found in shoulder patients, especially those with the forward head posture. In order to achieve full shoulder range of motion and postural correction, the extensibility of these muscles must be restored.

Patient Position

Supine with the shoulder abducted to 90° to 120° (less flexion with frozen shoulders).

Therapist Position

Alongside the patient at a 45° angle to the shoulder girdle. The patient may rest the arm on the therapist's knee to achieve better relaxation. The thumbs are placed underneath the muscle and the fingers grasp from above.

Procedure

Gently lift and bend the pectoral muscle away from the anterior chest wall. Small oscillations can be performed as well as a static hold. Be careful to not contact breast tissue.

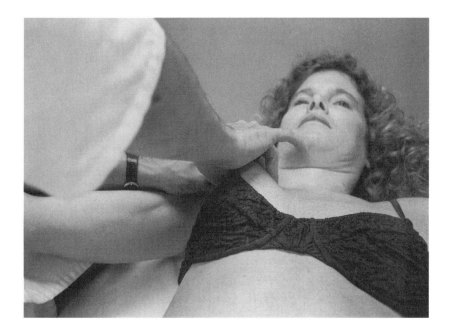

FIGURE 15.3

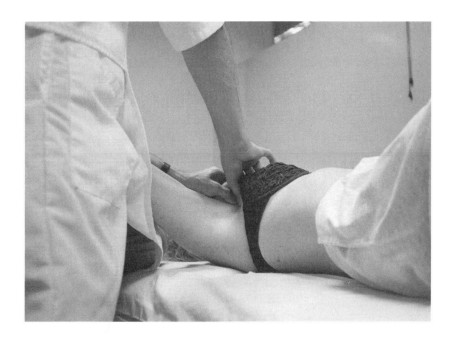

FIGURE 15.4

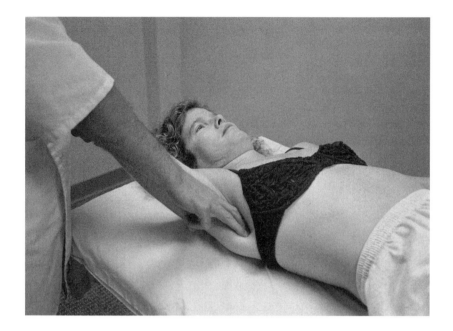

FIGURE 15.5

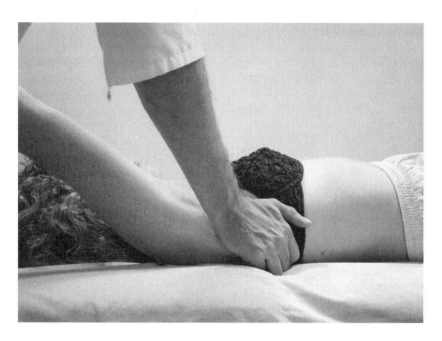

FIGURE 15.6

SUBSCAPULARIS TECHNIQUES (FIGS. 15.5, 15.6)

Rationale

The subscapularis muscle is often found to have significant restrictions in patients with decreased shoulder range of motion due to poor posture or immobilization. When full shoulder motion cannot be achieved, the therapist should recheck the subscapularis and the surrounding myofascia for trigger points or restrictions.

Patient Position

Supine with the arm abducted 30° to 60°. The arm may rest against the therapist for relaxation.

Therapist Position

Standing alongside the patient. One hand is placed from above into the belly of the subscapularis. The other hand may be used to stabilize the patient's arm, or it may be used to assist the upper hand in doing the mobilization.

Procedure 1

Small oscillations or sustained pressure can be used as a therapist applies moderate pressure into the subscapularis. The bottom hand may grasp from beneath to perform a muscle play technique.

Procedure 2

The patient's arm is elevated into flexion and gently distracted. The therapist places the palm of the hand along the lateral border of the scapula. Gentle stroking in a caudal direction is applied with the palm. If more specific fascial restrictions exist, the fingertips may be used to provide a static or oscillatory pressure.

ANTEROLATERAL FASCIAL ELONGATION (FIG. 15.7)

Rationale

This technique elongates the superficial anterior fascia, which is often restricted in patients with a protracted shoulder girdle position.

Patient Position

Supine with the shoulder elevated 120° to 160° depending on the area of restriction.

Therapist Position

At the top of the bed, grasping the patient's arm and providing a gentle upward distraction. The palm of the upper arm is placed just below the breast line. Be sure of proper draping and appropriate hand placement when performing this technique.

Procedure

The therapist applies a stronger tractioning force on the flexed arm while the lower arm tractions in the direction of the umbilicus. The direction of force may be changed to accommodate the existing restrictions. Lubricants should not be used to prevent shear force.

ROTATIONAL THORACIC LAMINAR RELEASE (FIG. 15.8)

Rationale

To mobilize the paravertebral and periscapular muscles into rotation. This is a deeper technique than those already described.

Patient Position

Sidelying with the head supported and the upper arm resting on the side of the body.

Therapist Position

Directly facing the patient with a pillow fit snugly between therapist and patient. The lower hand is placed along the paravertebral muscles near the medial border of the scapula. The upper hand rests on the glenohumeral joint.

Procedure

The fingers of the lower hand apply a deep pressure in a sweeping downward motion, while the upper hand retracts the shoulder girdle and

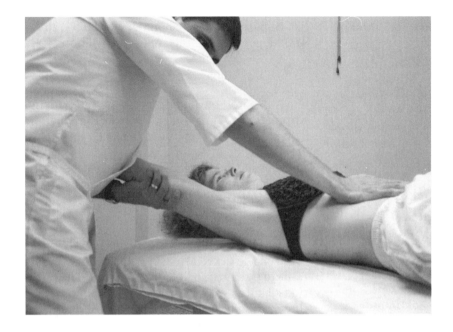

FIGURE 15.7

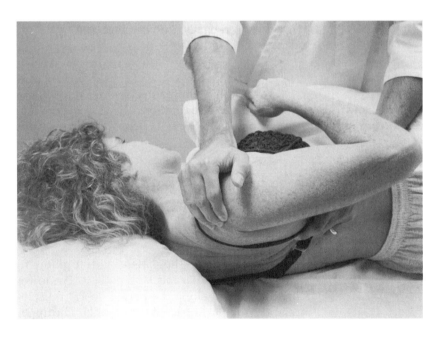

FIGURE 15.8

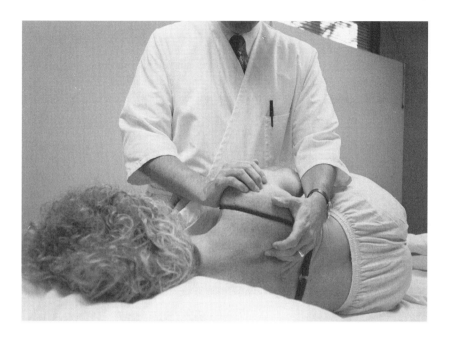

FIGURE 15.9

applies a rotational force through the thoracic spine.

SCAPULAR FRAMING (FIGS. 15.9 TO 15.11)

Rationale

A commonly performed technique that decreases tone in the periscapular muscles and prepares the scapulothoracic tissues for aggressive stretching.

Patient Position

Lying on the side facing the therapist, with a pillow separating the two. The patient's arm should be resting comfortably on the pillow.

Therapist Position

Standing facing the patient with the upper hand placed on the anterior acromion.

Procedure for Medial Border

Place the fingers of the lower hand gently along the medial border of the scapula. Gently retract the shoulder with the upper hand, and then stroke in a downward direction along the border of the scapula with the lower hand.

Procedure for Lateral Border

Place the palm of the lower hand over the acromion to stabilize the joint. The palm of the upper hand is placed over the lateral border of the scapula, and then strokes caudally with a firm pressure down the length of the border.

Procedure for Superior Border

Place the fingertips of both hands medial to the cervicothoracic junction over the upper trapezius. Stroke outward toward the acromion with a firm pressure. If needed, a gentle stretch performed with the palm of the hand can be given at the end of the stroke.

SCAPULAR MOBILIZATION (FIG. 15.12)

Rationale

To mobilize the scapula off the rib cage in order to stretch the surrounding myofascia. This technique should be done after there has been preparation of the tissues by scapular framing.

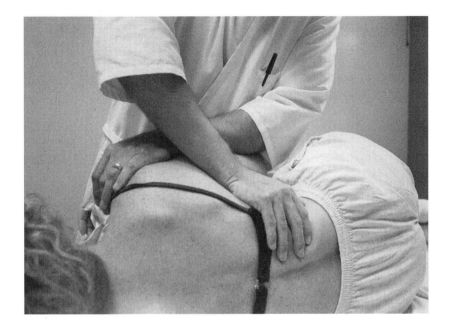

FIGURE 15.10

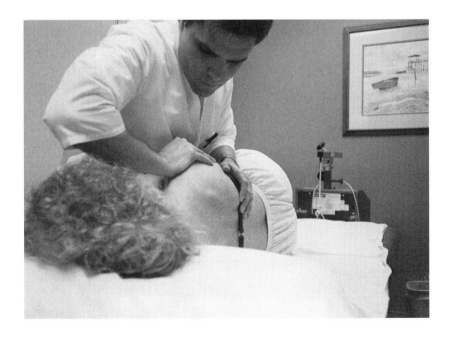

FIGURE 15.11

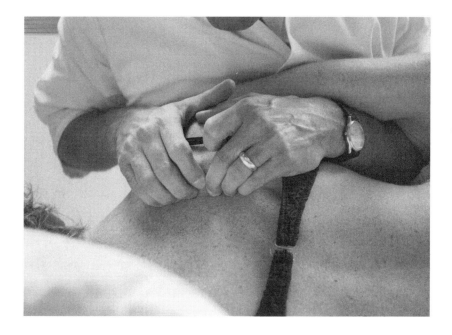

FIGURE 15.12

Patient Position

The patient is lying on the side facing the therapist, with a pillow separating the two.

Therapist Position

Standing directly in front of the patient with the top hand placed on the anterior shoulder joint. The fingers of the bottom hand lightly grasp the medial border of the scapula.

Procedure

Lift the scapula and shoulder girdle complex off of the thoracic rib cage. If the patient is larger, two hands may be needed.

SEATED PECTORAL AND ANTERIOR FASCIAL STRETCHES (FIGS. 15.13 TO 15.15)

Rationale

Sometimes patients are better able to relax in the seated position. These stretches can be used to elongate the anterior fascia and pectoral muscles to allow for better posture and improved shoulder range of motion.

Patient Position

Seated with the hands behind the head.

Therapist Position

Standing directly behind the patient with either the knee or hip stabilizing the thoracic region. As previously mentioned, a pillow should be placed between therapist and patient. The therapist grasps the patient just below the elbows.

Procedure 1

A posterior force towards the patient's head is applied while the patient takes deep breaths to improve anterior elongation. To incorporate the lateral fascia and muscles, the patient can be asked to lean or rotate to one side while the same force is applied. The patient's arms may also be fully extended for this technique.

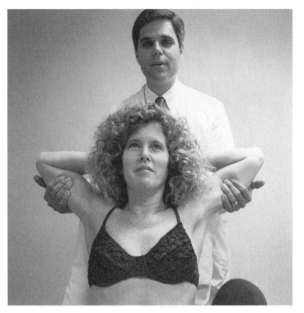

FIGURE 15.13

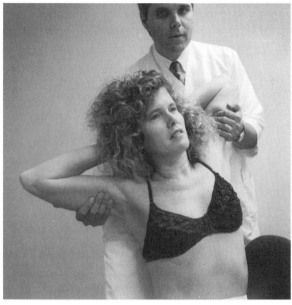

FIGURE 15.15

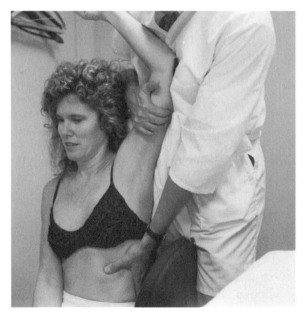

FIGURE 15.14

Procedure 2

The patient may have only one arm extended upwards, while the therapist places one hand along the lateral rib cage and the other just below the elbow. A traction force is then applied in opposite directions. A rotary component can also be added using the technique stated above.

CROSS-FRICTION OF SUPRASPINATUS AND BICEPS TENDON (FIG. 15.16)

Rationale

Cross-friction is used to increase local blood flow to enhance the rate of healing. It is very effective in treating tendonitis of the biceps or supraspinatus.

Patient Position

Supine with the arm abducted 30° and the elbow bent.

Therapist Position

At the patient's side supporting the arm with the bottom hand. The thumb of the top hand is in the bicipital groove.

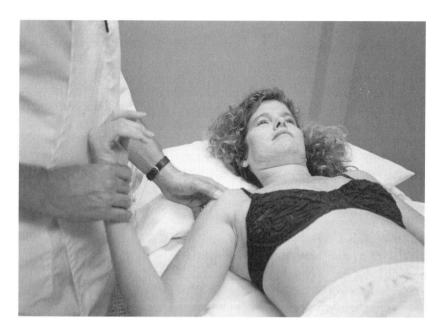

FIGURE 15.16

Procedure

The therapist may alternately laterally and medially rotate the shoulder to create some gentle friction. Direct friction over the bicipital groove is applied with the thumb. The second and third fingers with slight flexion at the distal interphalangeal joints may also be used if the patient is less acute. To friction the supraspinatus, the therapist abducts the shoulder 80° to 90° and palpates the notch formed by the acromion spine and the clavicle. The musculotendinous junction lies here. Use the same technique as described earlier.

CASE STUDY

A 34-year-old female patient presents at our clinic with an 8-week history of left shoulder pain following a fall. She has a history of a Bankart repair to the same shoulder in 1990 after an injury sustained in a motor vehicle accident. The orthopedist has ruled out injury to the prior repair as cause for her pain. On evaluation she presents with atrophy of the rhomboids and lower trapezius. Significant increase in tone is present in the upper trapezius, levator scapulae, and pectoral muscles. Cervical range of motion is limited by 25 percent into rotation and sidebending to the right. Left shoulder active range of motion is 100° of flexion, 90° of abduction, and 45° of external rotation. Passive range of motion is 100° of flexion, 90° of abduction, and 55° of external rotation with pain before end-range. There are multiple tender spots in the upper thoracic, scapulothoracic, and anterior chest wall regions. The acromioclavicular joint is painful to palpation and to internal rotation and adduction movements.

PATIENT PROBLEMS

1. Increased tone in the upper trapezius
2. Increased tone in the rhomboids
3. Increased tone in the levator scapulae
4. Increased tone in the pectorals
5. Decreased range of motion of the left shoulder
6. AC joint pain
7. Trigger points in the U/T and scapulothoracic regions

8. Restrictions in the anterior chest wall myo-fascia

9. Decreased cervical range of motion

From a myofascial standpoint, a good way to begin treatment of this patient would be to address these components prior to range of motion or strength. The previously discussed techniques might be incorporated into treatment of this patient in the following way.

1. Increased pectoral tone: pectoral muscle play
2. Restricted anterior chest wall: anterior fascial elongation with or without a rotary component
3. Periscapular restrictions: scapular framing, scapular mobilization, subscapularis release
4. Increased tone in upper thoracic region/upper trapezius: anterior/posterior lateral elongation of upper thoracic region
5. Increased tone in paravertebral muscles: rotational thoracic laminar release

After performing each myofascial technique, reassess the patient's range of motion to see what effect the treatment has made. Large increases in range can be achieved through the performance of myofascial techniques without ever performing true range of motion or joint mobilization of the glenohumeral joint. Once the myofascial restrictions are eliminated and the range of motion is improved, begin strengthening exercises if they are still required. Consider each patient's problems individually, continually reassessing the causes of limitation. Use these findings to guide your choice of treatment approach. If one approach is not working, consider a change in technique. Remember that the aforementioned techniques are only a small sample of available treatments.

In the case of this patient, myofascial treatment assisted in the ability to isolate the primary problem. On initial evaluation there was too much muscle guarding and myofascial restrictions to identify the cause of this patient's pain. After 4 treatment sessions using the discussed techniques, this patients pain centralized to the

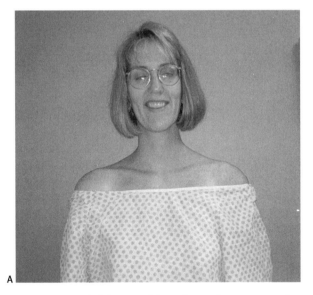
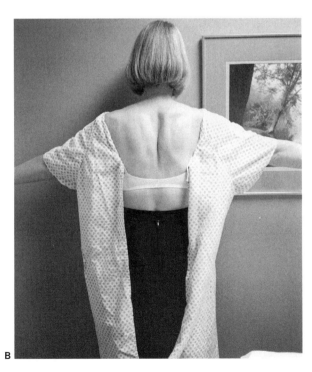

FIGURE 15.17 *A 34-year-old patient who presented with an 8-week history of left shoulder pain following a fall.* **(A & B)** *Presentation of the patient after the first four treatment sessions.*

acromioclavicular joint. This problem could not have been easily identified early on due to the protective muscular responses of the body. Once those protective mechanisms were removed, the problem became obvious. Figure 15.17 show, the presentation of the patient after the first 4 treatment sessions. At this point, the positions of the scapula and clavicle have moved closer to normal and the prominence of the acromioclavicular joint has become more obvious. The patient was referred back to the orthopedist for closer examination of the AC joint.

References

1. Cantu R, Grodin A: Myofascial Manipulation. Aspen Publishing, Gaithersburg, UD, 1992
2. Dicke E, Schliack H, Wolff A: A Manual of Reflexive Therapy. S Simon Publishing, Scarsdale, NY, 1978
3. Ham AW, Cormack DH: Histology. JB Lippincott, Philadelphia, 1979
4. Copenhaver WM, Bunge RP, Runge R et al: Bailey's Textbook of Histology. Williams & Wilkins, Baltimore, 1975
5. Warwick R, Williams PL: Gray's Anatomy. p. 32. 3rd British Ed. WB Saunders, Philadelphia, 1973
6. Cummings G: Soft Tissue Changes in Contracture. Stokesville Publishing, Atlanta, 1985
7. Grodin A, Cantu R: Myofascial Manipulation: Theory and Clinical Management. Forum Medicum, Berryville, VA, 1989
8. Woo S, Matthews JV, Akason WH et al: Connective Tissue Response to Immobility. Arthritis Rheum 18:257, 1975
9. Akeson WH, Woo SL, Amial D et al: The connective tissue response to immobilization: biomechanical changes in periarticular connective tissue of the rabbit knee. Clin Orthop 93:356, 1973
10. Akeson WH, Amial D, LaViolette D et al: The connective tissue response to immobilitiy: an accelerated aging response. Exp Gerontol 3:289, 1968
11. Akeson WH, Amial D, Mechanic GL et al: Collagen cross-linking alterations in joint contractures. Connective Tissue Res 5:15, 1977
12. Akeson WH, Amial D: Immobility effects of synovial joints: the pathomechanics of joint contracture. Biorheology 17:95, 1980
13. Evans E, Eggers G, Butler JK et al: Experimental immobilization and mobilization of rat knee joints. J Bone Joint Surg 42A:737, 1960
14. Amial D, Akeson WH, Woo S et al: Stress deprivation effect on metabolic turnover of medial collateral ligament collagen. Clin Orthop 172:265, 1983
15. Laban MM: Collagen tissue: implications of its response to stress in vitro. Arch Phys Med Rehabil 43:461, 1962
16. Neuberger A, Slack H: The metabolism of collagen from liver, bones, skin and tendon in normal rats. Biochem J 53:47, 1953
17. Frankel VH, Nordin M. Basic Biomechanics of the Skeletal System. p. 90. Lea and Febinger, Philadelphia, 1980
18. Wakim KG: The effects of massage on the circulation of normal and paralyzed extremities. Arch Phys Med Rehabil 30:135, 1949
19. Wolfson H: Studies on the effect of physical therapeutic procedures on function and structure. JAMA 96:2020, 1931
20. Martin GM, Roth GM, Elkins C, Krusen F: Cutaneous temperature of the extremities of normal subjects and patients with rheumatoid arthritis. Arch Phys Med Rehabil 27:665, 1946
21. Cuthbertson DP: Effects of massage on metabolism. Glasgow Med J 2:200, 1933
22. Ebner M: Connective Tissue Manipulation. Kreiger Publishing, Malabar, FL, 1985
23. Janda B: Central nervous motor regulation and back problems. p. 28. In IM Korr (ed): The Neurobiologic Mechanisms in Manipulative Therapy. Plenum Press, New York, 1978
24. Donatelli R, Wooden M: Orthopaedic Physical Therapy. p. 151. Churchill Livingstone, New York, 1989

16

Isokinetic Evaluation and Treatment

MARK S. ALBERT

MICHAEL J. WOODEN

Isokinetic exercise has become a popular form of resistive exercise in the physical therapy clinic. Since the late 1960s, the literature has consisted primarily of research data and clinical information relating to the knee. However, recent advances in equipment have made it possible to use positioning to apply isokinetics effectively to most other extremity joints, including the shoulder complex. The purposes of this chapter are to list some advantages of isokinetics in shoulder evaluation and treatment, to describe the adaptability of several dynamometers to shoulder diagonal patterns, to discuss principles of isokinetic testing and training with emphasis on shoulder positioning, and to describe considerations of test data interpretation.

Practical Advantages of Isokinetics

Isokinetic exercise, unlike isotonic exercise, offers totally accommodating resistance to a muscular contraction.[1-3] Because the speed of movement is constant, resistance to the movement varies according to the amount of force applied to the resistance arm. Therefore, in a maximum-effort isokinetic contraction, the muscle is loaded maximally at each point in the range of motion (ROM).[1-3]

With isotonic equipment or free weights, because the speed of movement is not preset, resistance to muscle contraction will vary according to gravity, positioning, lever arm lengths (in the equipment and in the patient's limbs), and cam sizes.[3] If, because of these factors, effective resistance occurs only at a certain point in the range, it is possible that the muscle is being strengthened only at that point. Consequently, isokinetic exercise offers the advantage of loading a muscle effectively throughout its ROM by fixing the speed of movement.

Isokinetics offers several other clinical advantages, such as the capacity for a wide range of speeds, both for testing muscle function and for rehabilitation or strength training.[4] This allows the clinician to determine at what velocities muscle torque deficits occur: at low speeds (so-called "strength" deficits), or high speeds ("power" and "endurance" deficits).[2] Testing and training at higher speed attempts to simulate normal activities in which angular velocities (as in walking, running, swimming, throwing, and other activities) are far in excess of most isotonic speeds.[3] Even the highest speeds of the MERAC (Universal Corp., Cedar Rapids, IA), at 500°/s, are not fast enough to match many activities, especially sports activities. However, exercising at different speeds may cause quantitative and qualitative recruitment of different muscle fiber types: therefore, most or all of the muscle can be loaded.[5-8]

Increases in speed of isokinetic concentric contraction are associated with decreases in both torque output and electromyographic activity of the muscle.[1,5-8] Therefore, compressive reaction forces at the joint should also decrease. In joints that exhibit an inflamed or painful response to exercise, increasing the speed may temporarily "spare the joint" by reducing joint reaction forces. Whether training solely at high speeds contributes to an increase of strength at low speeds is controversial, however.[4,5] Nevertheless, the use of higher speeds is an important safety factor in reactive joint conditions, provided that concentric isokinetic contraction is used.

Whether at fast or slow speeds, isokinetic resistance will accommodate to pain levels, further ensuring safety, because if the patient needs to decrease or stop the contraction suddenly because of pain, the resistance will decrease immediately, because resistance will never exceed the amount of force applied.[3] Unlike isotonic exercise, miminal momentum is produced with isokinetics. The use of submaximal effort isokinetics also enhances safety in cases of patient pain or reactive joint inflammation. Decreasing the force used in isokinetic resistance exercise will, in turn, decrease joint reaction forces as produced in submaximal effort. Submaximal effort training may also produce pain reduction selective recruitment of muscle fiber type (slow twitch or type I), and improved joint lubrication. In addition to the advantages already discussed, Davies[3] cites many other physiologic and clinical advantages of isokinetics. As with all types (or modes) of clinical muscle training, isokinetics possesses several disadvantages or precautions, which will be discussed in the next section. For example, a major physiologic limitation of Cybex systems prior to the 6000 model was an inability to exercise and measure muscle eccentrically. Because muscle generates the most amount of tension eccentrically[9] and because much of functional movement requires eccentric contraction, rehabilitation and testing of the glenohumeral joint in an eccentric mode have important applications and have received increasing emphasis

from clinicians and investigators.[10-13] Isotonic exercise incorporates eccentric muscle loading; however, for reasons previously stated, it does not fully accommodate for length–tension changes nor does it adequately control momentum or force vector problems. With the advent of recent technology in dynamometry, instruments such as the Kincom (Chattanooga Corp., Chattanooga, TN), Biodex (Biodex, Shirley, NY), and Lido (Loredan Biomedical, Davis, CA) have the capability of applying eccentric isokinetic loading with the inherent length–tension accommodation. Controversy exists as to the safety of robotic instruments when applied to human subjects, and continued research is needed to clarify this issue. A key concept to robotic testing and training involves thorough understanding of the alterations in the force–velocity curve that are produced by robotics.

Another consideration is that the resistance mechanism, at least on Cybex equipment, is uniaxial. Extremity joints, of course, are multiaxial, as their instantaneous centers of rotation change constantly through movement.[10-14] The extensive mobility of the shoulder and the multiple articulations within the shoulder complex further complicate the appropriate alignment of the machine axis with the changing, compromised axis of the patient's shoulder.

Other practical disadvantages of isokinetics in the clinic include the high cost of equipment, the amount of floor space required, and the time required to change positions and attachments to test the different movements. The latter is a particular problem with shoulder evaluation, because so many positions and motions are recommended. Testing of diagonal patterns reduces the time required for multiple dynamometer position changes, while assessing multiple muscle groups.

The testing and training protocols implemented before readiness for diagonal patterns require decisions about the positioning of the glenohumeral joint. To protect injured tissues while maintaining effective strengthening techniques, several important biomechanical principles warrant consideration. The 90° abducted position (90° AP) as described in the Cybex manual[4] can produce optimal external rotation torque and work values.[12,15] In addition, the proximity of the position may risk glenohumeral joint impingement.[15–18] The 90° AP also involves long-lever arm forces that are contraindicated in cases of joint instability and significant rotator cuff weakness.[19] The 90° AP is deleterious when restricted internal rotation ROM is present,[20] as torsion forces are transmitted from the scapula through the coracoclavicular ligaments into the acromioclavicular joint.

In contrast, the neutral position (elbow adducted close to the patient's chest wall) produces the optimal internal rotation torque values as well as high external rotation values. Two negative considerations of this position are the microvascular wringing out effect,[3,21] which deprives the active supraspinatus of necessary blood flow, and stress on the anterior capsular mechanism with forced stretching of the often inflexible subscapularis muscle (more often a significant problem in males).

Both Hinton[12] and Soderberg and Blaschak[15] suggest the need for multiple positions for testing and training and, not surprisingly, that no single patient or glenohumeral position is optimal for all clinical purposes. However, a compromise position that is safe from both vascular and biomechanical perspectives is the intermediate, or 45°, abducted position. Although Hageman et al.[22] found high concentric and eccentric torque values for both external and internal rotation at 45° AP, appropriate protection for both the anterior and posterior capsular and labral mechanisms also was found to exist. Interestingly, the 45° AP closely simulates the modified base position advocated by Davies[3] and can be readily adapted to conform to the plane of the scapula, which creates low capsular stress and produces peak isokinetic rotator cuff torque.[23,24] The 45° AP is also simply applied to all dynamometer setup capacities, with minor patient position or machine adjustments. Finally, the 45° AP positions conform closely to the natural, functional plane of motion (the plane of the scapula), and consequently provide a comfortable training position for most patients with pain, restrictions, and/or rotator cuff suppression.

Evaluation of Shoulder Diagonals

The Cybex II manual contains detailed information on testing all the cardinal plane movements of the shoulder.[4] Photographs and descriptions of positioning and machine settings allow for isolated testing of abduction, adduction, flexion, extension, and internal and external rotation. These procedures provide excellent information on specific muscles or muscle groups and are indicated for certain pathologies. The process of testing all of these movements as part of a comprehensive shoulder evaluation is quite time-consuming, however, and can be clinically unmanageable. Excessively high charges and questionable validity of multiple glenohumeral muscle measurement pose further arguments against multiple movement testing. The time management problem can be solved by evaluating overall muscle function with two diagonal movements, thus eliminating several lengthy steps.

In addition to its practical benefits, diagonal movement testing may also be more functional than cardinal plane movements, which fail to isolate and measure motion of the acromioclavicular, sternoclavicular, and scapulothoracic joints.[4] Of course, movement of these joints occurs throughout the range of glenohumeral motion. Resisted diagonal movement will load muscles that effect movement at all joints in the shoulder girdle. Knott and Voss,[25] pioneers in proprioceptive neuromuscular facilitation (PNF), first described "mass movement patterns" as being inherently diagonal in nature. These diagonals are dictated by anatomy—shapes of joints, lines of muscle pull, and soft tissue restrictions—and are those movements observed to be most used in everyday activities.[25] The movements to be described in this chapter are similar to the classic upper extremity PNF patterns.

Testing Procedure

The first diagonal movement described is the combination of extension, abduction, internal rotation (Ext/Abd/IR) and flexion, adduction, ex-

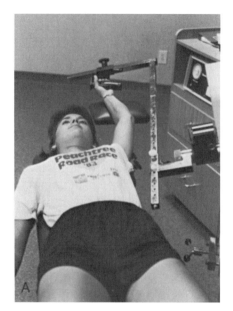

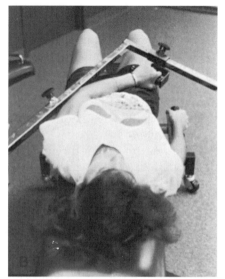

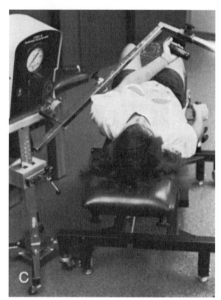

FIGURE 16.1 **(A)** *Initiation of the diagonal movement Ext/Abd/IR.* **(B)** *End of diagonal movement Ext/Abd/IR.* **(C)** *End of diagonal movement Flex/Add/ER.*

ternal rotation (Flex/Add/ER). Figure 16.1A shows the initiation of the Ext/Abd/IR movement, and Figure 16.1B shows the end of that same diagonal, blocked manually to prevent hyperextension. Figure 16.1C illustrates the end positions for the Flex/Add/ER movement.

For both movements, the patient is in-structed to try to keep the elbow straight and to rotate the arm internally or externally, depending on which movement is being performed. To allow for rotation, a swivel handle is used. It should be pointed out, however, that the rotational component cannot be resisted by the apparatus, as would be the case if manual resistance

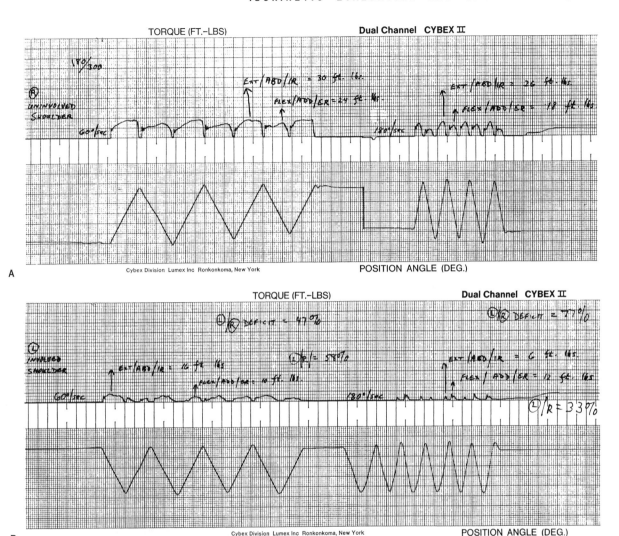

FIGURE 16.2 **(A)** *Torque curves of uninvolved shoulder for Ext/Abd/IR and Flex/Add/ER.* **(B)** *Torque curves of involved shoulder for Ext/Abd/IR and Flex/Add/ER.*

were used in PNF.[25] The dynamometer is tipped forward 15° to account for trunk movement and the forward-inclined plane of the scapula.[23,26]

Figure 16.2A is the normal torque curve for the diagonal Ext/Abd/IR and Flex/Add/ER in a postanterior dislocation patient who has recovered most of her ROM. The shoulder is tested at 60°/s (low speed) and 180°/s (high speed), the speeds recommended by Cybex for flexion and extension.[4] An athlete or unusually strong person can also be tested at higher speeds as long as measurable torque is being produced. Figure 16.2B represents the torque curve for the injured side in the same patient. The lower foot-pound readings for the "left involved shoulder" indicate strength deficits, at low and high speeds, ranging from 33 to 77 percent. Table 16.1 gives a summary of the torque measurements taken from Figure 16.2.

Not only can strength deficits be computed,

TABLE 16.1 *Summary of peak torque deficits*

DIAGONAL	SPEED	RIGHT UNINVOLVED (FT-LB)	LEFT UNINVOLVED (FT-LB)	DEFICIT (%)
Ext/Abd/IR	60°/s	30	16	47
	180°/s	26	6	77
Flex/Add/ER	60°/s	24	10	58
	180°/s	18	12	33

(Data from Figure 16.2)

but the shapes of the torque curves in Figure 16.2 can also be compared. The low-speed curves (60°/s) for the involved shoulder show a slower "rate of rise" than for the normal side. That is, the weaker side took longer to reach its peak torque. In addition, the duration of each Ext/Abd/IR and Flex/Add/ER contraction at low and high speed is shorter, as compared with the opposite side, indicating the inability to sustain tension. These variations in curve shape are further indications of muscle weak-

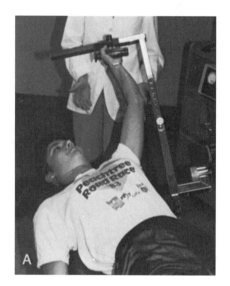

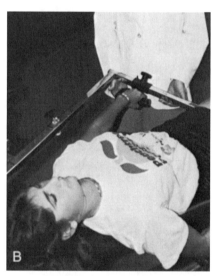

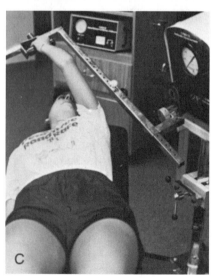

FIGURE 16.3 **(A)** *Initiation of diagonal movement Ext/Add/IR.* **(B)** *End of diagonal movement Ext/Add/IR.* **(C)** *Initiation of diagonal movement Flex/Abd/ER.*

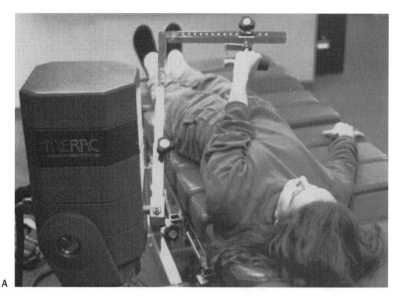

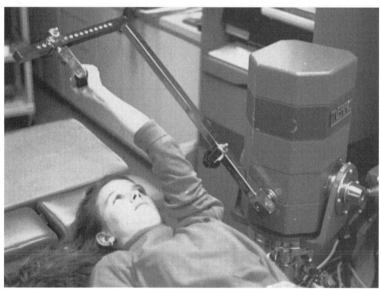

FIGURE 16.4 *MERAC isokinetic diagonal patterns.* **(A)** *Initiation of diagonal movement Ext/Add/IR.* **(B)** *End of diagonal movement Ext/Add/IR.*

ness that should improve after appropriate isokinetic training. Last, a comparison of the lower "position angle" scale indicates limitations at the extremes of ROM, although in this case the differences are slight.

This evaluation procedure can also be done for a second diagonal, the combination of Ext/Add/IR and Flex/Abd/ER. The sequence of these movements is illustrated in Figure 16.3. The start and finish positions for Ext/Add/IR are shown in Figure 16.3A and B, and Figure 16.4A and B, and initiation of Flex/Abd/ER is shown in Figure 16.3C. In this diagonal, the extreme of the flexion movement was blocked either manually or, as shown, using UBXT (Cybex, Ronkonkoma, NY) attachments. Torque deficit computation and shape of curve comparisons were done as previously described.

Interpretation of Isokinetic Test Parameters

Traditional clinical practice with isokinetics has focused on the knee, with consideration of a specific agonist to antagonist torque ratio (hamstring to quadriceps) as a key clinical parameter. Similarly, the glenohumeral joint presents a key clinical parameter with external rotation to internal rotation (ER/IR) torque ratios expressed as a percentage. Two studies[27,28] have reported ER/IR ratios of 80 percent or greater; however, most studies[3,12,13,15,18,29,33] have consistently demonstrated normative ratios of 60 percent to 70 percent Table 16.2. Consequently, the ER/IR ratio of 60 percent to 70 percent provides a basis for clinical description of normal force couple synergy and muscular tension capacity. The parameters of total work and endurance should also be examined, as they provide an additional perspective for clinical decision making and discharge status, and perhaps have greater functional significance than peak torque values.[19]

Because the upper extremity muscles are smaller in cross-sectional area than most lower extremity muscles, they tend to demonstrate smaller normative peak torque to body weight (PT/BW) relationships. The strongest muscle groups of the upper extremity also produce the highest PT/BW ratios: 45 percent to 56 percent for adductors and 25 to 26 percent for abductors, as consistently reported by Davies[3] and Alderink and Kuck.[13] No consensus regarding external rotation and internal rotation PT/BW ratios has been reported, with external rotation values ranging from 8 percent to 16 percent and internal rotation values ranging from 13 to 22 percent.[3,13,18]

The limited number of studies regarding shoulder isokinetic parameters and normative data have been performed with a variety of patient populations (mostly small numbers), differing test speeds and dynamometers, inconsistent methodology, and varied patient positions. Consequently, applying the normative data to a given population or to predicting functional progress or discharge status must be done with caution.

TABLE 16.2 *Comparisons of upper-extremity muscle torque*

STUDY	SUBJECTS	SPEEDS	FLEXION/ EXTENSION	ABDUCTORS/ ADDUCTORS	EXTERNAL ROTATION/ INTERNAL ROTATION
Cook et al.[27]	Male pitchers and nonpitchers	180°/s	70–81% 76–99%	NA	70–81% 81%[a]
Soderberg and Blaschak[15]	Males, nonathletes	60°, 180°, 300°/s	NA	NA	57–69%
Davies[3] (Ch. 12)	20 Males and females	60° and 300°/s	60% Males, 48% females	66% Males, 52% females	64%[a]
Ivey et al.[29]	31 Normals, mixed activity	60° and 180°/s	66% Males, 73% females	61% Males, 57% females	67%[a]
Alderink and Kuck[13]	24 Males, high school and college pitchers	90°, 120°, 180°, and 300°/s	48–55%	50–57%	66–76%[a]
Hinton[12]	26 Pitchers, high school	90° and 240°/s	NA	NA	56–62%[a]
Connelly-Maddux et al.[18]	21 Males, 20 females	60°/s	NA	NA	63% Males, 71% females

NA, not available.
[a] *Data from 90° shoulder abducted position.*

However, useful and consistent concepts have emerged from available isokinetic normative shoulder studies that provide general guidelines for clinical decision making.

Bilateral comparison testing, in which peak torque at the injured joint is expressed as a percentage of deficit compared with the uninvolved ("normal") side, is one method of interpretation of isokinetic test data commonly used in the clinical setting. Unfortunately, this method fails to account for differences in strength that may arise from hand dominance, sports activity, occupational demands, and preexisting injury. Common disagreements on whether strength differences occur between the dominant and nondominant sides provide a dilemma for clinical consideration. Ivey et al.,[29] Connelly-maddux et al.,[18] and Reid et al.[28] found no statistical difference between dominant and nondominant sides, while Alderinck and Kuck[13] concurred with the exception of shoulder adductors and extensors. In contrast, Cook et al.[27] and Coleman[30] described strength differences between sides in baseball throwers, and Davies[3] determined 10 to 25 percent differences between nondominant and dominant extremities. Perhaps, then, a small strength difference should be expected in a patient with vigorous and repetitive occupational or sports use of the dominant arm, but normal use in activities of daily living (ADLs) does not produce an expectation for greater peak torque of the dominant side.

When possible, industrial or sports pre-screening with isokinetic testing provides an ideal situation to establish "normal" values for a given individual that are useful if injury or dysfunction occurs.

Treatment Protocols

In general, isokinetic rehabilitation of the shoulder can be initiated when the joint complex has progressed to tolerance of resisted exercise through a given ROM. Fractures, dislocations, muscle tears, and other soft tissue injuries should be well healed, stable, and past the acute

TABLE 16.3 *Exercise progression based on the time/healing stages (earliest to latest)*

Multiple-angle isometrics (submaximal effort)
Multiple-angle isometrics (maximal), inertial
Short-arc concentric isokinetics (submaximal), inertial
Short-arc isotonics
Short-arc concentric isokinetics (maximal)
Full ROM concentric isokinetics (submaximal)
Full ROM isotonics
Full ROM concentric isokinetics (maximal)

(Adapted from Davies,[3] with permission.)

stage. Although full active ROM is not required, it should be painless at its extremes. In postsurgical cases, knowledge of the surgical procedure (review of the dictated surgical report is extremely helpful) is essential in determining direction of resisted movement. Table 16.3 reviews resistive exercise progressions that are effective preparatory stages for isokinetics and indicates the appropriate timing of isokinetic resistance modes.

Isokinetic training should be applied after consideration of patient position, dynamometer position, and attachments. In addition, the patient's scapular control, parameters of repetition, rest periods, speeds, allowable ROM for the particular pathology, and stage of healing should be considered.

Despite careful clinical planning with isokinetics, some patients will respond negatively with varied inflammatory responses of the tendon, capsule, and synovium, requiring immediate treatment. The use of cryotherapy postisokinetics is useful to prevent such symptomatic responses. Our clinical experience, in agreement with Engle and Canner,[19] indicates that each isokinetic training session should be followed by continual reassessment of program tolerance and results, and progression to more challenging training should be preceded by two or three trial sessions of fixed intensity.

In all cases of painful arc, joint restriction, and instability, appropriate use of stops to block movement is necessary, especially when using faster speeds in excess of 180°/s. Blocking may be produced manually or as a function of the dynamometer with mechanical or electronic technology. Each patient problem dictates individualized blocking; however, anterior glenohumeral instability problems require restriction of external rotation with abduction, while posterior instability requires restriction of internal rotation with flexion.

In choosing which speed to use in isokinetic rehabilitation, several criteria are used. The most simple determination is based on the evaluation. For the most part, low-speed torque deficits require low-speed training, whereas faster speeds are used for high-speed deficits. Often, however, deficits occur at both testing speeds, as the curves in Figure 16.2 indicate. In this case, a helpful guideline is the "25 percent rule." That is, if the strength deficit at the 60°/s testing speed is greater than 25 percent, rehabilitation at that speed is indicated. If the deficit is less than 25 percent at the lower testing speed, training should be at 180°/s or faster.

There are several exceptions to this rule. As mentioned previously, the need to reduce joint reaction forces may necessitate high-speed training even though major deficits at the low testing speed are found. The same is true for a painful joint when the patient will not tolerate movement at the indicated speed. Contractile pain is usually less at faster speeds, although occasionally slow-speed exercise is tolerated better. Other ways of lessening pain include submaximum effort and short-arc contraction, which avoids pain localized to a portion of the ROM. Some general guidelines for selecting speeds and pain-reducing protocols are listed in Table 16.4. Submaximum effort training is sometimes done for a few treatment sessions prior to actual testing of a patient who is not yet ready for the maximum effort contractions that are necessary for bilateral strength comparisons. Eccentric isokinetics also present a major contrast to concentric speed selection. Because of inherent force–velocity curve differences between eccentric and concentrics, eccentrics speeds for the shoulder must be much slower for both early and advanced applications. A useful clinical speed spectrum for a variety of diagnostic and patient con-

TABLE 16.4 *Guidelines for isokinetic speed and protocol selection in shoulder rehabilitation*

ISOKINETIC SPEED	PROTOCOL
60°/s	1. Strength deficit > 25% 2. Patient too weak to generate torque at higher speeds 3. High-speed movement too painful)
180°/s	1. Strength deficit < 25 2. Low-speed contraction too painful 3. Decrease joint reaction forces
Velocity spectrum protocol	Train at several speeds; simulate speeds used in normal activities
Short-arc contraction	To avoid painful ranges; possible instability at end range
Submaximum effort contraction	1. Not ready for maximum effort at any speed due to pain, inflammation, incomplete healing, etc. 2. Poor tolerance to initial test done at maximum effort

siderations is 30°/s to 180°/s with common starting speeds of 60°/s to 120°/s.

General Test and Warm-Up Considerations

Before maximal-effort isokinetic testing, it is important to provide a warm-up stimulus to increase intra-articular temperature and influence the viscoelastic properties of collagenous tissues to reduce strain potential. Warm-up sessions can consist of upper extremity repetitive, low-load isotonics, and/or submaximal aerobics for up to 5 minutes' duration, avoiding muscular fatigue. Apparatuses such as the Schwinn AirDyne (Schwinn Bicycle Co., Chicago, IL), UBE (Cybex, Ronkonkoma, NY), or the pulley mechanism of the Nordic Trak (Chaska, MN) can all provide the aerobic component. Warm-up repetitions are then provided on the dynamometer with 5 to 10 graduated efforts at 120°/s and five warm-ups at each test speed.

As a general rule, test speeds will vary from

60°/s to 300°/s.[27] Based on clinical experience, 60°/s is excessively slow for initial training and test speeds because of the production of large shear forces that are contraindicated in cases of acute injury, capsular sprains, and joint instability. Davies[3] and Soderberg and Blaschak[15] support early clinical training with intermediate speeds (120°/s to 180°/s) and gradual change to velocity spectrum rehabilitation protocol (VSRP) with increased velocities up to 300°/s and, finally, incorporating slow speeds 60°/s to 90°/s) during late-stage rehabilitation. As described by Wallace et al.,[31] 120°/s is easily controlled and tolerated by most individuals and provides the basis for our preferred initial warm-up speed.

Maximal effort testing of the glenohumeral joint after most traumatic injuries, arthroscopy, rotator cuff pathology, or arthrotomy should not be instituted until good tolerance of submaximal work has been demonstrated, at least 1 month after the procedure. Retest sessions should be scheduled at 1-month intervals to avoid negative reinforcement to the patient, owing to the predicted gradual changes in muscle physiology and force development that may manifest only 5 percent increases per week.[32]

Questions regarding numbers of repetitions and frequency of training sessions are difficult to answer because there is great variability among patients and the conditions requiring rehabilitation. A recommended starting protocol for low speed diagonal training is 60 repetitions (e.g., six sets of 10 repetitions) at 120°/s. To avoid overuse, patients work out no more than three times a week at regular intervals, with repetitions added depending on tolerance, until 90 repetitions are performed.

High-speed training can be progressed in a similar way at 180°/s, although Davies[3] recommends the use of several speeds at each session, using the VSRP.[3] Patients may build up to three sets of 10 at three different training speeds. Table 16.5 is an example of VSRP.

In general, when retesting shows strength deficits to be reduced to 10 percent or less, isokinetic training is discontinued. It is important to emphasize functional activities and ongoing

TABLE 16.5 *Velocity spectrum rehabilitation protocol*

REPETITIONS PER SPEED	VELOCITIES (°/s)
10	60–90–120–150–180–210–180–150–120–90–60

(Adapted from Davies,[3] with permission.)

home exercises at this stage to promote full recovery.

Updated Normative and Functional Considerations

Updated literature provides a clear consensus on isokinetic torque normative data trends, but, it remains difficult to make precise comparisons of isokinetic norms due to large methodologic variations in test devices, patient populations, patient test positions, and test speeds used. This section will review several areas of data important in clinical judgement and patient program management with respect to normative data for specific sports, sport-specific torque shifts expected as a result of training, limited perspectives on functional inferences (validity), and eccentric to concentric ratios for individual muscles.

SPORT-SPECIFIC NORMATIVE DATA

Although exact etiology is not yet proven, many studies concur that the propulsive phase (power or accelerative phase) of overhead upper extremity and shoulder motions produce a clear torque ratio shifts in many athletes, specifically in baseball, tennis, and swimming.[34–37] Athletic torque ratio shifts are most apparent for the external to internal rotation ratios and for the abduction to adduction ratios. Possible training induced changes create disproportionate increases in the torque levels of the propulsive muscles, the adductors, and internal rotators, without concomitant increases of external rotation or abduction.[13,34–36] McMaster et al.[34] found 52 percent

TABLE 16.6 *Sport-specific normative torque ratios*

STUDY	POPULATION	POSITION	ABD/ADD	ER/IR
Beach et al.[37]	28 Div. 1 swimmers	Prone 90° abd.	56%	70%
Chandler et al.[35]	24 College tennis players	Supine 90° abd.	NA	60–70%
McMaster et al.[34]	27 College swimmers	45° abd	Men 48%	45–57%
			Women 48%	57–74%
McMaster et al.[38]	15 Olympic-level water polo players	NA	65–68%	67–75%
Ng and Kramer[39]	20 Female college tennis players	Scapular plane	NA	78%
Wilk et al.[40]	83 Pro baseball players	Sitting, frontal plane	78–84%	65–75%
Wilk et al.[41]	150 Pro baseball pitchers	Sitting, 90° abd.	NA	61–65%
Wilk et al.[42]	50 Pro baseball pitchers	Sitting, frontal plane	NW 93–72%	
			W 77–89%	NA

Abbreviations: NW, nonwindowed data; W, windowed data.

greater torque for internal rotation and 43 percent greater torque for the adductors in comparing swimmers to nonswimmers, while Alderink and Kuck found similiar increases of 50 percent greater adduction in the throwing side for baseball players compared to nonthrowers.[13] Both Chandler et al.[35] and Brown et al.[36] demonstrated ER/IR ratios in the nondominant side of tennis and baseball players despite no differences in the external rotation torque between sides, which further demonstrates the torque shifts from increased internal rotation/adduction torque. Table 16.6 reviews sport-specific normative torque ratios and pertinent information on the tested populations and patient positions used in data sampling. Although few studies have reported on horizontal abduction to horizontal adduction, Weir et al.[43] established a 100 percent ratio in high school-aged wrestlers. In addition, Weir et al. demonstrated a significant increase in torque for both motions at slow speed as wrestlers aged from freshmen to senior years. This trend of increased torque as ages change from 14 to 18 is worthy of further study for other sports and certainly would be beneficial information for other muscle group torque ratios.

TORQUE RATIOS IN NORMALS

Normative data for athletes is important, but in most orthopedic/sports clinical settings, patients with shoulder complaints are not highly trained athletes, and expected torque ratios will more closely conform to predicted levels for normals. Tata et al.[44] demonstrated abduction/adduction ratios of 100 percent to 102 percent and external/internal rotation ratios of 78 percent to 87 percent for healthy males and females. Joy[45] found external/internal rotation ratios of 65 percent and abduction/adduction ratios of 70 percent to 81 percent for college-aged females. Although the variations in external rotation may be explained by the use of different dynamometers (Tata et al., Kincom, Joy, Biodex), the large variability between abduction/adduction ratios may be explained by the test positions used. Tata et al. used plane of scapular position, while Joy used a frontal plane position. Tata et al.'s study further suggested that the scapular plane is more clinically appropriate for testing and training, a viewpoint shared by the first author of this chapter for nonathletic patient cases. Finally, McMaster et al.[34] found external/internal rotation ratios of 65 to 78 percent and 58 to 74 percent for healthy males and females, respectively. McMaster's abduction/adduction ratios were 65 to 72 percent and 62 percent for males and females, respectively. This information, coupled with the data outlined in Tables 16.2 and 16.6, provides a comprehensive overview of male and female nonathletic and athletic norms for the agonist/antagonist ratios that are important parameters of muscle synergy in the shoulder complex.

ECCENTRIC TO CONCENTRIC TORQUE COMPARISONS

Although important clinical information is manisfested by the agonist/antagonist ratios, another isokinetic measurement parameter, the eccentric/concentric torque ratio from a single muscle, may provide guidelines regarding normal muscle function versus injury or dysfunction. Although extensive additional literature on this current topic is warranted, it appears that the relationship of eccentric and concentric function is important to injury prevention, assessment, and rehabilitation issues.[46] Generally, eccentric torque potentials exceed concentric torque levels in any given muscle, speed, or position consideration.[46] Therefore, the eccentric to concentric ratio will be expected to be minimally 100 percent. Ng and Kramer[39] found ratios of 119 percent and 127 percent for internal and external rotation, while Joy[45] found similiar levels of 129 percent and 123 percent, respectively. In addition, Joy delineated ratio of 131 percent and 117 percent for abduction and adduction, respectively. The actual peak performance of eccentric torque may not be sampled accurately at speeds of 180°/s or slower as in the above studies, but due to intrinsic characteristics of the isokinetic-eccentric loading, patient safety may preclude testing speeds above 180°/s. Mont et al.[47] determined tennis players' isokinetic performance for both external to internal rotation ratio and eccentric to concentric force ratio that appears widely variant from all other sampled studies and the first author's clinical experience.

FUNCTIONAL INFERENCES AND RELATIONSHIPS

Although controversy exists about functional inferences (or validity) from isokinetic measurements, much of the criticism of isokinetics relates to the common use of peak torque measurements in predicting a certain functional outcome or capacity such as running readiness after knee injury and throwing readiness after shoulder injury or surgery. Traditionally, peak torque at slow speeds 60°/s to 90°/s has been the primary clinical factor in readiness decisions. Athletic function for peripheral joints has been demonstrated to occur at extremely high speeds (above 240°/s for lower-extremity kinetic chain and above 1000°/s for the upper extremity kinetic chain) as a result of the summation of momentum through a series of joints. Therefore, it is apparent that slow-speed peak torque measures have limited value in predicting fast joint speed behaviors or most functional activities.

Clearly, the prediction of functional athletic capacity from isokinetic measures in the lower extremity dictates testing peak torque at 240° and faster,[48–50] which is paralled by the studies dealing with isokinetic prediction of upper extremity functions. Mont et al.[47] demonstrated 11 percent increases in both internal and external rotation from 180°/s training, which related to 11 percent increases in serving velocity in advanced tennis players. Mont et al. found both concentric and eccentric training methods to be equally effective. Wooden et al.[51] demonstated throwing velocity increases in junior and senior high school baseball players of 2 MPH using 500°/s individualized dynamic, variable resistance (IDVR) on the Merac system. This type of resistance is not directly classified as either isokinetic or isotonic, but possesses features of both modes. Earlier studies have demonstrated throwing and serving velocity increases from isokinetic training of the external and internal rotators[8,11] and adductors.[52] Beach et al. demonstrated 240°/s to be the functional speed for swimming performance and demonstrated the predictive value of abductor and external rotator endurance to shoulder injury in competitive swimmers.

Therefore, although literature on isokinetic validity for common shoulder sport activity is scant, the use of peak torque at high speed for functional prediction and the value of isokinetic training on sports performance have been established.

CASE STUDY 1

HISTORY

Patient P.H. is a 53-year-old housewife who was involved in a horseback riding accident on March 11, 1995. She was thrown from her horse, sustaining a comminuted fracture of the right proximal humerus. Two days later she underwent ORIF for insertion of an intramodullary rod.

INITIAL EVALUATION

The patient was referred for physical therapy 3 weeks postsurgery, and presented with complaints of pain, stiffness, and weakness of the shoulder joint, with mild pain radiating to the forearm, and a general feeling of "heaviness" of the upper extremity. The patient also reported mild stiffness of the neck, which was resolving. Functional limitations included moderate difficulty with dressing and bathing, and severe limitations in housework, gardening and so on. The patient also could not sleep on the injured side. Significant findings included the following.

	PASSIVE ROM	JOINT REACTIVITY	MUSCLE STRENGTH
Flexion	140°	Moderate	2/5+
Abduction	125°	High	2/5+
External rot.	38°	High	2/5
Internal rot.	72°	Moderate	3/5

There was widespread ecchymosis of the upper arm to the elbow joint. Mild tenderness and hypomobility of the surgical scar were noted. There was also tenderness of the supraspinatus, infraspinatus, teres minor, and subscapularis muscles. Although these muscles were weak there was no significant atrophy. Right scapular mobility was normal. The cervical spine, elbow, and wrist regions were clear.

Treatments goals included full decrease in pain and reactivity, shoulder joint ROM to 90 percent of the left side and muscle strength increase to 80 percent of the left side. The main functional goal was pain-free resumption of all ADLs, and the ability to lie on the affected side.

TREATMENT

WEEK 1

The problems identified included significant weakness in all directions and limited motion in the capsular pattern with moderately high reactivity and irritability. Initially, the treatment consisted of the following modalities.

- Moist heat and interferential stimulation to promote pain relief and relaxation
- Grades 1 and 2 oscillating mobilizations to reduce pain and joint reactivity. These included a variety of physiologic and accessory movements, and were followed by gym ball exercises to increase ROM
- Manual resistance exercises in all planes
- Home exercise program (HEP) including pendulum and latex band resistive exercises

WEEK 2

Tolerance to treatment was generally good, and improvements in mobility, strength, and reactivity were noted. By the end of the second week the patient's HEP was expanded to include wand exercises for shoulder flexion and extension; for flexion, a 2-pound weight was attached. The patient was also using a gym ball at home.

WEEK 3

The patient reported decreases in pain and irritability, as well as a considerable improvement in case of ADL. The following objective improvements were noted:

	PASSIVE ROM	JOINT REACTIVITY	MUSCLE STRENGTH
Flexion	155°	Moderate	35+
Abduction	146°	Moderate	3/5+
External rot.	45°	Moderate	3/5
Internal rot.	80°	Low	3/5+

Based on these findings, treatment was altered as follows:

- Pain modalities were discontinued.
- Mobilizations were increased to grades 4 to 4+, respecting reactivity.
- Concentric isokinetic strengthening for internal and external rotation was begun within these parameters: 90°/s, patient supine with the shoulder in 30° abduction in the plane of the scapula (POS). Submaximum effort contractions were increased gradually to maximum effort over three treatment sessions
- Progressive resistive exercises (PREs) included weighted wand exercises and most of the "super seven" rotator cuff exercises with low resistance. These were also incorporated in the patient's HEP

WEEKS 4 AND 5

Vigorous mobilization, especially to increase external rotation, was continued along with maximum effort IKN exercise and PREs.

By the end of week 5 the patient reported significant improvement in strength and mobility, with minimal ADL restrictions. Overhead activities were still somewhat difficult. The patient was able to lie and sleep on the injured side. ROM and muscle strength were as follows.

	PASSIVE ROM	JOINT REACTIVITY	MUSCLE STRENGTH
Flexion	172°	Normal	5/5
Abduction	166°	Low	4/5+
External rot.	84°	Low	4/5+
Internal rot.	92°	Normal	5/5

Concentric isokinetice testing revealed the following deficits in mean torque.

	90° PER SECOND	180° PER SECOND
Flexion	14°	12%
Extension	No deficit	No deficit
Abduction	22%	19%
Adduction	No deficit	No deficit
Internal rot.	No deficit	No deficit
External rot.	24%	26%

DISCHARGE

External rotation and abduction were still moderately weak, but the patient's function was approaching normal limits. Physical therapy was discontinued at this time, but the patient was instructed to continue her HEP indefinitely, and to return if any further problems arose.

CASE STUDY 2

HISTORY

Patient A.P. is a 47-year-old male, employed as a freight and box handler in an industrial setting. He was injured on August 15,1994 when he slipped and fell backward onto his dominant right shoulder at work, and sustained a full-thickness rotator cuff tear of 4 cm by 4 cm. size. The patient denied any previous injury to the right shoulder or to the neck and presented to the orthopedist with complaints of inability to lift his arm, but had minimal pain.

INITIAL EVALUATION

The patient had surgery on September 7th and was seen in the clinic on September 14th with the following physical status:

1. R arm supported in sling
2. Difficulties with all ADLs, especially dressing and personal hygiene
3. Pain level at rest 3
4. Pain level to 5 to 7 with movements.
5. Strength as follows
   Elevation (self-selected plane) R/L, 2+/5
   Internal rotation   R/L, 3+/5
   External rotation   R/L, 2/5
   Extension   R/L, 3+/4
6. Mobility
   Elevation (supine, assisted) R/L, 78°/175°
   Internal rotation   R/L, L-3/T-6
   External rotation (60° elevated, supine)
                                 R/L, (−15°)/88°
7. Functional goals—pain-free, normal ADLs and return to work tasks including lifting of boxes above head up to 35 pounds

TREATMENT PROGRAM

Grouped in monthly progressions. All exercises given for the home program will be designated as HEP for home exercise program.

MONTH 1

PROGRAM

Active assistive ROM: Elevation and external rotation (HEP)
Electrical stimulation: High voltage, surged
Pendular exercises (HEP)
Shoulder extension isometrics and scapular adduction (HEP)
Serratus anterior: Manual resistance in supine
Ice massage

STATUS

Active external rotation (60° of abduction, supine): 5°
Active assisted elevation: 98°

MONTH 2

PROGRAM

D/C pendular exercises
Start actual external rotation (in supine to 45° (HEP)
Upper body ergometer (UBE): 6 minutes
Eagle row: 2 plates, continue electrical stimulation
Scapular mobilization in multiple planes
ShoulderEase brace applied in place of sling for daywear only
Hold–relax stretches for elevation and ext. rotation (in supine)
Passive concentric phase elevation to terminal, comfortable limits followed by active assisted negative phase elevation to 110°
Eagle chest press: 3 plates (elbow below shoulder height)
Increase row to 3 plates, then 4 on Eagle
Self-administered static External Rotation stretch 5 up 10 minute holds (HEP)
Prone shoulder extension (no weight, HEP)
Grades 2 and 3 inferior glides to humeral head

STATUS

Mild, episodic pain and stiffness of shoulder
Ability to do dressing and ADLs slowly
Active assisted elevation: 98°, active elevation to 80°
Active external rotation: 33°
External rotation strength: Grade 4 –

MONTH 3

PROGRAM

Begin manual resisted supine shoulder flexion and external rotation
Impulse shoulder extension (standing) with 10 pounds
Sidelying external rotation exercises with 3 pounds (HEP)
Plane of scapula Lido isokinetic internal/external rotation (supine), 6 sets of 10 repetitions at 120°/s, 3 sets of 10 at 180°
Electrical stimulation 12 minutes with med. frequency, 15/50 contract/rest time
Assisted concentric elevation from 110° to 150°, negative unassisted in reverse range, followed by unassisted negative elevation from 125° to 0°

STATUS

Minimal pain or stiffness with ADLs
Active elevation to 130° with controlled scapular position
Active external rotation to 56° in supine (90° of abduction)

MONTH 4

PROGRAM

Added Impulse "punching" pattern (extended elbow from 90° abducted position) for serratus anterior and theraband for the same motion at home (HEP)
Impulse shoulder flexion with fixed elbow flexion "bowling" pattern and theraband simulation exercise (HEP)
Eagle pull downs added with 3 plates
Lido continued as above
Arm lifts into flexion added with 2 pounds

STATUS

Grade 4 supraspinatus

Mobility: Elevation 155°, external rotation—R/L = 75°/88°

No pain with light lifting and all ADL'sReturned to light duty work status with physician restriction of no more than 5-pound lifts

MONTH 5

PROGRAM

Same program with increased effort on Lido isokinetics and on inertial patterns as listed

STATUS

Elevation to 165°

Supraspinatus strength: Grade 5 −

Isokinetic testing results: Plane of scapula supine internal/external rotation

90°/s	23% deficit in ER	Peak torque
	52% better in IR	Peak torque
	44% deficit in ER	Total work
	90% better in IR	Total work
240°/s	41% deficit in ER	Peak torque
	6% better in IR	Peak torque
	33% deficit in ER	Total work
	61% better in IR	Total work

MONTH 6

The patient was seen for three visits during this month for the same program with continued counseling on the maintenance of his home program and protection of his arm/shoulder relative to safe biomechanics.

Despite the external/internal rotation torque imbalances and external rotation deficits, the patient had achieved nearly normal ROM and control, resolved pain, no apprehension with lifting or exertional activities, and was discharged.

Summary

A method of evaluating and treating shoulder girdle muscle weakness and joint dysfunction has been described. Diagonal movements relate closely to normal activity and provide time-saving and practical means of applying isokinetics to the shoulder. For specific weakness of a muscle or small muscle group (e.g., in rotator cuff tears), the isolated movements described in the isokinetic manual may be more helpful. Similarly, certain injuries or surgical repairs may necessitate isolation of movement to a cardinal plane with blocked motion as appropriate.

Both isokinetic testing and training sessions should be preceded by warm-up techniques. Clinical decisions with isokinetics include timing of application, number of repetitions, amount of patient effort, and importantly, the patient and glenohumeral positioning used. Although both the neutral and 90° AP have specific advantages, it appears that the 45° position offers the optimal compromise of physiologic, safety, and strengthening goals for clinical training.

Normative data for the shoulder indicate a strength/torque hierarchy as follows: adductors and extensors followed by flexors and abductors and, finally, the internal and external rotators. Side-to-side torque differences tend to be minimal unless specific vigorous preferred activities, such as baseball pitching, are involved. Peak torque to body weight ratios range from 45 to 46 percent for the strongest adductor group to a variable 8 to 22 percent for the external and internal rotators, respectively. A clinically important value for normal shoulder function and synergism is the ER/IR ratio, which should be 60 to 70 percent for most test positions at slow speed.

Although clinically useful normative data exist, this new area of isokinetic practice needs continued research. Similarly, existing clinical protocols and positions require additional research investigation, with the goal of improved patient care and potentially new uses for isokinetic technology as applied to the dynamic stabilizer system that is so critical to functional capacity of the human upper extremity.

References

1. Moffroid M, Whipple R, Hofkosh J et al: A study of isokinetic exercise. Phys Ther 49:735, 1969
2. Laird C, Rozier C: Toward understanding the ter-

minology of exercise mechanics. Phys Ther 59: 287, 1979

3. Davies G: A Compendium of Isokinetics in Clinical Usage: Workshop and Clinical Notes. S & S Publishers, LaCrosse, WI, 1984

4. Cybex: Isolated Joint Testing and Exercise: A Handbook for Using Cybex II and the UBXT. Cybex, Ronkokoma, NY, 1983

5. Moffroid M, Whipple R: Specificity of speed of exercise. Phys Ther 50:1693, 1970

6. Barnes WS: The relationship of motor unit activation to isokinetic muscular contraction at different contractile velocities. Phys Ther 60:1152, 1980

7. Thorstensson A, Grimby G, Karlsson J: Force velocity relations and fiber composition in human knee extension muscles. J Appl Physiol 40:12, 1976

8. Smith M, Melton P: Isokinetic versus isotonic variable resistance training. Am J Sports Med 9: 275, 1981

9. Rasch P, Burke R: Kinesiology and Applied Anatomy. 3rd Ed. Lea & Febiger, Philadelphia, 1967

10. Jobe FW, Tibone JE, Perry J, Moynes D: EMG analysis of the shoulder in pitching. A preliminary report. Am J Sports Med 11:3, 1983

11. Ellenbecker TS, Davies GJ, Rowinski MJ: Concentric versus eccentric isokinetic strengthening of the rotator cuff: objective data versus functional test. Am J Sports Med 16:64, 1989

12. Hinton RY: Isokinetic evaluation of shoulder rotational strength in high school baseball pitchers. Am J Sports Med 16:274, 1988

13. Alderink GJ, Kuck DJ: Isokinetic shoulder strength of high school and college age baseball pitchers. J Orthop Sports Phys Ther 7:163, 1986

14. Williams P, Warwick R: Gray's Anatomy. 3rd Ed. WB Saunders, Philadelphia, 1980

15. Soderberg GJ, Blaschak MJ: Shoulder internal and external rotation peak torque production through a velocity spectrum in differing positions. J Orthop Sports Phys Ther 8:518, 1987

16. Elsner RC, Pedegrana LR, Lang J: Protocol for strength testing and rehabilitation of the upper extremity. J Orthop Sports Phys 4:229, 1983

17. Einhorn AR, Jackson DW: Rehabilitation of the shoulder. p. 103. In Jackson DW (ed): Shoulder Surgery in the Athlete. Techniques in Orthopedics. Aspen Publications, Rockville, MD, 1985

18. Connelly-Maddux RE, Kibler WB, Uhl T: Isoki-netic peak torque and work values for the shoulder. J Orthop Sports Phys Ther 1:264, 1989

19. Engle RP, Canner GC: Posterior shoulder instability: approach to rehabilitation. J Orthop Sports Phys Ther 10:488, 1989

20. Kibler WB, Chandler TJ: Functional scapular instability in throwing athletes. Unpublished study, Lexington, KY, 1988

21. Rathbun JB, McNab I: The micro-vasculature pattern of the rotator cuff. J Bone Joint Surg 52:540, 1970

22. Hageman PA, Mason DK, Rylund KW, et al: Effects of position and speed on eccentric and concentric isokinetic testing of the shoulder rotators. J Orthop Sports Phys Ther 11:64, 1989

23. Johnston T: The movements of the shoulder joint. A plea for the plane of the scapula as the plane of reference for movement occurring at the humeroscapular joint. Br J Surg 2:252, 1952

24. Greenfield B, Donatelli R, Wooden M, Wilkes J: Comparison of isokinetic shoulder rotation strength in plane of scapula vs. frontal plane. Am J Sports Med 18:124, 1990

25. Knott M, Voss D: Proprioceptive Neuro-muscular Facilitation: Patterns and Techniques. 2nd Ed. Harper & Row, New York, 1968

26. Gardner E, Gray D, O'Rahilly R: Anatomy: A Regional Study of Human Structure. 2nd Ed. WB Saunders, New York, 1963

27. Cook EE, Gray VL, Savinar-Nogue E, Medeiros J: Shoulder antagonist strength ratios: a comparison between college-level baseball pitchers and nonpitchers. J Orthop Sports Phys Ther 8:451, 1987

28. Reid DC, Salboe L, Burnham R: Current Research of Selected Shoulder Problems. In Donatelli R (ed): Physical Therapy of the Shoulder. Churchill Livingstone, New York, 1987

29. Ivey FM, Calhoun JH, Rusche K, et al: Isokinetic testing of shoulder strength: normal values. Arch Phys Med Rehabil 66:384, 1985

30. Coleman AE: Physiological characteristics of major league baseball players. Phys Sports Med 10:51, 1982

31. Wallace WA, Barton MJ, Murray WA: The power available during movement of the shoulder. In Bateman, Welsh (eds): Surgery of the Shoulder. BC Decker, Philadelphia, 1984

32. Cote C, Simoneau JA, LaGasse P, et al: Isokinetic strength training protocols: do they induce skeletal muscle fiber hypertrophy? Arch Phys Med Rehabil 69:281, 1988

33. Loredan Co: Lido isokinetic normative values for shoulders. Unpublished clinical study, Davis, CA, 1987

34. McMaster WC, Long SC, Caiozzo VJ: Shoulder torque changes in the swimming athlete. Am J Sports Med 20:323, 1992

35. Chandler TJ, Kibler WB, Stracener EC et al: Shoulder strength, power, and endurance in college tennis players. Am J Sports Med 20:455, 1992

36. Brown LP, Niehues SL, Harrah A et al: Upper extremity range of motion and isokinetic strength of the internal and external shoulder rotators in major league baseball players. Am J Sports Med 16:577, 1988

37. Beach ML, Whitney SL, Dickoff-Hoffman SA: Relationship of shoulder flexibility, strength and endurance to shoulder pain in competitive swimmers. JOSPT 16:262, 1992

38. McMaster WC, Long SC, Caiozzo VJ: Isokinetic torque imbalances in the rotator cuff of the elite water polo player. Am J Sports Med 19:72, 1991

39. Ng LR, Kramer JS: Shoulder rotator torques in females tennis and non-tennis players. JOSPT 13:40, 1991

40. Wilk KE, Andrews JR, Arrigo CA: The Abductor and adductor strength characteristics of professional baseball pitchers. Am J Sports Med 23:307, 1995

41. Wilk KE, Andrews JR, Arrigo CA et al: The strength characteristics of internal and external rotator muscles in professional baseball pitchers. Am J Sports Med 21:61, 1993

42. Wilk KE, Arrigo CA, Andrews JR: Isokinetic testing of the shoulder abductors and adductors: windowed and non-windowed data collection. JOSPT 15:107, 1994

43. Weir JP, Wagner LL, Housh TJ et al: Horizontal abduction and adduction strength at the shoulder of high school wrestlers across age. JOSPT 15:183, 1992

44. Tata GE, Ng LR, Kramer JF: Shoulder antagonist strength during concentric and eccentric muscle actions in the scapular plane. JOSPT 18:654, 1993.

45. Toy BJ: Concentric and eccentric shoulder strength evaluation of college aged females. JAT 30:S37, 1995

46. Albert MS (ed): Eccentric Muscle Training In Sports and Orthopedics. Churchill-Livingstone, New York, 1991

47. Mont MA, Cohen DB, Campbell KR et al: Isokinetic concentric versus eccentric training of shoulder rotators with functional evaluation of performance enhancement in elite tennis players. Am J Sports Med 22:513, 1994

48. Johansson C, Lorentzon R, Fagerlund M et al: Sprinters and marathon runners. Doers isokinetic knee extensor performance reflect muscle size and structure.? Acta Physiol Scand 130:663, 1987

49. Kannus P: Peak Torque and total work relationship in the thigh muscles after anterior cruciate ligament injury. JOSPT 10:97, 1988

50. Krebs DE: Isokinetic, electrophysiologic and clinical function relationships following tourniquet-aided knee arthrotomy. Phys Ther 69:1989

51. Wooden MJ, Greenfield B, Johanson M: Effects of strength training on throwing velocity and shoulder muscle performance in teenage baseball players. JOSPT 15:223, 1992

52. Bartlett LR, Storey MD, Simons BD: Measurement of upper extremity torque production and its relationship to throwing speed in the competitive athlete. Am J Sports Med 17:89, 1989

17

Instabilities

ANGELO J. MATTALINO

Evaluation, diagnosis, and treatment of shoulder instability is a complex and constantly evolving process. The quality of diagnostic tests as well as our understanding of its pathology and patho-mechanics have greatly improved in recent years. Better diagnostic tools have led to better presurgical visualization of shoulder pathology. Arthroscopic evaluation has advanced the understanding of the pathology and the dynamics of shoulder instability. Arthroscopic surgery and open surgical techniques to correct shoulder instability patterns are evolving and still improving.

The shoulder joint has great mobility₁ with stability throughout its range of motion. Glenohumeral stability is maintained via static and dynamic influences. Negative intra-articular pressure and dynamic compression forces by muscular forces, primarily by the rotator cuff musculature, are examples of these influences. It has been estimated that 40 percent of the dynamic forces are contributed by the rotator cuff musculature and that removal of the labrum reduces these forces by half. Rehabilitation addressing neuromuscular conditioning can strongly influence shoulder stability.[1] Surgical repair and/or reconstruction of capsulolabral anatomy can help restore stability.

Bankhart initially described the detachment of the labrum and the inferior glenohumeral ligament complex from the anterior aspect of the glenoid.[2] Since this initial report, scientific experimentation has further delineated the role of the inferior glenohumeral ligament complex as the primary stabilizer resisting anterior transla-tion when the shoulder is at 90° of abduction. Plastic deformation of the glenohumeral ligaments has been found to contribute to the abnormal translation of the humeral head. Capsular laxity, insufficiency of the glenoid labrum, and weakness of the rotator cuff musculature can jeopardize glenohumeral joint stability and lead to abnormal humeral head translation and progressive rotator cuff pathology.[3]

The inferior glenohumeral ligament (posterior band) is the primary contributor to posterior stability of the shoulder when in 90° of abduction.[4] Inferior translation of the glenohumeral joint is affected by the superior glenohumeral ligament in the adducted position,[5] the inferior glenohumeral ligament complex at 45° and 90° of abduction, and the rotator cuff interval portion of the anterior-superior shoulder capsule.[6] The understanding of these pathomechanics is crucial in making clinical rehabilitative and surgical decisions.

Pathomechanics

There are three categories of stability factors about the glenohumeral joint: anatomic, dynamic, and static. The anatomic category includes the labrum, which adds depth to the glenoid surface, "changing a saucer to a bowl." The negative atmospheric pressure within the glenohumeral joint is another important anatomic contributor to stability. Injury to the labrum is thought to disrupt this atmospheric seal, thus contributing to instability.

Static support is provided by the capsuloligamentous structure about the glenohumeral joint. The inferior glenohumeral ligament is most important in preventing anterior and inferior translation. The middle glenohumeral ligament contributes static stability by resisting external rotation and abduction. The static stabilizing structures work in conjunction, each playing their role during specific points in the range of motion of the shoulder, and together providing an encapsulating network throughout glenohumeral joint range of motion.

The rotator cuff mechanism contributes "dynamic" support by compressing the surfaces of the glenohumeral joint. In particular the supraspinatus and the deltoid musculature are the dominate compressive contributors at 90° of abduction. The subscapularis is considered the most important in decreasing displacement, but its dynamic support is negated with the shoulder in abduction and external rotation, which are inherent in the "cocking" phase of throwing.

The infraspinatus muscle helps supplement this dynamic deficit of the subscapularis, by helping to decrease anterior translation of the glenohumeral joint during extremes of external rotation. Remember that the long head of biceps is also felt to contribute to anterior stability during abduction and external rotation by supplying a "strap" effect of the anterior aspect of the glenohumeral joint.[7]

Clinical Examination

Decision making is very dependent upon the clinical subjective and objective findings. Physical examination in the clinic and operating room under anesthesia dictates the need for and type of surgery to be performed. The magnitude and direction of instability patterns can be determined by an astute examiner.

Patient History

Listening to the patient is crucial. Certain information should be obtained if not volunteered by the patient. The dominant hand should be deter-

mined along with occupational and/or recreational demands required of the affected shoulder. Description and location of symptoms, frequency, and what activities worsen and relieve the symptoms, should be obtained. Onset of the problem and specific description of any traumatic event should be determined, in particular any history of shoulder dislocation and total number of dislocations and subsequent reductions.

Objective Examination

The normal unaffected shoulder should be examined first to use as comparison to discern the level of pathology. Palpation for areas of tenderness is recommended, anteriorly over the long head biceps tendon, rotator cuff insertions, and bony landmarks of the AC, SC, scapulothoracic, and glenohumeral joints. A neurologic exam to discern any motor and/or sensory deficits is performed.

Range of motion should be compared, beginning with forward flexion, abduction, and extension. Internal and external rotation should be measured at 0° and 90° of abduction, both sitting and supine. Noting the vertebral levels reached by the patient's thumbs is an excellent maneuver to compare internal rotation. Decreased external rotation is often encountered in shoulder instability patients.

Strength levels need to be determined and compared to the unaffected shoulder. Weakness secondary to pain should be discerned from true structural weakness, using local anesthesia if necessary. Abduction and rotator cuff strength should be determined as described elsewhere in this book.

Instability Testing

When testing for instability, it is essential to compare bilateral shoulders and check for natural laxity in other joints.

The *load and shift* test can determine both

anterior and posterior glenohumeral joint instability. The patient is placed in the supine position. Axial loading of the glenohumeral joint is accomplished or provided with one hand at the elbow (flexed at 90°) and the other hand placed just distal to the humeral head, both anteriorly and posteriorly. Next, the examiner should feel for "play" posteriorly and/or anteriorly in the glenohumeral joint, much like the Lachman test for the knee. Feel for a "clunk" as the humeral head potentially translates anteriorly and/or posteriorly; a positive "clunk" test can be indicative of a labral tear.[8] Variation in the degree of horizontal adduction and abduction may allow the examiner to reproduce familiar symptoms for the patient. This test has a grading system:

1. Trace, defined as a small amount of humeral head translation.

2. Grade I, defined as the humeral head riding up the glenoid but not over the rim.

3. Grade II, defined as the humeral head gliding up and over the glenoid rim and then reducing with applied stress.

4. Grade III, defined as the humeral head gliding up and over the glenoid rim with persistent dislocation even after the stress is removed.[8]

The *apprehension test* is performed by applying abduction and external rotation to the shoulder; then the examiner's hand placed posterior to the shoulder applies force in an anterior direction. One should observe the patient for signs of pain and/or apprehension of reproducing the symptoms of instability.

Jobe has described the *subluxation relocation test* to test for subtle instability of the glenohumeral joint. The examiner applies posterior force to the glenohumeral joint after anterior translation has been performed, with the shoulder in 90° of abduction and 90° of shoulder external rotation. Patients with anterior instability might report pain or apprehension with the shoulder in external rotation and abduction with the anteriorly directed force. This apprehension and/or pain dissipates with a subsequent force directed posteriorly.

Neer has described the Sulcus sign test for detection of inferior instability.[9] With the patient in the sitting position, palpate the glenohumeral joint laterally and apply an inferiorly directed dislocation force to the humerus. A positive test will produce a palpable and/or visible divot in the lateral aspect of the shoulder.

A thorough and complete musculoskeletal examination of the neck, cervical spine, and elbow should also be performed to rule out referred symptoms.

Imaging Studies for Shoulder Instability

Standard radiographic studies can be taken in the clinic to evaluate shoulder instability. This author prefers these views: (1) scapular AP view with the humerus in internal rotation, (2) scapular AP view with the humerus in external rotation, (3) prone axillary view, and (4) Stryker notch view. The AP view with humerus in internal rotation may reveal the Hill-Sachs lesion on the posterior lateral aspect of the humeral head, usually considered to indicate evidence of prior episodes of glenohumeral instability and/or frank dislocation. Either AP view may show evidence of subtle changes indicating periosteal bone build-up in the interior region of the glenoid. This finding can indicate prior capsular injury at this area. The axillary view can reveal the bony Bankhart lesion at the anterior aspect of the glenoid rim.[10] Studies have found the Stryker notch view to be very helpful in revealing the Hill-Sachs defect.[11]

To further delineate the extent of pathology due to shoulder instability, more invasive diagnostic imaging can be performed. Arthrography and CT scans have been used in the past with consistency in diagnosing labral pathology, capsular redundancy, Bankhart lesions, Hill-Sachs defects, and intra-articular loose bodies. The use of magnetic resonance imaging has been beneficial in identifying rotator cuff pathology, but it is not as reliable in diagnosing labral pathology. MRI can underestimate capsulolabral redundancy and injury without concurrent effusion. In this author's experience, intra-articular gadolinium-enhanced MRI has been reliable in evaluating soft tissue pathology in patients with shoulder instability. Gadolinium is injected intra-articularly via fluoroscopy to produce capsular distention and improved labral-capsular contrast depicted on MRI images, thus improving the sensitivity to identification of labral and capsular pathology.

Surgical Intervention for Shoulder Instability

The role of surgical intervention in the case of shoulder instability is to repair or reconstruct the pathology and stabilize the glenohumeral joint with minimal surgical morbidity.

As exemplified by the many different surgical procedures that have evolved over the years, no one procedure has consistently corrected shoulder "instability" without some associated morbidity, that is, limited range of motion. Though some of these procedures provide consistent "stable" results, occasionally patients are unable to return to their preinjury level of activity due to certain postoperative physical limitations. The throwing athlete, for example, may have postoperative stability but may be unable to regain the external rotation necessary to be an effective pitcher. Thus arises the most recent controversy of open versus arthroscopic surgical reconstruction for shoulder instability. Proponents of open reconstruction state that they can provide more reliable reconstructions than arthroscopic repair. Open reconstructive procedures have been traditionally recommended for athletes involved in contact sports such as football and rugby.

Proponents of arthroscopic stabilization procedures state that they can provide stability without compromising range of motion, in particular the external rotation needed.

I recognize the pros and cons of both approaches and thus employ them as individually indicated. Open reconstructive procedures such as capsular shift and open Bankhart repair are recommended to individuals who have a history of multiple frank dislocations.

For the overhand athlete, particularly the throwing athlete, I favor arthroscopic stabilization. Most recently I have combined the laser capsulorraphy technique with anterior stabilization both done arthroscopically, with good preliminary results, when an early, aggressive rehabilitation protocol is followed (see case study 1).

Thus, when deciding which surgical techniques to employ, it is crucial to be mindful of a patient's expectations. I emphasize that a successful surgical reconstruction is based not only on obtaining stability and a low reoccurrence rate, but on the return to preinjury level of activities, for example, baseball pitching.

OPEN RECONSTRUCTION TECHNIQUES

More than 100 open surgical procedures have been described in the orthopedic literature. They basically involved capsular tightening, muscle transfer, bone block transfer, and/or osteotomy. Presently, the two most consistently employed are the open Bankhart reconstruction and the anterior capsulolabral reconstruction.

Open Bankhart Reconstruction

The anatomic repair of the capsular-periosteal separation at the anterior glenoid neck is referred to as the open Bankhart repair.[2,12] The Bankhart reconstruction attempts to anatomically correct the primary stabilizer of the shoulder and the inferior glenohumeral ligamentous complex (Fig. 17.1). The anterior capsule is entered anteriorly in a vertical fashion where the capsule attaches to the glenoid medially. The anterior glenoid neck is debrided to exposed cortical bone. The glenoid periosteal tissue and the medially and superior shifted capsule are reattached to the glenoid margin. The attachment is classically achieved through drill holes and more recently with other bony fixation devices—bioabsorbable tacs, Suretac transglenoid sutures, or

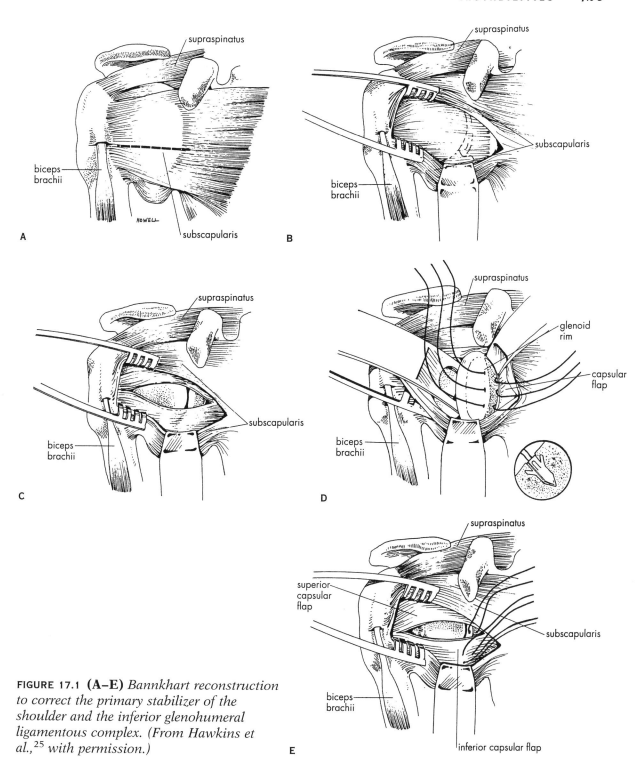

FIGURE 17.1 (A–E) *Bannkhart reconstruction to correct the primary stabilizer of the shoulder and the inferior glenohumeral ligamentous complex. (From Hawkins et al.,[25] with permission.)*

suture anchors, according to preference of the surgeon.

Open Capsular Shift Procedures

The anterior capsulolabral reconstruction is felt to better address the capsular redundancy in shoulder instability, in particular multidirectional instability. It is also thought to cause less resultant range of motion deficits, in particular, less deficiency of external rotation with abduction, because the subscapularis is not detached.[13] Rather than detaching the subscapularis tendon, it is split in line within its fibers at its upper two thirds and lower one third junctions. The capsule is then reflected from the subscapularis in a medial to lateral direction. The capsule is then split similar to the incision in the subscapularis tendon (Fig. 17-2). The capsule is

then incised from the glenoid margin forming a T-shaped incision. Shifting of the inferior leaf of the capsule obliterates any redundancy of the capsule. The superior leaf is then shifted inferiorly, and they are both attached to the anterior glenoid by various types of fixation devices at the preference of the surgeon. More sutures may be added to these redirected leafs for further tightening and/or reinforcement of the repair. Rehabilitation consists of progressive increases in range of motion and stretching, which allow the soft tissues to heal and promote normal joint arthrokinematics and upper extremity strength (see case study 2).

Open Repair of Posterior Instability

The reconstruction of the posteriorly unstable shoulder can be attempted with an anterior surgical approach. This involves more ag-

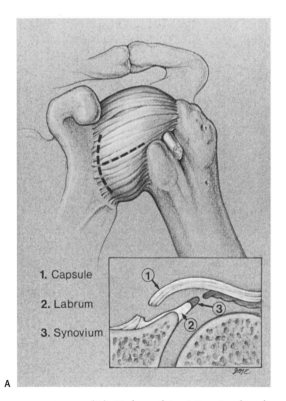
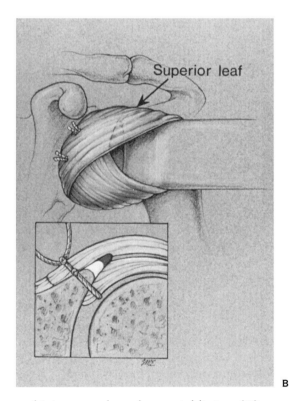

1. Capsule
2. Labrum
3. Synovium

Superior leaf

A   B

FIGURE 17.2 (A) *T-shaped incision in the glenohumeral joint capsule and synovial lining.* **(B)** *Superior shift of the inferior capsular flap and inferior shift of the superior capsular flap. (From Jobe et al.:,[26] with permission.)*

gressive inferior capsule detachment and superior advancement. The direct posterior approach can employ a posterior capsular shift and/or bony block of the posterior glenoid. The infraspinatus is dissected from the posterior capsule and cut diagonally from its insertion at the greater tuberosity. A similar T-shaped capsular incision is employed approximately 4 to 6 mm from its humeral insertion.

The inferior leaf of capsule is shifted superiorly and the superior leaf is shifted inferiorly, and then both are attached to roughened bone on the humerus. It has been recommended that the arm should be held in 10° to 15° of abduction and external rotation during the posterior capsular shift. The patient is placed in an abduction pillow/brace at about 20° of abduction for 4 to 6 weeks. Rehabilitation following a posterior capsular shift to stabilize the patient with posterior instability differs from protocols for rehabilitation following an anterior capsular shift. Internal rotation and horizontal adduction ranges of motion are limited initially, to protect the posterior capsule, and the use of a posterior glide mobilization is strictly contraindicated in the early stages of the rehab process. Progression of flexion, abduction, and external rotation range of motion is followed prior to the progression of internal rotation and horizontal adduction. Strengthening exercises that develop the anterior musculature, such as the subscapularis, are emphasized, as well as the scapular stabilizers. Closed-chain exercise with the shoulder in 90° of flexion are not indicated due to the stress imparted onto the posterior capsule.

Arthroscopic Techniques for Shoulder Instabilities

Arthroscopic evaluation of the shoulder is the best diagnostic tool for shoulder instability. Labral pathology, partial rotator cuff tears, capsular redundancy, and/or intra-articular loose bodies are often not seen on arthrography, CT scan, or MRI studies. Arthroscopy can be employed preceding open stabilization procedures.

Examination under anesthesia is the first stage of surgical treatment both open and arthroscopic procedures of shoulder instability. With muscular relaxation induced during anesthesia, the surgeon can more accurately discern the extent of instability patterns. The unaffected shoulder should be examined first, followed by the pathologic shoulder. The obvious reason is that patients often have inherent laxity, the extent of which should be determined prior to making surgical decisions on the affected shoulder. The clinical examinations addressed earlier in this chapter should now be repeated on bilateral shoulders, documenting any bilateral discrepancies in anterior, posterior, and inferior instability.

Next the anesthetized patient is positioned either in the lateral decubitus or "beach-chair" sitting position. Traction devices using 5 to 15 pounds of weight are preferred by many surgeons. Diagnostic arthroscopy is then begun in the usual fashion.[14,15] Arthroscopic debridement of labral tears, partial rotator cuff tears, chondral defects, removal of loose bodies, and/or any other pathology encountered is performed. At this point, the surgeon must decide that the clinical diagnosis of any instability pattern has been confirmed, and if so then proceed with either an arthroscopic or open stabilization procedure.

Many different arthroscopic stabilization techniques have evolved over the years, starting with the metal staple introduced by Johnson in the 1980s.[16] Present options for the arthroscopic surgeon vary from resorbable tacks, transglenoid suturing,[17,18] suture anchors,[19] metal stapling,[20] laser capsulorrhaphy,[19] and glenoid abrasion without internal fixation.[21]

Regardless of the specific stabilization technique employed by the surgeon, two steps should be followed prior to fixation. The first is preparation the capsuloligamentous complex, depending on the pathology encountered. If the capsule is redundant and/or reattached inferior to the anterior glenoid margin, it should be dissected free from its attachments (Fig. 17.3). Second, depending on the fixation technique selected, the capsuloligamentous complex is grasped and shifted superiorly and to the glenoid's anterior

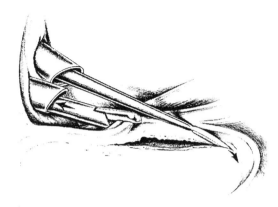

FIGURE 17.3 *The capsule-labrum complex is mobilized until the tissue is free. The tissue is moved with a grasper while using a banana knife or shoulder elevator. (From Esch and Baker,[22] with permission.)*

ridge. The glenoid neck is debrided and decorticated to exposed bleeding bone prior to reattachment of the capsular ligamentous tissue (Fig. 17.4). These two steps are the most crucial to a successful stabilization, no matter which of the fixation techniques is selected. Also, essential to a successful stabilization arthroscopically is good visualization during the arthroscopy. Visualization is dependent on proper portal placement and employing appropriately angled arthroscopy. These types of procedures are not for the novice or "occasional" arthroscopist!

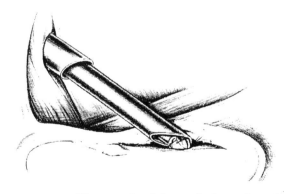

FIGURE 17.4 *The anterior labrum is decorticated with a burr or rasp to provide a bleeding bony surface. (From Esch and Baker,[22] with permission.)*

My preferred technique for arthroscopic stabilization is the Suretac biodegradable tac.[5,22] Though technically demanding, it should avoid the potential posterior complications associated with transglenoid drilling and/or posterior suturing. The surgical repair technique is similar to the transglenoid suture technique, with potential to repair Bankhart lesions and fixate the shifted and tightened inferior glenohumeral ligament complex (Fig. 17.5).

The biodegradable tac has a pullout strength of 100 N and a broad flat head with spikes on its underside to enhance capsular tissue purchase and control. The polyglyconate tac biodegrades, and its strength diminishes over the next 4 to 16 weeks; it is eventually reabsorbed by the synovial membrane (Fig. 17.6).[19] The capsuloligamentous tightening can be enhanced with the transglenoid suture technique used in conjunction or by employing the Holmium YAG laser capsulorraphy technique, if the surgeon feels optimal tightening of redundant tissue has not been accomplished. I have had short-term success with the combination of the Suretac and Holmium YAG Laser capsulorraphy techniques.

Laser

I have used lasers in arthroscopic procedures, beginning with the CO_2 laser system and presently with the Holmium YAG laser, which emits a wavelength of 2.1 mm and is transmitted through optical fibers in a saline medium. The Holmium YAG laser has been shown to produce a minimal amount of thermal necrosis and can precisely cut, resect, and ablate cartilaginous tissues.[18] Less postoperative pain and swelling, and accelerated reattainment of full range of motion, was observed in a clinical study comparing laser versus conventional meniscetomies in knee arthroscopy.[14] I have used the Holmium YAG laser effectively in the shoulder for debridement and resection of labral tears during shoulder arthroscopy.

The plastic deformation and redundant capsulaligamentous structure commonly found in

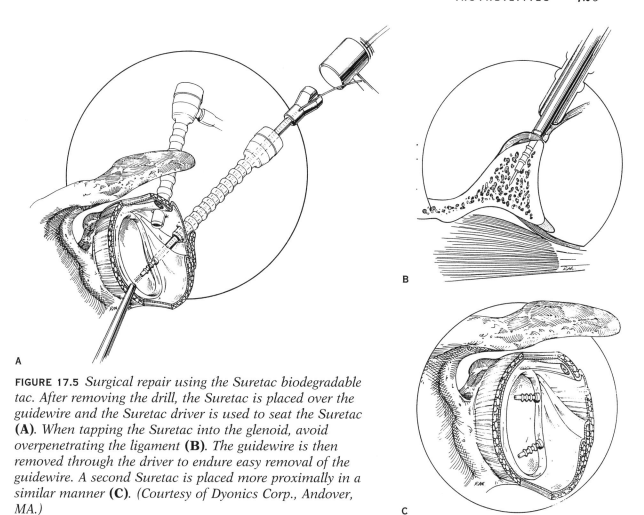

FIGURE 17.5 *Surgical repair using the Suretac biodegradable tac. After removing the drill, the Suretac is placed over the guidewire and the Suretac driver is used to seat the Suretac* **(A)**. *When tapping the Suretac into the glenoid, avoid overpenetrating the ligament* **(B)**. *The guidewire is then removed through the driver to endure easy removal of the guidewire. A second Suretac is placed more proximally in a similar manner* **(C)**. *(Courtesy of Dyonics Corp., Andover, MA.)*

the shoulder with pathologic instability has been the primary area of use for the Holmium YAG laser. The Holmium YAG laser can "shrink tissue" found in capsular redundancy and thus also decrease joint volume.[16] This tissue during arthroscopic observation becomes visibly shorter and causes apparent "tightening" of redundant capsuloligamentous structures, which can be controlled by the amount of energy delivered via the Holmium YAG laser. Reports on studies involving animal tissue suggest that the Holmium YAG laser energy can shorten glenohumeral ligaments.[14] A study demonstrated that significant capsular shrinkage can be achieved with the application of nonablative laser energy without det-

rimental effects to the viscoelastic properties of the capsular tissues.[18]

I have employed the laser-assisted capsular shift technique in conjunction with the Suretac anterior stabilization technique during shoulder arthroscopy for patients with shoulder instability. Early success has been observed in these cases, which are currently under clinical study. Fanton had excellent clinical results in 93 percent of 41 patients.[23] I feel that the laser-assisted capsular shift/capsulorrhaphy has potential in the treatment of certain shoulder instability patterns, particularly in the overhand athlete. Further laboratory and clinical outcome studies are needed to confirm the potential. The procedure

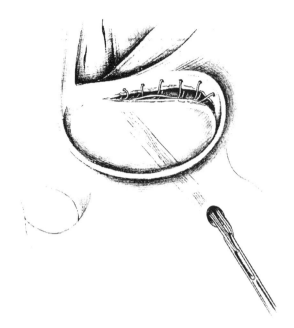

FIGURE 17.6 *Multiple sutures are passed through the single drill hold. (From Esch and Baker,*[22] *with permission.)*

is performed during shoulder arthroscopy, with anterior stabilization and/or Bankhart lesion repair with or without capsular shifting as indicated, using the Acufex Suretac system for fixation. The Holmium YAG laser is then employed under direct arthroscopic evaluation in a saline medium to perform capsulorraphy of the capsuloligamentous structures. The tissue shrinking described by other authors has been consistently observed.[24] Postoperative treatment is described in case study 1.

CASE STUDY 1
REHABILITATION FOLLOWING ARTHROSCOPIC ANTERIOR STABILIZATION WITH LASER CAPSULORRAPHY

SUBJECTIVE INFORMATION

The patient is an 18-year-old right-handed competitive volleyball player who reports a 1-year history of anterior instability in her left shoulder.

She initially incurred an anterior dislocation that required reduction, with 3 to 4 continued incidences of subluxation and feelings of instability with aggressive overhead movements during volleyball. Nonoperative physical therapy and continued exercises performed with the left shoulder did not reduce her feelings of instability. She underwent an arthroscopic anterior stabilization using Suretac bioabsorbable tacks and a laser capsulorraphy using the Holmium: Yag laser.

INITIAL POSTOPERATIVE MANAGEMENT

The patient is immobilized for the first 10 to 14 days in a sling, with removal of the sling only for range of motion of the elbow to prevent flexion contracture. The patient is given grip putty and instruction for distal range of motion for the elbow forearm and wrist. Ice is used to control postoperative pain.

INITIAL POSTOPERATIVE EVALUATION AND TREATMENT
(3 WEEKS POSTOP)

Examination of the patient shows moderate scapular winging and atrophy in the infraspinous fossa on the left. Capsular mobility of the uninjured shoulder shows 2+ anterior translation with a load and shift and supine capsular mobility test. The elbows passively hyperextend 15° bilaterally, and there is marked hyperextension of the MCP joints on both hands. The patient shows increased physiologic laxity of her upper extremities. The left postoperative shoulder shows only 1° of anterior translation, with further clinical testing deferred at this time due to the patient's acute postoperative nature. Passive range of motion of the left shoulder is initially 0° to 95° of flexion, 0° to 60° abduction, 0° to 15° of external rotation, and 55° of internal rotation with arm abducted 45°. The patient is able to volitionally contract the internal and external rotators on initial exam.

INITIAL TREATMENT *(WEEKS 3–4)*

Passive and active assistive range of motion of the left shoulder, gentle manual resistance, and multiple angle isometrics for shoulder IR/ER, bicep and tricep, and scapular protraction/retraction are emphasized. Range of motion limitations of 100° of flexion and abduction, and 45° of external rotation. Accessory glenohumeral joint mobilization is performed in the posterior direction; however, anterior glides are not performed to protect the anterior capsule. Modalities such as electric stimulation and heat/ice are used to facilitate ROM and control discomfort.

TREATMENT

WEEKS 4–10

Passive range of motion to terminal ranges of flexion and abduction is now initiated, with external rotation slowly progressed to 90°. Specific emphasis is placed on regaining internal rotation range of motion and joint mobilizations such as the posterior glide. For functional reasons, the shoulder is placed into horizontal adduction to further stretch the posterior capsule. The patient's current range of motion at 6 weeks postop is 0° to 160° of flexion, 0° to 125° of abduction, 0° to 55° of external rotation, and 0° to 45° of internal rotation. Strengthening exercises are progressed to isotonic PREs, emphasizing rotator cuff-dominant movement patterns and scapular stabilization. Closed-chain exercises are employed to enhance scapular co-contraction using therapeutic balls and wall push-ups.

WEEKS 10–16

Continued use of mobilization and stretching to restore full glenohumeral joint range of motion is combined with strengthening for the rotator cuff and scapular musculature. Isokinetic exercise in the modified base position for internal and external rotation is started at 12 weeks postop. Plyometric exercises consisting of chest passes and medicine ball catches are used to prepare the shoulder for the rapid concentric and eccentric loads inherent in sport activity. At 14 weeks postop, the patient's range of motion is 0° to 175° of flexion, 0° to 150° of abduction, 0° to 85° of external rotation, and 0° to 60° of internal rotation with 90° of abduction. An isokinetic test performed in the modified base position revealed 15 percent deficits in external rotation at speeds 90°, 210°, and 300°/s. Internal rotation strength on the left shoulder was only 5 percent weaker when compared to the right dominant arm. ER/IR unilateral strength ratios are 55 to 60 percent, and are approximately 10 to 15 percent below the desired 66 percent standard. The patient continues with rehabilitation on a three times weekly basis with continued emphasis on rotator cuff strengthening, as well as achieving a full functional range of motion. She is discharged at 16 weeks with a home exercise program of rubber tubing and isotonic rotator cuff exercises, and a general scapular program with closed-chain exercises. Her interval return to volleyball includes a 2- to 4-week period without overhead hitting or serving, with a gradual progression to these activities after pain-free practice activity has been demonstrated for the first 2 to 4 weeks.

CASE STUDY 2
REHABILITATION FOLLOWING OPEN CAPSULAR SHIFT

SUBJECTIVE INFORMATION

The patient is a 30-year-old male who initially dislocated his shoulder 2 years ago while snowboarding. Over the course of a 2-year period, the patient dislocated his right shoulder 12 to 13 times, with an increase in the ease of dislocation and greater difficulty in reducing the shoulder over time. The patient denies any neural symptoms postop or preop from the dislocations that occurred. He is involved in precarious sporting activities such as skiing, snowboarding, and mountain biking, and hopes to return to these activities following surgery. The injury and surgery occurred to his right arm and the patient is right handed. He was immobilized for 2 weeks following surgery without any movement or therapy. He presents to physical therapy with his shoulder in a sling.

INITIAL FINDINGS

The patient has a well-healed anterior incision, and is fully intact to light touch sensation immediately surrounding the incision. Mild atrophy of the deltoid and pectoralis major muscles is noted when compared bilaterally, with moderate infraspinatus atrophy. The patient's left shoulder shows 1° of anterior translation with a load and shift test, and no hypermobility is noted at the elbows or MCP joints. Initial PROM of the right shoulder is 90° of flexion, 50° of abduction, 0° of external rotation, and 50° of internal rotation. No further special testing of the shoulder is performed at this time due to the patient's acute postoperative nature.

INITIAL TREATMENT *(WEEKS 2–4)*

Sling immobilization continues until the fourth postoperative week. PROM is initiated within the ranges of 100° of flexion and abduction as tolerated, 0° of external rotation, and full internal rotation as tolerated. Gripping exercises with putty are used, and gentle manual resistance for the bicep, tricep, forearm, wrist musculature, scapulothoracic protractors, and retractors is performed with both support and protection of the glenohumeral joint. Submaximal isometrics for the internal and external rotators are initiated and performed as tolerated, with progression into manual resistance by the fourth postoperative week. By the fourth postoperative week, this patient has 120° of passive flexion, 90° of abduction, 20° of external rotation at 45° of abduction, and 50° of internal rotation.

TREATMENT

WEEKS 4–6

Continued use of passive and now active assistive and active range of motion is followed. Glenohumeral and scapulothoracic joint mobilization is used with avoidance of anterior glides to protect the healing anterior capsule. Rhythmic stabilization with the shoulder in varying degrees of flexion, with the patient in a supine position, is used to improve kinesthetic awareness and promote strength via the co-contraction of scapular musculature. Rotator cuff strengthening begins with no weight in patterns within the allowed ranges of motion. Low resistance and high repetition formats are followed. Shoulder shrugs, rows, and closed-chain pendulum exercises over a therapeutic ball are used to strengthen the scapular musculature. At 6 weeks postop, the patient has 145° of flexion, 110° of abduction, 45° of abduction, and 60° of internal rotation. He is tolerating rotator cuff strengthening exercises with light-resistance rubber tubing, and a 1.5-pound weight.

WEEKS 6–12

At this time the goals for the patient are for the gradual reattainment of full terminal ranges of motion. Continued passive stretching and glenohumeral joint mobilization are applied with particular emphasis on posterior glides to enhance both flexion and internal rotation range of motion, as well as caudal glides. The patient's strengthening program is advanced to include plyometric exercises initially with the therapeutic balls, and progressing to medicine balls. Weight-bearing protraction step-ups are used to enhance scapular stabilization. PREs for rotator cuff strengthening are advanced up to a 5-pound maximum level on this patient. At 12 weeks the patient is using a 5-pound weight for his isolated rotator cuff exercises, and is also using medium-level rubber tubing. A 6-pound medicine ball is controlled during the plyometric exercises. Range of motion at 12 weeks postop is 170° of flexion, 155° of abduction, 80° of external rotation with 90° of abduction, and 65° of internal rotation with 90° of abduction.

WEEKS 12–20

The continuation of range of motion and mobilization is combined with rotator cuff and scapular strengthening isotonic exercises. The initiation of isokinetic exercise in the movement pattern of internal and external rotation in the modified base position is recommended. The criterion for isokinetic exercise progression is the tolerance of a minimum of 3-pound isotonic rotator cuff exercises, and full range of motion within the isokinetic training ranges. An isokinetic test performed at 14 weeks postop on this patient shows external rotation strength to be 5 percent weaker on the postop extremity, and corresponding internal rotation strength to be 20 to 25 percent weaker across the three velocities tested.

WEEKS 20–28

An isokinetic evaluation at week 20 postop shows equal external rotation strength and 5 percent greater internal rotation strength at the three testing speeds. Pain-free isotonic and isokinetic training is currently tolerated by the patient. Independence is gained in the strengthening program. Active range of motion is 175° of flexion, 165° of abduction, 85° of external rotation, and 65° of internal rotation measured with 90° of internal rotation.

The patient is discharged to a home exercise program, and will use pulleys and capsular stretches (cross body for posterior capsule, and overhead stretching for interior capsule) to maintain range of motion. Interval sport programs are normally initiated at this time. Additional home exercise is given to this patient in the closed chain such as push-ups, push-ups with a plus, seated press-ups, and wall push-ups with partner overpressure, to attempt to prepare the patient's extremity for weight bearing and impact often incurred in his precarious sport activities such as skiing and snowboarding. No amount of preparation will be sufficient for violent trauma often incurred in these sporting activities. However, inclusion of plyometric and closed-chain exercise will allow progression of the patient's strengthening program beyond the standard open-chain rotator cuff and scapular exercises.

Traditional interval return programs, such as those for throwing and tennis, are discussed elsewhere in this book. Criteria for progression of the interval programs are adequate strength to perform the sport-related movement patterns in a pain-free manner without compensation from adjoining segments, adequate range of mo-

tion to prevent injury to adjoining segments (lack of glenohumeral joint ER, thus placing increased valgus stress on the elbow), a satisfactory clinical exam with respect to impingement, and instability testing (TSE).

References

1. Wilk KE, Arrigo C: Current concepts in the rehabilitation of the athletic shoulder. JOSP 18:365, 1993
2. Bankhart A: The pathology and treatment of recurrent dislocation of the shoulder joint. Br J Surg 26:22, 1938
3. Jobe FW, Kivitne RS: Shoulder pain in the overhand or throwing athlete: the relationship of anterior instability and rotator cuff impingement. Orthop Rev 18:963, 1989
4. Schwartz R, O'Brien S: Capsular restraints to the abducted shoulder: A biomechanical study. Orthop Trans 12:727, 1988
5. Warner J, Deng X, Warren R et al: Static capsuloligamentous restraints to superior-inferior translation of the glenohumeral joint. Am J Sports Med 20:675, 1992
6. Harryman D, Sidles J, Matsen F: The role of the rotator interval capsule in passive motion and stability of the shoulder. J Bone Joint Surg 74:53, 1992
7. Rodosky MW, Harner CD, Fue FH: The role of the long head of the biceps muscle and superior glenoid labral in anterior stability of the shoulder. Am J Sports Med 22:121, 1994
8. Hawkins R, Boker D: Clinical evaluation of shoulder problems. p. 149. In Rockwood CA, Matsen FA III (eds): The Shoulder. WB Saunders, Philadelphia, 1990
9. Neer C, Foster C: Inferior capsular shift for inferior and multi-directional instability of the shoulder. J Bone Joint Surg 62:897, 1980
10. Roukous J, Fegain J, Abbot H: Modified axially roentgenogram. Clinic Orthop 82:84, 1972
11. Pavlov H, Warren R, Weiss C et al: The roentgenographic evaluation of anterior shoulder instability. Clin Orthop 194:153, 1985
12. Bankhart A: Discussion on recurrent dislocation the shoulder. J Bone Joint Surg 30B:46, 1948
13. Rubenstein D, Jobe F, Gloosman R et al: Anterior capsulolabral reconstruction of the shoulder in athletes. J Shoulder Elbow 1:229, 1992

14. Bramhall J, Scarpinto D, Andrews JR: Operative arthroscopy of the shoulder. p. 105. In Andrews JR, Wilke K (eds): The Athlete's Shoulder. Churchill Livingstone, New York, 1994
15. Skyhar M, Altchek D, Warren R: Shoulder arthroscopy with the patient in the beach-chair position. Arthroscopy 4:256, 1988
16. Johnson LL: Symposium on Arthroscopy. Arthroscopy Association of North America annual meeting, San Francisco, March 1986
17. Caspari R: Arthroscopic reconstruction for anterior shoulder capsulorrhaphy. Techn Orthoped 3:59, 1988
18. Maki N: Arthroscopic stabilization: suture technique. Oper Techn Orthop 1:180, 1991
19. Wolf E: Arthroscopic Bankhart repair using suture anchors. Techn Orthop 1:184, 1991
20. Warner J, Warren R: Arthroscopic Bankhart repair using a cannulated absorbable fixation device. Oper Techn Orthop 1:192, 1991
21. Eisenberg J, Redler M, Hecht P: Arthroscopic stabilization of the chronic subluxating or dislocation shoulder without the use of internal fixation, abstracted. Arthroscopy 7:315, 1991
22. Esch J, Baker C: Anterior Instability. p. 99. In: Surgical Arthroscopy: The Shoulder and Elbow. JB Lippincott, Philadelphia, 1993
23. Fanton G, Thabit G: orthopaedic uses of arthroscopy and lasers. p. 47. Orthopaedic Knowledge Update Sports Medicine. AAOS, 1994
24. Hayashi K, Markel M, Thabit G et al: The effect of nonablative Laser energy on joint capsular properties: an in vitro mechanical study using a rabbit model. Am J Sports Med 23:482, 1995
25. Hawkins RJ, Bell RH, Lippitt SB: Atlas of Shoulder Surgery. Mosby-Year Book, St Louis, 1996
26. Jobe FW, Giangarra CE, Kvitne RS et al: Anterior capsulolabral reconstruction of the shoulder in athletes in overhand sports. Am J Sports Med 19:428, 1991

18

Rotator Cuff Repairs

JOSEPH S. WILKES

The causes of rotator cuff tears are varied and depend on the age of the patient as well as the precipitating activity. They may be traumatic or degenerative. Because of their locations—the supraspinatus primarily, and infraspinatus secondarily—they are the most frequently torn muscles of the rotator cuff Fig. 18.1.

Etiology

Previously it was believed that impingement was the primary cause of rotator cuff disorders, including tears.[1] Impingement occurs when the coracoacromial arch causes attrition of the tendon due to narrowing of the subacromial bursal space from either bony encroachment or enlargement of the tendon Fig. 18.2.[2]

Impingement is not the only cause of rotator cuff tears. Eccentric overload of the rotator cuff muscles, resulting in overuse and fatigue, causes fiber failure of the rotator cuff, and is probably the most common cause of tears in the young, athletic patient.[3] Tears in older patients are primarily the result of coracoacromial arch abrasion.[4] Instability patterns can also produce impingement syndrome, which causes rotator cuff tears secondarily. Fiber failure can also occur from chronic tendinitis. Other causes of rotator cuff tears are calcific tendinitis Fig. 18.3,[5] tumors,[6] and degenerative changes of the coracoacromial joint that produce inferior spurs Fig. 18.4.[7]

Eccentric overload patterns of the rotator cuff usually cause tearing of the undersurface of the rotator cuff because of repetitive deceleration stresses Fig. 18.5. Instability can cause fraying of either the upper or lower surface of the cuff depending on whether impingement or overload-type forces are placed on the rotator cuff.

Acute tears of the rotator cuff can occur from extrinsic overload, such as when a great force is applied to the abducted arm while the rotator cuff is active. Another example of extrinsic overload would be a situation in which a person was forced to catch himself during a fall by reaching overhead, thus placing a large distraction force on the arm. These mechanisms can injure the capsule and other muscles of the shoulder. An acute dislocation of the shoulder can not only disrupt the glenohumeral capsule but can tear the muscles about the shoulder, including those of the rotator cuff.

How the rotator cuff tear develops depends on the pattern of the abnormal forces applied to the rotator cuff. Patients with primary impingement have fraying of the upper surface of the rotator cuff that subsequently leads to rotator cuff tears and tendon ruptures Fig. 18.6. The subscapularis can also be involved in the impingement syndrome, and its integrity should be evaluated. The subscapularis should be used cautiously in a reconstruction procedure. Secondary impingement causes the same type of wear pattern.

Diagnosis

The diagnosis of a rotator cuff tear can be difficult because the signs and symptoms are similar to those of acute rotator cuff tendinitis. The clini-

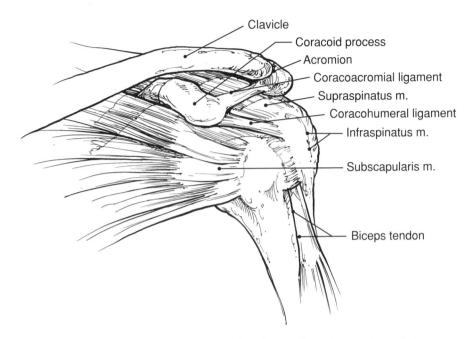

FIGURE 18.1 *Anterior-superior view of the shoulder shows the relationship of the osseous structures to the rotator cuff and the coracoacromial arch.*

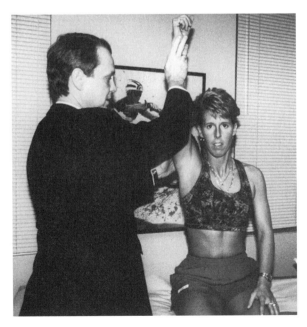

FIGURE 18.2 *The pain of impingement is reproduced with the arm in the fully abducted and flexed position.*

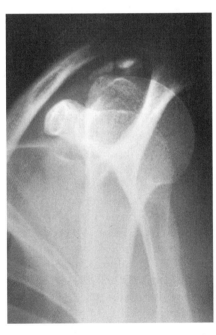

FIGURE 18.3 *Calcific deposit within the supraspinatus tendon.*

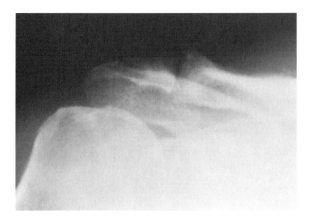

FIGURE 18.4 *Osteoarthritis of the AC joint. An inferior spur is impinging on the rotator cuff.*

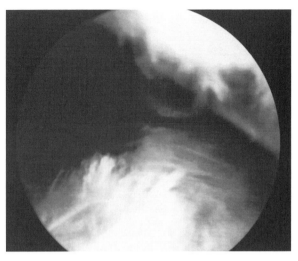

FIGURE 18.6 *Arthroscopic subacromial view shows fraying of the rotator cuff (grade II).*

cal history and physical examination are the most important components in making the diagnosis.[8] As part of the initial examination of a patient with a shoulder problem, routine radiographs frequently show sclerotic or cystic changes in the area of the greater tuberosity that may indicate advanced rotator cuff disease. If symptoms persist after a trial of conservative treatment, further noninvasive evaluation

should be undertaken to determine the status of the rotator cuff.

DIAGNOSTIC IMAGING TECHNIQUES

Currently, there are several imaging methods for confirming the presence, location, and size of a defect in the rotator cuff. The arthrogram, for many years, was the standard for documenting a rotator cuff tear Fig. 18.7.[9] The arthrogram is

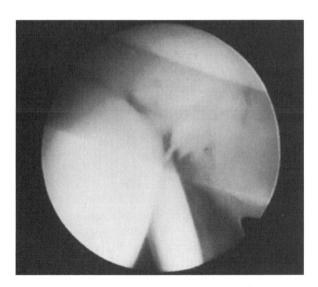

FIGURE 18.5 *Arthroscopic view of the inferior surface of the rotator cuff shows fraying of the undersurface.*

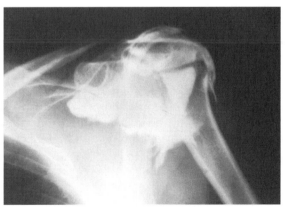

FIGURE 18.7 *Arthrogram of the shoulder with dye extravasation into the subacromial bursa indicating a tear of the rotator cuff.*

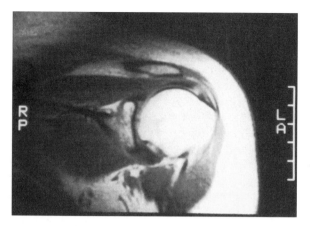

FIGURE 18.8 *MRI of the supraspinatus showing the compact space under the coracoacromial area and an abnormal signal in the supraspinatus tendon indicating a tear.*

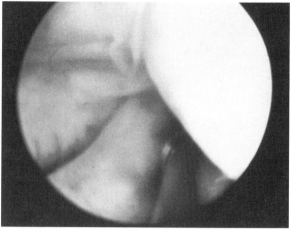

FIGURE 18.9 *Arthroscopic view of the glenohumeral joint shows the undersurface of the supraspinatus portion of the rotator cuff.*

extremely sensitive for full-thickness rotator cuff tears, with greater than 90 percent sensitivity and specificity,[10,11] an accuracy of 98 to 99 percent and an 8 percent incidence of false-negative results.[12] However, it usually cannot provide information about incomplete tears, tears on the superior surface, or advanced rotator cuff tendon disease. Arthrography requires insertion of a needle and dye into the glenohumeral joint. Extravasation of dye into the subacromial bursal area suggests a rupture. Ultrasonography is noninvasive and has approximately the same accuracy as the arthrogram.[13]

Recently, magnetic resonance imaging MRI has become well established in the evaluation of the rotator cuff tear. With newer technology, the sensitivity and specificity are greater than 90 percent in most studies.[13] Magnetic resonance imaging can detect not only the presence of full-thickness tears, but the presence of partial tears, their size, and their location with a high degree of accuracy as well Fig. 18.8.[12,14]

ARTHROSCOPIC EVALUATION

Arthroscopy can also play an important role in evaluating the rotator cuff for tears. Both the inferior and superior surfaces of the rotator cuff

along with the biceps tendon can be seen arthroscopically. The rotator cuff can be palpated with arthroscopic instruments to determine its integrity Fig. 18.9 and to differentiate partial- and full-thickness tears from chronic tendinitis. Arthroscopy can also help detect instabilities that may be associated with rotator cuff disorders. During the arthroscopic examination, the integrity of the anterior labrum and inferior glenohumeral ligament should be assessed and the shoulder joint examined for instability. SLAP (separation of the superior labrum anterior and posterior) lesions of the labrum can indicate glenohumeral dysfunction.

Surgical Treatment

Initially, most rotator cuff tears should be treated nonoperatively. The indication for surgical treatment is a documented partial- or full-thickness rotator cuff tear that has not responded to treatment and produces symptoms that interfere with the patient's normal functioning. However, acute, symptomatic tears in relatively young individuals should probably be repaired early.[15]

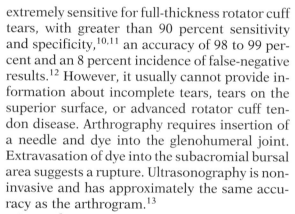

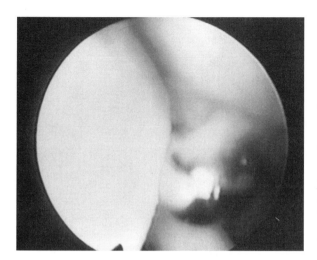

FIGURE 18.10 *Arthroscopic view of the glenohumeral joint with an arthroscopic motorized blade trimming the frayed rotator cuff ends.*

Arthroscopic evaluation of the rotator cuff can be combined with the surgical treatment of some tears. The partial-thickness tear with fraying on either the inferior or superior surface can be treated with debridement of the involved portion of the tendon Fig. 18.10. The debridement allows for freshening of the injured portion of the rotator cuff, thus stimulating a healing response. The remaining fibers hold the cuff in position to heal. Certainly, a patient with a more advanced partial-thickness tear (more torn fibers) of this type should proceed cautiously in the postoperative period with regard to activities. For a superior lesion, a coracoacromial decompression procedure should also be performed. The rehabilitation is similar to that following open repair of the rotator cuff, but the program is slightly accelerated. We are able to shorten the rehabilitation period in these patients because they have intact fibers remaining to protect the cuff's integrity.

During the arthroscopic evaluation, the intra-articular portion of the biceps tendon should be examined for injuries associated with rotator cuff lesions. Frequently, debridement or tenodesis of the long head of the biceps is indicated when there is a rotator cuff tear. Instability and labral abnormalities can also be evaluated at this time.

Small full-thickness rotator cuff tears (< 1 cm) can frequently be repaired by an arthroscopically assisted method. The same principles of repair are used as for an open repair. Under arthroscopic visualization, the greater tuberosity in the area of the involved tendon is burred down to a bleeding bony trough. Next, using an intra-articular suturing technique, sutures are passed through suture anchors in the greater tuberosity, and the rotator cuff is attached to the bone by tightening the suture Fig. 18.11.

Lesions larger than 1 cm should be repaired by an open technique. These lesions can be subdivided into small, medium, large, and massive tears. Small and medium tears are repaired through a superior lateral incision of the surgeon's choice Fig. 18.12A. Exposure of the rotator cuff tear is facilitated by a coracoacromial decompression. Small tears can generally be debrided and advanced to the bony bed without problems Fig. 12B and C. Medium and large tears frequently need moderate mobilization of the muscle bellies by tension to obtain good repair to the bony bed, or a V-Y repair can be done Fig. 18.13. Massive rotator cuff repairs require extensive mobilization of the muscle bellies and perhaps of the surrounding muscles, particularly of the subscapularis or infraspinatus, to allow coverage of the humeral head. In these patients, the biceps tendon is usually damaged or ruptured severely and a tenodesis can be done at the bicipital groove Fig. 18.14.[7,16–18]

Results

The results of rotator cuff repair are variable and seem to have a direct relationship to the patient's age and the severity of the tear.[19] Although it has been shown that repair of rotator cuff tears results in a significant increase in function for all patients, the degree of patient satisfaction with the repair depends on the size of the tear, associated pathology, and the age of the patient. Patients over the age of 65 years have a less favora-

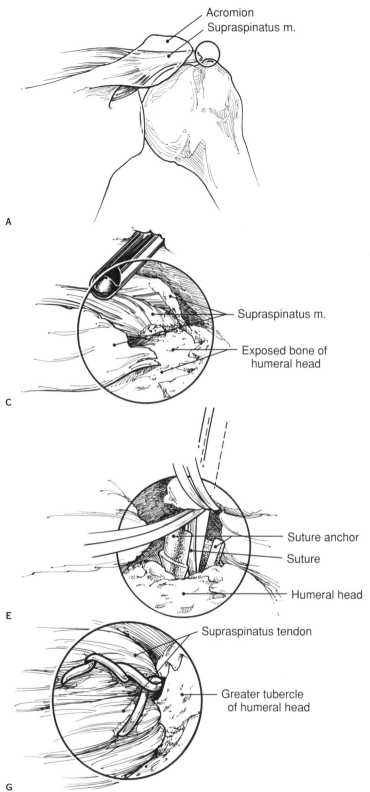

Acromion
Supraspinatus m.

A

Supraspinatus m.

Exposed bone of
humeral head

C

Suture anchor

Suture

Humeral head

E

Supraspinatus tendon

Greater tubercle
of humeral head

G

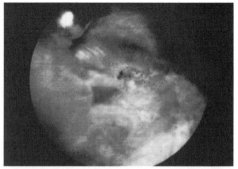

B

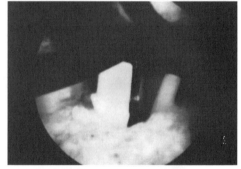

D

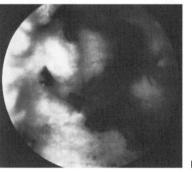

F

FIGURE 18.11 (A) *Arthroscopically assisted repair of a rotator cuff tear. The arthroscopic portal is in the subacromial bursa.* **(B)** *Subacromial bursal arthroscopic view of a tear of the rotator cuff.* **(C)** *Rupture of the tendinous insertion of the supraspinatus at its attachment to the humeral head.* **(D)** *Arthroscopic view of the greater tuberosity after preparation for rotator cuff repair.* **(E)** *Sutures are passed through suture anchors in the greater tuberosity.* **(F)** *Arthoroscopic view of the repaired rotator cuff.* **(G)** *Supraspinatus tendon is sutured to the humeral head.*

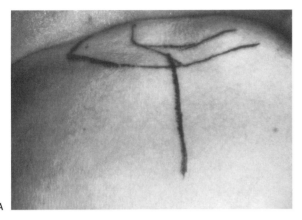

A

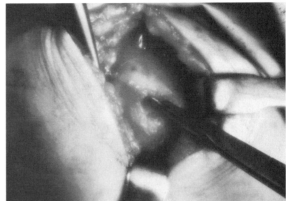

B

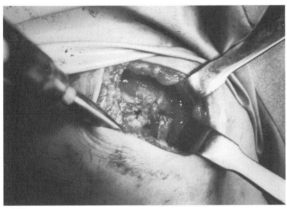

C

FIGURE 18.12 **(A)** *The acromion and clavicle are outlined for the intended superior lateral incision.* **(B)** *Small tear exposed with the open technique.* **(C)** *Small tear repaired by open technique.*

ble outcome than those under 65, although symptomatic patients of any age with complete rotator cuff tears have at least partial relief of their symptoms after a successful rotator cuff repair.[20]

CASE STUDY 1

A 46-year-old woman is a volleyball coach for a local college. She has participated in volleyball as an athlete and a coach for over 20 years. In early 1994, she noted increasing pain and discomfort in her right shoulder. She was treated with nonsteroidal anti-inflammatory medications and physical therapy without relief. An MRI was done in the fall of 1994, which showed an abnormal supraspinatus tendon with probable rotator cuff tear. When she first presented to

our office in April 1995, the patient had full range of shoulder motion, but she had a positive impingement sign and some weakness on abduction at 90°. She had no instability and her neurovascular examination was intact. Radiographic examination showed normal bony structures and joint spaces. A review of the MRI scan showed a grossly abnormal tendon and a probable tear in the supraspinatus of the rotator cuff. She was scheduled for arthroscopic examination of the shoulder.

At surgery, the diagnostic arthroscopy showed an intact biceps tendon and articular surfaces. She had a separation of the anterior superior labrum, but the inferior labrum was intact with no evidence of instability. When its inferior surface was viewed, the rotator cuff tendon was found to be abnormal and to have a tear Fig. 18.15. It was abnormal over a fairly large area, and it was thought that open repair was necessary. There-

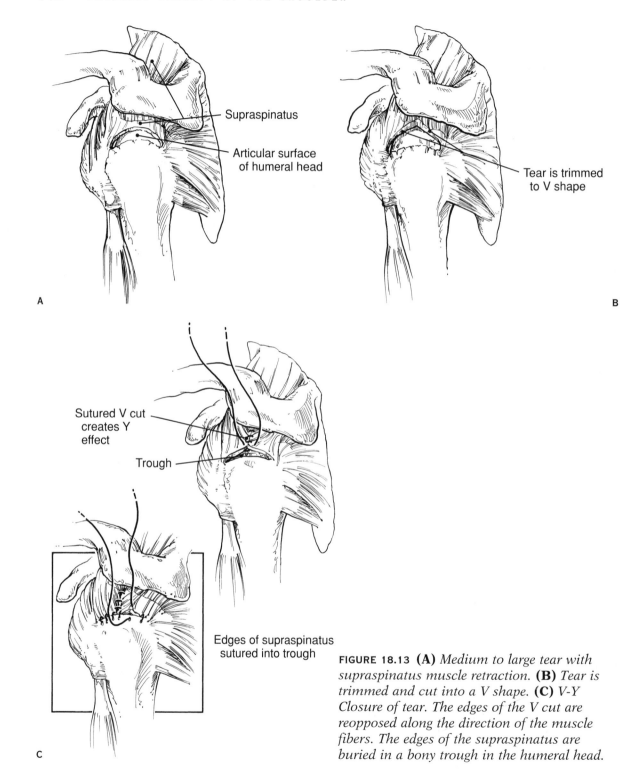

A

Supraspinatus

Articular surface
of humeral head

B

Tear is trimmed
to V shape

Sutured V cut
creates Y
effect

Trough

Edges of supraspinatus
sutured into trough

C

FIGURE 18.13 **(A)** *Medium to large tear with*
supraspinatus muscle retraction. **(B)** *Tear is*
trimmed and cut into a V shape. **(C)** *V-Y*
Closure of tear. The edges of the V cut are
reopposed along the direction of the muscle
fibers. The edges of the supraspinatus are
buried in a bony trough in the humeral head.

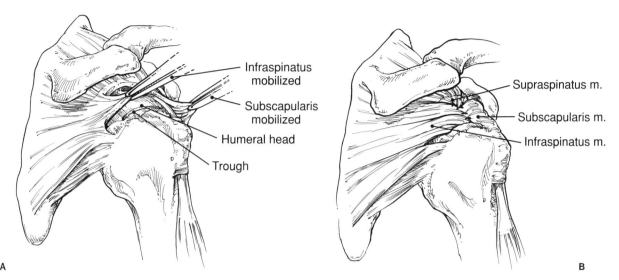

FIGURE 18.14 **(A)** *Massive tear of the rotator cuff with the "bald head" appearance of the humeral head. Mobilization of the infraspinatus and subscapularis and elevation of the supraspinatus muscle body to repair the rotator cuff.* **(B)** *Repaired massive tear after muscle mobilization.*

fore, an open incision in the anterolateral aspect of the shoulder was made exposing the rotator cuff, where a 2-cm superior tear was identified with some retraction of the tendon. The area was freshened, and the rotator cuff was repaired to a bony bed with advancement of the tendon back to the bone Fig. 18.16. After surgery, she was

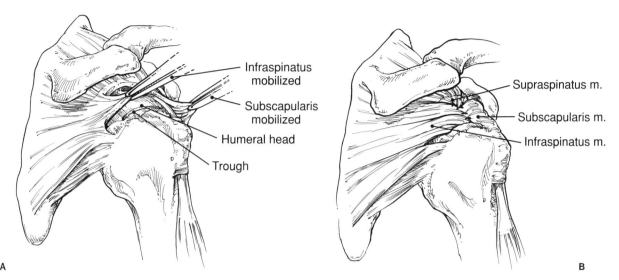

FIGURE 18.15 *Arthroscopic view of the inferior surface of the rotator cuff tear in Case Study 1.*

started on pendulum and passive range-of-motion exercises, which she continued for the first 4 weeks after surgery. At that time she had flexion to 90° and abduction to 60° but minimal external rotation. She began a structured program of physical therapy at 4 weeks after surgery and progressed satisfactorily over the next 6 to 8 weeks to full range of motion and full strength. At that point, 3 months after surgery, she was allowed to resume her normal activities.

CASE STUDY 2

A 48-year-old man was seen in the fall of 1994 with insidious right shoulder pain without a known precipitating injury. He had pain in the 60° to 120° arc of motion and some pain on forced abduction at 90° but he had good strength. He had no instability and had full range of motion. He began a trial of physical therapy and nonsteroidal anti-inflammatory medications, which allowed him to improve somewhat. He returned in the late spring of 1995 with recurrent

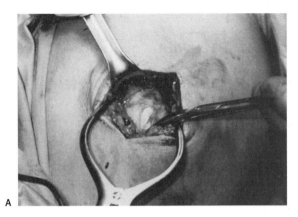
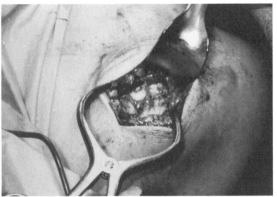

FIGURE 18.16 **(A)** *Appearance of the rotator cuff tear in Case Study 1 after exposure by open technique.* **(B)** *Repaired rotator cuff in Case Study 1.*

pain in the shoulder. His physical examination at that time was essentially unchanged. An MRI scan showed a probable rotator cuff tear. The patient underwent arthroscopic evaluation and was found to have no evidence of instability and an intact labrum. However, he had fraying of the undersurface of the rotator cuff and some fraying of the articular side of the subscapularis on the superior aspect Fig. 18.17A. Examination with the arthroscope in the subacromial bursa showed a 1-cm tear of the rotator cuff without retraction. The tear extended through approximately 80 percent of the supraspinatus tendon

Fig. 18.17B, which was slightly pulled away from the bone. After subacromial decompression, the bony bed on the greater tuberosity was freshened with a motorized arthroscopic blade through a third portal lateral to the acromion. Two sutures were placed through the supraspinatus tendon, and after drilling two holes in the greater tuberosity, the sutures were anchored into the bone with plastic suture anchors. With the shoulder in the abducted position, the sutures were digitally tied, pulling the rotator cuff tendon back down to the bony bed Fig. 18.18. Postoperatively, the patient was started on full passive range-of-mo-

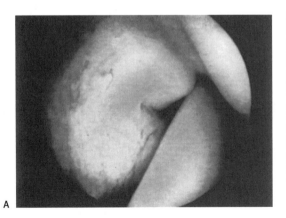
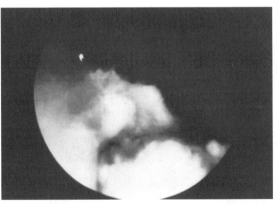

FIGURE 18.17 **(A)** *Arthroscopic view of the undersurface of the rotator cuff in Case Study 2.* **(B)** *Arthroscopic subacromial view of the superior surface of the rotator cuff showing an incomplete tear of the rotator cuff in Case Study 2.*

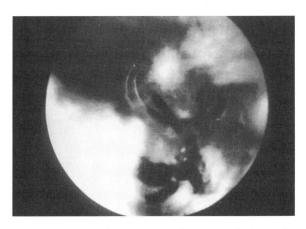

FIGURE 18.18 *Arthroscopic subacromial view of the repaired rotator cuff in Case Study 2.*

tion exercises. By 6 weeks, he had achieved full range of motion and had started strengthening exercises. By 10 weeks, he had excellent range of motion and was gaining strength with relief of postoperative pain. He was started on an increased exercise program.

References

1. Neer CS II: Anterior acromioplasty for the chronic impingement syndrome in the shoulder: a preliminary report. J Bone Joint Surg 54A:41, 1972

2. Nash HL: Rotator cuff damage: re-examining the causes and treatments. Phys Sportsmed 16:129, 1988

3. Fowler PJ: Shoulder injuries in the mature athlete. Adv Sports Med Fitness 1:225, 1988

4. Brewer BJ: Aging of the rotator cuff. Am J Sports Med 7:102, 1979

5. Hsu HC, Wu JJ, Jim YF et al: Calcific tendinitis and rotator cuff tearing: a clinical and radiographic study. J Shoulder Elbow Surg 3:159, 1994

6. Fallon PJ, Hollinshead RM: Solitary osteochondroma of the distal clavicle causing a full-thickness rotator cuff tear. J Shoulder Elbow Surg 3: 266, 1994

7. Bigliani LU, Rodosky MW: Techniques in repair of large rotator cuff tears. Tech Orthop 9:133, 1994

8. Hawkins RJ, Mohtadi N: Rotator cuff problems in athletes. p. 640. In DeLee JC, Drez DD Jr. (eds): Orthopaedic Sports Medicine: Principles and Practice. WB Saunders, Philadelphia, 1994

9. Brems J: Rotator cuff tear: evaluation and treatment. Orthopedics 11:69, 1988

10. Iannotti JP (ed): Rotator Cuff Disorders: Evaluation and Treatment. p. 14. American Academy of Orthopaedic Surgeons, Park Ridge, IL, 1991

11. Mink JH, Harris E, Rappaport M: Rotator cuff tears: evaluation using double-contrast shoulder arthrography. Radiology 157:621, 1985

12. Hawkins RJ, Misamore GW, Hobeika PE: Surgery for full-thickness rotator-cuff tears. J Bone Joint Surg 67A:1349, 1985

13. Burk DL Jr, Karasick D, Kurtz AB et al: Rotator cuff tears: prospective comparison of MR imaging with arthrography, sonography and surgery. Am J Roetgenol 153:87, 1989

14. Snyder SJ: Rotator cuff lesions: acute and chronic. Clin Sports Med 10:595, 1991

15. Hawkins RJ, Mohtadi N: Rotator cuff problems in athletes. p. 645. In DeLee JC, Drez DD (eds): Orthopaedic Sports Medicine: Principles and Practice. WB Saunders, Philadelphia, 1994

16. Ellman H, Hanker G, Bayer M: Repair of the rotator cuff. End-result study of factors influencing reconstruction. J Bone Joint Surg 68A:1136, 1986

17. Neviaser JS, Neviaser RJ, Neviaser TJ: The repair of chronic massive ruptures of the rotator cuff of the shoulder by use of a freeze-dried rotator cuff. J Bone Joint Surg 60A:681, 1978

18. Packer NP, Calvert PT, Bayley JI, Kessel L: Operative treatment of chronic ruptures of the rotator cuff of the shoulder. J Bone Joint Surg 65B:171, 1983

19. Hattrup SJ: Rotator cuff repair: relevance of patient age. J Shoulder Elbow Surg 4:95, 1995

20. Adamson GJ, Tibone JE: Ten-year assessment of primary rotator cuff repairs. J Shoulder Elbow Surg 2:57, 1993

19

Shoulder Girdle Fractures

MICHAEL J. WOODEN

DAVID J. CONAWAY

Shoulder pain, stiffness, and weakness after fracture are common problems presented to the orthopedic physical therapist. Fractures are always accompanied to some degree by soft tissue injury, leaving serious implications for rehabilitation well after the fracture has healed. Even if the fracture itself heals solidly, it is the soft tissue recovery that will determine the ultimate outcome of function.[1]

This chapter presents a brief overview of some of the more common shoulder girdle fractures. For each, general rehabilitation guidelines are offered. The effects of trauma and immobilization are also summarized.

Stages of Fracture Healing

As in any other body region, displaced fractures of the shoulder girdle must be immobilized to allow the fracture to progress through the stages of healing. Immediately following the fracture is the *acute, inflammatory stage*[2] of hematoma formation. In this stage of vasodilation and serous exudation, inflammatory cells are brought to the area to remove necrotic soft tissue and bone from the ends of the fragments. As the hematoma becomes more organized at the start of the *reparative stage,*[2] a "fibrin scaffold" is provided for the reparative cells, which differentiate and begin to produce collagen, cartilage, and bone. These cells, primarily osteoblasts, invade

the hematoma through capillary formation to form a callous of immature bone. Meanwhile, osteoclast cells resorb necrotic bone from the ends of the fragments. In the *remodeling stage,*[2] resorption and new bone formation continue as trabecular bone patterns are laid down in response to the stress applied. By this time, the immobilization, period should be ending so that the necessary "stress" is provided by remobilization of the limb.

The length of time required for each healing stage is influenced by many factors.[2] Some of these include the severity of the trauma, how much bone is lost, the presence of infection, which bone is fractured, how effective the immobilization is, and the patient's age, general health, and level of activity.

Effects of Immobilization on Soft Tissues

The combination of trauma to soft tissues and subsequent immobilization needed for bone healing contributes to stiffness of periarticular connective tissue structures and weakness of the surrounding musculature.[3] Much has been researched and written about changes in histologic, biochemical, and mechanical properties. To summarize, the most significant motion-limiting effects are as follows:

1. Loss of extensibility of capsule, ligaments, tendons, and fascia. Immobilization results in a decrease in water and glycosaminoglycan content. This contributes to an increase in aberrant cross-linking and a loss of movement between fibers.[4–6]

2. Deposition of fibrofatty infiltrates between joint structures acting as intra-articular "glue."[7]

3. Breakdown of hyaline articular cartilage.[8]

4. Atrophy and adaptive length changes in muscle.[9,10]

Conversely, it has been shown that movement tends to prevent or reduce these changes in connective tissue[4,11] and muscle.[9,10] The problem for us, as clinicians, is knowing when to begin active motion and when to progress to passive exercise. This requires close communication with the physician and an understanding of the stages of soft tissue healing. Evaluation of the direction of restriction, pain, and reactivity is essential in determining the readiness of movement.[12]

Clavicle Fractures

Clavicle fractures (Fig. 19.1) most commonly occur from a fall on the lateral aspect of the shoulder or, less commonly, onto the outstretched arm.[13] The clavicle typically fractures at the juncture of the middle one-third and distal

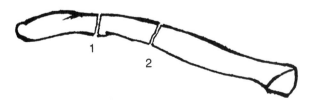

FIGURE 19.1 *Clavicle fractures at the (1) juncture of the middle and distal thirds and the (2) middle one-third.*

one-third (Fig. 19.2) and often in the middle one-third (Fig. 19.3).

The shoulder is immobilized for 14 to 21 days, either in a clavicle (or figure eight) brace or a sling. Badly comminuted, delayed union, or surgically repaired fractures will require more immobilization.

REHABILITATION

Active range of motion (ROM) exercises should begin within 14 to 21 days. Exercises should involve the shoulder girdle (elevation, depression, protraction, and retraction) and the shoulder joint (pendulum and wand exercises). In most cases, a home program is sufficient. In unusual cases of prolonged immobilization and excessive stiffness, passive mobilization may be necessary. Evaluation and treatment should include accessory and physiologic movements of the sternoclavicular, acromioclavicular, glenohumeral, and scapulothoracic joints. The latter is often overlooked, but may be particularly important because of immobilization in a retracted position.

Prolonged immobilization can also result in muscle weakness and even in visible atrophy. Resistive exercises can begin when the fracture appears solidly healed and when pain with movement is reduced.

Scapula Fractures

Scapula fractures are usually the result of a direct blow.[13] Most are nondisplaced; therefore, little or no immobilization is required.

NECK OF THE SCAPULA

The fracture line extends from the suprascapular notch to the lateral border (Fig. 19.4, no. 1). Downward displacement of the glenoid fragment is not usually severe.

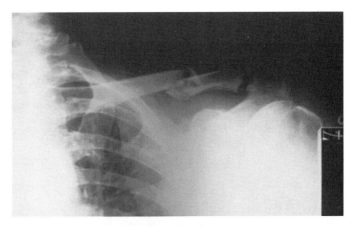

A

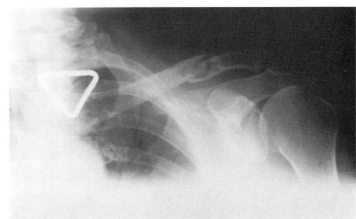

B

FIGURE 19.2 *Radiograph of clavicle fracture at the juncture of the middle and distal thirds* **(A)** *before reduction and* **(B)** *after reduction.*

BODY OF THE SCAPULA

Fragments are well protected by layers of muscle, even if comminuted (Fig. 19.4, no. 2).

CORACOID PROCESS

The fracture is usually not displaced, but occasionally is displaced downward (Fig. 19.4, no. 3).

ACROMION PROCESS

Again, this is not often displaced. If the fracture is communited or badly displaced, fragments can be removed surgically (Fig. 19.4, no. 4).

REHABILITATION

In most cases, active ROM exercises can begin within the first few days, and a home program will suffice. However, occasional prolonged immobilization because of severe displacement or surgical treatment may necessitate passive mobilization and muscle strengthening. All joints in the shoulder girdle complex should be evaluated, with particular emphasis on the scapulothoracic and its related musculature. If a direct blow to the scapula was the cause of injury, thoracic spine and rib mechanics should also be evaluated.

Fractures of the Humerus

Fractures of the upper humerus can involve the greater tuberosity, neck, or shaft (Fig. 19.5). Mechanisms of injury are varied, as are the needs for immobilization and surgery. The effects of trauma and immobilization on glenohumeral

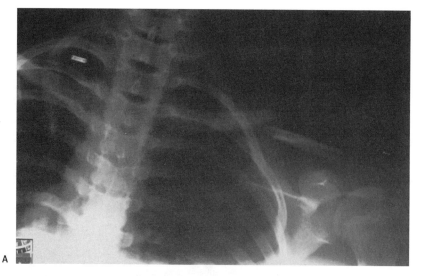

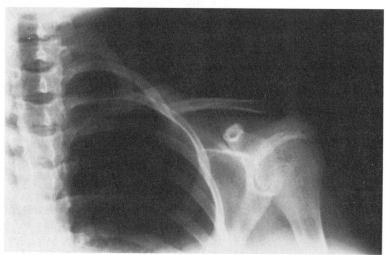

FIGURE 19.3 *Radiograph of clavicle fracture in the middle one-third* (**A**) *before reduction and* (**B**) *after reduction.*

joint soft tissues have especially significant implications for rehabilitation.

GREATER TUBEROSITY

Fractures of the greater tuberosity are usually the result of a fall on the shoulder, most commonly in elderly individuals.[13] In nondisplaced fractures (Fig. 19.6) splinting should be avoided so that active exercise can begin soon. An avulsed and displaced fragment must be reduced to avoid impingement with the acromion or coracoacromial ligament, which will result in pain-

ful, limited abduction.[13,14] These are often treated surgically with a fixation screw. Additional clearance acromioplasty or removal of the acromion may be necessary. Postoperative immobilization is from 14 to 21 days.

NECK OF THE HUMERUS

Humeral neck fractures are caused by a fall on the outstretched arm or the elbow, often in elderly, osteoporotic women.

Because shoulder joint stiffness is a common complication of humeral neck fractures, early movement is desirable. The immobilization re-

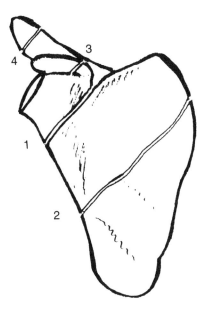

FIGURE 19.4 *Scapular fractures of the (1) neck, (2) body, (3) coracoid process, and (4) acromion process.*

quired depends on the severity of the displacement. In impacted and nondisplaced fractures (Fig. 19.7), the arm can come out of the sling frequently for exercise. If the fragments are displaced (Fig. 19.8), the arm may need to be immobilized in a sling held tightly to the chest for 14 to 21 days. Occasionally, an abduction splint is needed for as much as 4 weeks. Immobilization will be variable in cases of open reduction, internal fixation with plates or intramedullary rods.

SHAFT OF THE HUMERUS

Humeral shaft fractures usually involve the middle one-third, resulting from a direct blow or a twisting force that causes a spiral fracture (Fig. 19.9). As in other upper humerus fractures, early joint motion is desirable. However, immobilization is greatly variable, depending on the stability and whether casting or surgical fixation is used.

REHABILITATION

Because the glenohumeral joint is particularly susceptible to stiffness, early remobilization, when safe, is essential. Even while the arm is in a sling or cast, the patient should be taught

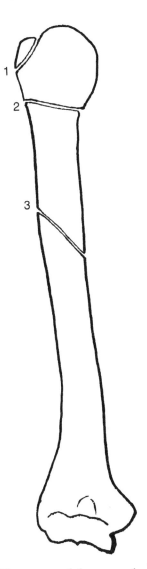

FIGURE 19.5 *Fractures of the upper humerus in the (1) greater tuberosity, (2) neck, and (3) shaft.*

careful active exercises or be seen frequently for active assistance-providing exercises. As the immobilization period ends, the exercises should be increased gradually in range and vigor.

Once the fracture is stable and reactivity is reduced at least to moderate (pain and end-range resistance are simultaneous[12,15]), careful passive mobilization can begin. Each movement should be tested for reactivity prior to mobilizing, be-

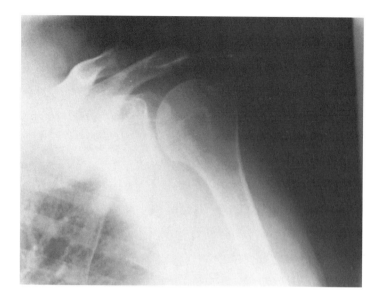

FIGURE 19.6 *Radiograph of non-displaced greater tuberosity fracture.*

cause some structures may be more inflamed and painful than others. For example, immobilizing the arm in a sling or in a position of adduction and internal rotation can result in a "capsular pattern" limitation.[16] In this capsular pattern, all movements at the glenohumeral joint, especially external rotation and abduction, will be restricted.[17] Therefore, mobilization should emphasize stretching the anterior and inferior portions of the capsule. During mobilization, pain should always be respected. When reactivity is moderate to high, grades I and II accessory mobilizations are used to reduce pain and promote relaxation. When reactivity is low to moderate, grades III and IV accessory and physiologic mobilizations are used to increase ROM.[18] Although most effort will be concentrated at the glenohumeral joint, other joints in the shoulder

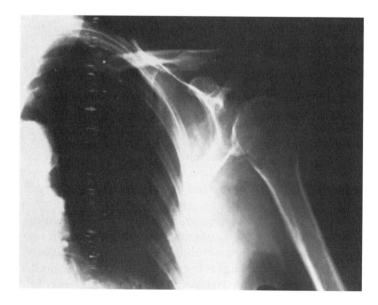

FIGURE 19.7 *Radiograph of impacted humeral neck fracture.*

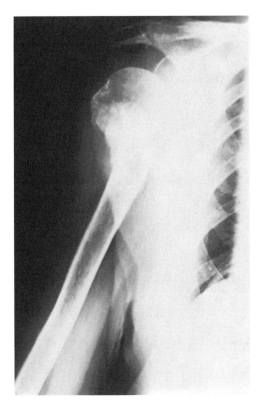

FIGURE 19.8 *Radiograph of displaced humeral neck fracture.*

girdle should be assessed after prolonged immobilization. The reader is referred to Chapter 13 for a detailed summary of shoulder joint and girdle mobilization techniques.

Immobilizing the shoulder girdle can result in significant muscle weakness. Muscles commonly involved are the upper and middle trapezius, the pectorals, and all muscles of the rotator cuff. To minimize weakness and atrophy, specific isometric exercises should be instructed early. After immobilization, if the fracture is stable, reactivity is not high, and ROM is at least 50 percent, submaximal effort progressive resistive exercises can begin, with progression to maximal effort as tolerated. Isokinetic devices are preferred, because "stops" can be used to protect the joint and because resistance can be applied to all planes of movement, including functional diagonals Chapter 16 outlines the use of shoulder isokinetics.

Summary

Fractures of the shoulder girdle are common and, because of soft tissue trauma and immobilization, often result in stiffness, especially at the glenohumeral joint. When possible, early movement is essential. After a period of immobilization, all joints of the shoulder complex should be assessed, regardless of the location of the fracture.

CASE STUDY

HISTORY

Patient O.C. is a 58-year-old woman who slipped and fell onto her right shoulder on June 11, 1994, sustaining a comminuted fracture of the proximal humerus, with anterior dislocation of the glenohumeral joint (Fig. 19.10A). This combined injury required open reduction to relocate the shoulder joint, as well as internal fixation of the fracture with an intramedullary rod (Fig. 19.10B). To facilitate shoulder joint range of motion as the patient began physical therapy, the rod was removed 1 month later on July 11, 1994. This kept the rod from impinging in the area of the supraspinatus. There was radiographic evidence of delayed healing, but the fracture was stable enough for the patient to begin physical therapy.

INITIAL EVALUATION

The patient was referred for physical therapy 6 weeks postinjury on July 25, 1994. She presented with complaints of severe shoulder pain (7 on a scale of 10), stiffness, and disability, indicating that she needed her husband's assistance with nearly all activities of daily living (ADL), including dressing, bathing, going to the toilet, and getting in and out of bed. She reported having been unable to move the upper extremity because of the pain.

Because of pain and high reactivity, range of motion (ROM) and accessory motions could not be assessed on the initial visit. Muscle strength was grossly 2/5, at best. The patient did tolerate moist heat and grades 1 and 2 oscillations to re-

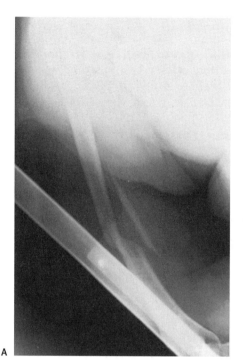
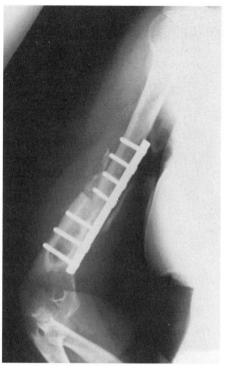

A

B

FIGURE 19.9 *Radiographs of spiral/oblique humeral shaft fracture* **(A)** *before surgical reduction and* **(B)** *after open reduction, internal fixation.*

duce pain, and was instructed in gentle pendulum exercises to be done at home.

TREATMENT

WEEKS 1 AND 2

Combinations of moist heat, narrow-pulse electrical stimulation, and oscillations were used to reduce pain and reactivity, and to promote relaxation. During this time the patient tolerated AAROM exercise. By the end of the second week, PROM and muscle strength were as follows.

	PROM	REACTIVITY	STRENGTH
Flexion	60°	Moderate	2/5+
Abduction	42°	High	2/5
External rot.	10°	High	2/5
Internal rot.	30°	Moderate	3/5

WEEKS 3 TO 6

The patient reported gradually decreased pain. She was better able to dress herself, and was able to get comfortable at night. During this time joint

reactivity continued to lessen, and the patient was more tolerant to passive glenohumeral ROM and mobilization techniques. To improve decreased scapulothoracic mobility, passive scapular distraction, elevation/depression, and protraction/retraction were begun. To increase functional muscle strength, glenohumeral and scapular proprioceptive neuromuscular facilitation (PNF) was begun. The patient's home exercise program (HEP) included pendulum and wand exercises in all planes, and low-resistance theraband strengthening exercises for shoulder elevation, abduction, adduction, and internal and external rotation. At the end of the sixth week, findings were as follows.

	PROM	REACTIVITY	STRENGTH
Flexion	120°	Low	3/5+
Abduction	98°	Moderate	3/5
External rot.	42°	Moderate	3/5+
Internal rot.	64°	Low	3/5+

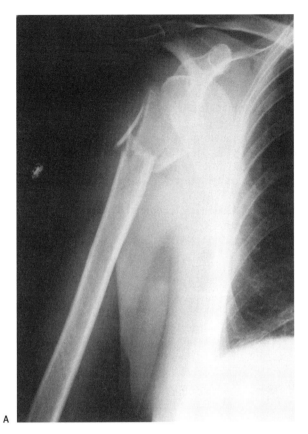

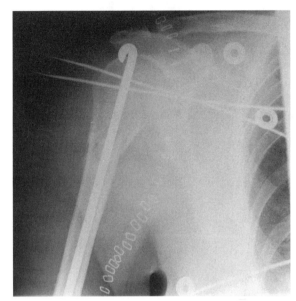

FIGURE 19.10 (A) *Patient O.C., comminuted fracture of the right humerus, with anterior dislocation of the glenohumeral joint.* **(B)** *After reduction, with the intramedullary rod in place.*

WEEKS 7 TO 10

By this time physical therapy frequency had been reduced to twice weekly, as ROM and function continued to improve. The passive mobilization program now included grades 4 to 6 physiologic and accessory movements with excellent tolerance. PREs included pull downs, military presses, and elbow curls. To promote further scapular strength and mobility, closed kinetic chain exercises included wall pushups, modified prone push-ups on 4-inch foam rolls, and the upper extremity ergometer with resistance to tolerance. Isokinetic internal and external rotation in the plane of the scapula at maximum effort was employed during the last 3 weeks of therapy.

DISCHARGE AND FOLLOW-UP

On October 31, 1994, after 10 weeks of therapy and 14 weeks after surgery, the patient reported only minimal, occasional pain. She was fully independent in her ADL, although overhead activities were still somewhat difficult. ROM and strength findings were as follows.

	PROM	REACTIVITY	STRENGTH
Flexion	175°	No pain	4/5+
Abduction	155°	No pain	4/5+
External rot.	90°	Low	4/5+
Internal rot.	85°	No pain	5/5

She was advised to continue her HEP indefinitely, and to return for reevaluation if any problems arose. The patient was seen for a follow-up visit by the surgeon on January 24, 1995. Radiographs revealed that some alignment was lost, but that overall position and healing were satisfactory (Fig. 19.11).

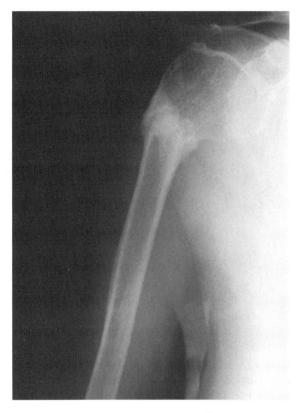

FIGURE 19.11 *Patient O.C., 7 months postinjury.*

References

1. Gradisar IA: Fracture stabilization and healing. p. 118. In Davies G, Gould J (eds): Orthopaedic and Sports Physical Therapy. CV Mosby, St. Louis, 1985

2. Cruess RL: Healing of bone, tendon and ligament. p. 147. In Rockwood CA, Green DP (eds): Fractures in Adults. JB Lippincott, Philadelphia, 1984

3. Engles M: Tissue response. p. 3. In Donatelli R, Wooden MJ (eds): Orthopaedic Physical Therapy 2nd Ed. Churchill Livingstone, New York, 1991

4. Akeson WH, Amiel D, Woo S: Immobility effects on synovial joints: the pathomechanics of joint contractures. Biorheology 17:95, 1980

5. Woo S, Matthews JV, Akeson WH et al: Connective tissue response to immobility: an accelerated aging response. Exp Gerontol 3:289, 1968

6. La Vigne A, Watkins R: Preliminary results on immobilization: induced stiffness of monkey knee joints and posterior capsules. Proceedings of a Symposium of the Biological Engineering Society, University of Strathclyde, Scotland University Park Press, Baltimore, 1973

7. Enneking W, Horowitz M: The intra-articular effects of immobilization on the human knee. J Bone Joint Surg 54A:973, 1972

8. Ham A, Cormack D: Histology. 8th Ed. JB Lippincott, Philadelphia, 1979

9. Tabary JC, Tabary C, Tardieu S et al: Physiological and structural changes in cat soleus muscle due to immobilization at different lengths in plaster casts. J Physiol (Lond) 224:221, 1972

10. Cooper R: Alterations during immobilization and regeneration of skeletal muscle in cats. J Bone Joint Surg 54A:919, 1972

11. Akeson WH, Amiel D, Mechanic GL et al: Collagen crosslinking alteration in joint contractures: changes in reducible crosslinks in periarticular connective tissue collagen after 9 weeks of immobilization. Connect Tissue Res 5:5, 1977

12 Wooden MJ: Mobilization of the upper extremity. p. 297. In Donatelli R. Wooden MJ (eds): Orthopaedic Physial Therapy 2nd Ed. Churchill Livingstone, New York, 1989

13. Adams JC: Outline of Fractures, Including Joint Injuries. 9th Ed. Churchill Livingstone, London, 1994

14. Turek SL: Orthopaedics: Principles and Their Applications. Vol. 2. 4th Ed. JB Lippincott, Philadelphia, 1980, p. 938

15. Paris SV: Extremity Dysfunction and Mobilization. Institute Press, Atlanta, 1980

16. Moran CA, Saunders SR: Evaluation of the shoulder: a sequential approach. p. 23. In Donatelli R (ed): Physical Therapy of the Shoulder. 2nd Ed. Churchill Livingstone, New York, 1991

17. Cyriax J: Textbook of Orthopaedic Medicine. Vol. 1. Diagnosis of Soft Tissue Lesions. Ballierre Tindall, London, 1978

18. Maitland GD: Peripheral Manipulation. 2nd Ed. Butterworth Publishers, London, 1978

Suggested Readings

Chapman MW (ed): Operative Orthopaedics. JB Lippincott, Philadelphia, 1988

Connolly JF (ed): DePalma's The Management of Fractures and Dislocations: An Atlas, 3rd Ed. WB Saunders, Philadelphia, 1983

Craig EV: Shoulder fractures in the athlete. In Petrone FA (ed): Athletic Injuries of the Shoulder. McGraw-Hill, New York, 1995

Crenshaw AH (ed): Campbell's Operative Orthopaedics. Vol. 3. WB Saunders, Philadelphia, 1970

Cruess R: Adult Orthopaedics. Churchill Livingstone, New York, 1984

DePalma AF: Surgery of the Shoulder. JB Lippincott, Philadelphia, 1983

Mueller KH: Intramedullary Nailing and Other Intramedullary Osteosyntheses. WB Saunders, Philadelphia, 1986

Park WH, Hughes SPF (eds): Orthopaedic Radiology. Blackwell Scientific Publications, London, 1987

Rang M: Children's Fractures. JB Lippincott, Philadelphia, 1974

Rockwood CA, Green DP, Bucholz RW (eds): Fractures in Adults, 3rd Ed. JB Lippincott, Philadelphia, 1991

Rockwood CA, Matsen FA: The Shoulder. WB Saunders, Philadelphia, 1991

Rodgers LF: Radiology of Skeletal Trauma. Churchill Livingstone, New York, 1982

Rowe CR: The Shoulder. Churchill Livingstone, New York, 1988

20

Total Shoulder Replacement

GEORGE M. MCCLUSKEY III

TIMOTHY UHL

The painful arthritic glenohumeral joint has been of interest to the orthopedic surgeon and physical therapist for a long time. The earliest reported arthroplasty for the painful shoulder joint was performed by a French surgeon, J.E. Pean, in 1892.[1] He substituted a platinum and rubber implant for the glenohumeral joint of a young man afflicted with tuberculosis. Dr. Charles Neer pioneered the development of shoulder prosthetic replacement from the early 1950s to the present. Neer's total shoulder prosthesis, redesigned in 1973, is the standard against which all new modifications must be judged. Recent advances in technique and prosthetic design, and a clearer understanding of the pathologic anatomy and kinematics of shoulder diseases, have led to a dramatic increase in the number of total shoulder replacements in this country. Unconstrained total shoulder replacement has consistently given good results with regard to pain relief and improved function.

This chapter will discuss various clinical conditions that often result in prosthetic replacement and some of their distinguishing clinical features. Principles of the postoperative rehabilitation required for patients undergoing replacement surgery will also be reviewed.

Clinical Considerations

HISTORY

Before patients can be considered for shoulder replacement, they must undergo a thorough evaluation of their overall medical history, their physical examination, and the details of the specific disease process involving the shoulder. Medically, they should be good candidates for anesthesia and surgery, because some medical conditions have a direct effect on the other joints, adjacent soft tissue structures, and organ systems of the patient. One example would be rheumatoid arthritis, which not only causes destruction of the shoulder joint surfaces, but affects surrounding muscles, tendons, and ligaments as well. Rheumatoid arthritis can also involve the lungs, immune system, and other vital structures. Another example is osteonecrosis, which can occur from the use of steroids to treat medical conditions, such as asthma.

Other factors in the history that are important considerations are the patient's age, work and recreational requirements, socioeconomic and educational background, family history, and handedness. A preoperative assessment of the

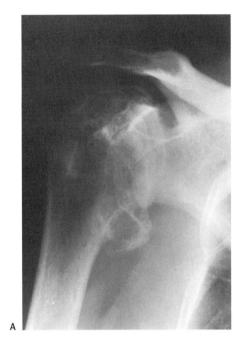

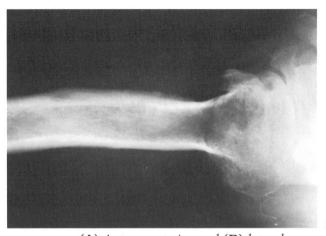

FIGURE 20.1 **(A)** *Anteroposterior and* **(B)** *lateral radiographic views show osteoarthritis in this patient. Hypertrophic spurring is seen along the humeral neck and glenoid along with posterior glenoid wear and concomitant posterior subluxation of the humeral head. The glenohumeral joint space is diminished from cartilage erosion.*

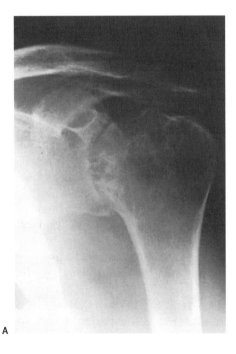

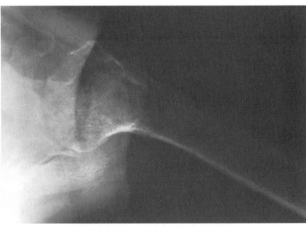

FIGURE 20.2 **(A)** *Anteroposterior and* **(B)** *lateral radiographic views of rheumatoid arthritis in this patient's shoulder. Osteopenia of the bone with degenerative cysts and central glenoid wear are visible along with erosion of bone and cartilage.*

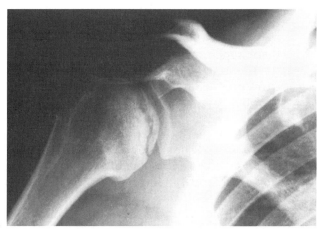

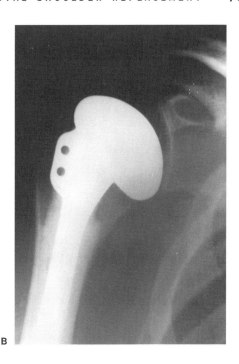

FIGURE 20.3 **(A)** *Anteroposterior radiographic view in a patient with stage 3 osteonecrosis of the humeral head showing avascular bone with subchondral collapse and crescent sign indicative of subchondral fracture.* **(B)** *Humeral head replacement was needed.*

patient's motivation and ability to understand and participate in a postoperative rehabilitation program is crucial.

The primary indication for a prosthetic replacement is pain. Commonly, patients complain of night pain, pain at rest, and pain provoked by activities of daily living, work, and recreation. Shoulder pain at rest is generally tolerated less well than that of the hip or knee.[2] Pain characteristics—location, character, frequency, duration, and radiation—are important to note. Additional causes of shoulder pain, including neurologic, cervical, and thoracic causes, should be investigated.

Limitations in motion and shoulder function are also indications for prosthetic replacement, but they should only be considered secondary indications. Evidence of advanced destructive joint disease on radiographs should only support the clinical diagnosis and decision. It is not in and of itself an indication for surgery in the absence of significant pain and dysfunction. For most patients who have degenerative lesions, restoration of shoulder motion and function to "near normal" is realistic. In some cases, severe

bone loss, soft tissue retraction, scarring, and nerve injuries preclude the possibility of significant functional improvement, and the goals of surgery become pain relief and prosthetic stability. These patients are placed in a "limited goals" rehabilitation program postoperatively.

PHYSICAL EXAMINATION

A general physical examination must include a detailed examination of both shoulders. A systematic method of recording joint motion should be used. In general, patients with glenohumeral arthritis have restricted active and passive ranges of shoulder motion with a predominance of scapulothoracic motion. Limited external rotation is more sensitive than forward elevation in determining the degree of restricted joint motion in arthritic shoulders.[2] Patients with rotator cuff tears may be differentiated from those with arthritic shoulders because they usually retain full passive motion while active motion and strength are limited.

Posterior joint line tenderness is a characteristic finding in patients with glenohumeral arthr-

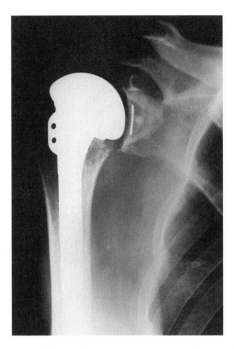

FIGURE 20.4 *Stage 4 osteonecrosis requires a total shoulder replacement. The glenoid component is made of polyethylene and the humeral component is modular, allowing the surgeon to mix and match stem and head sizes.*

recognized preoperatively and addressed at the time of surgery, especially when a defective rotator cuff is repaired concomitantly with prosthetic replacement.

Glenohumeral instability can be secondary to trauma, arthritis, or congenital abnormalities. Previous operations performed for instability can cause subluxation or dislocation of the opposite side of the shoulder joint from overtightening or soft tissue contracture on the operated side (as with posterior subluxation from an anterior contracture following surgery for anterior instability). Soft tissue balancing of the rotator cuff, deltoid, capsule, and glenohumeral ligaments, and proper alignment of prosthetic components regarding height and version, are necessary for a stable shoulder replacement.

Patients with glenohumeral arthritis should exhaust all nonoperative treatment options before shoulder replacement. Options include modification of activities, exercises to regain motion and strength, modalities, medications,

itis. It is often associated with crepitation in the glenohumeral joint with gentle rotation of the shoulder. Crepitation and tenderness at the anterolateral aspect of the acromion and subacromial space is more common in rotator cuff and impingement lesions.

A standardized muscle grading system allows the surgeon to record and compare preoperative and postoperative changes in strength effectively. Muscle atrophy and nerve injury that cause muscle weakness must be considered. The strength and overall function of the rotator cuff and deltoid are especially important in the preoperative assessment, particularly when the plan is to use a nonconstrained-type prosthesis. If the rotator cuff is severely compromised or irreparably torn, shoulder replacement results are less predictable with regard to pain relief and functional improvement. Impingement syndrome and acromioclavicular joint arthritis must be

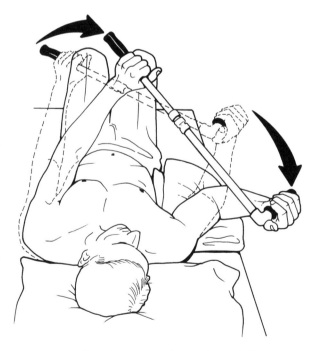

FIGURE 20.5 *Passive external rotation of the shoulder using a stick with arm supported on a pillow.*

and injections. Therapy programs should be individualized for each patient and should emphasize good communication between the patient, surgeon, and therapist. The patient should be informed about the diagnosis and goals of rehabilitation. Preoperative exercises to maximize passive range of motion and to condition shoulder muscles prepare the patient for postoperative rehabilitation.

Indications

The disease processes that are considered indications for shoulder replacement include osteoarthritis,[3] rheumatoid arthritis,[4] osteonecrosis,

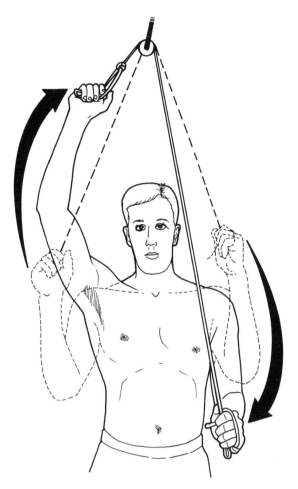

FIGURE 20.7 *Elevation of the arm with assistance of a rope and pulley system in the plane of the scapula.*

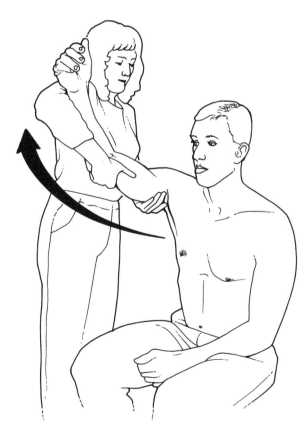

FIGURE 20.6 *Passive forward elevation in the plane of the scapula with the assistance of another person.*

arthritis of dislocation, post-traumatic arthropathy, cuff tear arthropathy,[5] and tumors.[6] Arthroplasty is also indicated for acute and chronic trauma and revision surgery.[2,7–9]

Absolute contraindications to shoulder prosthetic replacement include active infection, paralysis, extensive injury to both the rotator cuff and deltoid muscles, neurotrophic shoulder, and inappropriate patient motivation.[2] Although tearing of the rotator cuff and bone loss involving the humerus or glenoid can be problematic, they are not considered contraindications to shoulder replacement.

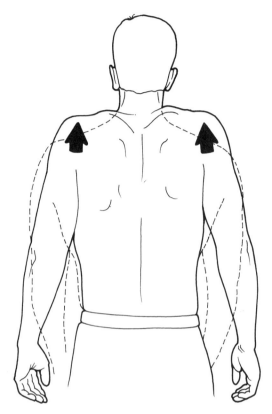

FIGURE 20.8 *Scapular stabilizing exercises of retraction and elevation.*

OSTEOARTHRITIS

Patients with primary osteoarthritis are ideal candidates for nonconstrained prosthetic replacement. The humeral head is enlarged with hypertrophic osteophytes around the margin of the articular cartilage that give good supporting structure for the prosthesis (Fig. 20.1). Also, the rotator cuff and biceps tendon are intact in 90 percent of these shoulders,[6] because the compression forces required to produce primary osteoarthritis in shoulders subjected to everyday activities require an intact rotator cuff. When biceps tendon ruptures do occur, they are usually unrelated to rotator cuff disease with its impingement but rather are due to bony excrescences along the bicipital groove entrance.

Pathologic findings involving the proximal humerus include loss or thinning of the articular cartilage and underlying subchondral sclerosis and cyst formation in the metaphyseal portion of the humerus. The large rimming osteophytes are characteristic radiographic findings in osteoarthritic shoulders. The osteophytes limit glenohumeral rotation and are covered with cartilage, making them appear larger at surgery when compared with their preoperative radiographic appearance.

In the osteoarthritic shoulder, there is usually complete loss of the normal glenohumeral joint space. The glenoid articular cartilage is characteristically worn eccentrically with minimal cartilage loss anteriorly and complete eburnation of articular cartilage posteriorly leading to progressive wear and bone loss. This posterior glenoid wear is characteristic, and when bone loss is extreme, may preclude use of the glenoid prosthesis or require bone grafting for prosthetic stability. Posterior subluxation of the humeral head occurs with progressive posterior glenoid wear and concomitant contracture of the anterior capsule and subscapularis. Special techniques can be used during prosthetic replacement to balance soft tissues and to regain near-normal glenohumeral version. They include subscapularis lengthening, release of contractures anteriorly, glenoid bone grafting, and proper orientation of prosthetic components. Restoration of the deltoid myofascial sleeve tension is critical for function of the cuff and deltoid muscles.

At surgery, loose osteochondral bodies are often found, especially in the subscapularis bursa, and should be removed. Acromial spurs and acromioclavicular arthritis with spurring should be assessed preoperatively by radiograph, and if clinically symptomatic, should be smoothed without detaching the deltoid muscle. When present, rotator cuff tears are repaired and bicipital lesions are treated appropriately.

RHEUMATOID ARTHRITIS

Rheumatoid arthritis not only affects the joint surfaces in the shoulder, but the muscles, bursae, ligaments, and tendons as well. Rotator cuff tears are found in 30 percent to 40 percent of patients with rheumatoid arthritis.[8-10] Neer has

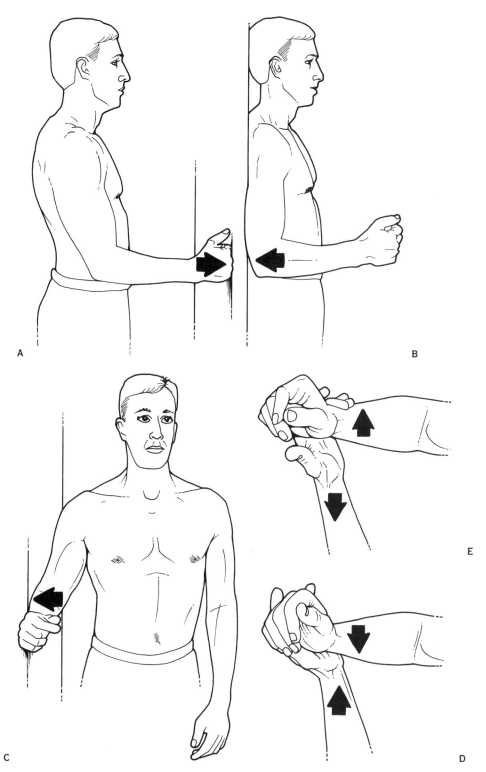

FIGURE 20.9 *Five-way isometrics for the glenohumeral joint with the elbow flexed at 90°.*
(A) *Flexion* **(B)** *Extension* **(C)** *Abduction* **(D)** *Internal rotation* **(E)** *External rotation.*

described three clinical varieties of rheumatoid arthritis that involve the shoulder—the dry, wet, and resorptive forms.[2] The dry form resembles osteoarthritis in that sclerosis, rimming osteophytes, and loss of joint space occur. It is sometimes referred to as "mixed arthritis." The wet and resorptive forms are characterized by severe bone loss, bone erosion secondary to pannus, and central glenoid wear with "centralization" of the humeral head (Fig. 20.2). Synovial proliferation and hypertrophy can be marked, requiring aggressive synovectomy as part of the operative procedure.

In rheumatoid shoulders, contracture and

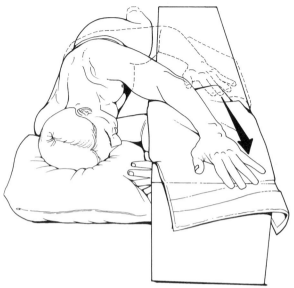

FIGURE 20.11 *Gravity-eliminated flexion in the sidelying position. A hardside suitcase with a towel draped over it works well to support the arm.*

shortening of anterior soft tissues is rare, and external rotation is easily achieved without subscapularis lengthening. Rotator cuff defects are usually repairable, and acromioplasty is seldom indicated. Occasionally, severe bone loss, erosion, and centralization of the humeral head make glenoid replacement and cuff repair inadvisable. These patients are placed in a "limited goals" rehabilitation program, which will be discussed later.

ARTHRITIS OF DISLOCATION

Degenerative arthritis that is the result of recurrent dislocations of the glenohumeral joint or of a surgical procedure for anterior or posterior dislocations that displaces the humeral head to a position opposite the surgical approach is referred to as arthritis of dislocation. In most shoulders, the head subluxates posteriorly following an anterior approach for a procedure to correct recurrent anterior dislocations. In others, a unidirectional surgical approach was used for a

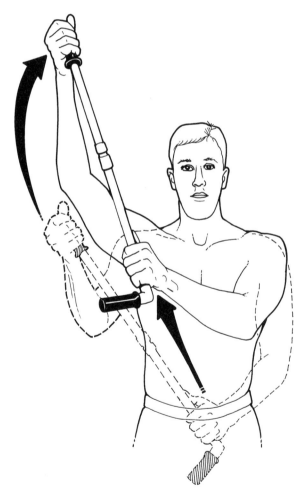

FIGURE 20.10 *Active assisted elevation with a stick in the plane of the scapula.*

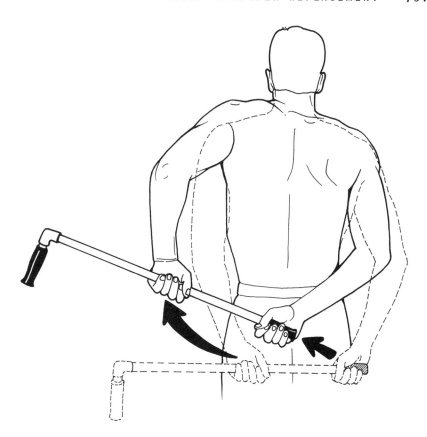

FIGURE 20.12 *Beginning internal rotation and extension exercise using a stick.*

multidirectional instability problem with residual inferior instability causing persistent symptoms. Most patients in this group are under the age of 45 at the time of the shoulder replacement.

Special problems encountered during arthroplasty in patients with arthritis of dislocation are often related to the initial procedure for instability. These problems include previous surgical scars associated with cutaneous neuromas, scarring and atrophy of the anterior deltoid, and subscapularis contracture that severely restricts external rotation.

Glenoid wear is usually pronounced when the humeral head is located eccentrically in the glenoid. Altering the version of the glenoid component is preferable to glenoid bone grafting in most shoulders. Stretching of soft tissues to accommodate a chronically subluxating or dislocating humeral head must be addressed with a capsulorrhaphy to balance soft tissues and to stabilize the prosthesis along with corresponding changes in the version of the humeral and glenoid prosthetic components. Modifications in the rehabilitation program are made depending on the degree and direction of instability noted preoperatively and intraoperatively.

Retained hardware is common in shoulders that have had previous surgery. Any intra-articular hardware, including any previously placed screws or staples, should be removed.

OSTEONECROSIS

Osteonecrosis or avascular necrosis can be the result of trauma, steroid use for systemic disease, alcohol abuse, or other causes. Only the femoral head has a higher incidence of nontraumatic osteonecrosis than the humeral head. Neer[2] and others[11,12] have divided osteonecrosis into four stages. Stages 3 and 4 of osteonecrosis usually require prosthetic replacement. In stage 3, the humeral head displays collapse of subchondral bone with a normal glenoid articular surface

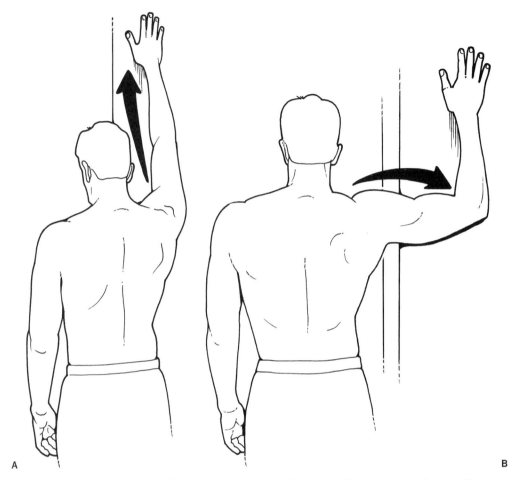

A   B

FIGURE 20.13 **(A)** *Terminal stretching for elevation.* **(B)** *External rotation with a wall.*

(Fig. 20.3). In these patients with an intact glenoid, humeral head replacement alone is indicated. Total shoulder replacement is reserved for patients with stage 4 osteonecrosis, with marked degenerative changes of the humeral head and glenoid articular surfaces (Fig. 20.4). The rotator cuff and biceps tendon are usually intact in these patients.

CUFF TEAR ARTHROPATHY

Neer described cuff tear arthropathy in 1975 as severe destruction of the glenohumeral joint with humeral head collapse and a massive rotator cuff tear in the absence of other known etiologic factors.[5] A combination of nutritional and mechanical factors contribute to this degenerative process. Gross instability of the glenohumeral joint develops, and the humeral head migrates cephalad causing wear into the acromion, acromioclavicular joint, and coracoid process. All patients treated with humeral head replacement or total shoulder replacement along with rotator cuff repair are placed in a limited goals rehabilitation program postoperatively with emphasis on pain reduction and stability instead of function.

POST-TRAUMATIC ARTHRITIS

Arthritis related to previous fractures or fracture-dislocations of the proximal humerus or glenoid is treated with prosthetic replacement in

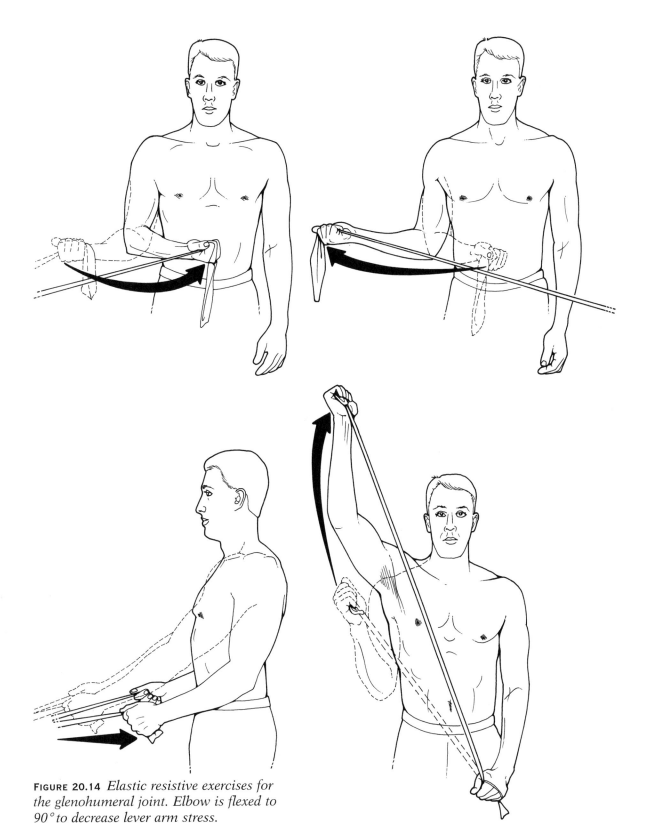

FIGURE 20.14 *Elastic resistive exercises for the glenohumeral joint. Elbow is flexed to 90° to decrease lever arm stress.*

469

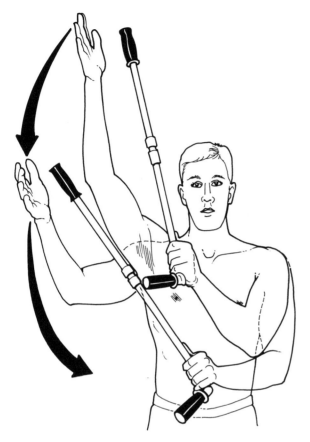

FIGURE 20.15 *Assisted elevation with stick followed by isometric hold at end range independently, followed by active eccentric lowering as tolerated (shown above). It is usually recommended to the patient to keep the stick close to the arm to aid in support in lowering, especially if the patient has a painful or weak arc.*

some patients. The procedure can be complicated by soft tissue scarring, bone loss, retracted tuberosities, malunion, nonunion, and nerve injuries. Retained hardware and deltoid deficiency from previous failed surgeries often complicate the situation further and elevate the risk for infection with subsequent procedures.

Special attention should be given to the repair of a torn, retracted, and scarred rotator cuff to maintain proper deltoid tension and restore normal humeral length and glenohumeral version.

Postoperative rehabilitation must be individualized for these patients, with close communication between the surgeon and therapist. Early restoration of passive motion prevents reformation of unwanted scar tissue that blocks motion. Patients with preoperative instability and dislocation must restrict motion in provocative positions to avoid prosthetic dislocations. One year of exercise is required to regain full motion and strength in these patients.

Rehabilitation

The rehabiliation of a patient who has had a total shoulder replacement should be like that of any other total joint replacement rehabilitation program. The primary reason for undergoing the surgery is pain relief, and the secondary goal is improvement of function. In our attempts to assist these patients in recovery, we must keep these goals in the correct order. It is very easy for the therapist to focus on the functional aspects too intently and sacrifice the primary goal of decreasing pain. This is not to say patients will not have any discomfort as they rehabilitate their shoulders; however, it should be monitored and minimized. Along with these goals, the immediate postoperative goals for rehabilitation are to prevent glenohumeral contracture while simultaneously protecting the prosthesis, rotator cuff, and deltoid. It is critical for the therapist, doctor, and patient to have reasonable and clear goals going into surgery.

CATEGORIES OF REHABILITATION

Rehabilitation after shoulder replacement should be individualized to the needs of the patient and related to the goals of the procedure. In general, however, there are three categories of rehabilitation programs: (A) programs for patients with a good rotator cuff and deltoid, (B) programs for patients with a poor rotator cuff and deltoid, and (C) limited goals programs.

The first two categories are designed to accomodate the patient's rotator cuff status and del-

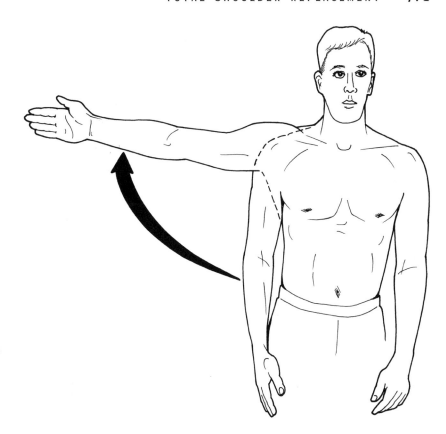

FIGURE 20.16 *Scaption is elevation of the arm in the scapular plane to strengthen the deltoid, supraspinatus, and trapezius.*

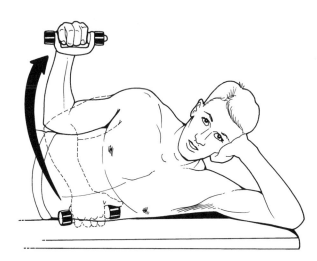

FIGURE 20.17 *Sidelying external rotation to strengthen the infraspinatus is usually performed with a small pillow under the elbow.*

toid integrity. The third category is included for those patients who have one or a combination of the following pathologies that leads to total shoulder arthroplasty: rheumatoid arthritis, previously failed rotator cuff repair, rotator cuff arthropathy, Erb's palsy, or previously failed total shoulder arthroplasty.

The following guidelines can be used by the clinician to develop an individualized rehabilitation program based on the status of the rotator cuff and deltoid musculature. It is important to listen to the patient's comments, as this will guide the rehabilitation progress. The time lines in Appendix 20.1 A–C are merely suggestions for rehabilitation progress. It is more important to listen to patients regarding their progress.

Patients in the limited goals program are placed in this category based on the recommendation of their surgeon. Pain relief is the primary goal of surgery for these patients. Full return of

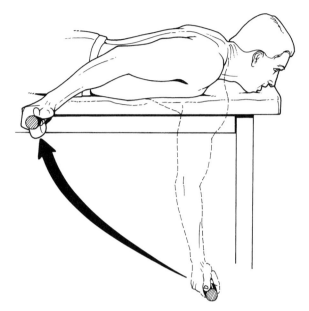

FIGURE 20.18 *Prone extension is used to strengthen the teres minor and posterior deltoid. If the patient is unable to lie prone, he or she can simply lean forward to a comfortable position and lean on the unaffected opposite arm for support.*

function is not an objective. Frequent communication between the surgeon and therapist is needed to determine the appropriate time for rehabilitation to begin. The time frame described in Appendix 20.1C is very conservative and should be modified according to individual needs and response to the rehabilitation program.

CRITICAL POINTS AND TECHNIQUES

Communication

Communication between surgeon and therapist, whether written or oral, is critical. The surgeon's opinion regarding the status of the repaired tissues and the prosthetic components guides the therapist in choosing a protocol and setting realistic goals for the patient. For example, if the surgeon had to antevert the glenoid component more than normal, the amount of external rotation the patient could expect to recover would be lessened. If full external rotation is forced in such a patient, the risk of shoulder dislocation would be high.

Lifting the Arm

The initial treatment session is by far the most important step in any shoulder rehabilitation program, because it sets the stage for the rest of the process. If this session is good, the patient develops trust and confidence in the therapist. However, if the session is bad because the patient resists the passive motion or has pain, the patient will associate pain with rehabilitation throughout the healing process.

Within the first minute or two, the therapist must determine the best way to approach each individual patient. Here is where the therapist's knowledge of the surgical procedure and its postoperative progress is needed. Having this knowledge gives the patient confidence in the therapist's expertise.

From a technical standpoint, the therapist and the patient should be in a comfortable position before performing the passive range of motion. Hand placement is also very important. In general, the more proximal placement of the therapist's hand on the patient's arm, the better. The patient will sense the therapist has better control of his or her arm and will not have a tendency to actively move it (see Fig. 20.6).

Performing External Rotation

When externally rotating the patient's arm, watch the position of the humerus. If the humerus is posterior to the midline of the body, the amount of external rotation will be lessened and more painful to achieve. In extension, stress will be placed on the sutures in the anterior structures.

Exercise Prescription

Most patients who have a total shoulder replacement are elderly and may have other medical problems; therefore, the volume of exercises should be kept at a reasonable level. Patients are generally very compliant in the early stages of rehabilitation because they do not want to jeopardize the results of their surgery and they want to get the arm moving again. Keep the number of repetitions low—in the 5 to 10 range—and the frequency at 2 to 4 times each day. Some patients

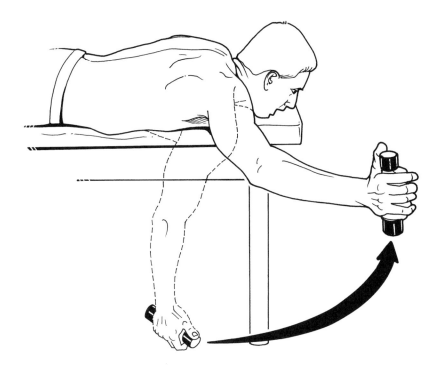

FIGURE 20.19 *Prone horizontal abduction is used to strengthen the supraspinatus. Watch for scapular substitution when supraspinatus is weak.*

will want to do more, but it is very easy to irritate the rotator cuff tendons when initiating passive range of motion, active assisted range of motion, and light resistive exercises. The patient's response after the first 2 to 3 days of new activities should serve as a guide for modifying the program to reach the patient's goals with minimal discomfort.

Resistive Exercise Progression

Resistive exercises typically follow this progression: isometric, gravity eliminated motions, active assisted range of motion, isometric hold at end range of active assisted range of motion with eccentric lowering, active range of motion, light elastic resistance below shoulder level, light dumbbell resistance, modified activities, and full return to activities.

Again, the patient's response to the exercises determines the progression of the program. For example, if a patient is moving the arm actively, comfortably, and biomechanically correctly, it would not be inappropriate to move directly from isometrics to active range of motion or light elastic resistance exercises, or both. On the other hand, if a patient is having pain with isometrics, switching to gravity eliminated activities might reduce the pain and still accomplish the goal of increasing strength and active range of motion.

Special Considerations

When osteoarthritis is the disorder necessitating total shoulder replacement, posterior glenoid wear and acromioclavicular joint involvement is common. From a rehabilitation standpoint, glenohumeral elevation in the pure frontal plane (flexion) is contraindicated because of the chance of posterior shoulder dislocation. Therefore, elevation activities for these patients are best performed in the plane of the scapula. Early in the rehabilitation process, excessive horizontal adduction can cause pain due to the freshly shaved ends of the acromion and clavicle.

Rheumatoid arthritis patients are generally much slower to recover than osteoarthritis patients. Because of the systemic nature of the disease process, other joints, such as wrist, hand,

and neck, are involved. Typical exercises for these patients must be modified to avoid aggravating these other joints. Osteopenia is often present, and many patients have rotator cuff tears. In these patients, rehabilitation must progress slowly and without force. If the patient is nonambulatory when undergoing total shoulder arthroplasty, transfers should not be done independently for approximately 5 to 6 months.

Avascular necrosis patients who often undergo a humeral head replacement only, are typically younger than the average total shoulder patient, and their musculotendinous structures are not involved. For these reasons, these patients often progress rapidly through the rehabilitation process as long as they are motivated and no complications arise.

Patients who develop arthritis after dislocation also have need of a modified postoperative program. By the time total shoulder arthroplasty is indicated in these patients, they have usually had 1 or 2 previous operations. They have shoulder stiffness and are apprehensive about unstable positions of the arm. The deltoid and subscapularis muscles of their shoulder are predisposed to retears because of the previous surgery. The surgeon's recommendation that these structures be protected for a longer period can delay rehabilitation.

Cuff tear arthropathy patients have massive rotator cuff tears and severe deterioration of the glenoid and humeral head. Surgeons often have to modify the version of the prosthesis and split the subscapularis muscle to obtain closure of the rotator cuff. These patients almost always are placed in the limited goals program.

Summary

The purpose of this chapter is to provide suggestions and guidelines for clinicians who are establishing individual rehabilitation programs for their total shoulder arthroplasty patients. Before such a program can be developed, however, a thorough understanding of the surgery and the purpose of the surgery is needed. Each surgeon will have his or her own philosophy, and the rehabilitation program should reflect that. It is a team approach that benefits the patient the most.

References

1. Pean JE, Bick EM (trans): The classic on prosthetic methods intended to repair bone fragments. Clin Orthop 54:4, 1973
2. Neer CS: Glenohumeral arthroplasty. p. 143. In: Shoulder Reconstruction. WB Saunders, Philadelphia, 1990
3. Neer CS: Replacement arthroplasty for glenohumeral osteoarthritis. J Bone Joint Surg 56A:1, 1974
4. Cofield RH: Unconstrained total shoulder prosthesis. Clin Orthop 173:97, 1983
5. Neer CS, Craig EV, Fukuda H: Cuff-tear arthropathy. J Bone Joint Surg 65A:1232, 1983
6. Post M, Grinblat E: Preoperative clinical evaluation. p. 41. In Friedman RJ (ed): Arthroplasty of the Shoulder. Thieme, New York, 1994
7. Neer CS, Kirby RM: Revision of the humeral head and total shoulder arthroplasties. Clin Orthop 170:189, 1982
8. Neer CS, Wetson KC, Stanton FJ: Recent experience in total shoulder replacement. J Bone Joint Surg 64A:319, 1982
9. Friedman RJ: Total shoulder arthoplasty in rheumatoid arthritis. p. 158. In: Shoulder Reconstruction. WB Saunders, Philadelphia, 1990
10. Friedman RJ, Thornhill TS, Thomas WH, Sledge CB: Nonconstrained total shoulder replacement in patients who have rheumatoid arthritis and class IV function. J Bone Joint Surg 71A:494, 1979
11. Ficat P, Arlet J: Necrosis of the femoral head. p. 53. In: Ischemia and Bone Necrosis. Williams & Wilkins, Baltimore, 1980
12. Springfield DS, Enneking WJ: Surgery of aseptic necrosis of the femoral head. Clin Orthop 130:175, 1978

APPENDIX 20.1

Rehabilitation Programs Following Total Shoulder Replacement

CATEGORY A *Postoperative Rehabilitation Program for Total Shoulder Arthroplasty—Good Rotator Cuff and Deltoid*

Day 1	Arm is positioned in a sling. Out of bed into chair and ambulating. Elbow, wrist, and hand active range of motion. Passive external rotation with a stick to pain tolerance and not beyond 30° (Fig. 20.5). Passive pendulum motions by therapist.	Weeks 4–6	Begin extension and internal rotation stretches (Fig. 20.12). Terminal stretching for elevation and external rotation (Fig. 20.13). Light elastic resistance exercises replace isometrics performed with elbow flexed to 90° and below shoulder level (Fig. 20.14). Flexion, extension, and abduction in the plane of the scapula (scaption) Internal and external rotation
Days 2–3	Family members are instructed in technique of passive forward elevation for rehabilitation at home (Fig. 20.6). Passive forward elevation in the plane of the scapula. When 120° of elevation is possible, the patient begins using a rope and pulley to elevate the arm (Fig. 20.7). Instruct patient in activities of daily living. Discharge from hospital.		Assisted elevation of arm with stick, wall, or rope and pulley with isometric hold at end range followed by active eccentric lowering to pain tolerance (Fig. 20.15).
Home Program	Passive external rotation with stick to 30°. Passive forward elevation with family member; progression to use of rope and pulley. Elbow, wrist, and hand active range of motion.	Weeks 10–12	Light dumbbell program replaces elastic resistance. Scaption—elevation in the plane of the scapula (Fig. 20.16). Sidelying or prone external rotation (Fig. 20.17). Prone extension (Fig. 20.18). Prone horizontal abduction (Fig. 20.19).
Precautions	No lifting with involved arm. Shoulder extension is limited. Elbow not to go behind midline of the body.		Upon obtaining 85 percent of normal active range of motion of the shoulder and a manual muscle testing score of at least four out of a possible five for anterior deltoid, internal, and external rotators, modified sport activities are allowed; short irons and putting for golf, and ground strokes in tennis.
Weeks 1–2	Review home program and modify as appropriate. Begin scapular stabilizing exercises within pain tolerance (Fig. 20.8). Retraction and protraction Elevation and depression Begin glenohumeral joint isometrics with elbow flexed (Fig. 20.9). Flexion, extension, abduction Internal and external rotation	Months 5–6	Full return to sport with full active and passive range of motion. Modified weightlifting program (elbow does not pass midline of body). Continue stretching and strengthening program independently. Isokinetic testing is allowed, if necessary.
Weeks 2–4	Begin active assisted elevation (Fig. 20.10) or gravity-eliminated active range of motion in elevation and external rotation (Fig. 20.11). Correct scapulohumeral rhythm should be maintained during these exercises. Activities of daily living to tolerance keeping the arm below shoulder level.		

CATEGORY B *Postoperative Rehabilitation Program for Total Shoulder Arthroplasty—Poor Rotator Cuff and Deltoid*

Day 1	In a sling with abduction pillow of varying size, or airplane splint.
	Out of bed into chair and ambulating.
	Elbow, wrist, and hand active range of motion.
Days 2–3	Passive pendulum with therapist to tolerance. Family member is instructed in technique of passive forward elevation for rehabilitation at home.
	May or may not begin passive external rotation with stick, to pain tolerance.
	Discharge from hospital.
Home Program	Passive pendulum.
	Elbow, wrist, and hand active range of motion.
	Passive external rotation with stick.
Precautions	No active range of motion activities for the shoulder.
	If in abduction pillow sling, do not let arm come into adduction, extension, or internal rotation.
Weeks 1–2	Passive forward elevation in the plane of the scapula. Instruct family member to 120°; progress to rope and pulley.
	Passive external rotation with stick to 30°.
Weeks 4–6	Begin scapular stabilizing exercises within pain tolerance.
	Begin glenohumeral joint isometrics with elbow flexed within pain tolerance.
Weeks 6–8	Begin active assisted range of motion exercises or gravity eliminated exercises for elevation and external rotation exercises with appropriate scapulohumeral rhythm as available.
	Begin terminal stretching for elevation and external rotation.
	Begin gentle internal rotation stretches.
Weeks 8–10	Replace isometric exercises with light elastic band exercises below shoulder level.
	Assisted elevation of arm with stick, wall, or rope and pulley with isometric hold at end range and active eccentric lowering.
Weeks 12–14	Replace light elastic band exercises with light dumbbell exercises.
	Focus on correct scapulohumeral rhythm with active range of motion of shoulder.

CATEGORY C *Limited Goals Program*

In Hospital	In sling with abduction pillow.
	Elbow, wrist, and hand active range of motion.
Weeks 2–3	Sutures removed.
	May or may not begin passive forward elevation in the plane of scapula with assistance of family member.
Week 6	Begin passive forward elevation if not started previously.
	Remain in sling for another 3 to 6 weeks for activities of daily living.
	Begin passive external rotation in limited range 10° to 20°.
	Begin scapular stabilizing exercises in pain tolerance.
Weeks 12–14	Begin isometrics.
	Begin gravity eliminated activities within pain tolerance.
Months 4–5	Begin light elastic resistance exercises.
	Progress to active elevation activities as pain allows.
Reasonable Outcomes	Active elevation to 120°. Active external rotation to 30°. Goal of pain-free use of arm below shoulder level.
Months 5–6	When 85 percent of available active range of motion is possible and anterior deltoid and internal and external rotator cuff strength reach four (out of a possible five) on manual muscle testing, modified sport and weightlifting activities are allowed as tolerated.
	Continue terminal stretching in elevation and in external and internal rotation.

Index

Page numbers followed by f indicate figures; those followed by t indicate tables.